THERAPEUTICS IN CARDIOLOGY

DEVELOPMENTS IN CARDIOVASCULAR MEDICINE

THERAPEUTICS IN CARDIOLOGY

edited by

A. BAYÉS DE LUNA
Department of Cardiology, University of Barcelona,
Hospital de la Santa Cruz y San Pablo, Barcelona, Spain

A. BETRIU
Department of Cardiology, Hospital Clinic, University of Barcelona, Barcelona, Spain

G. PERMANYER
Department of Cardiology, Hospital Vall d'Hebron, Barcelona, Spain

KLUWER ACADEMIC PUBLISHERS
DORDRECHT / BOSTON / LONDON

Library of Congress Cataloging in Publication Data

Therapeutics in cardiology.

    (Developments in cardiovascular medicine ;
81)
    Includes index.
    1. Heart--Diseases--Treatment. 2. Arrhyth-
mia--Treatment. I. Bayés de Luna, Antonio.
II. Series: Developments in cardiovascular
medicine ; v. 81. [DNLM: 1. Heart Diseases--
therapy. W1 De997VME v.81 / WG 200 T398]
RC683.8.T47 1988   616.1'206   87-24779
ISBN 0-89838-981-X (U.S.)

Published by Kluwer Academic Publishers
P.O. Box 17, 3300 AA Dordrecht, Holland.

Kluwer Academic Publishers incorporates the publishing programmes of
D. Reidel, Martinus Nijhoff, Dr W. Junk and MTP Press.

Sold and distributed in the U.S.A. and Canada
by Kluwer Academic Publishers,
101 Philip Drive, Norwell, MA 02061, U.S.A.

In all other countries, sold and distributed
by Kluwer Academic Publishers Group,
P.O. Box 322, 3300 AH Dordrecht, Holland.

Table of Contents

VI

VIII

Preface

Therapy in cardiology has advanced enormously in recent years. This has resulted in the organization of many meetings and the publication of numerous books dedicated to examining the latest aspects of, for instance, pharmacologic, electrical and surgical treatment. However, only a few of these meetings and publications have attempted to present an overall review of all advances that have taken place in the field of therapy.

In the last years the Spanish Society of Cardiology has shown a great interest in the continuous medical education in cardiology. The Society has organized various meetings and has published several books on the above-mentioned topics. Consequently, the Society has decided to publish this book, an update of the therapeutics in cardiology, of which a Spanish version is also available. World renowned experts and outstanding Spanish cardiologists were invited to review all aspects of therapy in cardiology.

We would like to thank the Spanish Society of Cardiology and the Catalan Cardiac Society for the generous assistance they have given us during all stages of book preparation. We also would like to express our appreciation to all the authors for their valuable contributions. Their combined efforts enable us to put this volume in the hands of the reader.

The book covers all the advances that have been made in the treatment of arrhythmias, arterial hypertension, heart failure, including terminal heart failure with the possibility of heart transplantation, valvular diseases, tetralogy of Fallot, as a representation of the progress made in the field of congenital heart disease, and every aspect of ischemic heart disease. We are confident that this book will help physicians to update their knowledge on therapeutic aspects of cardiology, in which progress has been both rapid and spectacular.

The editors

List of contributors

E. Alegría Ezquerra
  University Clinic, Cardiovascular Department, Faculty of Medicine,
  University of Navarra, 31080 Pamplona, Spain
  Co-authors: J.A. Arrieta, R. Huguet, J. Barba and D. Martinez-Caro
J.M. Almendral
  Department of Cardiology, G. Marañón Hospital, C. Ibiza 45,
  28009 Madrid, Spain
  Co-author: M.E. Josephson
E. Asin Cardiel
  Department of Cardiology, Centro Especial Ramón y Cajal, Carretera de
  Colmenar Viejo, km 9,100, 28034 Madrid, Spain
V. Bala Subramanian
  Department of Cardiovascular Research, Brunel University, Harrow
  Health Care Center, Harrow, United Kingdom
I. Balaguer Vintró
  Cardiovascular Epidemiology Section, Hospital de la Santa Cruz y
  San Pablo, San Antonio M. Claret 167, 08025 Barcelona, Spain
M. Ballester Rodés
  Department of Cardiology, Hospital de la Santa Cruz y San Pablo, San
  Antonio M. Claret 167, 08025 Barcelona, Spain
  Co-authors: M. Cladellas Capdevila, L. Abadal Berini, D. Obrador
  Mayol, M.J. Amengual Guedán, R. Bordes Prat, G. Pons Lladó,
  M. García-Moll, J.M. Padró Fernández, A. Arís and J.M. Caralps Riera
A. Bayés de Luna
  Department of Cardiology, University of Barcelona, Hospital de la Santa
  Cruz y San Pablo, San Antonio M. Claret 167, 08025 Barcelona, Spain
A. Betriu
  Department of Cardiology, Hospital Clinic, University of Barcelona,
  08036 Barcelona, Spain
  Co-authors: M. Heras and G. Sanz

B.R. Chaitman
Cardiology Division, Saint Louis University Medical Center, 1325 S. Grand Boulevard, Saint Louis, MO 63104, USA

J. Cinca
Intensive Care Unit, Hospital 'Valle de Hebrón', Paseo Valle de Hebrón 125, 08035 Barcelona, Spain
Co-authors: A. Moya, A. Bardáji and J. Figueras

I. Coma Canella
Coronary Unit, Municipal Health Center 'La Paz', Paseo de la Castellana 261, 28046 Madrid, Spain
Co-author: J. López Sendón

A. Cortina
Department of Cardiology, Hospital Virgen de Covadonga, Oviedo, Spain

J. Cosín Aguilar
Cardiovascular Investigation Center, Hospital La Fe, C. Campoamor 21, 46009 Valencia, Spain

C. Crexells
Cardiopulmonary Function Unit, Hospital de la Santa Cruz y San Pablo, Avda. Sant Antoni M. Claret 167, 08025 Barcelona, Spain

J.L. Delcán
Department of Cardiology, G. Marañón Hospital C. Ibiza 45, 28009 Madrid, Spain
Co-author: L. Martínez Elbal

M.A. DeWood
Division of Cardiology, Sacred Heart Medical Center, 101 West 8th Avenue, Spokane, WA 99220, USA
Co-authors: J.P. Shields, R. Berg Jr and R.N. Notske

J.Ma. Domínguez de Rozas
Department of Cardiology, Hospital de la Santa Cruz y San Pablo, San Antonio M. Claret 167, 08025 Barcelona, Spain
Co-authors: J. García Picart, J. Guindo Soldevila, R. Oter Rodríguez and A. Bayés de Luna

C.M.G. Duran
Department of Cardiology, National Hospital, Marques de Valdecilla 39008 Santander, Spain
Co-authors: I. Gallo, J.F. Nistal, A. Figueroa and J.L. Ubago

M. Facchini
Arrhythmia Research Unit, Clinical Physiology and Hypertension Center, Maggiore Hospital and Medical Clinic IV, Milano, Italy
Co-author: P.J. Schwartz

XVI

J. Farré Muncharaz
  Laboratory of Cardiac Electrophysics, Jimenez Diaz Foundation,
  Madrid, Spain
R. Frank
  Jean-Rostand Hospital, 39 Rue Jean-le-Galleau, 94200 Ivry, France
  Co-authors: G. Fontaine and J.L. Tonet
J. Froufe
  Coronary Unit, Municipal Health Center, Bilbao, Spain
  Co-authors: G. Hernando, J.M. Irigoyen, J. Solar and M. Peréz
F. Furlanello
  Department of Cardiology, Trent Hospital, 38100 Trent, Italy
V. Fuster
  Division of Cardiology, Mount Sinai Medical Center, 1 Gustave
  L. Levy Place, New York, NY 10029, USA
R. García Civera, Department of Cardiology. University Hospital Clinic.
  Avda. Blasco Ibanèz 17, 46010 Valencia, Spain
  Co-authors: R. Sanjuan, S. Morell, S. Botella, E. Gonzalez, E. Baldo,
  J. Llavador and V. Lopez Merino
F. García Cosío
  Department of Cardiology, Hospital de la Cruz Roja, c/ Reina
  Victoria 22, 28003 Madrid, Spain
  Co-author: J. Palacios Martinez
M. Garcia Moll
  Department of Cardiology, Hospital de la Santa Cruz y San Pablo,
  San Antonio M. Claret 167, 08025 Barcelona, Spain
P.C. Gillette
  Department of Pediatric Cardiology, South Carolina Children's Heart
  Center, 171 Ashley Avenue, Charleston, SC 29425, USA
T.B. Graboys
  Brigham and Women's Hospital and Harvard Medical School, Boston,
  MA 02115, USA
G. Hergueta Garcia de Guadiana
  Department of Cardiology, Provincial Hospital, Madrid, Spain
J.I. Herraiz Sarachaga
  Department of Pediatric Cardiology, Centro Especial Ramón y Cajal,
  Cra. de Colmenar, km. 9,100, 28034 Madrid, Spain
  Co-authors: J.C. Flores, R. Bermudez-Canete and M. Quero Jimenez
M. Iriarte Ezkurdia
  Department of Cardiology, General Hospital de Basurto, Bilbao, Spain
  Co-authors: J.M. Aguirre Salcedo, J. Boveda Romeo, E. Molinero de
  Miguel and J. Urrengoetxea Martinez

S.W. Jamieson
  Department of Cardiovascular Surgery, Stanford University Medical
  Center, Stanford, CA 94305, USA
R.A. Johnson
  Walla Walla Clinic, 55 W. Tietan, Walla Walla, WA 99362, USA
G. Lee
  The Western Heart Institute, St. Mary's Hospital and Medical Center,
  450 Stanyan Street, San Francisco, CA 94117, USA
  Co-authors: M.C. Chan, M.H. Lee, R.M. Ikeda, J.L. Rink,
  W.J. Bommer, R.L. Reiss, E.S. Hanna and D.T. Mason
T.H. LeJemtel
  Division of Cardiology, Department of Medicine, Albert Einstein
  College of Medicine, 1300 Morris Park Avenue, Bronx, NY 10461, USA
  Co-authors: R. Grose, J. Strain and E.H. Sonnenblick
V. López Merino
  Department of Cardiology and Functional Respiratory Research,
  Hospital Clinic University, Valencia, Spain
J. López Sendón
  Department of Coronary Diseases, Municipal Health Center 'La Paz',
  Paseo de la Castellana 261, 28046 Madrid, Spain
  Co-author: I. Coma Canella
F. Malpartida
  Department of Cardiology, University Clinic, Faculty of Medicine,
  University of Navarra, Pamplona, Spain
J. Márquez Montes
  c/ Ponzano 59, 28003 Madrid, Spain
  Co-authors: J.J. Rufilanchas, J. Alzueta, J. Ugarte, C. Hernandez,
  G. Linacero, J.J. Esteve, J. Arnau and D. Figuera
G.T. Meester
  Thorax Center, Erasmus University, P.O. Box 1738,
  3000 DR Rotterdam, The Netherlands
  Co-authors: R.W. Brower and H.J. ten Kate
M. Mirowski
  Department of Medicine, Sinai Hospital of Baltimore, Baltimore, MD
  21215, USA
  Co-authors: P.R. Reid, M.M. Mower, L. Watkins Jr, E.V. Platia,
  L.S.C. Griffith, T. Guarnieri and J.M. Juanteguy
R.J. Myerburg
  Division of Cardiology (D-39), University of Miami, School of Medicine,
  P.O. Box 01690, Miami, FL 33101, USA
  Co-authors: K.M. Kessler, L. Zaman, R.G. Trohman, N. Saoudi and

XVIII

A. Castellanos
F. Navarro Lopez
  Department of Cardiology, Hospital Clinic, University of Barcelona,
  08036 Barcelona, Spain
A. Oriol
  Department of Cardiology, Hospital de la Santa Cruz y San Pablo,
  San Antonio M. Claret 167, 08025 Barcelona, Spain
  Co-authors: C. Crexells and J.M. Augé
A. Pajaron Lopez
  Department of Cardiology, National Hospital 'Marqués de Valdecilla',
  39008 Santander, Spain
G. Permanyer Miralda
  Cardiology Division, Department of Medicine, Hospital 'Valle de
  Hebron', Paseo Valle de Hebrón 125, 08035 Barcelona, Spain
  Co-author: E. Galve Basilio
E. Piccolo
  Department of Cardiology, Mirano Hospital, Venice, Italy
L. Plaza Celemín
  Department of Cardiology, Hospital Victoria Eugenia
P. Puech
  Department of Cardiology, Hosptial Saint. Eloi, Montpellier, France
  Co-author: P. Gallay
K.P. Rentrop
  Mount Sinai School of Medicine, 1 Gustave L. Levy Place, New York,
  NY 10029, USA
  Co-authors: M. Cohen and S.T. Hosat
C. Ribeiro
  Cardiological Intensive Care Unit, Santa Maria Hospital, Lisbon,
  Portugal
G. Sanz
  Department of Cardiology and Coronary Unit, Hospital Clinic,
  University of Barcelona, Barcelona, Spain
  Co-author: G. Oller
J. Soler Soler
  Department of Cardiology, Hospital 'Valle de Hebron', Paseo Valle de
  Hebrón 125, 08035 Barcelona, Spain
E. Sowton
  Department of Cardiology, Guy's Hospital, St. Thomas Street,
  London SE1 9RT, United Kingdom
  Co-authors: P.M. Holt and J.C.P. Crick
J. Tamargo Menéndez. Pharmacological Department. Hospital Clinic,
  San Carlos. University City. Madrid 3, Spain

P. Théroux
  Montreal Heart Institute, 5000 East Belanger Street, Montreal, Quebec,
  Canada H1T 1C8
  Co-authors: X. Bosch, Y. Taeymans, A. Moise and D.D. Waters
L. Tomás Abadal
  Department of Cardiology, Hospital de la Santa Cruz y San Pablo,
  San Antonio M. Claret 167, 08025 Barcelona, Spain
V. Valle Tudela Department of Cardiology, 'Germans Trias' Hospital,
  Badalona, Spain
H.J.J. Wellens
  Department of Cardiology, University of Limburg, St Annadal Hospital,
  6214 PA Maastricht, The Netherlands
  Co-author: P. Brugada
P. Yuste Pescador
  Department of Cardiology, Centro Especial Ramón y Cajal,
  Cra de Colmenar Viejo km 9,100, 28034 Madrid, Spain
P. Zarco Gutierrez. Cardiopulmonary Department. Hospital Clinic,
  San Carlos. University City. Madrid 3, Spain

1. Severe Arrhythmias and Sudden Death

1.1 Introduction

PEDRO BRUGADA

Approximately every five minutes one sudden death occurs in the United States. One sudden death takes place every half-hour in as small a country as The Netherlands. If this prevalence of sudden death in industrialized countries holds true as an average, four to five-thousand sudden deaths occur yearly in the City of Barcelona and its surrounding area. But who are the victims? Where, how, when and why?

Sudden death is a major plague of our western society. Its incidence is five times higher than that of another abominable plague of our era: traffic accidents caused directly or indirectly by intoxication with alcoholic beverages. One person dies every twenty-three minutes under these circumstances in the United States. The causes here are clear, however, and preventive measures can be undertaken. But how may we prevent sudden death?

Sudden cardiac death is a multi-factorial problem. Although most sudden deaths occur in patients with coronary artery disease, it also occurs in patients with other or no structural heart diseases. Because of the variety of etiologies and pathophysiologic mechanisms of sudden death, preventive measures will have to vary accordingly. The most important remaining question is still, however, how to identify high-risk candidates for sudden cardiac death. Once identified, of course, adequate therapeutic measures should be undertaken to prevent sudden death. A very different problem is whether this is justifiable at a point in time when treatments designed to prevent (the first episode of) sudden death are still under investigation. One should not forget that screening of unselected populations is likely to create disease because of the false positive tests, and to increase patients' and physicians' stress if adequate therapeutic measures cannot be undertaken once a true positive candidate has been recognized. Also, whether it is financially possible to screen the general populations is not only a monetary problem. Bayessian analysis has taught us that most of our current tests will be inadequate in terms of predictive accuracy when applied to populations with a low prevalence of the disease sought. Any positive test, whether true of false, is likely to involve the patient in a cycle of diagnostic procedures in order to increase the security of the diagnosis. While this might be adequate in high-risk and symptomatic populations, one wonders how much disease would be created were the general population to be screened.

Major questions remain, therefore, about the future steps that society will have to undertake to have adequate diagnostic and therapeutic procedures to prevent sudden cardiac death. These and other aspects of sudden cardiac death will be discussed in this work. While we will be trying to increase our understanding of this problem, however, by the time the following articles have been read, thirty-six sudden deaths will have occurred in the United States, six in the Netherlands and two in the City of Barcelona.

1.2 Influence of Circadian Rhythm on the Electrophysiological Properties of the Human Heart

J. CINCA, A. MOYA, A. BARDAJI and J. FIGUERAS

Introduction

Experimental studies in dogs [1–4] have demonstrated that electrical stimulation of the sympathetic fibers of the heart accelerates intranodal conduction, shortens refractory periods and depresses the threshold for ventricular fibrillation. Stimulation of the parasympathetic fibers has the opposite effect. In the human being, few studies of this type are available. In a small series of patients, lengthening of intranodal conduction after electrical stimulation of the carotid sinus has been demonstrated [5]. In another series of patients, we observed variations in the electrical properties of the heart after anesthesia of the stellate ganglion [6].

Thus, fluctuations in neuro-vegetative tone that normally occur throughout the day in the human being may be accompanied by parallel changes in the electrical properties of the heart. The present study was designed to analyze the variations in electrophysiologic parameters that might occur in a 24-hour period. In the course of the study we developed a new technique for recording the His potential at the bedside of the patient during 24 hours.

Method

Patients

The study included 10 patients (7 men and 3 women), aged 17 to 55, in whom electrophysiologic study was indicated to ascertain the mechanism of tachycardia in six cases and that of syncopal episodes in four cases. All the patients had normal conduction intervals (AH<110 msec and HV<45 msec), a sinus recuperation time of less than 1500 msec and no bundle branch block. The patients presented normal nyctohemeral rhythm prior to the study.

Protocol

Once the basal study was completed according to the usual protocol [7], the patient was transferred to a room with natural illumination and connected to a polygraph (6-channel Elema Mingograf) and programmable stimulator (Devices LTD) that were located on the other side of a wall. The following parameters were determined at 1–2 hour intervals:

1. RR interval,
2. AH and HV intervals using a hexapolar electrocatheter that allowed simultaneous ventricular stimulation by the distal electrodes and recording of the bundle of His potential by a pair of intermediate electrodes,
3. QT interval at a fixed atrial stimulation rate, with a recording speed of 100 mm/sec and double voltage [8],
4. sinus recovery time (SRT) at atrial stimulation (coronary sinus) rates of 100, 120 and 130 beats/min,
5. ventriculo-atrial conduction [9],
6. refractory periods of the atrium, AV node, right ventricle and Kent fibers, and
7. axillary temperature.

Results are expressed as the percentage of change with respect to the maximum value of each parameter in the course of the study. The statistical significance of the results was evaluated with the Student test for paired samples.

Results

The endocavitary recordings remained stable throughout the study, as shown in Fig. 1. The patients tolerated well the 10–15 electrophysiologic tests performed in each of them. Body temperature showed a physiologic drop at dawn.

Sinus function

Sinus rate, expressed as RR interval duration, slowed progressively as the afternoon advanced, reaching a maximum at dawn (Fig. 2).

SRT at all three atrial stimulation rates was significantly lengthened ($p < 0.01$) in the period between 12.00 PM and 7.00 AM the next day, independent of the sleep-vigil state of the patient (Fig. 1). SRT corrected for heart rate (SRTc), obtained by subtracting the time length of the RR cycle previous to stimulation from the SRT, was accompanied by a marked dispersion of the results, which made the differences not significant.

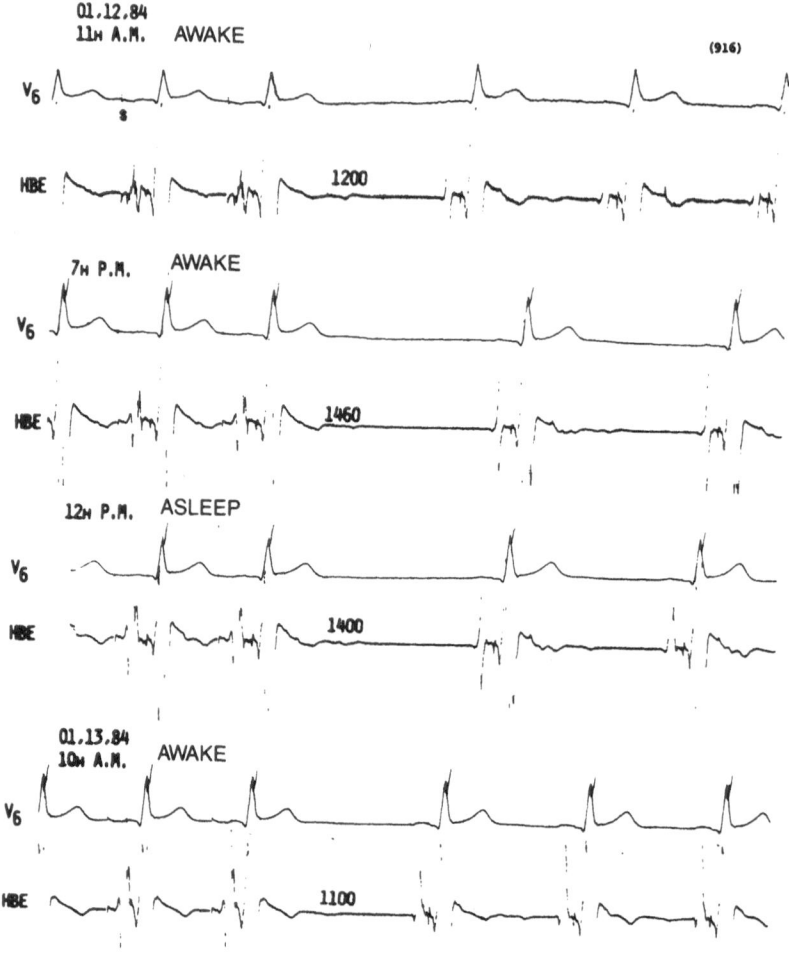

Fig. 1. Stability of the endocavitary recordings obtained at the patient's bedside in 24 hours. Representation of sinus recovery time (in msec) obtained sequentially at 11.00 AM (patient awake), 7.00 PM, 12.00 PM (patient asleep) and at 10.00 AM the next day. V6 = V6 lead of the conventional ECG; HBE = endocavitary lead in the area of the bundle of His.

AV conduction intervals

The AH and HV intervals showed a mean variation of ± 5.2% and ± 4.9%, respectively, in relation to the mean value of the group studied. However, neither of the two showed a significant tendency in the course of the study.

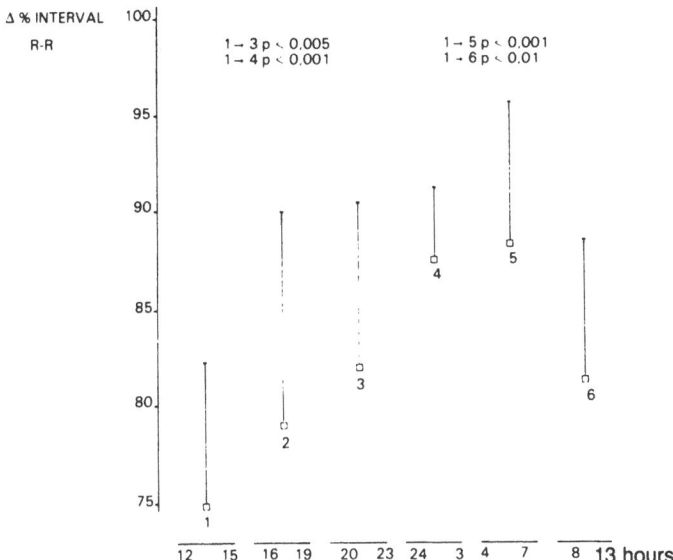

Fig. 2. Sequential changes of the sinus cycle (RR interval) in the course of 24 hours expressed as the percentage of variation with respect to the maximum value obtained during the study. The squares represent the mean value of all the cases and the bars correspond to the standard deviation. The time is divided into 3 hour intervals. In the upper part of the figure the statistical significance of the variations with respect to those obtained in the first study is shown (*value 1*).

Refractory periods and QT interval

The effective refractory periods of the atrium, AV node and right ventricle were significantly prolonged between 12.00 PM and 7.00 AM the next day (Figs 3 and 4).

The QT interval measured at a fixed rate showed parallel changes to those of the right ventricular refractory period, reaching significant lengthening at dawn (Fig. 5).

Discussion

The most relevant results of our study are:
1. demonstration that at dawn there is a significant lengthening not only of sinus cycle, but also of SRT, QT interval and the atrial, nodal and right ventricular refractory periods,
2. quantification of the degree of spontaneous variation in the electrophysiologic parameters, and

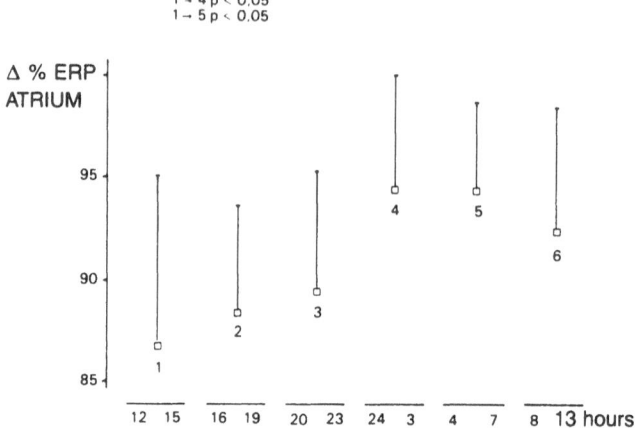

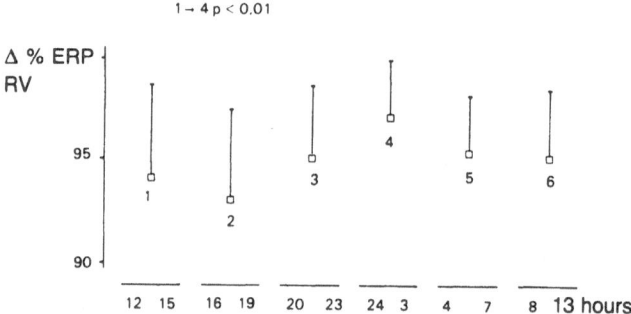

Fig. 3. Sequential changes of the effective refractory period (ERP) of the atrium and right ventricle (RV). Symbols as in Fig. 2.

3. description of a new technique that facilitates monitoring of the AH and HV intervals at the patient's bedside.

The nocturnal lengthening of the refractory periods could be due to an increase in vagal tone, since experiments in animals have shown that selective electrical stimulation of the vagus produces a slowing of the sinus rate [1, 2], nodal conduction [2] and the refractory periods of the node [2] and right ventricle [3]. In the human being, electrical stimulation of the carotid sinus has similar effects on the sinus rate and nodal conduction [5]. To summarize, our study would seem to indicate that the autonomic nervous system modulates not only sinus function but nodal conduction and atrial and ventricular myocardial refractoriness. The fluctuations in the electrical properties of these structures may have an effect on the characteristics of the reciprocating tachy-

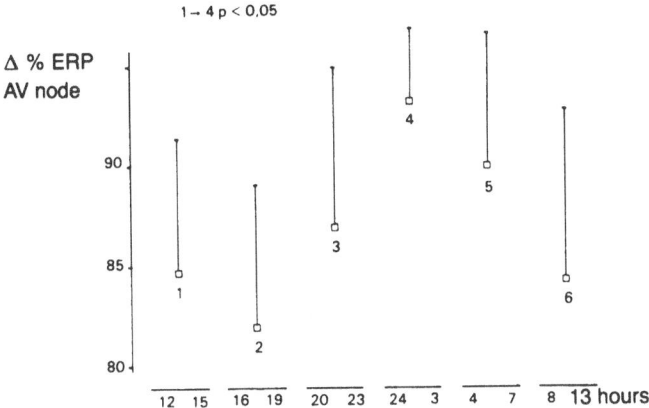

Fig. 4. Sequential variation of the effective refractory period (ERP) of the AV node.

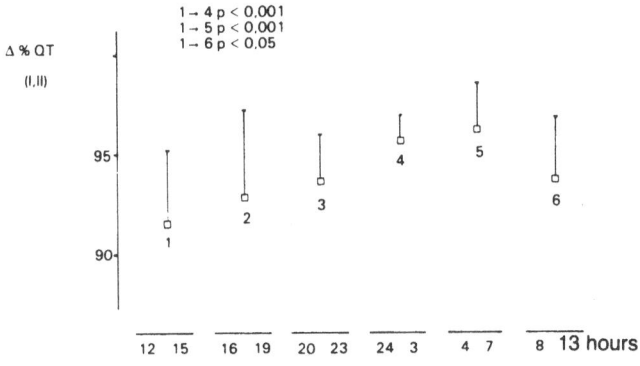

Fig. 5. Sequential variation of the QT interval measured in leads I and II of the ECG.

cardias, and their electrical inducibility or spontaneous appearance may therefore change in the course of the day.

The fact that the variations in nodal refractoriness were more marked than those observed in the conduction through this node (AH interval) is comparable to the difference that appears in these two parameters after vagal stimulation in dogs [10].

Application of our protocol probably did not significantly affect circadian pacemakers since body temperature continued to conform to normal circadian rhythm [11, 12]. Moreover, the sinus rate at night reached values similar to those of healthy individuals who showed normal nyctehemeral rhythm [13].

The parallel observed between the variations of the QT interval and the ventricular refractory period indicate that our technique for measurement of

QT is adequate and that it is useful to detect variations in ventricular refracto-riness induced by fluctuations in neuro-vegetative tone by conventional ECG. The use of formulas to correct QT values for heart rate frequently leads to inexact results [14, 15].

Correction of SRT for heart rate by simple subtraction produces a greater dispersion of the results and loss of the statistical significance of the variation of nocturnal SRT lengthening. The relation between SRT and sinus rate is probably complex and cannot be expressed by a simple mathematical sub-traction, requiring more complex formulas.

Our recording technique enables 24-hour monitoring of the electrophysi-ologic parameters at the patient's bedside and enabling a reduction of the number of electrocatheters needed for electrophysiologic study since the bundle of His potential can be recorded with the same catheter that stimulates the right ventricle.

Summary

To study the variability of the electrophysiologic parameters commonly used in cardiology, we made sequential determinations of these parameters at 1–2 hour intervals for 24 hours at the bedside of 10 patients with normal AV conduction intervals and sinus function.

The study showed that the electrophysiologic properties of the human heart are subject to circadian variations, characterized by significant slowing of the sinus rate, sinus recuperation time, refractory periods of the atrium, AV node and right ventricle, and the QT interval in the time period from 12.00 PM to 7.00 AM. The AH and HV conduction intervals can be adequately monitored at the patient's bedside.

References

1. Lazzara R, Scherlag BJ, Robinson MJ, Samet Ph: Selective in situ parasympathetic control of the canine sinoatrial and atrioventricular nodes. Circ Res 1973; 32: 393–401.
2. Spear JF, Moore EN: Influence of brief vagal and stellate nerve stimulation on pacemaker activity and conduction within the atrioventricular conduction system of the dog. Circ Res 1973; 32: 27–41.
3. Kolman BS, Verrier RL, Lown B: Effect of vagus nerve stimulation upon excitability of the canine ventricle. Role of sympathetic-parasympathetic interactions. Am J Cardiol 1976; 37: 1041–1045.
4. Haws ChW, Burgess MJ: Effects of bilateral and unilateral stellate stimulation on canine ventricular refractory periods at sites of overlapping innervation. Circulation 1978; 42: 195–198.
5. Borst C, Karemaker JM, Dunning AJ: Prolongation of atrioventricular conduction time by

12

electrical stimulation of the carotid sinus nerves in man. Circulation 1982; 65: 432–434.

6. Cinca J, Evangelista A, Montoyo J et al.: Electrophysiologic effects of unilateral right and left stellate ganglion block on the human heart. Am Heart J 1985; 109: 46–54.

7. Cinca J, Valle V, Gutierrez L, Figueras J, Rius J: Reciprocating tachycardia using bilateral anomalous pathways. Electrophysiologic and clinical implications. Circulation 1980; 62: 657–661.

8. Cinca J, Figueras J, Tenorio L et al.: Time course and rate dependence of the Q-T interval changes during noncomplicated acute myocardial infarction in human beings. Am J Cardiol 1981; 48: 1023–1028.

9. Cinca J, Valle V, Figueras J, Gutierrez L, Montoyo J, Rius J: Shortening of ventriculo-atrial conduction in patients with left sided Kent bundles. Am Heart J 1984; 107: 912–918.

10. Kralios FA, Millar CK: Sympathetic neural effects on regional atrial recovery properties and cardiac rhythm. Am J Physiol 1981; 240: H 590–596.

11. Moore-Ede MC, Czeisler ChA, Richardson GS: Circadian timekeeping in health and disease. Part 1. Basic properties of circadian pacemakers. New Engl J Med 1983; 309: 530–536.

12. Moore-Ede MC, Czeisler ChA, Richardson GS: Circadian timekeeping in health and disease. Part 2. Clinical implications of circadian rhythmicity. New Engl J Med 1983; 309: 530–536.

13. De Leonardis V, Cinelli P, Cappaci F, De Scalzi M, Citi S: Circadian rhythms in dynamic electrocardiography. J Electrocardiol 1983; 16: 351–354.

14. Browne KF, Zipes DP, Heber JJ, Prystowsky EN: Influence of the autonomic nervous system on the Q-T interval in man. Am J Cardiol 1982; 50: 1099–1103.

15. Ahnve S, Vallin H: Influence of heart rate and inhibition of autonomic tone on the Q-T interval. Circulation 1982; 65: 435–439.

1.3 Sudden Arrhythmic Death – Picture of the Possible Candidate

RONALD W.F. CAMPBELL

Introduction

Sudden arrhythmic death is not restricted to patients with coronary artery disease. It is variably expressed in other pathological conditions including the congenital long QT syndromes, aortic stenosis, cadiomyopathies, the pre-excitation syndromes, and mitral valve prolapse. Moreover, there is a small but important incidence in apparently normal individuals. Advances in diagnostic techniques and improved awareness of the risk of cardiovascular disease have helped define patient groups who are particularly susceptible to the complication of sudden arrhythmic death but, despite much effort, individual risk prediction is poorly developed.

Acute myocardial infarction

The highest risk situation for sudden arrhythmic death is probably in the first hours of acute myocardial infarction when there is a 20–30% incidence of ventricular fibrillation. The risk of this complication falls exponentially with time from the onset of symptoms [1]. Even in this relatively easily identified and well researched patient group, defining individual susceptibility to ventricular fibrillation has not proved practicable. Investigated factors have included the size and site of myocardial infarction [2], catecholamine levels [3], the QT interval [4], ventricular ectopic beat patterns [5–8], electrolyte levels [9] and QRS features detected by signal averaging techniques [10]. Although many of these features are associated with a modification of risk, none has proved of sufficient sensitivity or specificity to identify individuals who will develop ventricular fibrillation.

In acute myocardial infarction, the immediate prognosis of primary ventricular fibrillation is good (although may be somewhat poorer than has been believed in the past [11]) whilst that of secondary ventricular fibrillation is very bad.

Post acute myocardial infarction

Survivors of acute myocardial infarction are already a selected patient population. The overall mortality of acute myocardial infarction has remained little changed by the advent of coronary care units and rescue squads perhaps because the majority of deaths occur unnoticed or prior to the arrival of medical help. Following myocardial infarction the average annual mortality is 4–9% [11]. The following features have been observed to be associated with an increased risk of death:

a) Extensive coronary artery disease, particularly left main and three vessel disease [12–14]. It is controversial whether proximal left anterior descending disease has particular significance.
b) Poor left ventricular function (whether global or related to an aneurysm) and the size of the myocardial infarction [12–14]. These features may be reflected in the acute phase of infarction by persisting sinus tachycardia or left ventricular failure.
c) Late ventricular arrhythmias [14, 15].
d) Bundle branch block and axis shift particularly complicating anteroseptal myocardial infarction [16, 17].

The late prognosis for patients who have survived myocardial infarction complicated by primary ventricular fibrillation appears almost as good as that for patients whose acute event was not so complicated [18] but the outlook following secondary ventricular fibrillation is bad [19].

The value of antiarrhythmic drug therapy in reducing sudden death in survivors of acute myocardial infarction has been investigated in detail [20]. To date, there is no evidence that antiarrhythmic agents of the Vaughan Williams classes I or IV can improve prognosis by reducing sudden arrhythmic death. Indeed, it may be that such agents contribute to risk. A recent study has defined that Class I agents were almost certainly responsible for a proportion of out of hospital cardiac arrests [21].

β-adrenoreceptor blocking therapy has been shown to reduce mortality in survivors of acute myocardial infarction [22–24], the effect probably being applicable to both 'high' and 'low' risk populations. However, β-adrenoreceptor blockers may be of restricted application in patients with left ventricular dysfunction – a group particularly at risk.

Coronary artery disease (excluding AMI)

High risk sub-groups of patients with coronary artery disease can be identified.

Angina pectoris

Patients with angina who have extensive coronary artery disease, particularly left main disease [12], or who have impaired left ventricular function [25], or show frequent ventricular ectopic beats [2], are at increased risk of sudden death. The presence of these features can be relatively reliably inferred or confirmed from non-invasive tests – stress testing, dynamic electrocardiography, echocardiography and nuclear scintigraphy. At best, their detection identifies a patient *group* with a 20–30% annual mortality (that is, seven times that of unselected patients with angina pectoris).

It is unclear whether the severity of symptoms has any impact on prognosis. Neither is it known whether the use of β-adrenoreceptor blocking drugs in these patients reduces mortality, as is the case for survivors of acute myocardial infarction.

Survivors of out-of-hospital ventricular fibrillation

Data from out-of-hospital rescue squads has shown that patients surviving an out-of-hospital cardiac arrest, and who do not suffer an acute myocardial infarction, have a higher recurrence rate and associated poorer prognosis than patients who sustain infarction [26–28]. The hypothesis is that in the former, critical but reversible ischaemia creates the arrhythmia substrate which can be reproduced in further future ischaemic episodes. Patients whose ischaemia is sufficiently severe and long-lasting to produce permanent myocardial damage create the substrate only once.

The optimal method of reducing the substantial one year mortality for these patients is unknown. High dose antiarrhythmic therapy [29] may help but surgery and anti-ischaemic medications probably play as important a role.

The congenital long QT syndromes

The congenital long QT syndromes are significantly associated with sudden death [30]. A history of syncope (particularly at an early age), manifest ventricular arrhythmias, marked QT prolongation on the Valsalva manoeuvre and the use of management strategies other than β-blockers and surgery identify high risk patients. Surgical management (stellate ganglionectomy) or treatment with β-blockers improves prognosis.

Aortic stenosis

Sudden death is a long recognised complication of aortic stenosis [31] but there has been much debate as to whether this was for mechanical or electrical reasons. The latter seems most likely and is reflected in the fact that higher risk sub-groups are those patients with ventricular arrhythmias on their electrocardiogram. However, patients with large transvalvular pressure differences are also at increased risk of sudden death. There is no convincing evidence that mortality in this condition can be reduced by antiarrhythmic therapy.

Mitral valve prolapse

Mitral valve prolapse is an extremely common cardiac condition. Sudden arrhythmic death is a well recognised but relatively rare association [32]. The presence of resting ECG abnormalities – ST and T wave changes and QT prolongation – identifies a high risk group but this association is based on investigation of highly selected patients and the finding may not be applicable in other circumstances. So far, studies have been too small to better characterise the natural history of the condition. DCG and exercise stress testing is the best way to observe the ventricular arrhythmias which probably underlie the occasional event of sudden death. Antiarrhythmic therapy may be indicated on an individual basis but there is no evidence to support its more general use in an attempt to improve prognosis. The relation of the severity of symptoms to prognosis is unknown.

Cardiomyopathies

Sudden arrhythmic death is an increasingly recognised complication of a variety of cardiomyopathies, being associated with acute viral myocarditis [33], hypertrophic cardiomyopathy [34–36] and dilated idiopathic forms [37]. In all types, the presence of ventricular arrhythmias appears to be associated with an increased risk of sudden death. Very little is known regarding the risk modification (whether increased or decreased) by the use of antiarrhythmic therapy, but in patients with hypertrophic cardiomyopathy amiodarone may reduce risk while other agents do not [36].

Patients on antiarrhythmic therapy

Until recently, sudden death in patients taking antiarrhythmic therapy has been viewed as failure of that therapy to control an underlying life-threatening arrhythmia. Now there is increasing evidence that arrhythmogenesis – the creation of new arrhythmias or the aggravation of existing arrhythmias by drug therapy – may play an important part in causing sudden arrhythmic death. Numerous reports have identified the arrhythmogenic potential of antiarrhythmic compounds [38–43], and all such drugs should be considered to have this potential. Unfortunately, there are no good methods to predict arrhythmogenicity. Invasive electrophysiology studies have helped most to identify the problem but this time-consuming and resource-demanding technique is applicable to only highly selected patient groups. It behoves us all to consider this risk of antiarrhythmic therapy should prompt consideration of the wisdom of prescribing for the control of relatively trivial arrhythmic events.

Apparently normal individuals

Sudden death in, apparently, normal individuals may be due to a variety of causes but cardiac arrhythmias are probably responsible for the majority. Most victims are not free of disease but have sub-clinical forms of coronary artery disease, hypertrophic cardiomyopathy etc. Identifying those at particular risk within this population is not easy. The general risk factors for the development of coronary artery disease – a family history, abnormal lipids, hypertension etc – are helpful in large populations but are poor individual predictors. Apparently normal individuals with high frequency ventricular arrhythmias [44] appear to have an increased risk of cardiovascular events and of sudden cardiac death. The relative risk ratio may be no more than one and a half to three times that of truly normal individuals. Whether low frequency ventricular arrhythmias have a similar but lesser role is unknown and, even if proven, probably would be of little clinical relevance [45].

Conclusions

Were it available, accurate individual risk prediction of sudden arrhythmic death would have important consequences for clinical practice. However, apart from certain unusual circumstances, risk assessment for patients is very restricted and, for the present, applicable only to patient groups. In most pathological conditions, the severity of disease correlates well with prognosis but there remain many incidents of sudden arrhythmic death in patients with trivial disease. Natural history studies which are difficult to undertake and have little of the glamour of interventional research, are badly needed if risk prediction is to be refined. In addition, we must better assess the contribution

18

of drug therapy to sudden arrhythmic death; more harm than good may be done when antiarrhythmic therapy is prescribed.

References

1. Adgey AAJ, Allen JD, Geddes JS, James RGG, Webb SW, Zaida SA, Pantridge JF: Acute phase of myocardial infarction. Lancet 1971; 2: 501–504.
2. Bigger JT, Dresdale RJ, Heissenbuttal RH, Weld FM, Wit AL: Ventricular arrhythmias in ischaemic heart disease: Mechanism, prevalence, significance and management. Prog Cardiovasc Dis 1977; 4: 255–299.
3. Opie LH: Metabolism of free fatty acids, glucose and catecholamines in acute myocardial infarction. Am J Cardiol 1973; 36: 938–953.
4. Ahnve S, Lundman T, Shoaleh-Var M: The relationship between QT interval and ventricular arrhythmias in acute myocardial infarction. Acta Med Scand 1978; 204: 17–19.
5. Lown B, Fakhro AM, Hood WB, Thorn GW: The coronary care unit. New perspectives and directions. J Am Med Ass 1967; 199: 188–198.
6. Lie KI, Wellens HJJ, Downar E, Durrer D: Observations on patients with primary ventricular fibrillation complicating acute myocardial infarction. Circulation 1975; 52: 755–759.
7. El-Sherif N, Myerburg PJ, Scherlag BJ, Befeler B, Aranda JM, Castellanos A, Lazzara R: Electrocardiographic antecedents of primary ventricular fibrillation. Br Heart J 1976; 38: 415–422.
8. Campbell RWF, Murray A, Julian DG: Ventricular arrhythmias in first 12 hours of acute myocardial infarction. Natural history study. Br Heart J 1981; 46: 351–357.
9. Dyckner T, Helmers C, Lundman T, Webster PO: Initial serum potassium level in relation to early complications and prognosis in patients with acute myocardial infarction. Acta Med Scand 1975; 197: 207–210.
10. Kertes PJ, Glabus M, Murray A, Julian DG, Campbell RWF: Delayed ventricular depolarisation-correlation with ventricular activation and relevance to ventricular fibrillation in acute myocardial infarction. Eur Heart J 1984; 5: 974–983.
11. Kertes P, Hunt D: Prophylaxis of primary ventricular fibrillation in acute myocardial infarction. The case against lignocaine. Br Heart J 1984; 52: 241–247.
12. Humphries JO: Expected course of patients with coronary artery disease. In Rahimtoola SH (ed) Coronary artery bypass surgery. Philadelphia. FA Davis Co 1977, pp 340–352.
13. Sanz G, Castaner A, Betriu A, Magrina J, Roig E, Coll S, diol Pare JC, Navarro-López F: Determinants of prognosis in survivors of myocardial infarction. N Engl J Med 1982; 306: 1065–1070.
14. Multicenter Postinfarction Research Group: Risk stratification and survival after myocardial infarction. New Engl J Med 1983; 309: 331–336.
15. Moss AJ: Clinical significance of ventricular arrhythmias in patients with and without coronary artery disease. Prog Cardiovasc Dis 1980; 23: 33–52.
16. Lie KI, Liem KL, Schuilenberg RM, David GK, Durrer D: Early identification of patients developing late in-hospital ventricular fibrillation after discharge from the coronary care unit. A 5.5 year retrospective study of 1897 patients. Am J Cardiol 1978; 41: 674–677.
17. Hauer RNW, Lie KI, Liem KL, Durrer D: Long-term prognosis in patients with bundle branch block complicating acute anteroseptal infarction. Am J Cardiol 1982; 49: 1581–1585.
18. Geddes JS, Adgey AAJ, Pantridge JF: Prognosis after recovery from ventricular fibrillation complicating ischaemic heart disease. Lancet 1969; 2: 273–275.
19. Goldberg R, Szklo M, Kennedy H, Tonascia J: Short and long-term prognosis of myocardial

infarction complicated by ventricular fibrillation or cardiac arrest (Abstract). Circulation 1978; 58 (Suppl 2): 89.

20. May GS, Eberlein KA, Furberg CD, Passamani ER, DeMets DL: Secondary prevention after myocardial infarction: a review of long term trials. Prog Cardiovasc Dis 1982; 24: 331–352.

21. Ruskin JN, McGovern B, Garan H, DiMarco JP, Kelly E: Antiarrhythmic drugs: a possible cause of out-of-hospital cardiac arrest. N Engl Med J 1983; 309: 1302–1306.

22. The Norwegian Multicenter Study Group: Timolol-induced reduction in mortality and rein-farction in patients surviving acute myocardial infarction. New Engl J Med 1981; 304: 801–807.

23. B-Blocker Heart Attack Trial Research Group: A randomized trial of propranalol in patients with acute myocardial infarction. JAMA 1982; 247: 1707–1714.

24. Hjalmarson A, Herlitz J, Malek I, Ryden L, Vedin A, Waldenstrom A, Wedel H, Elmfeldt D, Holmberg S, Nyberg G, Swedberg K, Waagstein F, Waldenstrom J, Wilhelmsen L, Wilhelmsson C: Effect on mortality of metropolol in acute myocardial infarction. A double blind randomized trial. Lancet 1981; 2: 823–827.

25. Kannel WB, Feinlieb M: Natural history of angina pectoris in the Framingham study. Prognosis and survival. Am J Cardiol 1972; 29: 154.

26. Ruskin JN, DiMarco JP, Garan H: Out-of-hospital cardiac arrest. N Engl J Med 1980; 30: 607–613.

27. Liberthson RR, Nagel EL, Hirschman JC, Nussenfeld SR, Blackbourne BD, Davis JH: Pathophysiologic observations in prehospital ventricular fibrillation and sudden cardiac death. Circulation 1974; 49: 790–798.

28. Cobb LA, Werner JA, Trobaugh GB: Sudden cardiac death. Mod Con Cardiovasc Dis 1980; 49: 37–42.

29. Castellanos A: Antitthythmic drug therapy in survivors of pre-hospital cardiac arrest: com-parison of effects on chronic ventricular arrhythmias and recurrent cardiac arrest. Circulation 1979; 59: 855–863.

30. Schwartz PJ: The idiopathic long QT syndrome. The need for a prospective registry. Eur Heart J 1983; 4: 529–531.

31. Chizner MA, Pearle DL, DeLeon AC: The natural history of aortic stenosis in adults. Am Heart J 1980; 99: 419–424.

32. Campbell RWF, Godman MJ, Fiddler GI, Marquis RMM, Julian DG: Ventricular arrhyth-mias in syndrome of balloon deformity of mitral valve. Definition of possible high risk group. Br Heart J 1976; 38: 1053–1057.

33. Fiddler GI, Campbell RWF, Pottage A, Godman MJ: Varicella myocarditis presenting with unusual ventricular arrhythmias. Br Heart J 1977; 39: 1150–1153.

34. Maron BJ, Savage DD, Wolfson JK, Epstein SE: Prognostic significance of 24 hour ambula-tory electrocardiographic monitoring in patients with hypertrophic cardiomyopathy: a pro-spective study. Am J Cardiol 1981; 48: 252–257.

35. McKenna WJ, England D, Doi YL, Deanfield JE, Oakley CM, Goodwin JF: Arrhythmia in hypertrophic cardiomyopathy: I Influence on prognosis. Br Heart J 1981; 46: 168–172.

36. McKenna WJ: Arrhythmia and prognosis in hypertrophic cardiomyopathy. Eur Heart J 1983; 4 (Suppl F): 225–234.

37. Webb Peploe M: Dilated cardiomyopathy. Eur Heart J 1984; 5 (Suppl A): 161–164.

38. Winkle RA, Mason JW, Griffin JC, Ross D: Malignant ventricular tachyarrhythmias associ-ated with the use of encainide. Am Heart J 1981; 102: 854–864.

39. Nicholson MR, Campbell RWF, Julian DG: Ventricular tachycardia-management with encainide (Abstract). Circulation 1981; 64: 37.

40. Kenelly BM: Comparison of lidoflazine and quinidine in prophylactic treatment of arrhyth-mia. Br Heart J 1977; 39: 540–546.

41. Denes P, Gabster A, Huang SK: Clinical, electrocardiographic and follow-up observations in patients having ventricular fibrillation during Holter monitoring. Role of quinidine therapy. Am J Cardiol 1981; 48: 9–16.
42. McGovern B, Garan H, Kelly, Ruskin JN: Adverse reactions during treatment with amiodarone hydrochloride. Br Med J 1983; 287: 175–180.
43. Nathan AW, Hellestrand KJ, Bexton RS, Banim SO, Spurrell RAJ, Camm AJ: Proarrhythmic effect of the new antiarrhythmic agent flecainide acetate. Am Heart J 1984; 107: 222–228.
44. Cullen K, Stenhouse NS, Wearne KL, Cumpston GN: Electrocardiographic and 13 year cardiovascular mortality in Bussleton study. Br Heart J 1982; 47: 209–212.
45. Campbell RWF: Ventricular ectopic activity and its relevance to aircrew licencing. Eur Heart J 1984; 5 (Suppl A): 95–98.

1.4 Sudden Death in Cardiomyopathies

F. GARCÍA COSÍO and J. PALACIOS MARTINEZ

Introduction

Sudden death has traditionally been considered a sign of fury of the gods and a reason for meditation, although, in another light, it could also be seen as the death for the virtuous. It is a tragic and final event that, like many other biological phenomena, modern medicine has not ceased to analyze with the curious and bold gaze that has paved the way for so many therapeutic advances. Nowadays, sudden death (SD) translates in the mind of the physician into an abrupt cessation of cardiac function, generally due to arrhythmia.

In recent years, the instruments that the engineers have placed at the service of cardiology have permitted an increasingly more extensive study of the mechanisms involved in the cardiac arrhythmias and SD. First, the mechanisms of cardiac arrest were studied in patients in coronary units, resulting in their successful treatment. The next step was the creation of mobile therapeutic units, that take the reanimation measures used in the hospital to the patients out of hospital, thus enabling recovery of considerable number of patients with cardiac arrest [1, 2].

However, the most important efforts have been directed toward prevention. The means to detect patients likely to suffer fatal arrhythmia are being sought, mainly by prolonged ambulatory monitoring of the cardiac rhythm [3] and electrophysiologic study of how the arrhythmias are precipitated by programmed cardiac stimulation [4, 5]. The most common cause of SD in the industrialized countries is undoubtedly coronary disease, and most of the data accumulated are from this selected group of patients. It is therefore important to remember that there are certain circumstances peculiar to coronary disease, such as the complication of stable causes of arrhythmia, scar tissue or transitory ischemic phenomena that make such observations on SD in coronary disease not necessarily applicable to patients with cardiomyopathies.

Most cases of SD recorded with the Holter method [6–9] or by mobile units [2] show ventricular fibrillation; nonetheless, some patients display asystolia, which seems to have a worse prognosis [2]. In coronary atherosclerosis, a large amount of data have been accumulated that relate SD with repetitive ventricular arrhythmias detected by the Holter system. Most of the information on the problem of SD in the cardiomyopathies is in this line of possibilities.

The cardiomyopathies have recently been reclassified [10], but the existence of such a structured classification should not cause us to forget that there are still many unanswered questions in this field. For instance, an apparently well defined group, such as that of the dilated cardiomyopathies (DCM), probably includes a variety of processes with similar functional repercussions on the myocardium. Nonetheless, since the concept of DCM has evidently been accepted, we will limit ourselves to reviewing the available information on factors predisposing to SD in this syndrome.

Hypertrophic cardiomyopathy (HCM) has been extensively studied, probably because definition of its hemodynamic and echocardiographic features has made its detection and the compilation of numerous experiences easier. We will analyze HCM separately because its peculiarities make it difficult to compare with other types of cardiomyopathy.

The data available on other types of cardiomyopathy and specific myocardial diseases are not sufficient for an accurate analysis to be made as in DCM and HCM, and will not be considered.

Sudden death in dilated cardiomyopathy

Fifty per cent of the deaths that occur in this syndrome are sudden [11], presumably arrhythmic. We know of no studies that offer an anatomo-electrophysiologic correlation to explain the pathogenesis of arrhythmias in DCM, but it seems theoretically acceptable that the diseased myocardial fibers would have abnormal electrophysiologic properties which may include increased dispersion of the refractory periods, slow conduction of early impulses, or abnormal automaticity. Moreover, the dilated myocardium may be subject to abnormal pressures and, possibly, an inadequate blood supply [12–14] that could contribute to the appearance of electrophysiologic abnormalities. In fact, an association between the degree of impairment of left ventricular mechanical function and the incidence of ventricular arrhythmias has been observed in DCM [15, 16].

Three recent studies have analyzed the relationship between chronic repetitive ventricular arrhythmias and SD in DCM. The studies of Von Olhausen et al. [15] and Huang et al. [17] could not establish a correlation, but in that of Meinertz et al. [16] this relation was evident. Methodologic analysis of these communications clarifies the possible causes of the discrepancy. In the first two studies, the number of sudden deaths registered is small, making detection of the possible relation difficult. Moreover, the patients with severe ventricular arrhythmias received antiarrhythmic treatment, thus modifying the natural history of the group. On the contrary, the study by Meinertz et al. [16] included a larger number of patients who were followed up clinically and there was no pharmacologic intervention in the arrhythmias recorded. In this group, it was observed that 75% of the cases of SD had had 20 episodes or more of paired extrasystoles or of ventricular tachycardia runs daily, a figure not reached by any who died from heart failure. The presence of serious impairment of the mechanical function was also a significant factor, since only patients with a left ventricular ejection fraction of less than 40% died, and in 83% of cases only repetitive ventricular arrhythmias with important hemodynamic depression was predictive of sudden death.

The presence of chronic ventricular arrhythmias therefore seems to be an indicator of cardiac rhythm instability, but it is evident that an important number of SD are not predictable on the basis of this single datum. Does this mean that Holter studies should be repeated more frequently? In principle, it would seem advisable to study patients with serious hemodynamic involvement several times a year. However, it should be kept in mind that SD may be due to asystolia, atrioventricular block (AV) or rapid supraventricular arrhythmias, without disregard to the emboligenic potential of DCM, especially in the presence of atrial fibrillation [11, 18].

Can the natural course of the disease be altered by suppresion of these arrhythmias? There is no definite answer to this question, but we follow the recommendations of Graboys et al. [19], who apparently have managed to prevent sudden death by pharmacologic suppression of repetitive ventricular arrhythmias with aggressive treatment.

With what periodicity should Holter study be repeated in these patients? Studies should undoubtedly be weekly or biweekly when drugs or dosages are being changed in order to help find the ideal regimen. However, we do not have precise information on the evolution of arrhythmias with treatment which would allow us to establish specific recommendations for follow-up. Probably, control every three or six months would be sufficient if the patient's clinical course remains stable.

When a patient with DCM has sustained ventricular tachycardia, or it is demonstrated in a pharmacologic study after cardiac arrest, drug treatment should rely on chronic suppression tests of tachycardia induced by programmed cardiac stimulation [20].

Sudden death in hypertrophic cardiomyopathy

In HCM 60% or more of deaths are sudden. The intrinsic drama of the event is compounded by the fact that many patients are young and asymptomatic, and some are even athletes [21]. The natural history of this disease has been thoroughly studied by the groups of Bethesda and London [22, 23], and even before studies had been made of the incidence of arrhythmias family groups with special malignancy and a greater tendency to SD were defined [23, 24].

Obstruction of the left ventricular outflow tract was initially considered a key factor in the disease and it was thought that changes in the degree of obstruction could account for syncope and SD. At the end of the 70s, Holter studies demonstrated that there is a high incidence of arrhythmias in HCM, unrelated to the degree of obstruction [25–27]. Finally, a relation between repetitive ventricular arrhythmias and sudden death was demonstrated [28, 29].

The mechanism implicated in the ventricular arrhythmias may be related to the anatomic disposition of the muscle fibers or to the presence of macroscopic cracks in muscular masses [30], but there could also be electrophysiologic abnormalities peculiar to the myocardium of these hearts [31, 32]. On the other hand, myocardial blood flow is deficient in HCM, and ischemia may be another cause of ventricular arrhythmias [14, 33]. Some patients show areas of myocardial infarction where ventricular arrhythmias might originate [34].

Then again, not all cases of SD in HCM can be predicted from the presence of ventricular arrhythmia. Other arrhythmias are frequent, such as sinus bradycardia, atrial fibrillation and AV reentrant tachycardia [25–27]. Given the abnormal characteristics of the myocardium, with its impaired distensibility that makes ventricular filling difficult, it is possible that arrhythmias that in other circumstances would be well tolerated could have serious or fatal consequences in HCM [35].

For this reason, it is interesting to reconsider a study by James that describes the state of the cardiac conduction tissue in 22 patients with HCM who died suddenly [30]. In 12 cases there were *sinus node* lesions consistent in fibrosis, fatty degeneration or vascular obstruction, in 7 of them severe or massive. The *AV node* was abnormal in most cases, with predominance of a pattern of fragmentation and dispersion of the nodal tissue similar to the fetal structure. In 3 cases there were cysts or lacunae. The *bundle of His* was abnormal in more than half of the cases, with conspicuous focal fibrosis in the trunk or branches in 6, reduced trunk diameter in 3, a disperse, fetal type structure in 3 and cysts in 2 patients. *Anomalous connections* were also found between AV node and septal myocardium. Confronted with this accumulation of abnormalities, James theorized that the arrhythmia mechanism in HCM may be varied and that electrophysiologic studies of these patients should reveal frequent abnormalities.

In our laboratory, we studied 12 patients with HCM using clinical electrophysiology techniques for evaluation of AV conduction and sinus automaticity (the findings in the first 10 cases were the object of a previous publication [36]). The patients were part of a prospective HCM study and were not selected on the basis of the incidence of arrhythmia or arrhythmia-related symptoms (Table 1). We only excluded patients with serious hemodynamic impairment which could have been associated to poor tolerance to programmed cardiac stimulation.

The findings were surprising (Table 2). There were signs of sinus dysfunction in 3 cases, double nodal pathways in 3 and bifascicular block in 3 patients (2 of whom developed progressive prolongation of the HV interval with atrial stimulation, culminating in second degree block at high frequencies). Three patients showed an increase in AV node conduction that, although limited by HV block in 2 cases, produced a 1 : 1 AV conduction with an atrial rate of 250/min in the third. One patient had an anomalous left AV connection that only conducted retrogradely and which was responsible for the AV reentrant tachycardias. The study was completely normal in one case. Although some of the anomalies detected undoubtedly have little significance as isolated findings, in the group considered as a whole they are striking and suggest the existence of a correlation with James' [30, 36] anatomic findings.

A reexamination of the arrhythmias detected in HCM confirms the supposition that the arrhythmogenic mechanisms involved in this disease are complex. In 33 cases studied in our service, for which we had at least one 24-hour Holter

Table 1. Clinical data of 12 patients with hypertrophic cardiomyopathy and results of electrophysiologic studies.

Case	Age	Sex	Angina	Palpitation	Syncope	Obstruction	Clinical arrhythmias
1	18	M	−	−	+	−	Atrial fib.
2	30	M	+	−	−	−	−
3	25	M	+	−	−	−	−
4	31	F	−	−	−	P	−
5	9	F	+	−	+	P	−
6	51	M	+	−	−	B	−
7	30	M	+	+	+	P	Sustained ventr. tachy.
8	30	M	+	+	+	P	Reentrant AV tachycardia
9	23	F	+	+	−	B	−
10	33	M	−	−	−	B	−
11	35	F	−	−	−	−	−
12	63	F	+	−	−	B	−

P: on provocation.
B: basal.

recording in 30, aside from the increased incidence of repetitive ventricular arrhythmias (Table 3), we found noteworthy that of the atrial arrhythmias. Although it has been reported by other authors [25–27], the fact generally receives less comment than the ventricular arrhythmias. The presence of high ventricular rates during atrial tachyarrhythmia would be poorly tolerated in HCM, and these rates could become very high if atrial fibrillation, which is frequent, were to be associated with a superconductive AV node, a fetal feature commonly observed in our electrophysiologic studies. In cases of superconductive AV node, not only does poor hemodynamic tolerance have to be considered, but also the possible production of serious ventricular arrhythmias [37]. If we also take into account the increased incidence of embolism in

Table 2. Electrophysiologic findings related to sinus function and AV conduction in 12 cases of hypertrophic cardiomyopathy.

Secondary pauses in SRT	3
Double antegrade nodal pathway	3
Basal HV of more than 55 msec	4
Progressive prolongation of HV and second degree HV block with atrial stimulation	2
Superconductive AV node	3
δ wave and short PR	1
δ wave and normal PR	2
Antegrade preexcitation	0
Exclusively retrograde Kent bundle (QRS if δ wave)	1
No anomaly	1

Table 3. Incidence of arrhythmia in 33 cases of hypertrophic cardiomyopathy (clinical manifestations and Holter recordings).

Bradycardia or sinus pauses	2
Nonsustained atrial tachycardia	12
Paroxysmal atrial fibrillation	9
Sustained atrial fibrillation	6
Ventricular extrasystoles	
Monomorphic, less than 30/hour	8
Monomorphic, more than 30/hour	2
Multiform	4
Paired	3
Runs of 3 or more	3
Sustained ventricular tachycardia	1
Sustained AV reentrant tachycardia	1
Systemic embolism in patients with paroxysmal or sustained atrial fibrillation	5
Fatal embolisms	2

HCM with atrial fibrillation [21–23], confirmed in our cases, we must inevitably consider that atrial fibrillation may have a role in the incidence of SD in HCM.

In the experience of some authors [26, 38], sinus bradycardia has important consequences, requiring pacemaker implantation in some patients. We had this experience in one case. It should also be considered that sinus bradycardia with AV dissociation is a common cause of intolerance to verapamil treatment in HCM [39], which may be related to the prevalence of subclinical sinus dysfunction we detected. Finally, the potential that bradycardia has for facilitating ventricular arrhythmias in predisposed subjects is well known [40]. This effect may have appeared in one of our patients (case 1, Table 1) who had subclinical sinus dysfunction and suffered an episode of ventricular fibrillation.

Although the incidence of heart block in HCM does not seem to be very high, bundle branch block patterns are often observed and advanced AV block has been reported [38, 41]. AV block is likely to be a potential cause of SD, but the arrhythmic associations can be complex. In one of our cases (case 7, Table 1), the patient had bifascicular block and developed second degree HV block during atrial stimulation; however, the patient's syncopal episodes were due to sustained ventricular tachycardia that was controlled for 8 years by anti-arrhythmic treatment.

Reentrant AV tachycardias are common in HCM and their origin may be intranodal or due to anomalous AV fibers [35, 36, 38, 42]. The resulting rapid rates may cause syncope (case 8, Table 1), and, possibly, SD [35]. In this respect, it is interesting to remember that ventricular preexcitation is impossible to diagnose unequivocally in HCM using only the electrocardiogram because these patients can have δ waves, with or without short PR, in the absence of antegrade preexcitation [35, 38, 43]. These δ waves would be due to the intraventricular conduction disorders characteristic of this disease.

In summary, the ventricular arrhythmias are common in HCM, and the repetitive forms are associated with an increased incidence of SD, but there may be other arrhythmogenic mechanisms that contribute to the production of fatal arrhythmias. The treatment of arrhythmias in HCM should always be based on Holter recordings, not only to detect repetitive ventricular arrhythmias, but also atrial and atrioventricular arrhythmias, bradycardia and AV block. In particular, bradycardia can be precipitated by treatment with beta-blocking agents or verapamil and may require implantation of a pacemaker.

Nonsustained ventricular arrhythmias detected by Holter ECG should be treated with antiarrhythmic drugs, following the indications of Graboys et al. [19] and lending due attention to the possible appearance of bradyarrhythmia as a side effect. In cases of sustained ventricular tachycardia, the best tactic is probably to characterize the arrhythmia by means of programmed cardiac stimulation and serial pharmacologic suppression tests of the arrhythmia [20]. Another alternative may be treatment with high doses of amiodarone, without considering its effects on the precipitability of the arrhythmia, which does not seem to have any relationship with the drug's prophylactic effectiveness [44, 45].

A recently published study by McKenna et al. [46] poses new questions: one of the authors' HCM patients had an episode of syncope with undetectable arterial pulse, but the electrocardiogram disclosed simple sinus tachycardia. With this in mind, we should not overlook the possible role of hemodynamic factors (abrupt increase in obstruction, sudden decline in distensibility or contractility) in the pathogenesis of SD in HCM.

References

1. Nagel EL, Liberthson RR, Hirschman JC, Nussenfeld SR: Emergency care. Circulation 1975; 51–52 (Suppl III): 216–218.
2. Longstreth WT, Diehr P, Inui TS: Prediction of awakening after out-of-hospital cardiac arrest. New Engl J Med 1983; 308: 1378–1382.
3. Cosio, FG: Utilidad de la monitorización cardiaca ambulatoria por el método Holter. Med Clin 1983; 81: 732–735.
4. Josephson ME, Horowitz LN, Spielman SR, Greenspan AM: Electrophysiologic and hemodynamic studies in patients resuscitated from cardiac arrest. Am J Card 1980; 46: 948–955.
5. Morady F, Scheinman MH, Hess DS, Sung RJ, Shen E, Shapiro W: Electrophysiologic testing in the management of survivors of out-of-hospital cardiac arrest. Am J Card 1983; 51: 85–89.
6. Panidis I, Morganroths J: Holter monitoring during sudden cardiac death: clues to its etiology and prevention (Abstract). Circulation 1982; 66 (Suppl II): 25.
7. Nikolic G, Bishop RL, Sihgh JB: Sudden death recorded during Holter monitoring. Circulation 1982; 66: 218–225.
8. Denes P, Gabster A, Huang SK: Clinical, electrocardiographic and follow-up observations in patients having ventricular fibrillation during Holter monitoring. Role of quinidine therapy. Am J Card 1981; 48: 9–16.
9. Lewis BH, Antman EM, Graboys TB: Detailed analysis of 24 hour ambulatory electrocardiographic recordings during ventricular fibrillation or torsade de pointes. JACC 1983; 2: 426–436.
10. Report of the WHO/ISFC task force on the definition and classification of cardiomyopathies. Br Heart J 1980; 44: 672–673.
11. Johnson RA, Palacios I: Dilated cardiomyopathies of the adult. New Engl J Med 1982; 307: 1051–1058 and 1119–1126.
12. Weiss MB, Ellis K, Sciacca RR, Johnson LL, Schmith DH, Cannon PJ: Myocardial blood flow in congestive and hypertrophic cardiomyopathy. Relationship to peak wall stress and mean velocity of circumferential fiber shortening. Circulation 1976; 54: 484–494.
13. Thompson DS, Naqui N, Juul SM, Swanton RH, Wilmshurst P, Coltart DJ, Jenkings BS, Webb-Peploe MM: Cardiac work and myocardial substrate extraction in congestive cardiomyopathy. Br Heart J 1982; 47: 130–136.
14. Pasternac A, Noble J, Strenlens Y, Elie R, Henschke C, Bourassa MG: Pathophysiology of

chest pain in patients with cardiomyopathies and normal coronary arteries. Circulation 1982; 65: 778–789.

15. Von Olhausen K, Schafer A, Mehmel HC, Schwarz F, Senges J, Kubler W: Ventricular arrhythmias in idiopathic dilated cardiomyopathy. Br Heart J 1984; 51: 195–201.

16. Meinertz T, Hofman T, Kasper W, Treese N, Bechtoldt H, Steinen U, Pop T, Leitner VE-R, Andersen D, Meyer J: Significance of ventricular arrhythmias in idiopathic dilated cardiomyopathy. Am J Card 1984; 53: 902–907.

17. Huang K, Messer JV, Denes P: Significance of ventricular tachycardia in idiopathic dilated cardiomyopathy: Observations in 35 patients. Am J Card 1983; 51: 507–512.

18. Fuster V, Gersh BJ, Giuliani ER, Tajik AJ, Brandenburg RO, Frye RL: The natural history of idiopathic dilated cardiomyopathy. Am J Card 1981; 47: 525–531.

19. Graboys TB, Lown B, Podrid PJ, De Silva J: Long-term survival of patients with malignant ventricular arrhythmia treated with antiarrhythmic drugs. Am J Card 1982; 50: 437–443.

20. Farré J, Grande A, Hernandez-Antolin R, De Pablos L, Lopez-Minguez JR, Del Amo L, De Rabago P: Tratamiento de las arritmias ventriculares malignas. In: Sociedad Española de Cardiología (ed) Avances en cardiología. Científico Médica, Barcelona, 1983; 103–118.

21. Maron BJ, Roberts WC, McAllister HA, Rosing DR, Epstein SE: Sudden death in young athletes. Circulation 1980; 62: 218–229.

22. Braunwald E: The natural history of idiopathic hypertrophic subaortic stenosis. In: Wolstenholme GEW, O'Connor M (eds) Hypertrophic obstructive cardiomyopathy. J. & Churchill, London, 1971; 30–41.

23. McKenna W, Deanfield J, Faruqui A, England D, Oakley C, Goodwin JF: Prognosis in hypertrophic cardiomyopathy: role of age and clinical, electrocardiographic and hemodynamic features. Am J Card 1981; 47: 532–538.

24. Maron BJ, Lipson LC, Roberts WC, Savage DD, Epstein SE: 'Malignant' hypertrophic cardiomyopathy: Identification of a subgroup of families with unusually frequent premature death. Am J Card 1978; 41: 1133–1140.

25. Savage DD, Seides SF, Maron BJ, Myers DJ, Epstein SE: Prevalence of arrhythmias during 24 hours electrocardiographic monitoring and exercise testing in patients with obstructive and nonobstructive hypertrophic cardiomyopathy. Circulation 1979; 59: 866–875.

26. Canedo MI, Frank MJ, Abdulla AM: Rhythm disturbances in hypertrophic cardiomyopathy. Prevalence, relation to symptoms and management. Am J Card 1980; 45: 848–855.

27. McKenna WJ, Chetty S, Oakley CM, Goodwin JF: Arrhythmia in hypertrophic cardiomyopathy: exercise and 48 hour ambulatory electrocardiographic assessment with and without beta-adrenergic blocking therapy. Am J Card 1980; 45: 1–5.

28. McKenna W, England D, Doi YL, Deanfield JE, Oakley C, Goodwin JF: Arrhythmia in hypertrophic cardiomyopathy. I: Influence in prognosis. Br Heart J 1981; 46: 168–172.

29. Maron BJ, Savage DD, Wolfson JK, Epstein SE: Prognostic significance of 24 hour electrocardiographic monitoring in patients with hypertrophic cardiomyopathy: A prospective study. Am J Card 1981; 48: 252–257.

30. James TN, Marshall TK: De subitaneis mortibus. Assymetrical hypertrophy of the heart. Circulation 1975; 51: 1149–1166.

31. Coltart DJ, Neldfrum SJ: Hypertrophic cardiomyopathy: an electrophysiological study. Br Med J 1970; 4: 217–218.

32. Cosio FG, Moro C, Alonso M, Saenz de la Calzada C, Llovet A: The Q waves of hypertrophic cardiomyopathy. An electro-physiologic study. New Engl J Med 1980; 302: 96–99.

33. Thompson DS, Naqui N, Juul SM, Swanton RH, Coltart DJ, Jenkins BS, Webb-Peploe MM: Effects of propanolol on myocardial oxygen consumption, substrate extraction and haemodynamics in hypertrophic obstructive cardiomyopathy. Br Heart J 1980; 44: 488–498.

34. Maron BJ, Epstein SE, Roberts WC: Hypertrophic cardiomyopathy and transmural myocar-

dial infarction without significant atherosclerosis of the extramural coronary arteries. Am J Card 1979; 43: 1086–1102.

35. Goodwin JF, Krikler DM: Arrhythmias as a cause of sudden death in hypertrophic cardiomyopathy. Lancet 1976; 2: 937–940.

36. Cosio FG, Vidal JM, Palacios J, Tascon J: Estudio electrofisiológico de la función sinusal y la conducción aurículo-ventricular en la miocardiopatía hipertrófica. Rev Esp Card 1982; 35: 339–345.

37. Benditt DG, Pritchett ELC, Smith WM, Wallace AG, Gallagher JJ: Characteristics of atrioventricular conduction and the spectrum of arrhythmias in Lown-Ganong-Levine syndrome. Circulation 1978; 57: 454–465.

38. Gullotta SJ, Gupta RD, Padmanabham VT, Morrison J: Familial occurrence of sinus bradycardia, short PR interval, interventricular conduction defects, recurrent supraventricular tachycardia and cardiomegaly. Am Heart J 1977; 93: 19–29.

39. Epstein SE, Rosing DR: Verapamil: its potential for causing serious complications in patients with hypertrophic cardiomyopathy. Circulation 1981; 64: 437–441.

40. Han J: Mechanisms of ventricular arrhythmias associated with myocardial infarction. Am J Card 1969; 24: 800–813.

41. Karinv I, Sherf L, Salomon M: Familial cardiomyopathy. With special consideration of electrocardiographic and vectorcardiographic findings. Am J Card 1964; 13: 734–749.

42. Ingham RE, Mason JW, Rossen RM, Goodman DJ, Harrison DC: Electrophysiologic findings in patients with idiopathic hypertrophic subaortic stenosis. Am J Card 1978; 41: 811–816.

43. Cosio FG, Sanchez A, Vidal JM, Iglesias J, Garcia Martinez J: Preexcitation patterns in hypertrophic cardiomyopathy. Am Heart J 1981; 101: 233–234.

44. Morady F, Suave MJ, Malone P, Shen EN, Schwartz AB, Bhandari A, Keung E, Sung RJ, Schinman MM: Long-term efficacy and toxicity of high-dose amiodarone therapy for ventricular tachycardia or ventricular fibrillation. Am J Card 1983; 52: 975–979.

45. Waxman HL, Buxton AE, Marchlinski FE, Flores BT, Rogers DP, Josephson ME: Amiodarone for sustained ventricular tachyarrhythmias: Electrophysiologic study is not predictive of clinical efficacy (Abstract). Circulation 1983; 68 (Suppl III): 382.

46. Mc Kenna WJ: Arrhythmia and prognosis in hypotrophic cardiomyopathy. Eur Heart J 1983; 4 (Suppl F): 225–234.

1.5 Sudden Death in the Wolff-Parkinson-White Syndrome

HEIN J.J. WELLENS and PEDRO BRUGADA

Sudden death may occur in the young patient with the Wolff-Parkinson-White syndrome [1–16]. The purpose of this article is to discuss the mode of sudden death, the recognition of the possible candidate and the prevention of such an event.

Mode of sudden death

In the human heart the refractory period of the AV node protects the ventricle against very high rate supraventricular rhythms. In the presence of an accessory atrio-ventricular (AV) pathway the ventricular rate during supraventricular rhythms not only depends on the refractory period of the AV node but also on the refractory period of the accessory AV pathway. If the refractory period of the latter is very short atrial flutter and atrial fibrillation can become life-threatening arrhythmias. Indeed, in patients with the Wolff-Parkinson-White syndrome deterioration of atrial fibrillation to ventricular fibrillation has been reported [1, 8, 10, 12, 16]. As shown in Table 1 several factors determine the ventricular rate during atrial fibrillation.

An important role is played by the duration of the refractory period of the accessory AV pathway. Three groups of investigators [17–19] found a correlation between the duration of the refractory period of the accessory AV pathway and the ventricular rate during atrial fibrillation. There was an excellent correlation between the shortest R-R interval during atrial fibrillation and the duration of the refractory period of the accessory pathway [18, 19]. Theoretically therefore the most dependable way to identify the high risk patient with the WPW-syndrome would be the determination of the duration of the antegrade refractory period of the accessory pathway during programmed electrical stimulation of the heart. Because the duration of the refractory period of the accessory pathway might shorten on increasing heart rate several atrial pacing rates should be used during the study. This should preferable be followed by the induction of atrial fibrillation to ascertain the ventricular rate during this arrhythmia. Also, because the refractory period of the accessory pathway may shorten by sympathomimetic stimulation as occurs during exercise or isoprenaline administration [20] the antegrade refractory period of the accessory pathway should be determined under these circumstances. While the determination of the antegrade refractory period of the accessory pathway during programmed stimulation of the heart is an excellent method to recognize the high risk patient there are exceptions to this rule. As recently reported by our group [21] in the patient with atrial fibrillation and a relatively long antegrade refractory period of the accessory pathway the ventricular rate may be much higher than expected because of re-entry in the bundle branch system following ventricular activation over the accessory pathway. This reentry mechanism may result in a new QRS-complex with a short coupling interval. If this occurs frequently the ventricular rate during atrial fibrillation may be much higher than suspected from atrio-ventricular conduction over the accessory pathway alone.

It should be stressed however, that in general a good correlation exists between the antegrade refractory period of the accessory pathway and the ventricular rate during atrial fibrillation. As pointed out by Klein et al. [10] all 25 patients developing ventricular fibrillation during atrial fibrillation showed the shortest R-R interval to be 250 msec or less. The same authors showed that apart from a very short R-R interval during atrial fibrillation, a history of both atrial fibrillation and reciprocal tachycardia and the presence of multiple

Table 1. Factors determining ventricular rate during atrial fibrillation in Wolff-Parkinson-White syndrome.

Accessory pathway
1. Refractory period.
2. Input, transmission and output characteristics which are influenced by the width, length and type of tissue of the accessory pathway.
3. Concealed conduction:
   – in atrio-ventricular direction,
   – in ventriculo-atrial direction.
4. Reentry.

Atrio-ventricular nodal pathway
1. Refractory period.
2. Input, transmission and output characteristics.
3. Concealed conduction.
4. Reentry.

Ventricle.
1. Refractory period.
2. Intramural or bundle branch reentry.

accessory pathways were helpful in identifying the patient prone to the development of ventricular fibrillation. It is of importance that several of them were receiving digitalis at the time of occurrence of their ominous arrhythmia. In our own experience ventricular fibrillation usually develops during exercise or anxiety, indicating that additional sympathomimetically-induced shortening of the antegrade refractory period of the accessory pathway leads to very high ventricular rates during atrial fibrillation resulting in ventricular fibrillation.

Recognition of the high risk patient

Because sudden death can be the first manifestation of the WPW syndrome [7, 9] information as to the duration of the antegrade refractory period of the accessory pathway is of importance in the asymptomatic patient. The following three findings point to a relatively long refractory period:

1. *Intermittent preexcitation:* in our experience patients showing intermittent AV conduction over their accessory pathway never have a short refractory period of this structure in antegrade direction.
2. *The ajmaline or procainamide test:* we have demonstrated that failure to produce complete block in the accessory pathway in antegrade direction by the intravenous injection of 50 mg ajmaline given over a three minute period indicates as antegrade refractory period of the accessory pathway of 270 msec or less [22] (see Table 2). The same was found after the intravenous administration of procainamide [23] when 10 mg/kg bodyweight was injected over a 5 minute period. Complete antegrade block occurred in the accessory pathway when the refractory period was 270 msec or longer.
3. *The effect of exercise:* Levy et al. [24] showed that the development of complete block in the accessory pathway during exercise corresponded to a relatively long antegrade refractory period of the accessory pathway. On using this test, however, one should realize that exercise shortens conduction time through the AV node thereby increasing the degree of ventricular

Table 2. Effect of 50 mg ajmaline given intravenously in relation to the length of the antegrade refractory period of the accessory pathway in 100 consecutive patients with the WPW-syndrome.

	Antegrade block in AP	
	+	−
ERP AP>270 msec	43/47	4/47
ERP AP≤270 msec	8/53	45/53

Abbreviations: ERP = effective refractory period; AP = accessory pathway.

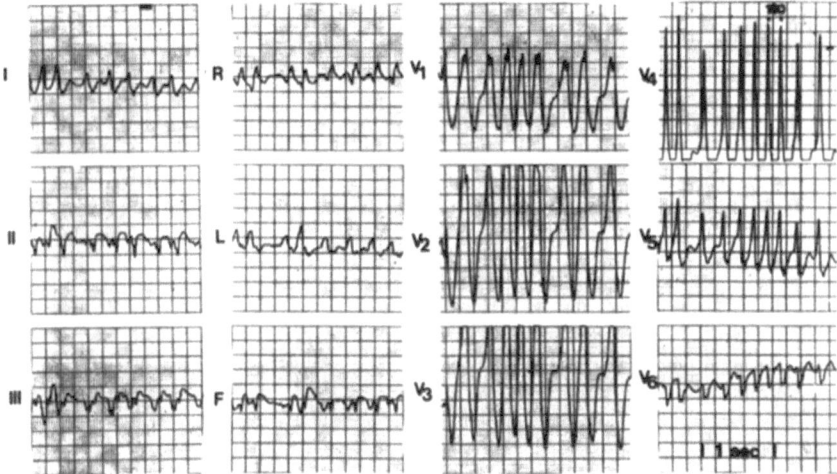

Fig. 1. Atrial fibrillation in a patient with a left-sided accessory pathway. The rapid ventricular rate is the consequence of the short antegrade refractory period of the accessory pathway.

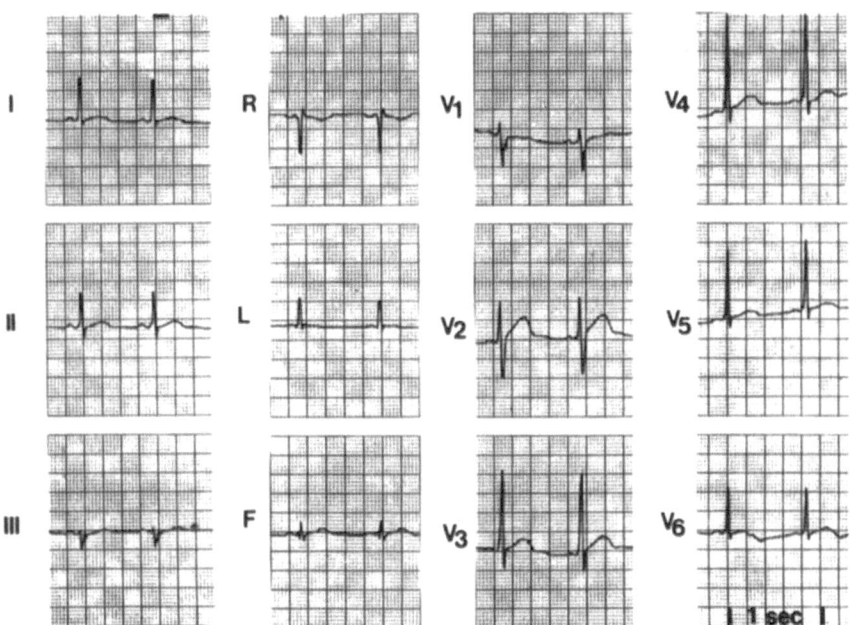

Fig. 2. The same patient during sinus rhythm. Note that little contribution to ventricular activation occurs from atrio-ventricular conduction over this left-sided accessory pathway.

excitation over the AV node-His axis. Especially in left laterally located accessory pathways this may falsely give the impression of antegrade block in the accessory pathway.

The degree of preexcitation during sinus rhythm has no predictive value as to the length of the refractory period of the accessory pathway. This is an important point because as shown in Figs 1 and 2 patients with little evidence of preexcitation during sinus rhythm may have life-threatening ventricular rates during atrial fibrillation.

Prevention of sudden death

Since the mode of death unique to the WPW-patient is based on the presence of an accessory pathway with a short refractory period, the most logical form of therapy would be the administration of an agent that would lengthen the duration of the refractory period of the accessory pathway. Previously we have reported on the relation between the initial length of the refractory period of the accessory pathway and the effect of drugs [25]. It was found that patients with an antegrade refractory period equal to or more than 270 msec responded to administration of quinidine, procainamide, ajmaline and amiodarone by marked prolongation of the antegrade refractory period of their accessory pathway. Of importance, however, in relation to the treatment of the WPW-patient at risk was the observation of no or only slight lengthening of the antegrade refractory period of the accessory pathway following the administration of these drugs when the duration of the antegrade refractory period of the accessory pathway was less than 270 msec. In the latter group of patients, of the drugs investigated, amiodarone gave the greatest amount of lengthening of the duration of the antegrade refractory period of the accessory pathway. We also found that the effect of chronic oral amiodarone administration could be predicted from the results of the ajmaline or procainamide test [26]. Those data indicate that the effect of most antiarrhythmic drugs on the duration of the antegrade refractory period of the accessory pathway is least in patients who are most in need of prolongation of the refractory period of that structure. With some of the newer drugs like lorcainide and encainide the relation between the initial duration of the antegrade refractory period of the accessory pathway and the effect of the drug is however less clear [27, 28].

The symptomatic patient

In the WPW-patient with documented ventricular fibrillation or atrial fibrillation with high ventricular rates surgical interruption of the accessory pathway should be considered. As pointed out by Gallagher et al. [29] this can be done

36

with excellent results. We study the effect of Amiodarone on the antegrade refractory period of the accessory pathway only in the patient with a septal location of the bypass. The duration of the refractory period of the accessory pathway and the ventricular response to electrically induced atrial fibrillation are determined before and after at least 28 days of chronic oral administration of amiodarone. Since the effect of amiodarone on the duration of the refractory period of the accessory pathway may be individually different, we insist upon a study with and without amiodarone in the symptomatic patient. If in the patient with a septally located bypass the results of amiodarone therapy are unsatisfactory we refer the patient for surgical interruption of the accessory pathway.

The asymptomatic patient

As described, intermittent preexcitation, the production of AV block in the accessory pathway by ajmaline or procainamide and possibly the disappearance of preexcitation on exercise identify the patient with WPW not at risk for sudden death in case of atrial fibrillation. If the WPW electrocardiogram is repeatedly present and antegrade conduction over the accessory pathway cannot be blocked by ajmaline, we determine the duration of the refractory period of the accessory pathway during a programmed stimulation study. In the asymptomatic patient with a short refractory period of the accessory pathway we do not routinely prescribe amiodarone because of the side effects of the drug. These patients are being followed to get better knowledge about the natural history of this subgroup of patients. Such knowledge should inform on the real danger of sudden death in the patient with an accessory pathway and a short refractory period, and thus provide a more realistic basis for treatment.

References

1. Dreifus LS, Haiat R, Watanabe Y: Ventricular fibrillation: A possible mechanism of sudden death in patients with Wolff-Parkinson-White syndrome. Circulation 1971; 43: 520.
2. Laham J: Actualités electrocardiographiques 1969: Le syndrome de Wolff-Parkinson-White. Paris, Librairie Malione, SA, 1969.
3. Kaplan MA, Cohen KL: Ventricular fibrilation in the Wolff-Parkinson syndrome. Am J Cardiol 1969; 24: 259.
4. Okel BB: The Wolff-Parkinson-White syndrome: Report of case with fatal arrhythmia and autopsy findings of myocarditis, interatrial lipotamous hypertrophy and prominent right moderator band. Am Heart J 1968; 75: 673.
5. Castillo-Fenoy A, Goupil A, Offenstadt G, et al.: Syndrome de Wolff-Parkinson-White et mort subite. Ann Med Intern 1973; 124: 871.
6. Lem CH, Toh CCS, Chia BL: Ventricular fibrillation in type B Wolff-Parkinson-White syndrome. Aust NZJ Med 1974; 4: 151.

7. Coumel PH, Slama R: Syndrome de Wolff-Parkinson-White. Rev Prat 1975; 25: 1821.

8. Dreifus LS, Wellens HJJ, Watanabe Y, et al.: Sinus bradycardia and atrial fibrillation associated with the Wolff-Parkinson-White syndrome. Am J Cardiol 1976; 38: 14.

9. Gallagher JJ, Pritchett ELC, Sealy WC, et al.: The pre-excitation syndromes. Progr Cardiovasc Dis 1978; 20: 285.

10. Klein GJ, Bashore TM, Sellers TD, et al.: Ventricular fibrillation in the Wolff-Parkinson-White syndrome. N Engl J Med 1979; 301: 1080.

11. Martin-Noel P, Denis B, Grundwald D, et al.: Deux cas mortels de syndrome de Wolff-Parkinson-White. Arch Mal Cœur 1970; 63: 1647.

12. Ahlinder S, Granath A, Holmer S, et al.: The Wolff-Parkinson-White syndrome with paroxysmal atrial fibrillation changing into ventricular fibrillation, successfully treated with external heart massage. Nord Med 1963; 70: 1336.

13. Fox TT, Weaver J, March HW: On the mechanism of the arrhythmias in aberrant atrioventricular conduction (Wolff-Parkinson-White). Am Heart J 1952; 43: 507.

14. Touche M, Touche S, Jouvet M, et al.: Eléments de prognostic dans le syndrome de Wolff-Parkinson-White. Presse Mèd 1968; 76: 567.

15. Duvernoy WFC: Sudden death in Wolff-Parkinson-White syndrome. Am J Cardiol 1977; 39: 472.

16. Cosio FG, Benson DW, Anderson RW, et al.: Onset of atrial fibrillation during antidromic tachycardia: Association with sudden cardiac arrest and ventricular fibrillation in a patient with Wolff-Parkinson-White syndrome. Am J Cardiol 1982; 50: 353.

17. Castellanos A Jr, Myerburg RJ, Craparo K, et al.: Factors affecting ventricular rates during atrial flutter and fibrillation in pre-excitation (Wolff-Parkinson-White) syndrome. Br Heart J 1973; 35: 811.

18. Wellens HJJ, Durrer D: Wolff-Parkinson-White syndrome and atrial fibrillation: Relation between refractory period of the accessory pathway and ventricular rate during atrial fibrillation. Am J Cardiol 1974; 34: 777.

19. Campbell RWF, Smith RA, Gallagher JJ, et al.: Atrial fibrillation in the pre-excitation syndrome. Am J Cardiol 1977; 40: 514.

20. Wellens HJJ, Brugada P, Roy D, et al.: Effect of isoproterenol on the anterograde refractory period of the accessory pathway in patients with the Wolff-Parkinson-White syndrome. Am J Cardiol 1982; 50: 180.

21. Kuck KH, Brugada P, Wellens HJJ: Observations on the antidromic type of circus movement tachycardia in the Wolff-Parkinson-White syndrome. JACC 1983; 5: 1003.

22. Wellens HJJ, Bär FW, Gorgels AP, et al.: Use of Ajmaline in identifying patients with the Wolff-Parkinson-White syndrome and a short refractory period of their accessory pathway. Am J Cardiol 1980; 45: 63.

23. Wellens HJJ, Braat SHJG, Brugada P, et al.: Use of Procainamide in patients with the Wolff-Parkinson-White sydrome to disclose a short refractory period of the accessory pathway. Am J Cardiol 1982; 50: 921.

24. Levy S, Broustet JP, Clémenty J, et al.: Syndrome de Wolff-Parkinson-White: Corrélations entre l'exploration électrophysiologique et l'effet de l'épreuve d'effort sur l'aspect électrocardiographique de préexcitation. Arch Mal Cœur 1979; 72: 634.

25. Wellens HJJ, Bär FW, Dassen WR: Effect of drugs in WPW syndrome. Importance of initial length of effective refractory period of accessory pathway. Am J Cardiol 1980; 46: 665.

26. Brugada P, Dassen WR, Braat SH, et al.: Value of the ajmaline/procainamide test to predict the effect of chronic oral Amiodarone on the anterograde effective refractory period of the accessory pathway in the Wolff-Parkinson-White syndrome. Am J Cardiol 1983; 52: 70.

27. Bär FW, Farré J, Ross D, et al.: Electrophysiological effects of lorcainide: a new antiarrhythmic drug. Br Heart J 1981; 65: 292.

28. Abdollah H, Brugada P, Green M, et al.: Clinical efficacy and electrophysiologic effects of intravenous and oral encainide in patients with accessory atrioventricular pathway and supraventricular arrhythmias. Am J Cardiol 1984; 54: 544.
29. Gallagher JJ, Sealy WC, Cox JL, et al.: Results of surgery for preexcitation caused by accessory atrioventricular pathways in 267 consecutive cases. In: Josephson ME, Wellens HJJ (eds) Tachycardias; mechanism, diagnosis, treatment. Lea and Febiger, Philadelphia, 1984; 259.

1.6 Conclusions

C. RIBEIRD

The study and treatment of the arrhythmias has grown to include diverse fields. Clinical, electrophysiologic and pharmacologic studies have enabled us to specify the place the arrhythmias occupy in clinical practice.

In most cases of sudden death, there are few doubts that the terminal event is a phenomenon of lethal cardiac electrical instability. However, this phenomenon is always surrounded by an aura of mystery and apprehension.

The authors of this chapter have commented on a large variety of factors that contribute to the pathogenesis of sudden death. It has been demonstrated that the subject is not static, but instead offers a dynamic substrate that can suffer modifications due to changes in autonomic nervous tone, blood flow, basal heart rate, pH, electrolyte balance, tissue oxygenation and humoral mediators.

As a contribution, Dr Cinca has published a report on 'Circadian influences on the electrophysiologic properties of the human heart'. The objective of his study was to investigate whether there are circadian alterations in the electrophysiologic cardiac parameters, that is AV conduction time, and the refractory periods of the atrium, AV node and right ventricle. Dr Cinca found that there is a nocturnal prolongation in cardiac refractory periods and the QT interval, reduction in the repetitive ventricular responses and difficulty in inducing reciprocating tachycardia at this time of the day.

Dr Campbell did not reach optimistic conclusions: although the population *groups* at risk can be identified, the prediction of *individual* risk is imperfect. Likewise, factors that modify the risk are poorly understood, and Dr Campbell concluded that to reduce the risk of sudden death a better knowledge of the physiopathology of ventricular tachycardia and fibrillation is needed.

However, Dr Campbell thought that it was important to define two groups: apparently normal individuals and patients with clinical problems. When commenting on the apparently normal individuals, Dr Campbell insisted on the following points:
- elevated rate of ventricular arrhythmias,
- occult coronary heart disease,
- family history of sudden death,
- hyperlipidemia,

– important tobacco abuse.

When we consider these points, we become aware of the difficulties involved in determining the degree of individual risk.

In the terrain of individuals with clinical problems and a propensity to sudden death, Dr Campbell emphasized the fact that the majority of the victims of sudden death have coronary heart disease, although sudden death can appear in small children, young athletes, persons with a prolonged QT interval, mitral prolapse, etc.

The most conspicuous factors modifying risk are, among others:

– β-blocking treatment in chronic ischemic heart disease,
– surgical treatment of left main coronary artery disease,
– surgical treatment of some ventricular aneurysms.

However, attention must be given to some medical acts that are antagonistic, such as the proarrhythmic effect of the antiarrhythmic drugs.

Considering the clinical situations that might lead to sudden arrhythmic death, aside from those already mentioned, two fundamental diseases appear:

– cardiomyopathies,
– preexcitation syndromes.

It is known that hypertrophic cardiomyopathy often produces ventricular tachyarrhythmias that, if malignant, can be an important cause of sudden death. Dr García Cosío has defined various subgroups at risk for sudden death.

Dr Wellens and Dr Brugada have reported new findings that should be added to the already numerous contributions they have made to cardiology in relation to a classic problem: Wolff-Parkinson-White syndrome.

2. The Pharmacological Treatment of Severe Arrhythmias

2.1 Introduction

A. BAYÉS DE LUNA

If there were no danger of sudden death (SD), ventricular arrhythmias (VA) would have little importance in practice. If we consider SD to be death that presents within an hour of the onset of the first symptoms, there is one SD per minute in the United States [1, 2]. Although in Spain there are no exact statistics on the number of SD, the estimation in that there are more than 30,000 per year. Eighty to ninety per cent of the SD are of cardiac origin and of these 80–90% are due to ventricular fibrillation precipitated by premature ventricular complexes (PVC). For this reason, anything related to PVC treatment is important. No study [3] has demonstrated that empirical administration of an antiarrhythmic drug reduces the risk of SD.

On the other hand, most of the antiarrhythmic drugs can aggravate an already existent arrhythmia or induce the appearance of a new one (e.g. *torsade de pointe*) [4]. This is another important issue that has led us to believe [5] that it is inopportune to empirically treat patients for PVC. At least the effect of the different drugs must be controlled with repeat Holter recordings.

It is thus important to consider whether all patients with PVC should be treated. Approximately 3% of patients who have suffered an acute myocardial infarction die of SD within the first year after the event. In view of the fact that in the United States there are one million new infarctions each year, theoretically up to 30,000 people could be saved. However, to do so, one million patients would have to be treated, possibly aggravating already existent arrhythmias or provoking the appearance of new ones in a number of cases. As there is no antiarrhythmic drug that is highly effective and innocuous, we should only treat postinfarction patients or those who have other heart diseases with a risk of SD [5].

Recent epidemiologic studies [5–7] have demonstrated that the two parameters that most affect the mortality of postinfarction patients are: complex type PVC (types 3 to 5 of Lown's classification) and heart failure. It thus seems appropriate to treat PVC of types 3 to 5 of the Lown classification and those of type 2 (more than 30 per hour) in postinfarction patients. Treatment is probably also indicated in patients with other heart diseases, especially if they have poor ventricular function, uncreated sympathetic tone, ischemic episodes or long QT. On the other hand ventricular arrhythmias that occur in apparently healthy individuals should be considered to be benign.

Symptomatic ventricular tachycardia and ventricular fibrillation outside the acute phase of infarction are considered as a malignant ventricular arrhythmia (MVA). This affects a limited number of patients, probably no more than 2–3% of the postinfarction cases, some instances of dilated cardiomyopathy and other forms of severe heart diseases. Those patients who present with these arrhythmias and do not die as a consequence of them have a 30% mortality rate within the first year [8]. These cases must be adequately, not empirically, treated to avoid recurrence of the arrhythmia. It is mandatory that an individualized and controlled therapy be undertaken.

There are three approaches to monitoring treatment. Myerburg and Castellanos recommend determining *plasma concentrations* [9]; this serves to obtain a therapeutic level that, independent of the presence or not of extrasystoles, has been demonstrated to be effective in the reduction of the incidence of SD. The other two approaches, *acute testing* (AT) [8], introduced by Lown and his team, and *intracavitary electrophysiologic studies* (IES) [10], defended fundamentally by Josephson, have also demonstrated their usefulness, although there are more studies corroborating the efficacy of IES than of AT.

AT can only be performed if the Holter recording evidences frequent and reproducible PVC, and it is considered the most appropriate means of choosing a treatment. If the Holter ECG shows few PVC or they are not reproducible, treatment can rely on IES or plasma concentrations. These two procedures are used by some groups unguided by the Holter results.

These aspects will be dealt with in this chapter. Dr P. Puech will treat the aspects related to a special type of malignant ventricular arrhythmia defined by the French school, the *'torsades de pointe'*. Drs Almendral, Graboys and Myerburg, of the groups of Philadelphia (Josephson), Boston (Lown) and Miami (Castellanos), pioneers in the use of electrophysiologic studies, acute testing and plasma concentrations in the control of antiarrhythmic therapy, will describe their experiences in these fields.

We think that the future of the Mirowski technique and the catheter procedures is very promising, considering that the ideal antiarrhythmic has yet to be found. These techniques will probably soon be of daily use in the treatment of the malignant arrhythmias.

Lastly Dr Domínguez de Rozas will discuss the value of empirical treatment with amiodarone in patients with malignant ventricular arrhythmias.

References

1. Julian DC: Toward preventing coronary death from ventricular fibrillation. circulation 1976; 54: 360–366.
2. Wenger NK, Mock MB, Burgkist I: Ambulatory ECG recording. Current Probl Cardiol 1980; 5: 1–42.
3. Julian DG: Prevention of sudden death. In: Harrison DC (ed) Cardiac arrhythmias. A decade of progress. GK Hall Med Publ, Boston, 1981; 111.
4. Velebit V, Podrid P, Lown B, Cohen B, Graboys T: Aggravation and provocation of ventricular arrhythmias by antiarrhythmic drugs. Circulation 1982; 65: 886–894.
5. Bayes de Luna A, Serra Grima JR, Oca F: ECG de Holter. Ed Científico-Médica, Barcelona, 1983.
6. Ruberman V, Weinblatt E, Goldberg J, Frank CW, Shapiro S: Ventricular premature beats and mortality after acute myocardial infarction. N Engl J Med 1977; 279: 750–757.
7. Harrison DC (ed): Cardiac arrhythmias. A decade of progress. GK Hall Med Publ, Boston, 1981.
8. Graboys TB, Lown B, Podrid PJ, De Silva R: Long term survival of patients with malignant ventricular arrhythmias treated with antiarrhythmic drugs. Am J Cardiol 1982; 50: 437–445.
9. Myerburg RJ, Kessler K, Kiem I, et al.: Relationship between plasma levels of procainamide suppression of PVC and prevention of recurrent ventricular tachycardia. Circulation 1981; 64: 280–288.
10. Horowitz LN, Josephson ME, Kastor JA: Intracardiac electrophysiologic studies as a method for the optimation of drug therapy in chronic ventricular arrhythmias. Prog Cardiovasc Dis 1980; 23: 81–89.

2.2 Torsades de Pointe

P. PUECH and P. GALLAY

Torsades de pointe were described by Dessertenne as a variety of non-sustained polymorphous ventricular tachycardia in subjects presenting bradycardia due to atrio-ventricular block [1]. The name 'torsades de pointe' is now universally accepted and is preferred to other synonyms referring to the same aspect of the waves in the ectopic ventricular complexes: ventricular pseudo-fibrillation [2], transitory ventriculation [3], transitory recurrent ventricular fibrillation [4], paroxistic ventricular fibrillation [5], cardiac ballet [6], ventricular fibrilloflutter [7], polymorphious ventricular tachycardia [8], multiform ventricular tachycardia [9] and helicoidal tachycardia [10].

Considering only the morphology of ventricular complexes in tachycardia, torsade de pointe may belong to either of two groups:
1. The usual type which corresponds to the torsade de pointe 'stricto sensu' according to the original French description appearing on a lengthened QT and induced by a ventricular extrasystole with late coupling (on the peak of the T or U wave) and generally permanent.
2. The ventricular tachycardias with morphology of torsade usually with a normal QT between crises and with slightly early coupling of the initial extrasystole. This difference is not purely academic, but corresponds to different therapeutic etiologies and therapeutics.

The general characteristics of torsade de pointe are electrical, clinical and evolutive. Electrically, the torsade are seen as a succession of ectopic complexes of long amplitude and variable polarity, with progressive and cyclic rotation (in general from 5 to 10 complexes) and rapid complexes (points) in relation to the isoelectric line. The characteristic appearance of waves in the tracing is not always evident in a single lead; therefore, simultaneous recording of various leads, especially in the frontal plane, show the helicoidal aspect of the tracing. In contrast to ventricular fibrillation, the depolarization and repolarization phases are clearly individualized. The P waves, usually visible in the surface tracings, appear to be dissociated and slower in selective atrial recordings. The mean ventricular frequency is of 220/min, but there are important variations, as the torsade may be relatively slow (160/min) or very fast (280/min) and present with an irregular rhythm. The duration of each torsade is of some seconds and it is usually necessary to have a minimum of 6 ventricular complexes in succession to identify the characteristic aspect of the torsade. Isolated or grouped ventricular extrasystoles, frequently forming aborted torsade of 3–5 polymorphic complexes, are recorded in the interval between torsade.

Clinically, the torsade which is prolonged provoke a cardio-circulatory failure generating syncope, specially if the torsade is produced in a standing position.

Their evolution is characterized by the spontaneous resolution with frequent recurrent crisis. If left untreated, torsade de pointe may degenerate into ventricular fibrillation.

Premonitory appearances of torsade de pointe are sometimes seen, especially in the usual type with inter-critical long QT. The appearance of a ventricular bigeminism with prolonged QT in the basal rhythm is a frequent forerunner of torsade; thus, lengthening of diastole associated to a post-extrasystolic pause prolongs the repolarization of the following complex which is demonstrated by exaggerated deformation of the final part of the Y wave on which the triggering ventricular extrasystole will fall [11]. The inscription of giant T waves (in AV blocks in particular) and above all the alternance of the T wave (especially in the syndromes of congenital long QT) are also frequent forerunners of torsade.

Torsades de pointe and long QT

Etiology

The principal causes of torsade are extreme bradycardias, hypokalemia and IA type antiarrhythmic drugs. Torsade de pointe represents between 10 and 15% of the causes of Adams-Stokes crisis in the course of atrio-ventricular blocks. The block is usually advanced and permanent, but the torsade may appear in the course of a paroxysmal AV block or during the temporal accentuation of the bradycardia, for example, after the administration of atropine [12] or anticholinergic substances [13] in case of infrahisian block. Torsades de pointe in the course of sinusal bradycardias are much more rare [14].

Hypokalemia is the most frequent cause of the torsade de pointe seen in clinical practice [4, 14, 15] with numerous causes for the loss of potassium (laxatives, diuretics, chronic diarrheas, primary or secondary hyperaldosteronism. Certain β-lactam antibiotics used in high dosis for severe infection (carboxipenicillin) provoke marked hypokalemia-producing torsades de pointe [16]. Figure 1 is an example of this.

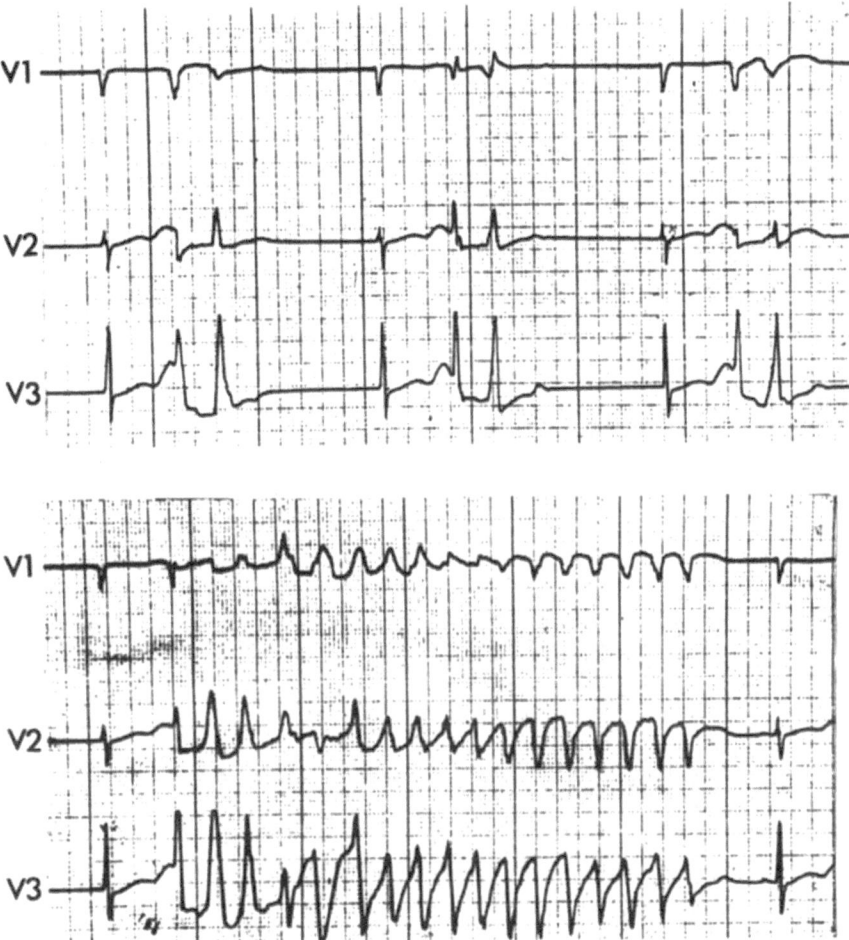

Fig. 1. Female of 71-years-old. Hypokalemia of 2.7 mE/L is due to carboxipenicillin treatment. Above: couplets of premature ventricular contraction with coupling interval of 680 msec, the basical rhythm is junctional escape rhythm. Below: torsades de pointe.

Quinidine has long been recognized as a triggering factor in torsade de pointe [5]. The 'quinidine syncopes' are always in linear relationship with the dosis, and the plasmatic concentration during the torsades is frequently within therapeutic limits, thus suggesting an idiosyncratic phenomenon [17] or pre-disposing factors [11]. Other class IA antiarrhythmic drugs (disopyramide, procainamide) may be responsible for the torsades de pointe [18, 24], some being fatal [25].

The causes of torsade de pointe are multiple. Hypomagnesemia has been included among the metabolic factors, especially in chronic alcoholics [26, 27].

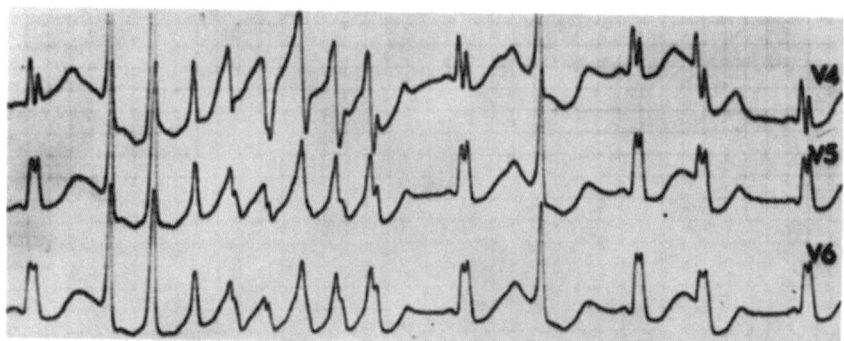

Fig. 2. Female of 80-years-old. Prenilamine provokes marked hypokalemia (2.9 mEq/L) producing torsades de pointe.

Hypokalemia is an exceptional cause and rarely isolated [28, 29].

Within the group of drugs that can trigger torsades de pointe, IB or IC type antiarrhythmic drugs are rarely found (lidocaine, aprindine [30]) which affect ventricular repolarization (JR interval) only slightly if at all. The lengthening of repolarization under sotalol explains the appearance of torsade with this β-blocker [31, 32] with a greater frequency than with amiodarone [18, 33–37]. It is also frequently associated with other factors, particularly bradycardia and/or hypokalemia. Other drugs in use in cardiology such as prenilamine [38–41], lidoflacine [42, 43] or bepridil [44] provoke torsades de pointe as do other vasodilators for cerebrovascular use such as vincamine [45, 46] and phenoedil [47, 48]. Of the psychotropic drugs, phenotiacin [22, 49], tricyclic antidepressives [50, 51] and tetracyclines [52] may provoke torsade de pointe. Quinidine torsades may be related to those observed with the use of chloroquine [53]. Very fast slimming drugs may alter the QT and give rise to sometimes fatal arrhythmias among which torsades de pointe can be seen. From among the exogenic intoxications, poisoning by organophosphorate insecticides is the most well-known [54, 55] with arsenic poisoning being rare.

Acute encephalic accidents and especially encephalomeningeal hemorrhage are often accompanied by severe disturbances of ventricular repolarization, although the torsade-type arrhythmias appear to be infrequent [8, 26, 56]. In mitral valve prolapse the QT interval is sometimes lengthened, favouring the appearance of torsades [57]. The frequence of associated factors favouring the appearance of the torsades de pointe stands out. The predominance of these, brought about by drugs in the female sex, is notable [28, 38, 44] (personal observations), with perhaps the statistically longer QT interval being a predisposing factor as well as the frequent use of laxatives. The existence of a hypokalemia in the course of the antiarrhythmic-antianginal treatment (Fig. 2) and the bradycardia caused by certain antiarrhythmic drugs may precipitate the torsades de pointe. The existence of a cardiomegaly is a factor favouring quinidine torsades [11, 58]. Digital drugs which alone do not provoke torsade de pointe, might facilitate the appearance of these in subjects treated with antiarrhythmic drugs of the IA type [11], perhaps secondary to the cellular depletion of potassium, therefore shortening the potential of subendocardic action and also increasing the dispersion of repolarization among the subendocardic and subepicardic layers.

The congenital syndromes of long QT (Jerwell-Lange-Nielson and Romano-Ward) are complicated by severe arrhythmias with torsade de pointes possibly degenerating into ventricular fibrillation [59].

Mechanism

There is an experimental model of arrhythmia which is similar to torsade de pointe as seen in clinical practice. On preparations of endocardic fibres isolated from the ventricle of the dog, cesium (5 mM) lengthens the duration of the action potential of the Purkinje fibres and provokes the appearance of early post-potentials by the slow rhythm [60]. When the postpotentials appear in phase 3 for a relatively high potential level (between -65 and -80 mV) these may produce a sustained activity [60] as a result of the low concentration of potassium [61]. This abnormal activity in phase 3 is abolished by the low concentration of TTX suggesting the intervention of an entry current of sodium in these postpolarizations. In the animal model, the intravenous injection of cesium chloride (1 to 1.5 mg/kg) lengthens the QT interval (QU) and produces ventricular arrhythmias, including torsade de pointe-type polymorphous tachycardias.

Electrophysiological studies in man

The recording of monophasic action potentials (MAP) on different zones of the right ventricle in subjects with long QT [62] shows that ventricular repolarization is of variable duration according to the topography of MAP. In the zones in which the MAP is very long, there is a hump in the late part of phase 3, so that when there is an arrhythmia the initial extrasystole arises from this abnormal portion of action potential. The delay in repolarization and the arrhythmia which reprocedes for this motive disappear with ventricular stimulation.

Programmed ventricular stimulation gives different results depending on whether it is carried out some time after an episode of torsade or in the evolutive period. Except during crisis, torsades are not reproducible [68] although it seems possible to trigger them at times in the critical phase [64–66].

Magnesiotherapy

A deficit of magnesium is rarely seen. The supply of magnesium, which was recently described [66], undoubtedly has its own electrophysiological effect through the ATP-ase dependent Mg pump which acts on the active trans-membrane Na-K exchange (K penetration in the cell).

The emergency treatment, an intravenous bolus of 1–2 g of magnesium sulphate, often has a spectacular effect on the torsade (personal observation). In case of necessity this may be continued by a perfusion of 1 mg/min/24 hours of $MgSO_4$.

Further experimentation will allow to determine to what degree magnesiotherapy could prevent cardiac stimulation from being used for the emergency treatment of torsades de pointe.

Cardiac acceleration

The well-known effect of shortening of the action potential by accelerating the stimulation frequency and the improved resynchronization this implies, with the refractory periods being less disperse, explains the beneficial action of the tachycardiac procedures in the treatment of the torsade de pointe with long QT.

Perfusion of isoprenaline is only of minor help, and its action is demonstrated above all in the torsade de pointe in severe bradycardias. The potentially beneficial effect of isoprenaline runs the risk of being lessened by facilitating the production of extrasystoles and by reducing the arrhythmic cycle and leading to ventricular fibrillation.

For these reasons, transitory electrical stimulation is the treatment of choice, adjusting the stimulation frequency to the threshold of disappearance of the arrhythmia [14]. Theoretically, atrial stimulation is preferable, as it provides good ventricular synchronization, but in reality, in a context of emergency and keeping in mind the risk of displacement of the atrial electrode, ventricular stimulation is usually used.

In conclusion, torsades de pointe with long basal QT appear when the repolarization is prolonged in an asynchronic manner. It is possible that the rarity of the torsade in patients treated with amiodarone is related to the fact that the repolarization is delayed in a uniform way, thus preventing ventricular desynchronization. The appearance of postpotentials in phase 3, for a relatively high level of repolarization of membrane, reflects an abnormal automatism, a factor that triggers the arrhythmia. This initial event is followed by a polymorphic tachycardia. The focal origin of this self-maintained tachycardia from two opposite focii of very similar frequencies or reincorporation with the variable circuit and slow conduction can not at present be evaluated [67].

Treatment

Antiarrhythmic drugs

Antiarrhythmic drugs which prolong the repolarization (class IA and III) are accepted as being contra-indicated. It is preferable to avoid all types of anti-arrhythmic drugs, although isolated successes with substances with little or practically no effect on repolarization have been published, as in case of the antiarrhythmic drugs of group IB (lidocaine, diphenylhydantoin), IC (pro-paphenon) [9], or verapamil [53]. The non-constant positive results may be explained by the reduction or supression of inductor extrasystoles, without aggravating the lengthening of the QT.

Action of the causal factor

Suppression of the substance or substances which may influence ventricular repolarization could be sufficient to make the torsade disappear, if the elim-ination of the incriminating product is rapid and if there is no associated metabolic factor, in particular hypokalemia.

Correction of the metabolic disturbances is imperative. In the case of hypokalemia, either demonstrated or simply suspected, it is necessary to administrate intravenous potassium in high dosis (12 to 20 g/24 hours) under electrocardiographic control.

Definitive cardiac stimulation completely prevents the risk of recurrent torsades de pointe in permanent or paroxysmal atrio-ventricular blocks.

Congenital long QT syndrome

The imbalance in the sympathetic innervation of the heart explains the length-ening of the QT and the factors frequently observed to precipitate the syn-copes by torsades de pointe (effort, emotion, stress). Treatment with β-blockers, with the exclusion of sotalol, constitutes the most appropriate long-term treatment. Left-sympathectomy has given variable results.

Torsades de pointe and normal QT

Acute ischaemic torsades de pointe

A ventricular tachycardia with the aspect of torsades in the course of acute myocardial infarction is rare [9, 68]. In a recent study, Vidal et al. [69] calculated 2.2% within the first 72 hours of myocardial infarction. Prinzmetal

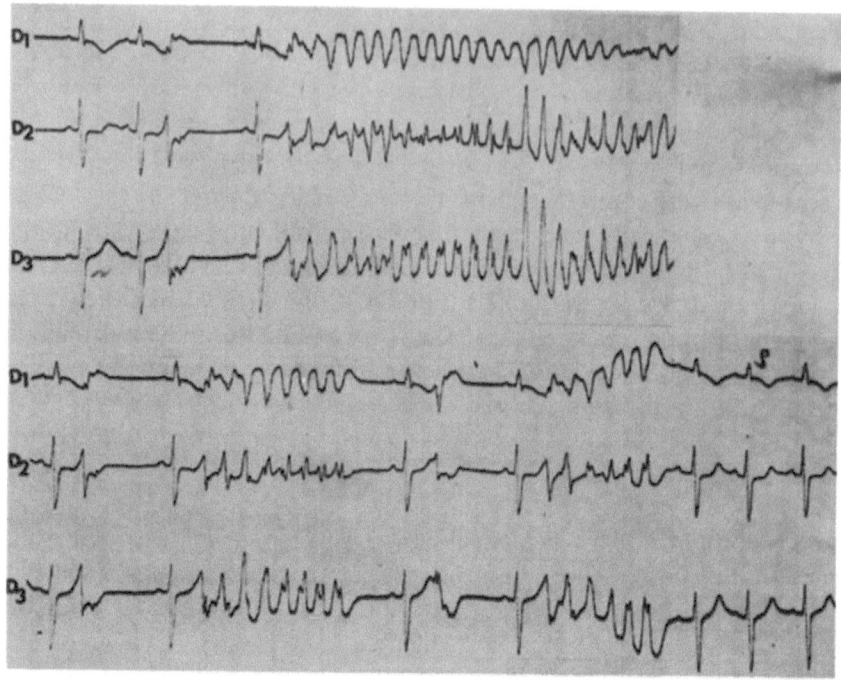

Fig. 3. Male of 58-years-old. Torsades in the course of the acute myocardial infarction. Intermittent bygeminal premature ventricular contraction leading to torsades de pointe with relatively low coupling interval. QT interval variations (normal or mildly prolonged).

angina, which may be accompanied by alternans in repolarization, has on occasion been found to be the origin of the torsades, with ischaemia very rarely being the only inducing factor [70].

The QT interval is usually normal. It is sometimes transiently or permanently lengthened [71, 72]. The triggering extrasytole has an early coupling (Fig. 3), and the cycle of the tachycardia is generally short (fast torsades). The transformation of torsades into authentic ventricular fibrillation is particularly frequent.

The treatment of ischaemic torsades is frequently difficult. Isoprenaline is formally contra-indicated. Antiarrhythmic IA and IB drugs are usually not effective. Propaphenon gave a high percentage of success in the series of Zilcher et al. [9]. Amiodarone or tosilate of bretilium perfusions are sometimes efficient. Calcium antagonists are indicated in the case of Prinzmetal angina. Endocavitary stimulation presents unconstant results and the often high frequency of stimulation required may be poorly tolerated from a hemodynamic point of view. Stimulation is sometimes even dangerous, precipitating the appearance of ventricular fibrillation. No study on the effects of intravenous magnesiotherapy for this indication have yet been published.

Recurrent torsade de pointe

Tachycardias with morphology of torsade with normal or somewhat prolonged QT have been observed, with relatively early coupling of the initial extrasystole, usually in patients with chronic coronary heart disease and also in several cardiomyopathies [73].

These tachycardias can generally be reproduced by means of ventricular stimulation [64, 68, 73] and can be transformed into monomorphic ventricular tachycardias either spontaneously or under stimulation, or using class IA (quinidine or procainamide) antiarrhythmic drugs. Therefore, this type of torsade may be considered as a variety of polymorphous ventricular tachycardia, much more similar in its mechanism to common ventricular tachycardia than to the torsade de pointe with long QT. This relationship with the recurrent ventricular tachycardias is reinforced by the usual efficacy of class IA antiarrhythmic drugs in this type of torsade. The role of other antiarrhythmic drugs in the long-term treatment of the recurrent ventricular tachycardias also stands out.

Catecholaminic torsades de pointe

Disturbances of the polymorphous ventricular rhythm comparable to torsade de pointes have been seen in young individuals [74]. In this population, 7 to 13 year old, the circumstances of appearance of the polymorphous tachycardia are very particular, suggesting the influence of a catecholaminic discharge: stress, emotion or effort. The tachycardias may be reproduced by an exercise test or perfusion of isoprenaline. Keeping these elements in mind, treatment with β-blocking agents is particularly indicated.

Idiopathic torsades de pointe

Torsade de pointe are occasionally seen in subjects whose intercritical ECG was normal and with absent heart disease or evident triggering circumstances.

In some observations, the torsade de pointe has a familial character. Some of these observations are similar to the Romano-Ward syndrome to an extent that a familial investigation often reveals a long QT in other members of the family. On the other hand, a normal QT at rest may be prolonged on carrying out an exercise test. However, the QT may be permanently normal in very rare cases of familial torsade de pointe, the peculiarity of which is derived from the fact that they may be induced by programmed ventricular stimulation [75]. Very little is yet known regarding isolated idiopathic torsade de pointe.

In two personal recent observations, these idiopathic torsades were triggered by the endocavitary stimulation (recurrent crisis leading to ventricular fibrillation), were refractory to the administration of potassium and responded well to high dosis of intravenous magnesium. This type of torsade is possibly responsible for certain sudden deaths in subjects without apparent heart disease.

References

1. Abinader EG, Shahar J, P. Puech: Possible female preponderance in prenylamine – induced 'Torsades de pointes' Tachycardia. Cardiology, 1983; 70: 37–40.
2. Azpitarte Almagro J, Casero A, Melgares R: Torsade de pointes inducida por disopiramida. Presentación de un caso de evolución fatal. Rev Esp Cardiolog 1984; 37: 145–148.
3. Bardy GH, Ungerleider RM, Smith WM, Ideker RE: A mechanism of Torsades de pointes in a canine model. Circulation 1983; 67: 52–59.
4. Bauman JL, Bauernfeind RA, Hoff JV, Strasberg B, Swiryn S, Rosen KM: Torsades de pointes due to quinidine: observations in 31 patients. Am Heart J 1984; 107: 425–430.
5. Bennett KR: Torsade de pointes and mitral valve prolapse. Am J Cardiol 1980; 45: 715.
6. Bens JL, Duboisset, Quiret JC, Lesbre J Ph, Bernasconi P: Syncopes par torsades de pointe induites ou favorisées par la prénylamine. Arch Mal Cœur 1973; 66: 1247–1254.
7. Botti G, Bonatti V: Pathogenesis of ventricular arrhythmias in long QT syndromes. In: Masoni A, Alboni P (ed) Cardiac electrophysiology today. Academic Press, London and New-York, 1982; 291–305.
8. Brachmann J, Scherlag BJ, Rosenstraukh LV, Lazzara R: Bradycardia-dependent triggered activity: relevance to drug-induced multiform ventricular tachycardia. Circulation 1983; 68: 846–856.
9. Brochier M, Fauchier JP: Torsades de pointes et ré-entrées provoquées par les antiarrhythmiques. Arch Mal Cœur 1978; 71: 477–482.
10. Castellanos A, Salhanick L: Electrocardiographic pattern of procainamide toxicity. Am J Med Sci 1967; 253: 52–60.
11. Coumel Ph, Fidelle J, Lucet V, Attuel P, Bouvrain Y: Catecholamine-induced severe ventricular arrhythmias with Adams-Stokes syndrome in children. Report of four cases. Br Heart J 1978; 40 (suppl): 28–37.
12. Damiano BP, Rosen MR: Effects of pacing on triggered activity induced by early after depolarizations. Circulation 1984; 69: 1013–1025.
13. Dany F, Merle L, Goudoud JC, Liozon F, Blanc P, Bouvot JC, Nicot G, Dangoumau J: Les accidents cardiaques de la vincamine. Therapie 1981; 36: 55–64.
14. Dessertenne F: La tachycardie ventriculaire à deux foyers opposés variables. Arch Mal Cœur 1966; 59: 263–272.
15. Evans TR, Curry PVL, Fitchet DH, Krikler DM: 'Torsades de pointes' initiated by electrical stimulation. J Electrocardiol 1976; 9: 255–258.
16. Fauchier JP, Lanfranchi S, Ginies G, Raynaud R: Syncopes par 'torsades de pointe' au cours d'un traitement par la chloroquine. Ann Cardiol Angeiol 1974; 23: 341.
17. Fazekas T, Kiss Z: Torsade de pointes ventricular tachycardia associated with lidoflazine therapy. Eur Heart J 1984; 5: 343.
18. Fontaine G, Frank R, Lascault G, Tonet JL, Fillette F, Grosgogeat Y: Torsades de pointes favorisées par stimulations ventriculaires à rythme lent. Arch Mal Cœur 1983; 76: 918–924.
19. Forfar JC, Gribbin B: Torsade de pointes after amiodarone with drawal of wild hypokalaemia on repolarization. Eur Heart J 1984; 5: 510–512.

20. Fowler NO, Mc Call D, Chou T, Holmes JC, Hanenson IB: Electrocardiographic changes and cardiac arrhythmias in patients receiving psychotropic drugs. Am J Cardiol 1976; 37: 223–230.
21. Goldsmith S, From AHL: Arsenic-induced atypical ventricular tachycardia. N Engl J Med 1980; 303: 1096–1098.
22. Gonzalez-Hermosillo JA, Cardenas M, Hurtado BL, Vidal J: Taquicardia ventricular helicoidal ('torsades de pointes'). Arch Inst Cardiol México 1977; 47: 5.
23. Grenadier E, alpan G, Maor N, Keidar S, Binenboim C, Margulies T, Palant A: Polymorphous ventricular tachycardia in acute myocardial infarction. Am J Cardiol 1984; 53: 1280–1283.
24. Guillou M, Ceriou A, Blanc JJ, Boschat J, Granatelli D, Penther D: Torsades de pointes; responsabilité eventuelle d'un vasodilatateur périphérique, le fénoxédil. Nouv Presse Méd 1975; 4: 29.
25. Hanley SP, Hampton JR: Ventricular arrhythmia associated with lidoflazine: side-effects observed in a randomized trial. Eur Heart J 1983; 4: 889–893.
26. Herrmann HC, Kaplan LM, Bierer BE: QT prolongation and Torsades de pointes tachycardia produced by the tetracylic anti-depressant agent maprotiline. Am J Cardiol 1983; 51: 904–906.
27. Horowitz LN, Greespan AM, Spielman SR, Josephson ME: Torsades de pointes: electrophysiologic studies in patients without transient pharmacologic or metabolic abnormalities. Circulation 1981; 63: 1120–1128.
28. Isner JM, Sours HE, Paris AL, Ferrans VJ, Roberts WC: Sudden unexpected death in avid dieters using the liquid protein modified fast diet: observations in 17 patients ant the role of the prolonged QT interval. Circulation 1979; 60: 1401–1412.
29. Jenzer HR, Hagemeijer F: Quinidine syncope: Torsades de pointes with low quinidine plasma concentrations. Eur J Cardiol 1976; 4: 447–451.
30. Keren A, Tzivoni D, Gavish D, Levi J, Gottlieb S, Benhorin J, Stern S: Etiology, warning signs and therapy of Torsade de pointes. A study of ten patients. Circulation 1981; 64: 1167–1174.
31. Khan M, Logan KR, Mc Coomb JM, Adger AAJ: Management of recurrent ventricular tachy-arrhythmias associated with QT prolongation. Am J Cardiol 1981; 47: 1301–1308.
32. Kirkler DM, Curry PVL: 'Torsades de pointes' and atypical ventricular tachycardia. Brit Heart J 1976; 38: 117–120.
33. Kiss Z, Fazckas T: Arrhythmias in organophosphate poisonings. Acta Cardiol 1979; 34: 3223–2330.
34. Langou RA, van Dyke C, Tahan SR, Cohen RS: Cardiovascular manifestacions of tricyclic anti-depressant overdose. Am Heart J 1980; 100: 458–464.
35. Laprevotte-Heully MC, Lambert H, Larcan A: Syncopes par torsades de pointes. Rôle de la vincamine. A propos de 3 observations. Nouv Presse Méd 1974; 3: 13.
36. Lathour H, Puech P, Hertault J, Stefanou G, Grolleau R, Simorre R, Sat M: Syncopes après réduction de fibrillation auriculaire par choc électrique et hydroquinidine. Arch Mal Cœur 1966; 59: 533.
37. Leclercq JF, Maisonblanche P, Cauchemez B, Atuel P, Coumel Ph: Troubles du rythme ventriculaires polymorphes familiaux incessants avec anomalies de la repolarisation ventriculaire forme frontière du syndrome du QT long congenital? Arch Mal Cœur 1984; 77: 1013–1019.
38. Leclerq JF, Kural S, Valere PE: Bépridil et torsades de pointe. Arch Mal Cœur 1983; 76: 341–347.
39. Lestringant A: Torsades de pointe sous traitement par bêtalactamines. Thèse Montpellier, mai 1982.

40. Loeb HS, Pietras RS, Gunnar RM, Tobin JR: Paroxysmal ventricular fibrillation in two patients with hypomagnesemia. Treatment by transvenous pacing. Circulation 1968; 37: 210.
41. Lucet V, Dongoc D, Toumieux MC, Mercier JN, Fidelle J: Torsades de pointe chez l'enfant. Rôle possible du diphémanil. Presse Méd 1984; 13: 1979.
42. Ludomirsky A, Klein HO, Sarelli P, Becker B, Hoffman S, Taitelman U, Barzilai J, Lang R, David D, Disegni E, Kaplinsky E: QT prolongation and polymorphous ('Torsade de pointes') ventricular arrhythmias associated with organophosphorous insecticide poisoining. Am J Cardiol 1982; 49: 1654–1658.
43. Luomanmäki K, Keikkilä J, Hartikainem M: T wave alternons associated with heart failure and hypomagnesemia in alcoholic cardiomyopathy. Eur J Cardiol 1975; 3: 1167.
44. McCoomb JM, Logan KR, Khan MM, Geddes JS, Adgey AAJ: Amiodarone induced ventricular fibrillation. Eur J Cardiol 1980; 11: 381–385.
45. Mc Kibbin JK, Pololck WA, Barlow JB, Scott Millar RN, Obel IW: Sotalol, hypokalaemia, syncope and torsade de pointes. Br Heart J 1984; 51: 157–162.
46. McWilliam JA: Some applications of physiology to medicine. II, Ventricular fibrillation and sudden death. Br Med J 1923; 2: 215.
47. Mikolich JR, Jacobs WC, Fletcher GF, Cardiac arrhythmias in patients with acute cerebro vascular accidents. JAMA 1981; 246: 1314–1317.
48. Motte G, Laine JF, Sebag C, Davy JM: Torsades de pointe favorisées par l'atropine. Nouv Presse Méd 1982; 11: 3571–3572.
49. Motte G, Coumel Ph, Abitbol G, Dessertenne F, Slama R: Le synchrone QT long et syncopes par Torsades de pointes. Arch Mal Cœur 1970; 63: 831–853.
50. Navarro-López F, Cinca J, Sanz G, Periz A, Magrina J, Betriu A: Isolated T wave alternans. Am Heart J 1978; 95: 369–374.
51. Neuvonen PH, Elonen E, Vuorenmaa T, Laasko M: Prolonged QT interval and severe tachyarrhythmias, common features of sotalol intoxication. Eur J Clin Pharmacol 1981; 20: 85–89.
52. Normand JP, Kahn JC, Mialet G, Bardet J, Bourdarias JP, Mathivat A: Torsades de pointes induites ou favorisées par la prénylamine. Ann Cardiol Angeiol 1974; 23: 527–533.
53. Olshansky B, Martins J, Hunt S: N-acetylprocainamide causing torsades de pointes. Am J Cardiol 1982; 50: 1439–1441.
54. Pernot C, Henry M, Aigle JC: Syndrome cardio-auditif de Jerwell et Torsades de pointes. Arch Mal Cœur 1972; 65: 261.
55. Puech P, Bosc E, Grolleau R, Cabasson J, Mellet JM, Ferriere M: Troubles du rythme cardiaque liés aux fénoxédil. Ann Cardiol Angeiol 1976; 25: 297–302.
56. Puritz R, Henderson MA, Baxer SN, Chamberlain DA: Ventricular arrhythmias caused by prenylamine. Br Med J 1977; 2: 608–609.
57. Ranquin R, Parizel G: Ventriculor fibrillo-flutter (torsade de pointe): an established electro-cardiographic and clinical entity. Angiology 1977; 28: 115–118.
58. Salvador M, Thomas C, Mazeno M, Conte J, Meriel P, Lesbre P: Troubles du rythme directement induits ou favorisées par les déplétions potassiques. Arch Mal Cœur 1970; 63: 230–257.
59. Santinelli V, Chiariello M, Santinelli C, Condorelli M: Ventricular tachyarrhythmias complicating amiodarone therapy in the presence of hypokaliemia. Am J Cardiol 1984; 53: 1462–1463.
60. Sawaya JJ, Rubeiz GA: Prinzmetal's angina with Torsades de pointe ventricular tachycardia. Acta Cardiol 1980; 35: 47.
61. Scagliotti D, Strasberg B, Hai HA, Kehoe R, Rosen K: Aprindine-induced polymorphous ventricular tachycardia. Am J Cardiol 1982; 49: 1297, 1300.
62. Schwartz SP, Hallinger LN: Transient ventricular fibrillation. Amer Heart J 1954; 48: 390–404.

58

63. Sclarovsky S, Lewin RF, Krakoff O, Strasberg B, Arditti A, Agmon J: Amiodarone induced polymorphous ventricular tachycardia. Am Heart J 1983; 105: 6–11.
64. Sclarovsky S, Strasberg B, Lewin RF, Agmon J: Polymorphous ventricular tachycardia: clinical features and treatment. Am J Cardiol 1979; 44: 339.
65. Selzer A, Wray HW: Quinidine syncope, paroxysmal ventricular fibrillation occuring during treatment of chronic atrial arrhythmias. Circulation 1964; 30: 17.
66. Slama R, Coumel Ph, Motte G, Gourdon R, Wayenberger M, Touche S: Tachycardies ventriculaires. Fontières morphologiques entre les dysrythmies ventriculaires. Arch Mal Cœur 1973; 66: 1401–1411.
67. Smirk FM: Cardiac ballet: repetitions of complex electrocardiographic patterns. Br Heart J 1969; 31: 426.
68. Soffer J, Dreifus LS, Michelson EL: Polymorphous ventricular tachycardia associated with normal and long QT intervals. Am J Cardiol 1982; 49: 2021–2029.
69. Strasberg B, Sclarovsky S, Erdberg A, Duffy CE, Lam W, Swiryn S, Agmon J, Rosen KM: Procainamide-induced polymorphous ventricular tachycardia. Am J Cardiol 1981; 47: 1309–1314.
70. Strasberg B, Welch W, Palileo E, Swiryn S, Bauernfeind R, Rosen KM: Familial inducible Torsade de pointes with normal QT interval. Eur Heart J 1983; 4: 383–391.
71. Tamura K, Tamura T, Yoshida S, Inui M, Fukuhara N: Transient recurrent ventricular fibrillation due to hypopotassemia with special note on the U wave. Jpn Heart J 1967; 8: 652.
72. Taylor GJ, Crampton RS, Gibson RS, Stebbins PT, Waldman MT, Beller GA: Prolonged QT interval at onset of acute myocardial infarction in predicting early phase ventricular tachycardia. Am Heart J 1981; 102: 16–24.
73. Tzivoni D, Keren A, Cohen AM, Loebel H, Zahavi I, Chenzbraun A, Stern S: Magnesium therapy for Torsades de pointes. Am J Cardiol 1984; 53: 528–530.
74. Veglia L, Scandifio T, Guenicchio G: 'Torsioni di punta' e amiodarone. G Ital Cardiol 1978; 8: 1025.
75. Vidal J, Hernández Guevara JL, Cárdenas M: Taquicardia ventricular helicoidal, 'Torsades de pointe' en el infarto agudo del miocardio. Arch Inst Cardiol México, 1983; 53: 237–245.
76. Wald RW, Waxman MB, Colman JM: Torsade de pointes ventricular tachycardia. A complication of disopyramide shared with quinidine. J Electrocardiol 1981; 14: 301–307.
77. Wellens HJ: Value and limitations of programmed electrical stimulation of the heart in the study and treatment of tachycardias. Circulation 1978; 57: 845–853.
78. Wellens HJ: Quoted by Fontaine et al. [18].
79. Wiggers CJ: Studies on ventricular fibrillation caused by electric shock. Am Heart J 1929; 5: 351.
80. Zilcher H, Glogar D, Kaindl F: Torsades de pointe: occurence in myocardial ischaemia as a separate entity. Multiform ventricular tachycardia or not? Eur Heart J 1980; 1: 63–71.

2.3 Non-invasive Assessment of Antiarrhythmic Drugs

THOMAS B. GRABOYS

Definition of efficacy of antiarrhythmic agents presents a complex management problem. If the aim of the antiarrhythmic therapy is suppression of malignant dysrhythmic events, then the process would understandably be much different if medication is being used to suppress a sporadic though non-threatening episode. While one may choose a drug for a given patient based upon reported effectiveness among groups of individuals with similar problems, it is at the present time impossible to predict whether that patient will respond favorably or adversely to the agent. Because arrhythmias are sporadic, the selection process must address the issue of a therapeutic objective, i.e., what is the endpoint which defines drug efficacy. A final consideration relates to whether there is an inherent advantage to a non-invasive approach to drug selection which can be applied by the clinician without the need to resort to invasive testing. The purpose of this chapter will be to address these issues.

For the physician confronted with an individual who is experiencing troublesome palpitations or non-sustained episodes of tachyarrhythmia, whether it be ventricular or supraventricular, the major clinical consideration is whether those dysrhythmias are manifestations of significant underlying structural heart disease and whether they are potentially compromising for the patient. If there is no evidence of associated heart disease, and these are merely sporadic symptoms that seem to be causally related to dysrhythmia, chronic daily therapy is rarely necessary. If the events are infrequent, selection of an antiarrhythmic drug becomes an empiric matter based upon certain 'historical precents'. One approach is to have the patient self administer a group of medications (so-called therapeutic 'cocktail') during an episode of dysrhythmia [1]. Table 1 lists several typical 'cocktails' we have utilized for sustained arrhythmia.

If the frequency of these events is such that chronic therapy is indicated, but yet they are not felt to be threatening, or the patient has not experienced pre-syncope or frank loss of consciousness, the approach may also be an empirical trial of antiarrhythmic drugs which have historically been effective for that particular dysrhythmia. However, among individuals who have had so-called malignant ventricular arrhythmia, defined as hemodynamically compromising ventricular tachycardia or non-infarction-related ventricular fibrillation, or for individuals who have a high density of repetitive and complex ventricular premature beats in the setting of a recent acute myocardial infarction, our approach has been to hospitalize such patients and undertake a systematic management approach as defined in this chapter.

Non-invasive selection of antiarrhythmic drugs for patients having experienced malignant ventricular arrhythmia

The essentials of this approach have been detailed elsewhere [2] and are based upon
1. the relationship of advanced or complex forms of ventricular premature beats (VPBs) to recurrent arrhythmia and
2. that the suppression of such forms is associated with improved survival and freedom from recurrent arrhythmia.

We employ four phases which begin with a 48 hour observation period (Control; Phase 0) during which the patient undergoes continuous ambulatory ECG monitoring, maximal Bruce protocol exercise treadmill testing, and evaluation of left ventricular function after cessation of antiarrhythmic drugs.

Table 1. Oral single dose antiarrhythmic combination therapy to treat sustained tachyarrhythmias.*

Dysrrhythmia	Drug combination
Atrial fibrillation	Quinidine (600 mg) β-blocker Sedative
Atrial flutter	Digoxin (0.5–0.75 mg) β-blocker
Supraventricular tachycardia	Verapamil (160 mg) or Digoxin (0.75–1.0 mg)
Ventricular tachycardia	Procainamide (1.5 g) or Quinidine (600 mg) or Mexiletine (400 mg)

* Non-hemodynamically compromising in otherwise healthy persons.

Approximately 75% of patients who have a history of recurrent malignant arrhythmia will demonstrate a sufficient density and reproducibility of ventricular premature beats to qualify for antiarrhythmic drug testing utilizing their level of ambient ventricular ectopic activity as a standard against which to assess drug efficacy. Several features of this so-called Control or Phase 0 time frame are worthy of note. First it allows the physician an opportunity to determine whether exercise provokes, suppresses, or has no effect on ambient ventricular ectopy. This is of practical import because a number of antiarrhythmic agents may paradoxically aggravate arrhythmia only during exercise. The basis of this may be enhanced reentry occasioned by drug-induced intraventricular conduction disturbance or a direct negative inotropic effect on the heart. The advantage of having a baseline ventricular function study provides an opportunity to assess whether a given antiarrhythmic drug or group of drugs adversely affects ventricular function.

Phase 1: acute drug testing

The aim of this phase is to screen available antiarrhythmic drugs to determine which agents are seemingly effective, ineffective or perhaps adversely affect the patient's arrhythmia [4]. Rapid assessment of drug efficacy can be achieved by administering a large single oral dose of a given antiarrhythmic, e.g. quinidine 600 mg, procainamide 1.5 g or metoprolol 100 mg. The patient undergoes programmed monitoring of the heart rhythm over a 3–5 hour period with hourly bicycle exercise and serum blood determinations of the tested drug. A drug is deemed effective if there is a 50% reduction in total VPBs or a 90% reduction in repetitive forms including total ablation of salvos of ventricular tachycardia (Fig. 1). One distinct advantage of Phase 1 testing is that after a 24 hour washout period we can then proceed to a second acute drug test and hence rapidly screen five or six drugs in one week's time.

A legitimate concern is whether there is concordancy between an acute drug test and more chronic drug administration. In general, for those drugs which have suitable pharmacokinetics to allow for acute testing, there is approximately an 85% concordancy-discordancy rate between the results of Phase 1 and 2 testing [5]. Selection of a suitable oral dose was initially an arbitrary one of fifty percent of the usual 24 hour total dose. If a drug is seemingly ineffective during acute oral administration and yet the serum drug level does not reach so-called therapeutic levels, we would proceed to Phase 2 testing, assuming that the drug had not been given an adequate trial. However, if therapeutic levels were achieved after the acute oral dose and the drug was ineffective, then it is a reasonable conclusion that chronic administration will not be effective in suppressing arrhythmia. These considerations notwithstanding,

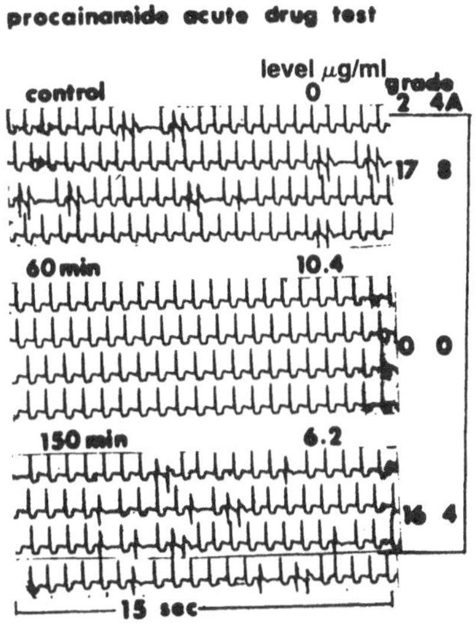

62

Fig. 1. Example of acute drug study (Phase 1). After administration of 1.5 gm of procainamide, trendscription monitoring demonstrates abolition of ventricular arrhythmia correlating with peak serum drug level.

we feel confident that the value of acute drug testing at a minimum resides in the finding of either drug intolerance or an aggravation of arrhythmia during this important observation period.

Phase 2: short-term drug maintenance

After a number of drugs have been tested and several have been found to be effective, the patient then enters Phase 2 studies. The aim of this phase is to assess efficacy of a given drug with a dosing program that would simulate chronic drug administration. A further aim is to determine patient tolerance of the antiarrhythmic agent during longer drug exposure. This phase may require 48–96 hours of drug administration or perhaps longer if there appears to be an active metabolite (e.g. lorcainide-norlorcainide) or the need to attain adequate serum levels which have been shown to suppress repetitive forms (e.g. procainamide). Drug efficacy is then determined by means of 24 hour ambulatory electrocardiographic monitoring as well as maximal exercise stress testing (Fig. 2). Typically a patient will undergo 3 chronic drug trials in hopes that we can find two agents which are independently effective.

CONTROL　　　　　　　　**MEXILITINE**

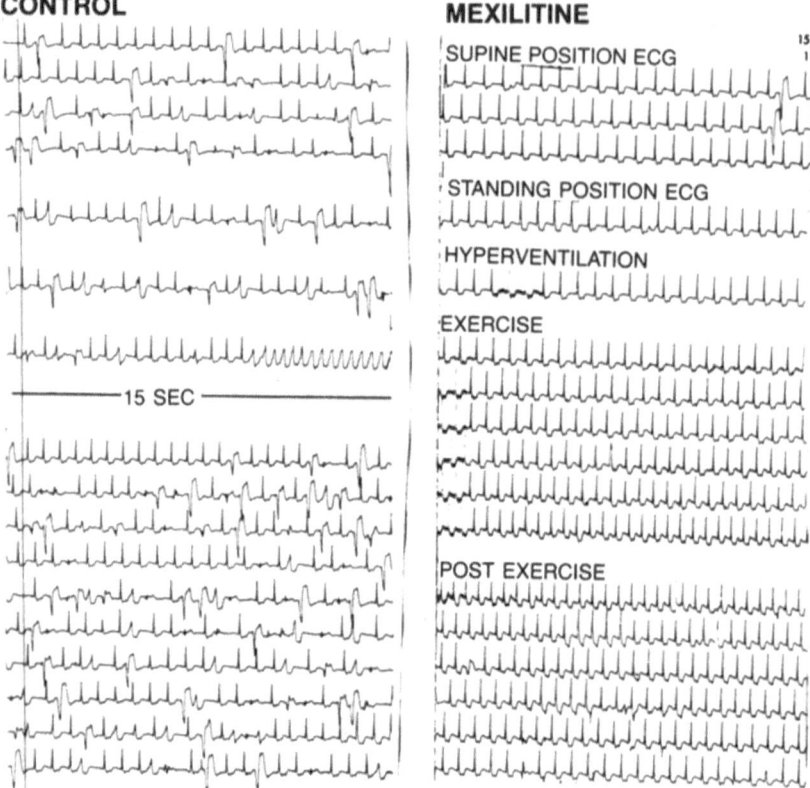

Fig. 2. Example of control exercise study (left panel) and Phase 2 administration of antiarrhythmic drug demonstrating successful ablation of exercise-induced ventricular tachycardia.

Phase 3: long-term antiarrhythmic drug maintenance

This is the outpatient phase of the drug trial during which time we define long-term drug efficacy and safety. Again, ambulatory ECG monitoring and maximal treadmill testing are carried out approximately every 6 months for the first year and then yearly thereafter depending on the particular drug or group of drugs being administered.

Other considerations in the selection of an effective antiarrhythmic drug program

Among patients who have experienced malignant ventricular arrhythmia, it has been our practice to administer two or more antiarrhythmic drugs in a so-called 'fail safe' fashion. Thus, if one medication is not absorbed or a dose is missed, protection is still accomplished by the other antiarrhythmic drug. We have found that a membrane-active drug in combination with a β-blocker has much to offer in terms of therapeutic synergism and in addition, such combinations may allow the use of lower and hence, better tolerated dosages of the membrane-active drug, yet still achieving a particular therapeutic objective [6, 7].

Successful long-term management requires important attention to the details of precise recordkeeping, potential drug-drug interactions, particularly involving diuretics; maintenance of serum potassium in excess of 4.0 and preferably closer to 4.5 mEq/L; and an attempt to decompress the complex psychosocial issues which may serve as a potential trigger for recurrent arrhythmia among these patients. Obviously in those individuals with coronary heart disease, definition of an aggressive anti-ischemic program will work in concert to provide more effective antiarrhythmic control.

It is important to emphasize the combined utility of exercise testing to ambulatory ECG monitoring for exposure of arrhythmia in these patients. We recently reported our experience among 263 patients who underwent 1377 maximal treadmill tests [8]. Complications of the testing occurred in 24 patients (9.1%) during 32 tests (2.3%). These complications included cardiac arrest, precipitation of intervention-required ventricular tachycardia or bradycardic mediated cardiac arrest. This low incidence of serious complications underscores the safety of the technique in a high risk population.

Final comments

Approximately 30% of patients referred to us will have insufficient ambient ventricular arrhythmia or non-reproducibility of ventricular premature beats such that monitoring-exercise testing cannot be used to select or gauge antiarrhythmic drug efficacy. In such patients we proceed to electrophysiologic study, but it is our view that this avenue should be reserved for a minority of patients, particularly if he or she exhibits a high density of spontaneous arrhythmia. Invasive electrophysiologic studies have a number of methodologic problems which include: lack of standardized protocols, reproducibility and difficulty in defining a given endpoint; lack of consensus as to the number of pulses or currents delivered; pacing rate or site of stimulation necessary to evoke a given response. Perhaps most important is consideration of how to assess ongoing protection from recurrent arrhythmia if adjustment of the drug dose or discontinuation of the drug is required. It is simply not practical to rehospitalize patients for repeat electrophysiologic study. However, if monitoring and exercise testing are utilized, then such methods provide a basis for ongoing assessment of drug efficacy.

Acknowledgment

This study was supported in part by the Rappaport International Program in Cardiology.

References

1. Margolis B, De Silva RA, Lown B: Episodic drug treatment in the management of paroxysmal arrhythmia. Am J Cardiol 1980; 45: 621–626.
2. Lown B, Podrid PJ, De Silva R, Graboys TB: Sudden cardiac death: Management of the patient at risk. Curr Probl Cardiol 1980; 4: 1.
3. Podrid PJ, Graboys TB: Exercise stress testing in the management of cardiac rhythm disorders. Med Clin North Am 1984; 68: 1139–1152.
4. Velebit V, Podrid PJ, Lown B, Cohen B, Graboys TB: Aggravation and provocation of ventricular arrhythmia by antiarrhythmic drugs. Circulation 1982; 65: 886.
5. Gaughan CE, Lown B, Lanigan J et al.: Acute oral testing for determining antiarrhythmic drug efficacy. I. Quinidine. Am J Cardiol 1976; 38: 677.
6. Low B, Graboys TB: Management of the patient with malignant ventricular arrhythmias. Am J Cardiol 1977; 39: 910.
7. Graboys TB, Lown B, Podrid PJ, De Silva R: Long term survival of patients with malignant ventricular arrhythmia. Am J Cardiol 1982; 50: 437.
8. Young DZ, Lampert S, Graboys TB, Lown B: Safety of maximal exercise testing in patients at high risk for ventricular arrhythmia. Circulation 1984; 70: 184–190.

2.4 An Electrophysiological Approach to Drug Therapy of Ventricular Arrhythmias

JESUS M. ALMENDRAL and MARK E. JOSEPHSON

The rationale for using invasive electrophysiologic studies to guide drug therapy in tachyarrhythmias includes the accomplishment of 3 steps:
1. Ability to reproduce the clinical arrhythmia in the laboratory by programmed electrical stimulation.
2. Assessment of drug responses in the individual patient.
3. Ability to predict outcome in relation to both inducibility and drug response.

In this chapter we will review the application of this method to ventricular arrhythmias. They will be divided in 3 categories according to the clinical presentation: recurrent sustained ventricular tachycardia (VT), cardiac arrest and nonsustained VT.

Inducibility of the clinical arrhythmia

In the sustained ventricular tachycardia group

In 85 to 100% of patients presenting clinically with recurrent sustained VT, a uniform, sustained, morphologically similar arrhythmia can be induced by programmed electrical stimulation (Table 1) [1–6]. The incidence appears to be higher when the stimulation protocol includes a third extrastimuli [7], multiple right ventricular sites [8] and eventually the left ventricle [9]. Although the majority of cases in the reported series had coronary artery disease, patients with VT and no organic heart disease also appear to have a high incidence of inducibility [10]. In patients with cardiomyopathy, the results are more discordant, the inducibility rate ranging from 52 [10] to 100% [11, 12].

In the cardiac arrest group

In patients presenting clinically with out-of-hospital cardiac arrest, the initial arrhythmia causing the episode is usually unknown. However, in 60 to 90% a fast ventricular arrhythmia, that could have been the cause of the arrest, can be induced by programmed electrical stimulation (Table 2) [13–18]. The induced arrhythmia is sustained VT in the majority of cases, ventricular fibrillation in some 15% and VT degenerating to ventricular fibrillation in about 10% [14]. A relationship has been suggested between the initial documented rhythm at the time of the arrest and the chances of inducibility, being the arrhythmias less likely to be induced if the initial rhythm was ventricular fibrillation as opposed to VT [19]. On the contrary, in patients with inducible arrhythmias, similar incidence of inducible ventricular fibrillation and VT was found whether the initial documented rhythm was ventricular fibrillation or VT [14]. This may be semantics, however, since VT which degenerates to ventricular fibrillation is often classified as VT.

Table 1. Inducibility by PES in sustained VT.

Author	No patients	Inducible by PES	
		No	%
Fisher et al. [4]	19	18	95
Ruskin et al. [6]	22	22	100
Horowitz et al. [28]	20	20	100
Naccarelli et al. [10]	39[a]	27	69
Mason et al. [26]	186[b]	165	89
Buxton et al. [3]	102	101	99
Total	388	353	91

[a] Patients without coronary artery disease.
[b] Includes 38 patients with nonsustained VT (23 cases) or ventricular fibrillation (15 cases).
Abbreviations: PES: programmed electrical stimulation; VT: ventricular tachycardia.

Table 2. Inducibility by PES in cardiac arrest patients.

Author	No patients	Inducible by PES	
		No	%
Ruskin et al. [15]	60	45	75
Kehoe et al. [16]	44	28	64
Benditt et al. [17]	34	30	88
Morady et al. [18]	45	34	76
Roy et al. [14]	119	72	61
Total	302	209	69

Abbreviation: PES: programmed electrical stimulation.

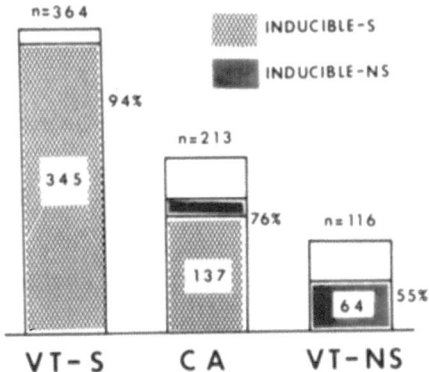

Fig. 1. This figure reflects our present experience regarding inducibility of ventricular arrhythmias. Note that the incidence of inducible ventricular tachycardia (VT) – either nonsustained (NS) or sustained (S) – is highest in patients presenting with sustained ventricular tachycardia, as compared to patients presenting with cardiac arrest (CA) or nonsustained ventricular tachycardia. n = number of patients.

In the nonsustained VT group

In patients presenting clinically with nonsustained VT, the chances of reproducing the clinical arrhythmia by programmed electrical stimulation are 63% [20]. This incidence seems to be related to the underlying heart disease: 75% in coronary patients, between 30 and 50% in patients with cardiomyopathy, mitral valve prolapse or no heart disease [10, 21]. Fig. 1 updates our present experience with these 3 groups of ventricular arrhythmias.

Assessment of drug responses

This is carried out by a programmed ventricular stimulation protocol, similar to that performed on the baseline study. However, there has been some controversy as to what can be considered a satisfactory drug response [22]. We consider satisfactory the absence of any inducible sustained tachyarrhythmia [23] in response to the complete electrical stimulationn protocol, provided a sustained tachyarrhythmia was induced in the baseline study. However, it has been suggested that a mere narrowing of the tachycardia zone or an increase in the number of extrastimuli required for the initiation of the tachyarrhythmia are indicators of a good drug response [4]. In contrast, other authors consider a drug prophylactic only if nonsustained tachycardia, longer than 3 to 6 beats, was also abolished [24, 25].

In the sustained VT group

The incidence of a satisfactory drug response, as judged by electrophysiologic testing, varies in different reported series (Table 3), ranging from 20 to 80%. There seems to be a tendency towards a lower incidence of drug-responders in the more recent series as compared to older ones. This has previously been pointed out [26] and attributed to the addition of a third extrastimulus to the stimulation protocol. In fact, a retrospective study found that, in patients with sustained VT inducible with single or double ventricular extrastimuli in the baseline state, the addition of a third extrastimulus during serial drug testing will reduce to less than half the number of patients considered drug-responders [27]. However this study included both sustained VT and nonsustained VT and did not take into consideration clinical outcome. We have not found the number of ventricular extrastimuli to be a major problem since recurrences are noted even if VT induction changed from 2 to 3 ventricular extrastimuli. We believe the major change is patient selection. Now we are getting drug refractory patients – earlier studies often were dose failures.

The above mentioned studies only include drugs considered conventional in the U.S.A.; that excludes amiodarone, which will be discussed separately. Procainamide is the single most effective drug in preventing the initiation of sustained VT [28], provided high doses are used [29]. Quinidine and disopyramide have also been reported to have a reasonable likelihood of success [30, 31], whereas lidocaine, diphenylhydantoin and mexiletine are only occasionally effective [28, 32]. Recent studies from our group show that sustained VT in the setting of idiopathic dilated cardiomyopathy is inducible but the likelihood of drug responsiveness rather low (Fig. 2) [12].

It would be valuable if drug response to electrophysiologic testing could be predicted by clinical and/or electrocardiographic variables. If so, serial drug

Table 3. Drug responses in sustained VT, as judged by PES.

Author	No inducible by PES	Drug responders	
		No	%
Ruskin et al. [6]	22	17	77
Naccarelli et al. [10]	24[a]	9	37
Mason et al. [26]	129[b]	50	39
Waxman et al. [36]	126	51	40
Total	301	127	42

[a] Patients without coronary artery disease.
[b] Includes 38 patients with nonsustained VT (23) or ventricular fibrillation.
Abbreviations: PES: programmed electrical stimulation; VT: ventricular tachycardia.

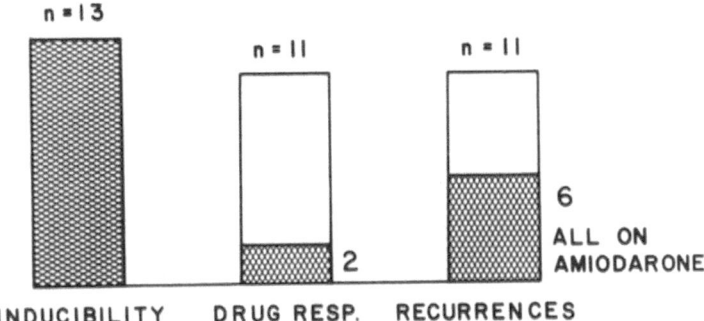

VT-S IN DILATED CARDIOMYOPATHY

Fig. 2. This figure compares inducibility, drug responsiveness and clinical recurrences in our patients with idiopathic dilated cardiomyopathy and sustained ventricular tachycardia. Note the low incidence of drug responders (2/11 patients) and the high incidence of clinical recurrence (6/11 over a mean follow-up period of 21 months). It is of interest that all patients that recurred were receiving amiodarone.

testing could be avoided in patients unlikely to be drug-responders. However, one study found no single variable independently predictive of responsiveness [33]. In another study, univariate analysis disclosed 4 factors, age less than 45 years, ejection fraction greater than 50%, hypokinesia as the only contraction abnormality, and absence of organic heart disease, associated with successful medical treatment [34]. However, in this and in another study [35], only when constructing a function incorporating multiple variables, the majority of patients were correctly classified [34, 35]. Even these latter studies are biased by patient selection.

Trying to avoid multiple serial drug testing, another issue has been raised, whether the electrophysiologic response to one antiarrhythmic agent is predictive to that of the others. It has been found that the response to procainamide predicted the response to other class IA agents, since only 7% of 145 drug regimens tested in patients inducible on procainamide, had prevented inducibility [36]. Another study found concordant responses for quinidine and procainamide but not for either of these drugs and disopyramide [33].

In the cardiac arrest group

Disparate incidences of drug responsiveness have been reported in different cardiac arrest series studied with serial electrophysiologic testing (Table 4). Interestingly enough, when pooling those series together the incidence of drug responsiveness is similar to the reported sustained VT studies (Table 3).

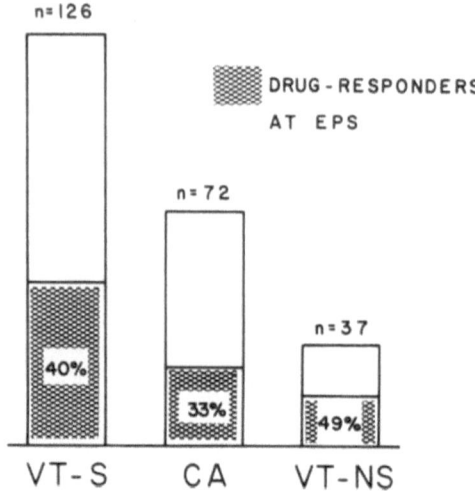

n=126

DRUG - RESPONDERS

AT EPS

n=72

n=37

40%

33%

49%

VT-S   CA   VT-NS

Fig. 3. The incidence of drug responders as assessed by electrophysiologic studies (EPS) in the 3 clinical subgroups is summarized. Note that there are no substantial differences among these 3 groups. Abbreviations as in previous figures.

In the nonsustained VT group

Only 2 reported series have focused on the electrophysiologic evaluation of drugs in this group of patients [10, 37]. The incidence of drug responders in the laboratory was 71% (5/7) in one series [10] and 49% (18/37) in the other [37]. However, the results in these 2 studies are probably consistent since coronary patients were excluded in the first series [10] and the incidence of drug responders found to be significantly higher in patients without underlying heart disease (7/8, 88%) in the latter study [37]. Moreover, the predictive

Table 4. Drug responses in cardiac arrest patients as judged by PES.

Author	No inducible by PES	Drug responders	
		No	%
Ruskin et al. [15]	45	34	76
Kehoe et al. [16]	28	5	18
Benditt et al. [17]	30	9	30
Morady et al. [18]	34	9	26
Roy et al. [14]	72	24	33
Total	209	81	39

Abbreviation: PES: programmed electrical stimulation.

accuracy of drug failure by programmed electrical stimulation was not addressed.

Fig. 3 summarizes the incidence of drug responders in our laboratory for all 3 groups of ventricular arrhythmias. Note that it is similar regardless of clinical presentation.

Electrophysiologic predictability of outcome

In the sustained VT group

The crucial step to the electrophysiologic approach is the correlation between drug response in the laboratory and clinical outcome. Unfortunately, there are no controlled studies addressing this issue. However, several non-controlled studies have been reported (Table 5), involving small number of patients with rather short follow-ups, and using mainly type IA antiarrhythmics [6, 10, 25, 28, 34, 38]. It has to be realized that the results could be partially biased because some of the non-responders to conventional antiarrhythmics were operated on or received experimental drugs.

These studies consistently found a significantly lower incidence of both recurrence [6, 10, 25, 28, 34] and sudden death [38] in the patients whose arrhythmias were rendered noninducible by drugs than in the ones treated with drugs on which they were still inducible. One study performed an actuarial analysis and found a significantly lower percentage of patients free of

Table 5. Outcome in relation to drug response to PES: patients with recurrent sustained VT.

Author	Drug responders				Non-responders[a]			
	No	Follow-up[a] (months)	Recurrence		No	Follow-up (months)	Recurrence	
			No	%			No	%
Ruskin et al. [6]	17	8	2	12	5	3	4	80
Mason et al. [25]	26	8[b]	8	31	16	8[b]	13	81
Naccarelli et al. [10]	9	12[b]	0	0	15	12[b]	6	40
Horowitz et al. [28]	13	3–27	0	0	7	< 1	7	100
Spielman et al. [34]	29	18	4	15	14	11	9	64
Total	94		14	15	57		39	68

[a] Excluding surgery or drugs considered experimental in U.S.A.

[b] Mean follow-up of the series.

[c] This study excludes patients with coronary disease.

Abbreviations: PES: programmed electrical stimulation; VT: ventricular tachycardia.

recurrences in the 'non-responders' [25]. The difference persisted significant for more than 2 years of follow-up [25]. When pooled them together (Table 5) the recurrence rates were 15% and 68% for 'responders' and 'non-responders' respectively.

In the cardiac arrest group

The results tend to be similar in the cardiac arrest group. Table 6 reflects the data from 5 previously reported series. Again, just the number of patients on each category suggests some bias on the results: while more than half of the inducible patients are 'non-responders' (Table 4), the number of 'non-responders' drops to half of that of the responders when considering patients treated with conventional agents (Table 6). The introduction of alternate modes of therapy, mainly surgery, experimental drugs and, in recent years, implantable electronic devices, probably accounts for these findings, and reflects the resistance of physicians to discharge patients with a history of cardiac arrest on regimens that do not prevent inducibility. However, this undoubtedly represents an uncontrolled variable and a potential bias on the results and conclusions.

In the nonsustained VT group

Few data are available on this group of patients. In a series excluding coronary patients, no symptomatic events occurred during a 12 month follow-up on 5

Table 5. Outcome in relation to drug response to PES: patients with cardiac arrest.

Author	Drug responders				Non-responders[a]			
	No	Follow-up[a] (months)	Recurrence		No	Follow-up (months)	Recurrence	
			No	%			No	%
Ruskin et al. [15]	34	18	2	5	11	15	4	36
Kehoe et al. [16]	5	14	0	0	9	9	7	78
Benditt et al. [17]	9	18	1	11	5	18	2	40
Morady et al. [18]	9	20	3	33	_[b]	–	–	–
Roy et al. [14]	24	_[c]	4	17	9	_[c]	3	33
Total	81		10	12	34		26	47

[a] Excluding surgery or drugs considered experimental in U.S.A.
[b] Most patients received amiodarone.
[c] Not specifically stated for these patients; 18 months for the whole series.
Abbreviation: PES: programmed electrical stimulation.

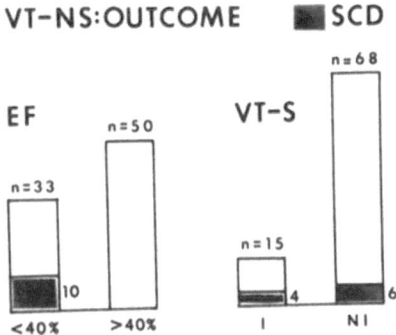

Fig. 4. In this figure the incidence of sudden cardiac death (SCD) in patients with nonsustained ventricular tachycardia is represented. Two factors, an ejection fraction (EF) of less than 40%, and the presence of an inducible sustained (I) sustained ventricular tachycardia (VT-S) were independent predictors of a bad prognosis (133). NI = noninducible.

inducible patients treated with drugs that rendered them non-inducible [10]. Three of 34 patients treated with an electrophysiology guided regimen died suddenly in a non-controlled study, including 40% of coronary patients [20]. However no data are available to assess the risk of untreated nonsustained VT versus treated. Some data from our laboratory [20] suggest that some patients with nonsustained VT need not be treated, since they have a good prognosis (Fig. 4).

Amiodarone

Amiodarone is a rather unique antiarrhythmic because of its frequent success in the clinical setting despite failure in preventing inducibility by programmed electrical stimulation [39–42].

Most of the studies have found that in 60 to 90% of patients with inducible ventricular arrhythmias, the arrhythmia will remain inducible on amiodarone [39, 43–45]. This figure would not be particularly surprising compared to most if not all of the available antiarrhythmics. However, it has been shown that amiodarone prevents clinical recurrences in about two-thirds of patients presenting with recurrent VT [39, 40, 43, 46, 47] and even a higher percentage of patients with cardiac arrest [18, 48]. This striking dissociation between clinical and electrophysiological responses is not well understood. Amiodarone produces a marked reduction in total and complex ectopy [49] and it has been suggested that may control VT by eliminating the triggers instead of acting on the reentrant circuit.

Efforts have been made to correlate laboratory findings with clinical outcome; however, this has led to rather conflictive results. Some studies have found that patients rendered noninducible by amiodarone have a good prognosis [39, 50, 51]. However, our results [40, 43] show a comparable incidence of recurrences in the group of patients rendered noninducible. Correlations have been reported between ease of inducibility [44, 45], clinical tolerance of the induced VT [51] or the conjunction of multiple variables [52] and clinical outcome, but are awaiting further confirmation. Most of these series report on patients studied by programmed electrical stimulation 2 to 6 weeks after starting on amiodarone. Recent studies from our laboratory suggest that, although VT usually remain inducible after 3 months of therapy, electrophysiologic studies performed at that time may be more predictive of outcome [53].

Acknowledgments

This study was supported in part by grants from the American Heart Association, Southeastern Pennsylvania Chapter, Philadelphia, PA, and grants from the National Heart, Lung, and Blood Institute, Bethesda, MD.
We acknowledge Maria Coscia for preparing the manuscript.

References

1. Wellens HJJ, Duren DR, Lie KI: Observations on mechanisms of ventricular tachycardia in man. Circulation 1976; 54: 237–244.
2. Josephson ME, Horowitz LN, Fashidi A, Kastor JA: Recurrent sustained ventricular tachycardia. 1. Mechanisms. Circulation 1978; 57: 431–440.
3. Buxton AE, Waxman HL, Josephson ME: Electrical stimulation techniques to predict and assess antiarrhythmic drug efficacy in patients with ventricular arrhythmias. In: Van Durme JP, Bogaert MG, Julaina DG, Kulbertus HE (eds) Chronic antiarrhythmic therapy. AB Hassle, Molndal, Sweden, 1983; 151–163.
4. Fisher JD, Cohen ML, Mehra R, Altschuler M, Escher DJW, Furman S: Cardiac pacing and pacemakers. II. Serial electrophysiologic-pharmacologic testing for control of recurrent tachyarrhythmias. Am Heart J 1977; 93: 658–668.
5. Mason JW, Winkle RA: Electrode-catheter arrhythmia induction in the selection and assessment of antiarrhythmic drug therapy for recurrent ventricular tachycardia. Circulation 1978; 58: 971–985.
6. Ruskin JN, Garan H: Chronic electrophysiologic testing in patients with recurrent sustained ventricular tachycardia. Am J Cardiol 1979; 43: 400.
7. Buxton AE, Waxman HL, Marchlinski FE, Untereker WJ, Waspe LE, Josephson ME: Role of triple extrastimuli during electrophysiologic study of patients with documented sustained ventricular arrhythmias. Circulation 1984; 69: 532–540.
8. Doherty JU, Kienzle MG, Buxton AE, Marchlinski FE, Waxman HL, Josephson ME: Discordant results of programmed ventricular stimulation at different right ventricular sites in patients with and without spontaneous sustained ventricular tachycardia: a prospective study of 56 patients. Am J Cardiol 1984; 54: 336–342.
9. VandePol CJ, Farshidi A, Spielman SR, Greenspan AM, Horowitz LN, Josephson ME:

Incidence and clinical significance of induced ventricular tachycardia. Am J Cardiol 1980; 45: 725–731.

10. Naccarelli GV, Prystowsky EN, Jackman WM, Heger JJ, Rahilly GT, Zipes DP: Role of electrophysiologic testing in managing patients who have ventricular tachycardia unrelated to coronary artery disease. Am J Cardiol 1982; 50: 165–171.

11. Poll DS, Buxton AE, Doherty JU, Marchlinski FE: Ventricular tachyarrhythmias in congestive cardiomyopathy: importance of presenting arrhythmia on the response to programmed stimulation (Abstract). Circulation 1985; 70 (Suppl III): III 34.

12. Poll DS, Marchlinski FE, Buxton AE, Doherty JU, Waxman HL, Josephson E: Sustained ventricular tachycardia in patients with idiopathic dilated cardiomyopathy: electrophysiologic testing and lack of response to antiarrhythmic drug therapy. Circulation 1984; 70: 451–456.

13. Josephson ME, Horowitz LN, Spielman SR, Greenspan AM: Electrophysiologic and hemodynamic studies in patients resuscitated from cardiac arrest. Am J Cardiol 1980; 46: 948–955.

14. Roy D, Waxman HL, Kienzle MG, Buxton AE, Marchlinski FE, Josephson ME: Clinical characteristics and long-term follow-up in 119 survivors of cardiac arrest: relationship to inducibility at electrophysiologic testing. Am J Cardiol 1983; 52: 969–974.

15. Ruskin JN, Garan H, DiMarco JP, Kelly E: Electrophysiologic testing in survivors of prehospital cardiac arrest: therapy and long-term follow-up (Abstract). Am J Cardiol 1982; 49: 958.

16. Kehoe RF, Moran JM, Zheutlin T, Tommasco C, Lesch M: Electrophysiologic study to direct therapy in survivors of prehospital ventricular fibrillation (Abstract). Am J Cardiol 1982; 49: 928.

17. Benditt DG, Benson DW, Klein GJ, Pritzker MR, Kriett JM, Anderson RW: Prevention of recurrent sudden cardiac arrest: role of provocative electropharmacologic testing. JACC 1983; 2: 418–425.

18. Morady F, Scheinman MM, Hess DS, Sung RJ, Shen E, Shapiro W: Electrophysiologic testing in the management of survivors of out-of-hospital cardiac arrest. Am J Cardiol 1983; 51: 85–89.

19. Myerburg RJ, Sung RJ, Conde C, Mallon SM, Castellanos A: Intracardiac electrophysiologic studies in patients resuscitated from unexpected cardiac arrest outside the hospital (Abstract). Am J Cardiol 1977; 39: 275.

20. Buxton AE, Marchlinski FE, Waxman HL, Flores BT, Cassidy DM, Josephson ME: Prognostic factors in nonsustained ventricular tachycardia. Am J Cardiol 1984; 53: 1275–1279.

21. Buxton AE, Waxman HL, Marchlinski FE, Josephson ME: Electrophysiologic studies in nonsustained ventricular tachycardia: relation to underlying heart disease. Am J Cardiol 1983; 52: 985–991.

22. Swerdlow CD, Winkle RA, Mason JW: Prognostic significance of the number of induced ventricular complexes during assessment of therapy for ventricular tachyarrhythmias. Circulation 1983; 68: 400–405.

23. Josephson ME, Horowitz LN: Electrophysiologic approach to therapy of recurrent sustained ventricular tachycardia. Am J Cardiol 1979; 43: 631–641.

24. Ruskin JN, DiMarco JP, Garan H: Out-of-hospital cardiac arrest. Electrophysiologic observations and selection of long term antiarrhythmic therapy. N Engl J Med 1980; 303: 607–613.

25. Mason JW, Winkle RA: Accuracy of the ventricular tachycardia-induction study for predicting long-term efficacy and inefficacy of antiarrhythmic drugs. N Engl J Med 1980; 303: 1073–1077.

26. Mason JW, Swerdlow CD, Winkle RA, Griffin JC, Ross DL, Keefe DL, Clusin WT: Programmed ventricular stimulation in predicting vulnerability to ventricular arrhythmias and their response to antiarrhythmic therapy. Am Heart J 1982; 103: 633–639.

27. Swerdlow CD, Blum J, Winkle RA, Griffin JC, Ross DL, Mason JW: Decreased incidence of

antiarrhythmic drug efficacy at electrophysiological study associated with the use of a third extrastimulus. Am Heart J 1982; 104: 1004–1011.

28. Horowitz LN, Josephson ME, Farshidi A, Spielman SR, Michelson EL, Greenspan AM: Recurrent sustained ventricular tachycardia. 3. Role of the electrophysiologic study in selection of antiarrhythmic regimens. Circulation 1978; 58: 986–997.

29. Greenspan AM, Horowitz LN, Spielman SR, Josephson ME: Large dose procainamide therapy for ventricular tachyarrhythmias. Am J Cardiol 1980; 46: 453–462.

30. DiMarco JP, Garan H, Ruskin JN: Quinidine for ventricular arrhythmias: value of electrophysiologic testing. Am J Cardiol 1983; 51: 90–95.

31. Lerman BB, Waxman HL, Buxton AE, Josephson ME: Disopyramide: evaluation of electrophysiologic effects and clinical efficacy in patients with sustained ventricular tachycardia of ventricular fibrillation. Am J Cardiol 1983; 51: 759–764.

32. Waspe LE, Waxman HL, Buxton AE, Josephson ME: Mexiletine for control of drug-resistant ventricular tachycardia: clinical and electrophysiological results in 44 patients. Am J Cardiol 1983; 51: 1175–1181.

33. Swiryn S, Bauernfeind RA, Strasberg B, Palileo E, Iverson N, Levy PS, Rosen KM: Prediction of response to class I antiarrhythmic drugs during electrophysiologic study of ventricular tachycardia. Am Heart J 1982; 104: 43–50.

34. Spielman SR, Schwartz JS, McCarthy DM, Horowitz LN, Greenspan AM, Sadowski LM, Josephson ME, Waxman HL: Predictors of the success or failure of medical therapy in patients with chronic recurrent sustained ventricular tachycardia: a discriminant analysis. JACC 1983; 1: 401–408.

35. Swerdlow CD, Goug G, Echt DS, Winkle RA, Griffin JC, Ross DL, Mason JW: Clinical factors predicting successful electrophysiologic-pharmacologic study in patients with ventricular tachycardia. JACC 1983; 1: 409–416.

36. Waxman HL, Buxton AE, Sadowski LM, Josephson ME: The response to procainamide during electrophysiologic study for sustained ventricular tachyarrhythmias predicts the response to other medications. Circulation 1983; 67: 30–37.

37. Buxton AE, Waxman HL, Marchlinski FE, Josephson ME: Electropharmacology of non-sustained ventricular tachycardia: effects of class I antiarrhythmic agents, verapamil and propranolol. Am J Cardiol 1984; 53: 738–744.

38. Swerdlow CD, Winkle RA, Mason JW: Determinants of survival in patients with ventricular tachyarrhythmias. N Engl J Med 1983; 308: 1436–1442.

39. Heger JJ, Prystowsky EN, Zipes DP: Clinical efficacy of amiodarone in treatment of recurrent ventricular tachycardia and ventricular fibrillation. Am Heart J 1983; 106: 887–894.

40. Waxman HL, Groh WC, Marchlinski FE, Buxton AE, Sadowski LM, Horowitz LN, Josephson ME, Kastor JA: Amiodarone for control of sustained ventricular tachyarrhythmias: clinical and electrophysiologic effects in 51 patients. Am J Cardiol 1982; 50: 1066–1074.

41. Nademanee K, Hendrickson J, Kannan R, Singh BN: Antiarrhythmic efficacy and electrophysiologic actions of amiodarone in patients with life-threatening ventricular arrhythmias: potent suppression of spontaneously occurring tachyarrhythmias versus inconsistent abolition of induced ventricular tachycardia. Am Heart J 1982; 103: 950–959.

42. Heger JJ, Prystowsky EN, Jackman WM, Naccarelli GV, Warfel KA, Rinkenberger RL, Zipes DP: Amiodarone: clinical efficacy and electrophysiologic effects during long-term therapy for recurrent ventricular tachycardia or ventricular fibrillation. N Engl J Med 1981; 305: 539–545.

43. Waxman HL, Buxton AE, Marchlinski FE, Flores BT, Rogers DP, Josephson ME: Amiodarone for sustained ventricular tachyarrhythmias: electrophysiologic study is not predictive of clinical efficacy. Circulation 1983; 68 (Suppl III): III–382.

44. Borggrefe M, Breithardt G, Seipel L: Value of serial electrophysiological testing in the

treatment of ventricular tachyarrhythmias with amiodarone. Circulation 1983; 68 (Suppl III): III–381.

45. McGovern B, Garan H, Malacoff RF, DiMarco JP, Sellers TD, Ruskin JN: Predictive accuracy of electrophysiologic testing in the treatment of ventricular arrhythmias with amiodarone. Circulation 1982; 66 (Suppl II): II–223.

46. Heger JJ, Prystowsky EN, Miles WM, Zipes DP: Antiarrhythmic, electrophysiologic and adverse effects of amiodarone during treatment of recurrent ventricular tachyarrhythmias. Circulation 1983; 68 (Suppl III): III–280.

47. Kaski JC, Girotti LA, Messuti H, Rutilzky B, Rosenbaum MB: Long-term management of sustained recurrent symptomatic ventricular tachycardia with amiodarone. Circulation 1981; 64: 273–279.

48. Nademanee K, Singh BN, Cannom DS, Weiss J, Feld G, Stevenson WG: Control of sudden recurrent arrhythmic deaths: role of amiodarone. Am Heart J 1983; 106: 895–901.

49. Nademanee K, Singh BN, Hendrickson JA, Intarachot V, Cannom DS, Lopez B, Feld G, Weiss J, Stevenson W: Amiodarone in refractory life-threatening ventricular arrhythmias. Ann Int Med 1983; 98: 577.

50. Horowitz LN, Spielman SR, Greenspan AM, Webb CR, Kay HR: Utility of electrophysiologic testing of amiodarone for ventricular tachyarrhythmias. Circulation 1983; 68 (Suppl III): III–382.

51. Horowitz LN, Spielman SR, Greenspan AM, Webb CR, Kay HR: Ventricular arrhythmias: use of electrophysiologic studies. Am Heart J 1983; 106: 881–886.

52. Naccarelli GV, Fineberg N, Zipes DP, Heger JJ, Duncan G, Prystowsky EN: Amiodarone: discriminant analysis successfully predicts clinical outcome in patients who have ventricular tachycardia induced by programmed stimulation. Circulation 1982; 66 (Suppl II): II9–223.

53. Kadish AH, Marchlinski FE, Doherty JU, Buxton AE: Amiodarone: correlation of serial electrophysiologic studies with outcome (Abstract). Circulation 1984; 69 (Suppl II): II 531.

2.5 Application of Plasma Level Determinations to Antiarrhythmic Drug Management
Integration with Various End-points of Therapy

ROBERT J. MYERBURG, KENNETH M. KESSLER, LIAQAT ZA-
MAN, RICHARD G. TROHMAN, NADIR SAOUDI and
AGUSTIN CASTELLANOS

Therapeutic effectiveness of antiarrhythmic agents, defined as the prevention of lethal or potentially lethal arrhythmias, must incorporate considerations of 3 elements:
1. the forms and/or frequency of chronic ventricular arrhythmias, as well as the characteristics of arrhythmias labeled as 'potentially lethal';
2. the clinical settings in which various forms of ventricular arrhythmias occur; and
3. the validity of end-points used to guide antiarrhythmic therapy.

The interactions between these 3 factors are complex, and in most clinical settings no uniformly accepted algorithms have been developed for application to patients at risk for unexpected potentially lethal arrhythmias. The absence of important elements of information necessary to test the hypothesis that antiarrhythmic drugs will alter propensity to potentially lethal arrhythmias, plus the lack of uniform patient populations and study designs, have resulted in failure to develop uniform conclusions about management. In this chapter, several current approaches to treatment of patients at risk will be reviewed, and the place of plasma level monitoring of antiarrhythmic drugs will be discussed in respect to each method.

End-points of antiarrhythmic therapy for ventricular arrhythmias

Strategies for the use of antiarrhythmic drugs in patients at risk for potentially lethal arrhythmias have included
1. suppression of ventricular ectopic activity,
2. therapy guided by data acquired during programmed electrical stimulation studies, and
3. empiric therapy with or without plasma level monitoring.

Each approach has accumulated a body of information supporting its use, but each also has persisting unresolved issues and controversy about its application.

Suppression of premature ventricular contractions

Suppression of ventricular ectopic activity was originally interpreted to mean quantitative or near-quantitative eradication of premature ventricular contractions. For many patients at risk for potentially lethal arrhythmias, quantitative suppression of premature ventricular contractions is a goal which is difficult to achieve [1, 2]. Further, the data necessary to confirm the assumption that premature ventricular contraction suppression per se, as the primary end-point of therapy, equates with protection against potentially lethal arrhythmias in chronic heart disease, is still lacking. Conversely, it is not yet known that *failure* to suppress premature ventricular contractions by adequate quantities of antiarrhythmic drugs indicates persistence of risk [3]. Other confounding information include the observations.

1. that antiarrhythmic drug pharmacodynamics differ in acute and chronic clinical settings, when measured in terms of the concentrations of antiarrhythmic agents required for suppression of premature ventricular contractions [4] (Fig. 1),
2. that high frequency premature ventricular contractions may persist at concentrations of antiarrhythmic agents which can be demonstrated to prevent episodes of recurrent ventricular tachycardia [4] (Fig. 2) or ventricular fibrillation [5], and
3. that patients may remain at risk for potentially lethal forms of ventricular arrhythmias even with quantitative suppression of premature ventricular contractions [6].

All of these observations highlight the conclusion that the relationships between forms of ventricular arrhythmias)e.g., PVC's versus salvos versus ventricular tachycardia/fibrillation), the frequency for ventricular ectopic activity, and the influences of antiarrhythmic therapy on these two methods of analysis require further clarification.

A therapeutic end-point which is based on eradication of specific forms of ventricular ectopic activity assumed to identify high risk for potentially lethal arrhythmias, as opposed to quantitative suppression of premature ventricular contractions, may be a more achievable end-point of therapy. Lown and co-workers suggested in 1977 that therapy directed to the suppression of the more advanced grades of ventricular ectopic activity constituted a satisfactory therapeutic end-point for management of patients at risk for potentially lethal arrhythmias [2]. More recently, Graboys and co-workers [7] published further data in support of this approach, suggesting that eradication of Lown Class 4-B and Class 5 ventricular ectopy, documented by ambulatory monitoring and exercise testing, provided a satisfactory end-point of therapy even if premature ventricular contraction suppression was <50%. Using this method, these investigators demonstrated a dramatic difference in outcome, with approxi-

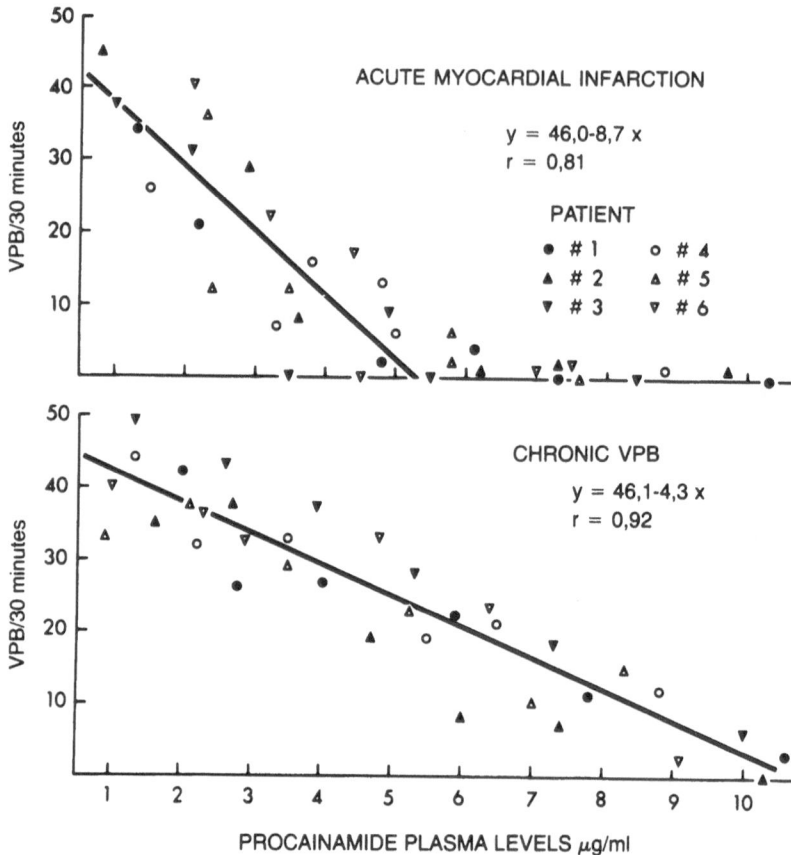

Fig. 1. Comparison of effectiveness of procainamide in suppressing premature ventricular complexes (PVCs) in acute myocardial infarction and in chronic ischemic heart disease. *Top:* plasma levels of procainamide and total PVC count on 30-minute segments of a Holter monitor tape in six acute myocardial infarction patients. *Bottom:* similar data for six patients with stable chronic ischemic heart disease. The frequency of PVCs at minimum plasma levels of procainamide is similar in both groups of patients (y-intercepts = 46.0 and 46.1 PVCs/30 minutes, respectively). However, the slopes are significantly different in the two patient groups (p<0.02), suggesting that PVCs in acute myocardial infarction are more sensitive to suppression by procainamide at comparable plasma levels than are PVCs in the setting of chronic ischemic heart disease. Linear regressions were calculated for all points producing 95% or less PVC suppression. The individual data for each of the six patients in each group are indicated by the six symbols in the top panel. (Reprinted with permission of the American Heart Association, Inc. from [4])

mately 90% of the patients in whom advanced forms persisted dying within 3 years, and a 90% survival rate in those patients in whom this end-point was achieved.

82

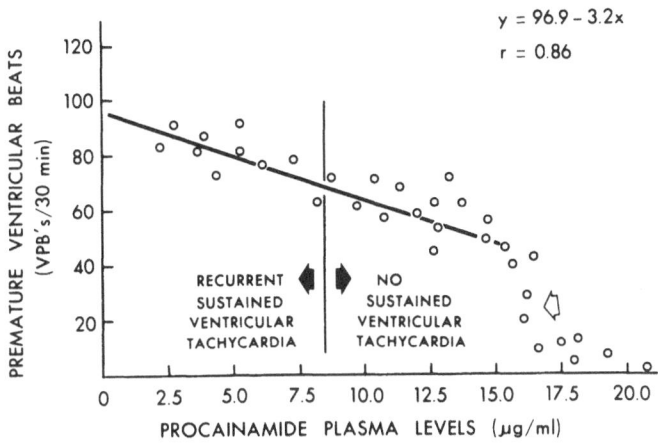

Fig. 2. Plasma levels of procainamide, frequency of premature ventricular complexes (PVCs) and protection against sustained ventricular tachycardia (VT) in a patient having frequent episodes of recurrent sustained ventricular tachycardia. The threshold plasma level of procainamide for protection against sustained VT was 8.2 μg/ml. Between 2.0 and 15.0 μg/ml, there was uniform, dose-related suppression of PVCs, which had achieved suppression of only 31% of baseline PVC frequency at the plasma level that protected against sustained VT. In the range between 15.0 and 20.0 μg/ml (open arrow), the relationship between plasma levels and frequency of PVCs changes, departing from the linear regression line constructed for data points at lower plasma levels. This suggests a PVC suppression threshold effect beginning in the range of 12.5–15.0 μg/ml, a considerably higher plasma level than required for protection against VT. No single nonlinear analysis fit the data. (Reprinted with permission of the American Heart Association, Inc. from [4].

Therapy guided by programmed electrical stimulation

The second end-point listed above, programmed electrical stimulation for the purpose of identifying risk of potentially lethal arrhythmias and for evaluating efficacy of antiarrhythmic intervention, has received considerable attention in recent years. This approach to management assumes that induction of specific ventricular arrhythmias in the clinical electrophysiology laboratory is predictive of risk for the clinical occurrence of such arrhythmias, and that the ability to prevent induction by the use of antiarrhythmic drugs indicates protection against the spontaneous clinical arrhythmias. This approach was initially applied to patients with chronic recurrent ventricular tachycardia [8–11], and several major studies have suggested that this is a successful method for management of such patients. A number of controversies concerning predictive accuracy of protocols and the proper role of this technique persist, but are beyond the scope of this writing. In addition, this method of guilding long-term therapy has also been applied to patients who have survived prehospital cardiac arrest [12, 13], although debate continues about which patients benefit optimally from this approach, compared to the others [7, 14–16]. Patients in whom the mechanism of prehospital cardiac arrest is hypotensive sustained ventricular tachycardia are least controversial [15, 17]. Although ventricular fibrillation is a far more common mechanism of prehospital cardiac arrest identified at initial contact by emergency rescue systems [17], and even bradyarrhythmic events are more common than documented sustained ventricular tachycardia [17, 18], there is a 70–80% probability of inducing ventricular tachycardia in the laboratory among patients in this subgroup [13, 17]. A response to a particular therapeutic regimen, suggested by loss of inducibility during programmed stimulation in the presence of drug therapy, is accepted as predictive of long-term efficacy of management with a specific agent [8–11, 19].

When the electrical mechanism of prehospital cardiac arrest is documented to be ventricular fibrillation, attempts to induce sustained ventricular tachycardia or ventricular fibrillation in the clinical electrophysiology laboratory by programmed stimulation studies are less uniformly successful. In our experience [17] and that of Ruskin et al. [20], approximately 30% of the ventricular fibrillation survivors are inducible into either sustained ventricular tachycardia or ventricular fibrillation during baseline programmed electrical studies. It is assumed that inducibility has the same prognostic significance as does inducibility in recurrent ventricular tachycardia patients, although no properly controlled studies have been carried out to test this assumption. Furthermore, data from Ruskin et al. [12] and Josephson et al. [13] both suggest that prevention of inducibility by specific antiarrhythmic therapy is protective against recurrent cardiac arrest during long-term management of these patients.

The remaining 70% of patients who have prehospital cardiac arrest due to ventricular fibrillation are either non-inducible (30%) or inducible into various non-sustained forms (40%) – repetitive ventricular responses, salvos, non-sustained ventricular tachycardia [20]. Some investigators have suggested that inducibility of non-sustained forms in this patient population indicate high risk for recurrent cardiac arrest, and that prevention of induction of such forms by antiarrhythmic therapy indicates protection [12]. These data are based on relatively small numbers of patients, and more extensive studies of carefully defined clinical groups are required to reach definitive conclusions. Our data, although not yet conclusive, supports the hypothesis that inducibility of non-sustained ventricular tachycardia indicates high risk for recurrent cardiac arrest, but we believe that the case for suppression of induced non-sustained forms as an end-point of therapy is yet to be proved.

A second area of major controversy involves the subgroup of ventricular fibrillation survivors who are not inducible in the electrophysiologic laboratory, even into non-sustained forms. Some investigators have suggested

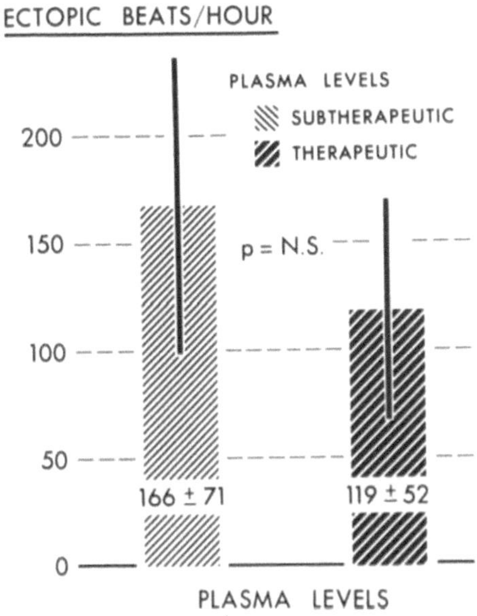

84

Fig. 3. Frequency of ventricular ectopic beats recorded from 24-hour Holter monitor tapes in long-term survivors of prehospital cardiac arrest. Frequency recorded when trough levels of antiarrhythmic agents were subtherapeutic (light cross-hatching) compared with frequency at therapeutic levels (heavy cross-hatching). Black lines indicate ± SE. Data derived from 101 Holter monitor recordings (63 at therapeutic plasma levels and 38 at subtherapeutic levels), indicate insignificant decrease in ectopic beat frequency at therapeutic plasma levels compared with subtherapeutic levels. Both groups maintained high frequency of chronic ventricular ectopic beats. (Reprinted with permission of the American Medical Association, Inc. from [14].)

that non-inducibility may mean non-vulnerability, at least in some patients [12, 21], but data from ambulatory monitor recording suggests that many patients who are non-inducible still carry a significant risk [22], particularly if they have high grade ventricular ectopy on ambulatory recordings [2, 7]. Thus, this subgroup of patients should be treated with antiarrhythmic therapy guided by other techniques.

Empiric antiarrhythmic therapy

The difficulty in predictably suppressing ventricular ectopic activity in high risk patients (Fig. 3), plus the suggestion that patients may be protected against recurrent arrhythmias even when complex forms are not completely suppressed (Fig. 4), focuses on the pragmatic need for a third approach to antiarrhythmic therapy targeted to the prevention of potentially lethal arrhythmias. This empiric approach includes monitoring of plasma levels of

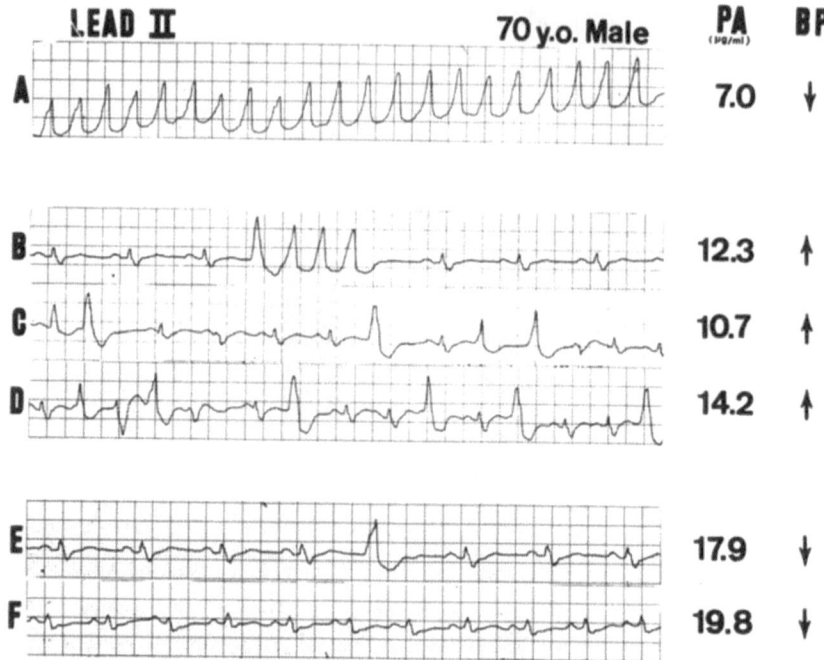

Fig. 4. Representative rhythm strips and corresponding plasma levels of procainamide (PA) in a patient who had recurrent sustained ventricular tachycardia. A. A run of ventricular tachycardia, associated with a fall in blood pressure (BP ↓) when the plasma level of procainamide was 7.0 μg/ml. B–D. Three representative strips at plasma levels above that required to prevent ventricular tachycardia, at which complex forms of ventricular ectopic activity still occurred. The patient remained normotensive during these periods (BP ↑). E, F. Almost complete suppression of premature ventricular complexes (PVCs) at higher plasma levels (17.9 and 19.8 μg/ml, respectively), but these levels resulted in myocardial depression and hypotension (BP ↓). (Reprinted with permission of the American Heart Association, Inc. from [4].)

antiarrhythmic agents, with dose-adjustment to a plasma level range which demonstrates efficacy on a statistical basis [1, 5, 14, 22], or dose ranging of certain antiarrhythmic agents in which meaningful plasma level monitoring is not technically feasible or practical. Our experience with empiric therapy, based on a plasma level monitoring and dose ranging, began in 1975, during long-term follow-up studies of prehospital cardiac arrest survivors. At that time, the use of programmed electrical stimulation studies in high risk patient populations was in its infancy; and at the same time, we began to observe the futility of attempts to quantitatively suppress chronic ventricular ectopic activity in survivors of prehospital cardiac arrest [1], as Lown et al. also observed in other high risk patients [2]. We began to test the use of plasma level monitoring itself as an end-point for therapy.

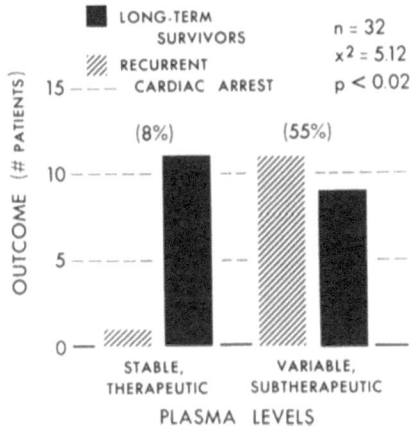

Fig. 5. Risk of recurrent cardiac arrest in survivors of prehospital cardiac arrest followed up until recurrent event (recurrent cardiac arrest (cross-hatched bars)), or for at least 24 months (long-term survivor group (solid bars)). Risk of recurrent cardiac arrest in patients maintaining stable therapeutic plasma levels of antiarrhythmic agents was 8% (1/12), while risk for recurrent cardiac arrest in patients whose plasma levels fell into subtherapeutic range, or fluctuated markedly between therapeutic and subtherapeutic ranges, was 55% (11/20) (n = 32; x^2 = 5.12; p<0.02). (Reprinted with permission of the American Medical Association, Inc. from [14].)

Since our initial 4 years of experience suggested clinical efficacy measured by a lower than expected incidence of recurrent cardiac arrest [5, 14] (Fig. 5), despite failure to predictably suppress ventricular ectopic activity, we continued to test this approach as a method of therapy. Continued studies to the present suggest that plasma level monitoring as a primary end-point yields an acceptable outcome compared to other methods [22]. Empiric therapy does carry with it a major uncertainty that we are dealing to a greater extent with statistical probabilities, as opposed to individual responses, than is the case with programmed electrical stimulation or specific complex form suppression. However, our observations during an 8-year study of survivors of prehospital cardiac arrest managed by this method demonstrated a 10% recurrent cardiac arrest rate during the first year of follow-up, followed by a 5%/year increment for each of the ensuing 3 years. The recurrent cardiac arrest rate becomes insignificant beyond the initial 36–48 months of follow-up [22]. This outcome contrasts to a 30% recurrent cardiac arrest rate during the first year of follow-up and an additional 15% during the second year among survivors of prehospital cardiac arrest in the time period from 1970–1973 [23, 24]. Thus, the cumulative 2-year recurrent cardiac arrest rate in the 1975–83 study is 15%, compared to 45% in the 1970–73 period (p<0.001) [22]. In the earlier study, antiarrhythmic therapy was inconsistent and used at dosages much below those considered standard today [23]. However, despite the fact that a number of key predictors of risk were similar in the two groups, including age, sex, percentage of patients with coronary artery disease, prior myocardial infarctions, low output states at the time of cardiac arrest, and the frequency of intraventricular conduction disturbances, other subtle population differences may confound the comparison between the two time periods. Nonetheless, a recurrent cardiac arrest rate of 10% at 1 year and 15% cumulative at 2 years, using plasma level monitored antiarrhythmic therapy with standard drugs, is an achievable end-point against which to compare other techniques.

Overview of the role of plasma level monitoring

Monitoring of plasma levels of antiarrhythmic agents may have applications in techniques of management beyond the use of empiric antiarrhythmic therapy. Specifically, matching plasma levels to the results of programmed electrical stimulation and of ambulatory monitor recordings during attempts to suppress complex forms of ventricular ectopic activity, may help guide the clinician in maintaining an end-point of therapy which appears useful. Metabolic fluctuations may influence the interpretation of monitored plasma levels, such as changes in the unbound fraction of antiarrhythmic drug concentrations during the evolution of acute myocardial infarction [25], or during long-term follow-up of high risk patients [26]. Nonetheless, levels identified to be protective against ventricular tachycardia induction in the electrophysiology laboratory, or levels which are associated with suppression of advanced forms of ventricular ectopy or ambulatory monitoring, may be used as a guide to continued protection during long-term follow-up of such patients.

Evaluation of the outcome of antiarrhythmic drug management, guided by any end-point, is complicated by the fact that all antiarrhythmic drugs have different ranges of 'therapeutic' plasma concentrations.

In order to compare patients who are receiving different drugs within specific study groups, we have developed a simple method for 'normalizing' plasma levels in respect to their known therapeutic ranges [22]. This method, shown in Table 1, separates the upper and lower values within the therapeutic range from values above and below that range for any drug for which meaningful plasma levels can be determined. A target score for therapy of groups of patients can be determined by identifying the levels at which an end-point of therapy can be achieved (e.g., prevention of inductibility in the electrophysiology laboratory; suppression of salvos or non-sustained ventricular tachycardia on ambulatory monitoring or exercise testing). For patients who require an epiric approach to therapy, our data suggests that a target score of 3 (upper half of therapeutic range) is appropriate, and a score of 4 (supratherapeutic levels) can be used if tolerated [22]. In an 8-year study of survivors of prehospital cardiac arrest, we have applied this technique and found that a mean normalized score of 2.63 ± 0.94 was observed in the long-term survivors, while a score of 1.33 ± 1.23 ($p<0.01$) was observed in patients who had recurrent cardiac arrests. In addition, plasma levels were below the target score of 3 at the last plasma level determination in 14 of 16 patients (87%) who had recurrent cardiac arrests, while levels were at or above a score of 3 in 24 of 34 patients (71%) who remained long-term survivors ($p<0.001$) [22].

For the management of individual patients whose therapy is guided by the results of programmed electrical stimulation, or by specific suppression of complex forms on ambulatory monitoring, the normalized scoring of plasma levels may be convenient, but is not essential. Simply matching plasma levels to a favorable end-point is sufficient. For example, Fig. 6 demonstrates data recorded from a patient monitored during an acute drug testing protocol. During a $2\frac{1}{2}$ hour monitoring period prior to a single oral dose of quinidine sulfate, the patient had approximately 10 ventricular ectopic beats/minute, and many salvos (sample in tracing A). Quinidine completely suppressed the ventricular ectopic beats for almost 2 hours when the plasma level was $2.0\,\mu g/ml$. When the ectopy returned, at approximately the same frequency, no forms more advanced than single beats were recorded until the quinidine plasma level fell below $1.3\,\mu g/ml$. Targeting to a plasma level of $1.8\,\mu g/ml$ suppressed the complex forms, with lesser suppression of the total frequency. If one accepts complex form suppression as an end-point of therapy [7], chronic management can be guided by dose adjustment to maintain the target level in this patient. It is also noteworthy that high plasma levels of another common drug, procainamide, was unsuccessful in controlling complex forms in this patient. A similar algorithm of matching plasma levels to end-points during programmed electrical stimulation evaluation has been demonstrated [9], and,

Table 1. Normalized plasma levels antiarrhythmic agents.

Score	Range	Examples of values for selected drugs in general use in the United States, 1980–83		
		Procainamide	Quinidine	Disopyramide
0	Nil	–	–	–
1	Subtherapeutic	$<4.0\,\mu g/ml$	$<2.3\,\mu g/ml$	$<2.0\,\mu g/ml$
2	Therapeutic lower half	$4.0–6.0\,\mu g/ml$	$2.3–3.6\,\mu g/ml$	$2.0–3.5\,\mu g/ml$
3	Therapeutic upper half	$6.1–8.0\,\mu g/ml$	$3.7–5.0\,\mu g/ml$	$3.6–5.0\,\mu g/ml$
4	Supratherapeutic	$<8.0\,\mu g/ml^*$	$<5.0\,\mu g/ml^*$	$<5.0\,\mu g/ml^*$

* Upper limits of supratherapeutic ranges are determined by tolerance, toxic and/or dose-related pro-arrhythmic effects. These limits are not predictable for individual patients, and must be guided by individual assessment of each patient.

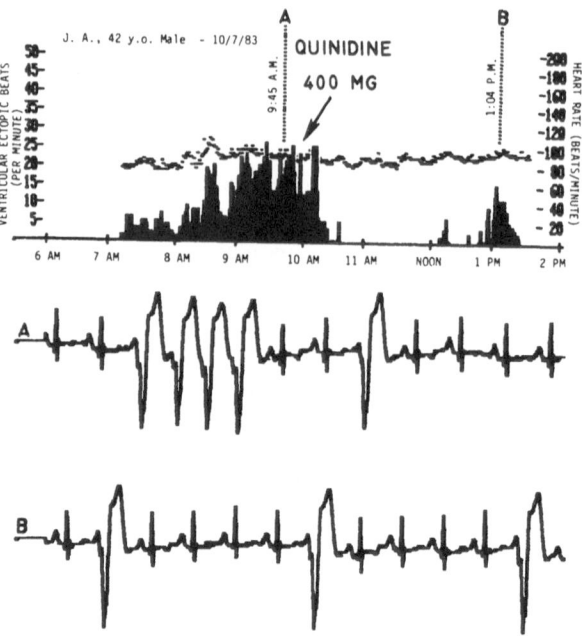

Fig. 6. Differential suppression of unifocal single premature ventricular contractions and salvos. The top panel demonstrates the frequency of ventricular ectopic beats (bars) and heart rate variations (dots) during a $6^{1}/_{2}$ hour computerized trend recording. The electrocardiagram labelled 'A' corresponds in time to line 'A' (9:45 a.m.) from the trend recording, and tracing 'B' corresponds to line 'B' (1:04 p.m.). Tracing A and B are representative of the most advanced forms recorded before and after a 400 mg oral dose of quinidine sulfate. After receiving quinidine, ventricular ectopy was completely suppressed for more than an hour but premature ventricular contractions then returned, achieving approximately the same mean frequency recorded before the drug. In contrast, salvos which had been frequent before quinidine did not return at the same time that single ventricular ectopics recurred; salvos were suppressed for an additional 2 hours after point 'B'. Corresponding plasma levels were a peak quinidine concentration of $2.0 \mu g/ml$ at the time of complete suppression, 1.3 to $1.8 \mu g/ml$ when single ventricular ectopics had returned, and less than $1.3 \mu g/ml$ when salvos returned. Differential sensitivity of complex forms, in relationship to changing plasma concentrations of quinidine, was observed in this patient.

in our experience, can be applied to long-term management after initial evaluation. In the latter case, however, any necessary *drug change* requires evaluation of the end-point for the new drug to maximize efficacy [19].

Conclusion

Plasma level monitoring of antiarrhythmic drugs has a role in the management of patients at risk for potentially lethal arrhythmias. Our original hypothesis was based on the proposal that this approach, used empirically, is useful because 'anti-fibrillatory/anti-tachycardia' effects may dissociate from 'anti-arrhythmic' effects (i.e., chronic PVC suppression). In addition, however, targeting of plasma levels may also be useful for long-term management of patients whose therapy is guided by more specific end-points: programmed electrical stimulation or complex form suppression. The problem of comparing plasma levels for different drugs used in groups of patients can be overcome by normalizing levels by a method we have tested in survivors of prehospital cardiac arrest.

Acknowledgments

This study was supported in part by a research grant from the NHLBI (HL28130), an NIH Institutional Research Training Grant (HL07436) (Dr Trohman), a Grant-in-Aid from the American Heart Association, Greater Miami Chapter (Dr Kessler), and funding from Ministère des Relations Exterieures and Fondation pour la Recherche Medicale, Rouen, France (Dr Saoudi).

References

1. Myerburg RJ, Briese FR, Conde CA, Mallon SM, Liberthson RB, Castellanos A: Long-term antiarrhythmic therapy in survivors of prehospital cardiac arrest: initial 18 months' experience. J Am Med Assoc 1977; 238: 2621–2624.
2. Lown B, Graboys TB: Management of patients with malignant ventricular arrhythmias. Am J Cardiol 1977; 39: 910–919.
3. Blackburn H, deBacker G, Crow R, Prineas R, Jacobs D: Epidemiology and prevention of ventricular ectopic rhythms. Adv Cardiol 1976; 18: 208–216.
4. Myerburg RJ, Kessler KM, Kiem I, et al.: Relationship between plasma levels of procainamide, suppression of premature ventricular complexes and prevention of recurrent ventricular tachycardia. Circulation 1981; 64: 280–290.
5. Myerburg RJ, Conde CA, Sheps DS, Appel RA, Kiem I, Sung RJ, Castellanos A: Antiarrhythmic drug therapy in survivors of prehospital cardia arrest: Comparison of effects on chronic ventricular arrhythmias and on recurrent cardiac arrest. Circulation 1979; 59: 855–863.
6. Herling IM, Horowitz LN, Josephson ME: Ventricular ectopic activity after medical and surgical treatment of recurrent sustained ventricular tachycardia. Am J Cardiol 1980; 45: 636–639.
7. Graboys TB, Lown B, Podrid PJ, DeSilva R: Long-term survival of patients with malignant ventricular arrhythmias treated with antiarrhythmic drugs. Am J Cardiol 1982; 50: 437–443.
8. Wellens HJJ, Bar FWH, Lie KI, Duren DR, Dohman HJ: Effect of procainamide, propranolol and verapamil on mechanism of tachycardia in patients with chronic recurrent ventricular tachycardia. Am J Cardiol 1977; 40: 579–585.

9. Horowitz LH, Josephson ME, Farshidi A, Spielman SR, Michelson EL, Greenspan AM: Recurrent sustained ventricular tachycardia. 3. Role of the electrophysiologic study in selection of antiarrhythmic regimens. Circulation 1978; 58: 986–997.

10. Mason JW, Winkle RA: Electrode-catheter arrhythmia induction in the selection and assessment of antiarrhythmic drug therapy for recurrent ventricular tachycardia. Circulation 1978; 58: 971–985.

11. Josephson ME, Horowitz LN: An electrophysiologic approach to the therapy of recurrent sustained ventricular tachycardia. Am J Cardiol 1979; 43: 631–642.

12. Ruskin JN, DiMarco JP, Garan H: Out-of-hospital cardiac arrest: electrophysiologic observations and selection of long-term antiarrhythmic therapy. N Engl J Med 1980; 303: 607–613.

13. Josephson ME, Horowitz LN, Spielman SR, Greenspan AM: Electrophysiologic and hemodynamic studies in patients resuscitated from cardiac arrest. Am J Cardiol 1980; 46: 948–955.

14. Myerburg RJ, Kessler KM, Zaman L, Conde CA, Castellanos A: Survivors of prehospital cardiac arrest. J Am Med Assoc 1982; 247: 1485–1490.

15. Myerburg RJ, Castellanos A: Antiarrhythmic drugs for the prevention of potentially lethal arrhythmias – assessment of current approaches. Int J Cardiol 1983; 4: 350–356.

16. Myerburg RJ, Zaman L, Luceri RM, Kessler KM, Hamburg C, Kayden D, Castellanos A: Prehospital cardiac arrest survivors: classification of risk groups on the basis of electrophysiologic testing. Ann NY Acad Sci 1985.

17. Myerburg RJ, Conde CA, Sung RJ et al.: Clinical, electrophysiologic and hemodynamic profile of patients resuscitated from prehospital cardiac arrest. Am J Med 1980; 68: 568–576.

18. Myerburg RJ, Estes D, Zaman L, Luceri RM, Kessler KM, Trohman R, Castellanos A: Outcome of resuscitation from bradyarrhythmic or asystolic prehospital cardiac arrest. J Am Coll Cardiol, in press.

19. Swerdlow CD, Winkle RA, Mason JD: Determinant of survival in patients with ventricular tachyarrhythmias. N Engl J Med 1983; 308: 1436–1442.

20. Ruskin JN: Personal communication.

21. Morady F, DiCarlo L, Winston S, Davis JC, Scheinman MM: Clinical features and prognosis of patients with out-of-hospital cardiac arrest and a normal electrophysiologic study. J Am Coll Cardiol 1984; 4: 39–44.

22. Myerburg RJ, Kessler KM, Estes D, Conde CA, Luceri RM, Zaman L, Kozlovskis PL, Castellanos A: Long-term survival after prehospital cardiac arrest – Analysis of outcome during an 8-year study. Circulation 1985; 70: 327–345.

23. Liberthson RR, Nagel EL, Hirschman JC, Nussenfeld SR: Prehospital ventricular defibrillation: Prognosis and follow-up course. N Engl J Med 1974; 291: 317–321.

24. Baum RS, Alvarez H, Cobb L: Survival after resuscitation from out-of-hospital ventricular fibrillation. Circulation 1974; 50: 1231–1235.

25. Kessler KM, Kissane B, Cassidy J, Pefkaros K, Hamburg C, Myerburg RJ: Dynamic variability of antiarrhythmic drug binding during the evolution of acute myocardial infarction. Circulation 1985; 70: 830–839.

26. Kessler KM, Lisker B, Conde C, Silver J, Ho-Tung P, Hamburg C, Myerburg RJ: Abnormal quinidine binding in survivors of prehospital cardiac arrest. Am Heart J 1984; 107: 665–669.

2.6 Amiodarone as Drug of First Choice in the Prevention of Sustained Ventricular Tachycardia (VT) and/or Ventricular Fibrillation (VF)

J.MA. DOMÍNGUEZ DE ROZAS, J. GARCÍA PICART, J. GUINDO SOLDEVILA, R. OTER RODRÍGUEZ and A. BAYÉS DE LUNA

Introduction

The prevention of sudden death in patients with malignant ventricular arrhythmias is one of the greatest challenges facing cardiology in the eighties. Drug selection by means of intracavitary electrophysiological studies (IES) introduced by Josephson et al. [1], the acute drug test (ADT) described by Lown et al. [2], and the determinations of plasma levels defended by Myerburg and Castellanos [3] are the most common pharmacological alternatives in use in hospitals in the search and choice of an efficient antiarrhythmic treatment, considering in general that empirical treatment is inadvisable in patients with malignant ventricular arrhythmias.

For all these techniques, due to the pharmacokinetics of amiodarone, this drug is usually not used as drug of first choice and is dependent on the failure of other antiarrhythmics. The reasons for this are the doubtful utility of electrophysiological tests in determining the response to amiodarone [4–7], the doubtful validity or uncertainty of the use of plasma level determinations of amiodarone [8–10], and the long latency period between administration of the drug and the moment of maximum efficiency [11]. For these reasons and due, possibly, to the lack of availability of the product for routine use in some countries, the majority of publications on amiodarone in the treatment of VT/VF has been limited to groups of patients selected following the failure of other antiarrhythmics [12–19], in which case we are probably confronted with patients with particularly uncontrolled ventricular arrhythmias. In spite of this, amiodarone is considered in many of these studies to be a highly effective antiarrhythmic in the control of malignant ventricular arrhythmias.

The aim of this study was to determine the validity of empirical treatment with amiodarone as drug of choice in the treatment of VT/VF in a general population of patients, not selected following the failure of other antiarrhythmics.

Method

Between January 1984 and January 1987, 33 patients with malignant ventricular arrhythmias were included in a study designed to evaluate systematic empirical treatment with amiodarone in the prevention of the recurrence of ventricular tachycardia or ventricular fibrillation.

The criteria needed for inclusion in the study were:
1. Less than 80 years old,
2. having presented an episode of sustained VT (a VT requiring medical intervention for its control) or VF,
3. arrhythmia not due to the acute phase of myocardial infarction (96 hours) or other correctable cause (electrolytic disturbances, drugs etc.),
4. absence of clear contraindication to amiodarone,
5. possibility of outpatient follow-up, and
6. having completed a minimum of 10 days with amiodarone.

On analyzing the results, the condition was deemed to be a VF when, in spite of an initial recording of VT, this was seen to degenerate into VF, requiring immediate electric cardioversion. Of the 33 patients initially included, only one could not be followed-up in out-patient control and was excluded from the analysis.

Final points of the analysis were:
1. failure of amiodarone,
2. patient's death,
3. suppression of amiodarone due to the appearance of colateral effects with functional alterations.

Failure of amiodarone was defined as sudden death or the relapse of arrhythmia with equal characteristics, after 10 days of treatment. The recurrence of arrhythmia with slower ventricular rate and hemodynamic tolerance was not considered to be a failure of the treatment, although it was the cause, in some patients, for an association with other antiarrhythmic drugs. The only case in which a Mirowski defibrillator had previously been placed was considered to be a failure of the amiodarone and was included in the results as a sudden death due to multiple hospital relapses of the arrhythmia with effective cardioversions and later death due to heart failure. The patients in whom the appearance of colateral effects (n = 3) was the motive for suppression of the drug were considered for analysis until the moment of suppression. After discharge, the patients were followed up in a specialized out-patient clinic with clinical, analytical and radiological controls, paying special attention to the appearance of toxic side effects. In case of death, direct information was obtained from relatives who lived with the patient, or from the medical center where he had attended. Sudden death was defined as either instant or occurring within six hours after having been seen with no worsening of the clinical situation.

Amiodarone was administered in doses of 1,200 mg/day for a week, followed by 600–800 mg/day for the rest of the month and 400–600 mg/day on continuation, for 5–6 days a week. The patients having arrhythmias that were considered to be of greater clinical severity (VF) were given higher doses. In 6 patients, other drugs were associated with amiodarone (mexiletine and propaphenone) for the first month. A study of left ventricular function with isotopes and/or angiography and periodic controls with Holter recording were carried out systematically whenever possible.

Holter recorded post-treatment was considered positive when any of the following were seen:

1. over 30 premature ventricular contractions (PVC)/hour,
2. presence of pairs of PVC, and/or
3. salvos of 3 or more PVC.

Of the total of 33 patients in the study, 32 were admitted directly to our Cardiology Intensive Care Unit due to arrhythmias. Only one patient initially attended at another centre and was referred to the out-patient clinic for later evaluation.

The group was made up of 25 males and 7 females. The diagnosis and clinical characteristics are summarized in Tables 1 and 2. The diagnosis in 22 patients was ischemic heart disease, operative rheumatic valulopathy in 2, dilated cardiomyopathy in 2, hypertrophic cardiomyopathy with family history of sudden death in one and with no detectable heart disease in 5 (in one case there was coexisting hypothyroidism). In the group with ischemic heart disease (n = 22), the arrhythmia was produced in 10 during the late hospitalization phase following acute myocardial infarction (16.2 ± 5.6 days) and in 12 following hospital discharge after the same illness, with an interval of over 40 days. Six patients were definite pacemaker wearers, though in no case had implantation of pacemaker been due to Stokes-Adams' crisis; in four cases pacemaker implantation was due to advanced AV block or marked sinusoidal depression, and in two cases it was based on the benefits obtained with the provisional

Table 1. Diagnosis.

	No of patients
Ischemic heart disease	22
Valvular heart disease	2
Idiopathic dilated cardiomyopathy	2
Hypertrophic cardiomyopathy	1
Primary hypothyroidism	1
Whithout cardiopathy or other pathology	4
Total	32

pacemaker for control of the ventricular arrhythmia. In one patient a Mirow-ski internal defibrillator was placed before treatment was begun. The type of arrhythmia bringing about inclusion in the study was VF in 15 and VT with a mean ventricular heart rate of 202 ± 41 in 17. The history of the arrhythmia previous to treatment was less than 15 days in 27 patients, to 1 month in 2 patients and to 12 months in 3. In functional class I-II (NYHA) there were 23 patients, and 9 were in class III-IV. The mean time of follow-up was 16.9 ± 11 months (3–58 months) and was only less than 6 months in 1 patient.

LVEF was obtained in 28 cases, 18 by means of isotopic ventriculography and angiographically in 10.

Twenty-four-hour Holter monitoring was performed on 30 patients following a minimum of 15 days' treatment. In the search for clinical predictors of the results, we analyzed the relationship between these and the following variables: age, sex, diagnosis, type of arrhythmia, number of episodes, number of cardioversions, coexistence of bundle branch block, result of the Holter monitoring, functional class and LVEF.

The statistical analysis was carried out by means of the Student-Fisher t-test

Table 2. Baseline characteristics.

Age	51.7 ± 17.5
Male/Female	25/7
NYHA	
I–II	23
III–IV	9
Fascicular blocks	
With	14
Without	18
Arrhythmia	
VF	15
VT	17
Interval from the first episode to admitance	
≤ 15 days	27
> 15 days	5
Number of episodes	
1	11
> 1	21
Number of defibrillations	2.1 ± 3.6
Permanent pacemaker	6
Other antiarrhythmic drugs added*	6
Holter post-treatment (n = 30)	
Positive	10
Negative	20
Mean ejection fraction (n = 28)	$39 \pm 20\%$

* Only during the first month.

for independent quantitive variables, chi-square with Yates' correction and Fisher's exact test for the qualitative variables.

Results

In the follow-up time of 16.9 ± 11 months, the global mortality was 37.5% (12 cases). All deaths were considered to be of cardiac origin (Table 3). The differentiation between sudden or non-sudden cardiac death according to the established criteria was possible in all but one case. The incidence of sudden

Table 3. Mortality: cause and time of death (n = 32).

	$\leqslant 6$ month	>6 month	Total
Sudden death	6	2	8
CHF*	3	–	3
Unknown	1	–	1
Total	10	2	12

* Congestive heart failure.

Table 4. Univariate predictors of mortality.

	All death (P)	Sudden death (P)
Age	NS	NS
Sex	NS	NS
Diagnosis (ischemic versus non-ischemic heart disease	NS	<0.05
NYHA (I–II versus III–IV)	<0.01	NS
Branch blocks	NS	NS
Arrhythmia (TV/FV)	<0.05	<0.05
Time since the first episode*	NS	NS
Number of episodes	NS	NS
Number of defibrillations	NS	NS
Other antiarrhythmic drugs added	NS	NS
Permanent pacemaker	NS	NS
Post-treatment Holter (results)	NS	NS
Ejection fraction	<0.05	NS

* Time since the first episode: >15 days versus ≤ 15 days.

Table 5. Mortality according to arrhythmia and LVEF.

	N	Death	Alive
VF (n = 11) p>0.05			
LVEF <30%	5	5[b]	0
LVEF≥30%	6	0	6
VT (n = 17) p = NS			
LVEF <30%	8	2[a]	6
LVEF≥30%	9	1[b]	8

[a] No sudden death.
[b] Sudden death.

death was 25% (8 cases). Of the total deaths, 83% ocurred within the first six months of inclusion in the study (Table 3).

In Table 4, we have summarized the degree of significance of the variables analyzed in respect to global death and sudden death. Predictive factors in global mortality were the worst functional class (NYHA III-IV; $p<0.01$) the type of arrhythmia (VF versus VT, $p<0.01$) and reduced LVEF (survivors 44.6 ± 19.7 versus 27.7 ± 7.5 in cases of exitus: $p<0.05$) (Table 4). No differences were seen in global and sudden death among the patients with definite pacemaker ($n = 6$). On the other hand, in the analysis of sudden death the predictive factors were the diagnosis (a greater incidence of ischemic heart disease, $p<0.01$) and the type of arrhythmia (VF versus VT: $p<0.05$).

When analyzed as a whole for all patients, LVEF was of no predictive value for sudden death. On the other hand, following the subdivision of the patients into groups of high risk and low risk, in agreement with the type of arrhythmia (VT or VF), the LVEF (established within an arbitrary limit of 30%) allowed the patients with maximum risk of sudden death to be separated within the group of VF. Of the 5 patients with VF and LVEF<30%, all died of sudden death. On the other hand, in the group with VF and LVEF≥30% all patients survived (Table 5). Within the VT group ($n = 17$) the incidence of sudden death was low: only one case in a patient with hypertrophic cardiomiopathy and family antecedent of sudden death.

Discussion

Although amiodarone has been widely used in the preventive treatment of VT/VF in recent years, its use appears to have been limited to the patients in whom conventional antiarrhythmic drugs have failed. In this respect our study is different from the majority of publications in that we used amiodarone as a drug of first choice in empirical and systematic treatment in a series of consecutive patients who had suffered an episode of VF or VT.

During a follow-up period of 16.9 ± 11 months we observed an incidence of therapeutic failure or sudden death of 25%, 83% of the deaths being produced during the first 6 months. This index of therapeutic failure is similar to that published by Di Carlo [20] and slightly inferior to that of Horowitz [5] and Fogoro [21] in more numerous series and in which conventional antiarrhythmic drugs had failed. Di Carlo [20] described cardiac arrest due to VT, VF and sudden eath in 25 of 104 patients (24%). Horowitz [5], including symptomatic VT as failure as well as VF or sudden death, found a somewhat higher number of failures, 38 of 100 patients. In Fogoro's study [21] and applying failure criteria similar to those of Horowitz, amiodarone proved to be ineffective in 23 of the 70 patients with VT/VF (32%). In agreement with these figures, and considering the possibility that patients in whom this treatment took place following the failure of conventional drugs may have arrhythmias of worse prognosis, the similarity of results in our study and those of the series published would advise against the administration of amiodarone as drug of first choice. However, the differences in the clinical characteristics of the patients studied should also be kept in mind before drawing definite conclusion. Swerdlow [22], Spielman [23] and Kerin [24] among others, have shown the existence of predictive clinical factors, the results of which are quite separate from the treatment or selection method used, and which invalidate any type of conclusion being drawn from a comparison among groups of patients with non-homogenous clinical characteristics. Swerdlow [22] observed that the worst functional class has a predictive value independent of the sudden death risk. In 166 patients treated with different antiarrhythmic drugs selected in agreement with the electrophysiological method, Spielman [23] found that factors correlating with the success of the treatment are: age under 45, LVEF superior to 50%, absence of heart disease and hypokinesia as the only anomaly of contraction. On the other hand, in patients with potentially malignant ventricular arrhythmias in whom selection of the antiarrhythmic drug is made in agreement with the result of the Holter monitoring, Kerin [24] observed that the capacity of the treatment to control the arrhythmia decreases with LVEF. Among patients with LVEF<40%, the incidence of accumulative sudden death in 1, 2, and 3 years was 57%, 71% and 79% respectively.

In light of the clinical variations considered, the analysis of our results allows us to define those patients in whom treatment with amiodarone as drug of choice have greater possibilities of success or failure.

In our study, the diagnosis (ischemic versus non ischemic heart disease) and the type of arrhythmias were the two variables of greater statistical significance in the identification of patients with a good or bad response to treatment.

Predictive value of the diagnosis is not a surprising finding and agrees with the results described by Wellens [25], who drew attention to the good prognosis of the idiopathic ventricular tachycardia (in patients without detectable heart disease) when compared to patients with ischemic heart disease. In our study we compare the incidence of sudden death among patients with ischemic heart disease and the rest of the patients in whom, although there may be different diagnoses, there is an unusually high number of idiopathic ventricular tachycardias (50% of total patients of this latter group).

We feel that the second factor found to have predictive value, the type of arrhythmia (VF versus VT), is no more than a logical consequence of the criteria chosen to define the initial arrhythmia. With such criteria, patients were subdivided into two groups depending on whether the arrhythmia produced circulatory arrest (VF) or not (VT). In another study carried out in 104 patients treated with amiodarone following the failure of conventional arrhythmic drugs, Di Carlo et al. [20] found that one predictive factor for failure of treatment was the antecedent of syncope or cardiac arrest, a parameter which in fact showed patients with arrhythmia as being more serious clinically, as was also seen in our group of patients with circulatory arrest.

In contrast to other studies which also analyze their results according to the different clinical parameters [20, 23, 26], the LVEF did not reach an independent predictive value in our study, although it was on the margin of significance. The reduced number of patients studied may explain this discordance of our results. However, the LVEF does add predictive value when its significance is analyzed following subdivision of the patients, in agreement with the type of initial arrhythmia (VF or VT). Coexistence of an LVEF inferior or, equal or superior to 30% enables patients in the worse prognosis group (VF) to be separated into better or worse response to treatment. All the cases with VF and LVEF inferior to 30% died due to sudden death. On the other hand, in the patients with VT the mortality was low and independent of the LVEF value.

In conclusion we may deduce that in the group of patients studied there are clinical variables (diagnosis, type of arrhythmia and LVEF), which enable identification of patients in whom treatment with amiodarone as drug of first choice has a greater chance of failure. In consequence, we consider that treatment with amiodarone as a drug of choice should be preceded by clinical characterization (including the LVEF determination) of the patient in arrhythmia with risk of sudden death, ruling out those patients in whom there coexists VF and an LVEF inferior to 30%. In contrast, in patients with sustained VT or those who have presented an episode of VF and have an LVEF equal or superior to 30%, amiodarone administered in an emperical form as drug of choice, constitutes a valid therapeutic alternative.

Summary

In 32 patients with sustained ventricular tachycardia (VT) or recuperated ventricular fibrillation (VF), we carried out empirical treatment with amiodarone as drug of first choice. The patients were followed up for 16.9 ± 11 months (3–58), and results of treatment were analyzed both globally and according to the clinical variables collected during follow-up. The incidence of global cardiac death was 37.5% (12 cases) and of sudden death 25% (8 cases). The worst functional class (NYHA III–IV; $p<0.01$), the type of arrhythmia (VF versus VT; $p<0.05$) and the lesser left ventricular ejection fraction (LVEF) ($p<0.01$) were the variables which correlated significantly with the global mortality. In sudden death patients, significant variables were the diagnosis (ischemic heart disease versus miscellaneous; $p<0.05$) and the type of arrhythmia (VF versus VT; $p<0.05$). The LVEF did not reach a significant value as an isolated variable. However, when patients were divided into high and low risk groups, according to the type of arrhythmia (VF versus VT), and LVEF<30% permitted identification of all patients with sudden death in the group of VF. In conclusion, we consider that treatment other than that used in this study should be selected for patients with VF and LVEF<30%. In patients with VT or an LVEF≥30% empirical treatment with amiodarone as drug of first choice is a valid therapeutic alternative.

References

1. Josephson ME, Horowitz LN: Electrophysiologic approach to therapy of recurrent sustained ventricular tachycardia. Am J Cardiol 1979; 43: 631–642.
2. Lown B: Management of patients at high risk of sudden death. Am Heart J 1982; 103: 689–697.
3. Myerburg RJ, Conde C, Sheps DS et al.: Antiarrhythmic drug therapy in survivors of prehospital cardiac arrest: Comparison of effects on chronic ventricular arrhythmias and recurrent cardiac arrest. Circulation 1979; 59: 855–863.
4. Veltri E, Reid P, Platia E, Griffith L: Results of late programmed electrical stimulation and longterm electrophysiologic effects of amiodarone therapy in patients with refractory ventricular tachycardia. Am J Cardiol 1985; 55: 375–379.
5. Horowitz L, Greenspan A, Spielman S, Webb Ch, Morganroth J, Rotmensch H, Sokoloff N, Rae A, Segal B, Kay H: Usefulness of electrophysiologic testing in evaluation of Amiodarone therapy for sustained ventricular tachyarrhythmias associated with coronary heart disease. Am J Cardiol 1985; 55: 367–371.
6. Kennedy E, Lerner E, Rosenfeld I, McPherson C, Bastford W, Gradman A: Accurate prediction of arrhythmia outcome with amiodarone: Use of discriminant analysis based on invasive and non invasive variables (Abstract). J Am Coll Cardiol 1985; 5: 481.
7. Zipes D, Prystowki E, Heger J: Amiodarone: electrophysiologic actions, pharmacokinetics and clinical effects. J Am Coll Cardiol 1984; 3: 1059–1071.
8. Siddoway L, McAllister C, Wilkinson G, Roden D, Woosley R: Amiodarone dosing: a

proposal based on its pharmacokinetics. Am Heart J 1983; 106: 951–955.

9. Haffajes C, Love J, Canada A, Leski L, Asdourina G, Alpert J: Clinical pharmacokinetics and efficacy of amiodarone for refractory tachyarrhythmias. Circulation 1983; 67: 1347–1355.

10. Haffajes C, Sofelt S, Benotti J, Sloan K, Alpert J: Amiodarone for VT-VF: Role of follow-up programmed ventricular stimulation, Holter monitoring and serum amiodarone levels in predicting outcome (Abstract). Circulation 1984; 70: II–436.

11. Rosenbaum MB, Chiale PA, Halpern MS et al.: Clinical efficacy of Amiodarone as antiarrhythmic agent. Am J Cardiol 1976; 38: 934–944.

12. Haffajes CI, Love JC, Alpert JS, Asdourian GK, Sloan KC: Efficacy and safety of long-term amiodarone in treatment of cardiac arrhythmias: dosage experience. Am Heart J 1983; 106: 935–942.

13. Morady F, Sauve MJ, Malone P et al.: Long-term efficacy and toxicity of high-dose amiodarone therapy for ventricular tachycardia or ventricular fibrillation. Am J Cardiol 1983; 52: 975–979.

14. Hager JJ, Prystowsky EN, Zipes DP: Clinical efficacy of amiodarone in treatment of recurrent ventricular tachycardia and ventricular fibrillation. Am Heart J 1983; 106: 887–892.

15. Peter T, Hamer A, Mandel WJ, Weiss D: Evaluation of amiodarone therapy in the treatment of drug-resistant cardiac arrhythmias. Long-term follow-up. Am Heart J 1983; 106: 943–950.

16. Nademaee K, Hendrickson JA, Cisnom DS, Goldreyer DN, Singh BN: Control of refractory life-treatening ventricular tachyarrhythmia by amiodarone. Am Heart J 1981; 101: 759–768.

17. Greene LH, Graham EL, Werner JA et al.: Toxic and therapeutic effects of amiodarone in the treatment of cardiac arrhythmias. JACC 1983; 2: 1114–1128.

18. Rakita L, Sobol MS: Amiodarone in the treatment of refractory ventricular arrhythmias. Importance and safety of initial high-dose therapy. JAMA 1983; 250: 1293–1295.

19. Torreu V, Tepper D, Flowers D et al.: QT prolongation and the antiarrhythmic efficacy of amiodarone. JACC 1986; 7: 142–147.

20. Di Carlo L, Morady F, Sauve M, Malone P, Davis J, Evans-Bell T, Winston S, Scheiman M: Cardiac arrest and sudden death in patients treated with amiodarone for sustained ventricular tachycardia or ventricular fibrillation: Risk stratification based on clinical variables. Am J Cardiol 1985; 55: 372–374.

21. Fogoros R, Anderson K, Winkle R, Swerdlow Ch, Mason J: Amiodarone: clinical efficacy and toxicity in 96 patients with recurrent, drug-refractory arrhythmias. Circulation 1983; 68: 88–94.

22. Swerdlow Ch, Winkle R, Mason J: Determinants of survival in patients with ventricular tachyarrhythmias. N Engl J Med 1983; 308: 1436–1442.

23. Spielman SR, Schwartz JS, McCarthy DM et al.: Predictors of the success or failure of medical therapy in patients with chronic recurrent sustained ventricular tachycardia: a discriminant analysis. JACC 1983; 1: 401–408.

24. Kerin N, Blevins R, Frumin H et al.: Effect of arrhythmia control on prevention of sudden death in coronary artery disease (Abstract). Circulation 1984; 70: II–267.

25. Wellens H, Bar F, Brugada P: Ventricular tachycardia – The clinical problem. In: Josephson ME (ed) Ventricular tachycardia. Mechanisms and management. Futura Publ, New York, 1982, pp 180–191.

26. Vlay S, Reid P, Griffith L, Kallman C: Relationship of specific coronary lesions and regional left ventricular dysfunction to prognosis in survivors of sudden cardiac death. Am Heart J 1984; 108: 1212.

Conclusions

A. BAYÉS DE LUNA

Conclusions

In the preceeding pages, the different pharmacologic approaches to the treatment of malignant ventricular arrhythmias (MVA) have been described. I do not think that it has been demonstrated which is of choice. In reality, the election depends partly on the possibilities of each hospital and the cost of these expensive techniques. It would be helpful if a long-term study were realized comparing the different approaches to determine which of them is the best [1–10]. Until this is done, the choice of procedure will be individual.

The algorithm in Fig. 1 summarizes the possible approaches. As we have already mentioned, different authors have obtained promising results by using acute drug test, plasma concentrations or intracavitary electrophysiological studies (IES). If none of these forms of treatment control can be practiced, or if no effective results are obtained, the best course could be an empirical treatment consisting of oral administration of a potent and minimally arrhythmogenic antiarrhythmic drug with frequent Holter controls to confirm its efficacy, changing to another drug if necessary. Amiodarone, propaphenone and flecainide are, probably, the drugs of first choice, but mexilitine, tocainide and disopyramide may be effective, as well as the traditional drugs quinidine and procainamide. In this sense the experience of Domínquez et al. with amiodarone is very promising. The most arrhythmogenic is probably quinidine and that which most depresses contractility in patients with left ventricular failure is disopyramide and flecainide. If pharmacologic treatment of MVA fails, non-pharmacologic treatment should be considered (pacemaker, defibrillator implantation, surgical or catheter ablation techniques) [11–13].

We think that the future of the Mirowski's technique and the catheter procedures are very promising, especially considering that the ideal antiarrhythmic has yet to be found.

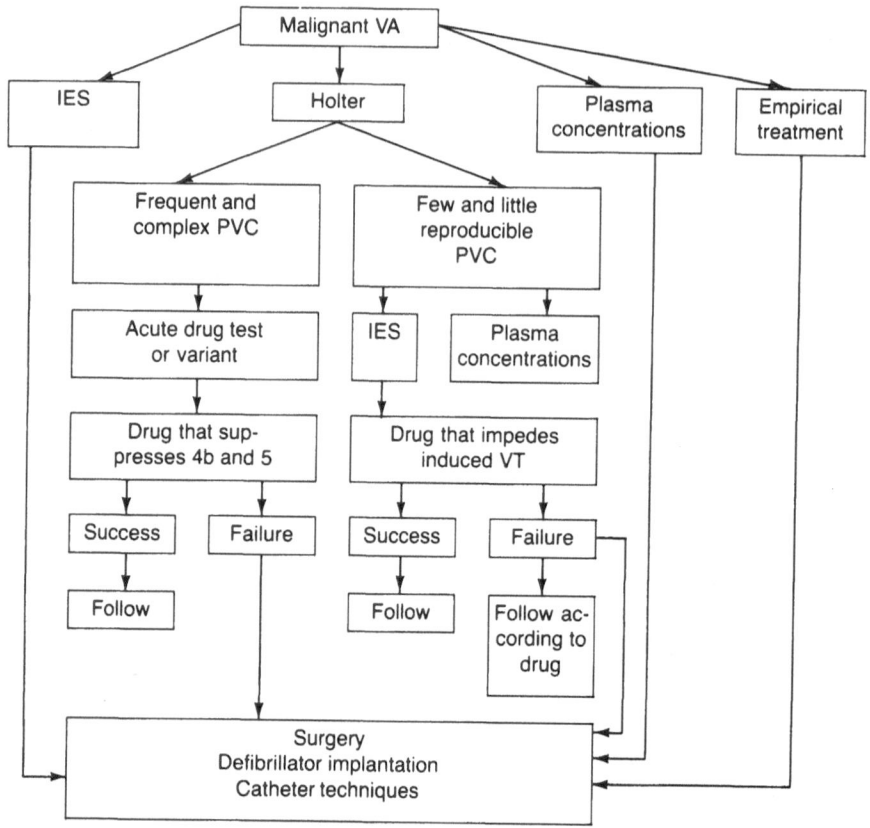

Fig. 1. Algorithm of possible approaches to the management of the ventricular malignant arrhythmias.

References

1. Julian DC: Toward preventing coronary death from ventricular fibrillation. Circulation 1976; 54: 360–366.
2. Wenger NK, Mock MB, Burgkist I: Ambulatory ECG recording. Current Probl Cardiol 1980; 5: 1–42.
3. Julian DG: Prevention of sudden death. In: Harrison DC (ed) Cardiac arrhythmias. A decade of progress. GK Hall Med Publ, Boston, 1981; 111.
4. Velebit V, Podrid P, Lown B, Cohen B, Graboys T: Aggravation and provocation of ventricular arrhythmias by antiarrhythmic drugs. Circulation 1982; 65: 886–894.
5. Bayés de Luna A, Serra Grima JR, Oca F: ECG de Holter, Editorial Científico-Médica, Barcelona, 1983.
6. Ruberman V, Weinblatt E, Goldberg J, Frank CW, Shapiro S: Ventricular premature beats and mortality after acute myocardial infarction. N Engl J Med 1977; 279: 750–757.
7. Harrison DC: Cardiac arrhythmias. A decade of progress. GK Hall Med Publ, Boston, 1981.

8. Graboys TB, Lown B, Podrid PJ, De Silva R: Long term survival of patients with malignant ventricular arrhythmias treated with antiarrhythmic drugs. Am J Cardiol 1982; 50: 437–445.

9. Myerburg RJ, Kessler K, Kiem I et al.: Relationship between plasma levels of procainamide suppression of PVC and prevention of recurrent ventricular tachycardia. Circulation 1981; 64: 280–288.

10. Horowitz LN, Josephson ME, Kastor JA: Intracardiac electrophysiologic studies as a method for the optimation of drug therapy in chronic ventricular arrhythmias. Prog Cardiovasc Dis 1980; 23: 81–89.

11. Fisher JD, Kim SG, Furman D et al.: Role of implantable pacemakers in control of recurrent ventricular tachycardia. Am J Cardiol 1982; 49: 194–199.

12. Geoffrey O, Hartzler MD: Electrode catheter ablation of refractory focal ventricular tachycardia. J Am Coll Cardiol 1983; 2: 1107–1113.

13. Mirowski M, Mower MM, Langer A, Heilman MS: The automatic implantable defibrillator: A new avenue. In: Kulbertus HE, Wellens HJJ (eds) Sudden death. Martinus Nijhoff, Dordrecht, Boston, Lancaster, 1980.

3. The Surgical Treatment of the Arrhythmias

3.1 Introduction

J. FARRÉ MUNCHARAZ

Although the arsenal of drugs now available for interrupting episodes of tachycardia, as well as for preventing recurrences, is considerable, a substantial number of patients is not adequately controlled with antiarrhythmic drugs. The next papers will deal with some of the non-pharmacologic alternatives presently available. The role of the cardiac pacemakers will be discussed elsewhere.

The use of non-pharmacologic therapeutic approaches to patients with tachycardia should pursue the objective of obtaining a better quality and/or life expectancy than that provided by antiarrhythmic agents. The selection of candidates for these alternative forms of treatment is based on considerations relative to the age of the patients, presence of organic heart disease, site of origin, mechanism and clinical consequences of the tachycardia, response to conventional antiarrhythmic drugs and those under development, the patient's capacity to follow a determined antiarrhythmic treatment and previous experience with the non-pharmacologic therapeutic modality selected.

Accessory bundle surgery is undoubtedly the least experimental of all forms of surgical treatment of tachycardias. In the hands of an expert and patient surgeon provided with a preliminary electrophysiologic study with electrocatheters and programmed stimulation as well as an accurate intraoperatory map, most of the atrioventricular accessory bundles can be successfully sectioned with almost no mortality and small morbidity. The long-term prognosis of these patients has yet to be defined, especially with respect to the possibility that they may develop tachycardias unrelated to the accessory bundle sectioned. Data obtained in our laboratory in a series of 64 consecutive patients with accessory bundles and tachycardia demonstrate that (excluding atrial flutter and fibrillation) there are multiple tachycardia mechanisms in 20% of the patients and that 77% of the tachycardias are unrelated to the single or most evident accessory bundle. Inadequate preoperative evaluation can therefore lead to unsatisfactory long-term results in this type of patients.

Surgery of the ventricular tachcyardias (VT), particularly in patients with post myocardial infarction scarring, can be performed with acceptable mortality and offers promising short- and long-term results. However, the long-term prognosis of these patients is unknown. It must be clarified whether we should act only on the zones linked to the clinical VT or on all the potential types of ventricular tachycardia that can be demonstrated in a patient. We also do not know if antiarrhythmic medication should be given to patients who have had endocardial resection and present nonsustained VT induced by programmed electrical stimulation in the postoperative electrophysiologic study. These unknowns, together with the progressive nature of ischemic heart disease, may justify placing implantable defibrillator electrodes during the operation, connecting them to batteries if the patient presents severe arrhythmias in the future or if sustained VT is induced in the postoperative electrical study. Until now, patients considered to be candidates for surgical treatment of recurrent sustained VT are those refractory to medical treatment. However, this concept is not clearly defined. If we assume that refractory VT is that which can be induced by electrical stimulation after diverse trials with antiarrhythmic drugs, between 65% and 75% of the patients with recurrent sustained VT after myocardial infarction could be considered candidates for non-pharmacologic forms of treatment. However, we know that in the case of amiodarone and perhaps propaphenone and other drugs, laboratory induction of sustained VT is not useful to predict the clinical recurrence of the arrhythmia. In our experience, 74% of the patients with sustained post infarction VT treated with oral amiodarone (400–800 mg/day) remain alive and without VT during a follow-up of 28 ± 17 months, the mortality being 15% and the proportion of cases in which treatment with this drug must be withdrawn 11%.

The implantable defibrillator is today something more than an idea since there are now nearly 400 patients carrying the unit developed by Dr Mirowski. This is a fascinating area in which important advances in the configuration and localization of the electrodes, the mode of function of the cardioverter/defibrillator and the physical dimensions of the device implanted are pending realization.

Finally, the techniques of electrical ablation by catheter have opened the era of therapeutic electrophysiology. In the forthcomming years we will see if it will be electrical energy, or another type, which will be channeled through a catheter to specifically injure areas essential for maintaining tachyarrhythmias. Many of these techniques, such as those that will be discussed today, will be history within 5 years. Important tasks are waiting to be done and we invite the reader to participate in them.

3.2 The Role of Left Stellectomy in the Prevention of Lethal Arrhythmias

MARIO FACCHINI and PETER J. SCHWARTZ

Introduction

It has progressively become evident that the sympathetic nervous system plays an important role in the genesis of malignant arrhythmias [1–5]. This role is likely to range from what seems to be an aggravating factor, as it occurs during acute myocardial ischemia, to what constitutes a more substantial pathogenetic mechanism, as in the case of the long QT syndrome [6].

According to these observations, there has been a widespread evaluation of anti-adrenergic drugs, namely β-blockers, in the prevention of sudden death, particularly in patients with a prior myocardial infarction [7]. This approach, although valid, does not take into account the importance of the α-adrenergic effects of catecholamines in modifying the electrophysiologic substrate of cardiac arrhythmias [8]. Also, the right and left cardiac sympathetic nerves have a different arrhythmogenic potential [9]. It is known in fact that unilateral sympathetic discharges may be more arrhythmogenic than a massive but homogeneous activation of the sympathetic nervous system.

In this chapter we will discuss the rational basis and the clinical role of left sympathetic cardiac denervation in the prevention of lethal arrhythmias.

Effects of left stellate ganglion stimulation

While right sided sympathetic nerve stimulation induces mostly sinus tachycardia and modifications of T wave morphology, stimulation of nerves originating from the left stellate ganglion produces a variety of rhythm disturbances. While most of these arrhythmias are supraventricular [10–12], sometimes the stimulation of left sided nerves can elicit ventricular tachyarrhythmias, such as ventricular tachycardia, even in intact hearts. This arrhythmogenic potential becomes more evident in a myocardium already unstable because of a recent myocardial infarction or an acute myocardial ischemia [13, 14]. In the experi-

A.B. 50 YEARS - DURING ANESTHESIA

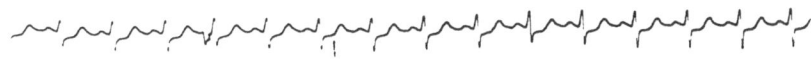

LEFT STELLATE GANGLION STIMULATION

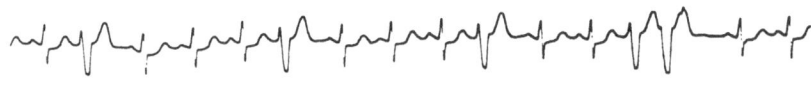

1 sec

Fig. 1. See text for explanation.

mental laboratory the specific interaction between a 2 min coronary occlusion and a brief (30 sec) electrical stimulation of left stellate ganglion consistently produces ventricular tachycardia and fibrillation, so to constitute a valuable method for the evaluation of anti-arrhythmic drugs [13, 15].

We have recently observed (Fig. 1) the appearance of premature ventricular beats by simply touching with a blunt instrument the left stellate ganglion of a patient with a recent anterior myocardial infarction. This observation was made just prior to perform a high thoracic left sympathectomy. Moreover the arrhythmogenic potential of left cardiac sympathetic nerves has been very well observed in man (long QT syndrome [6]).

Effects of left stellectomy: experimental data

A left sympathetic cardiac denervation can be produced experimentally not only by surgical ablation of the left stellate ganglion but also by a transient interruption of the nervous traffic by simply cooling the ganglion. The effects of left stellectomy are summarized in Table 1.

The antiarrhythmic effect of left stellectomy has been confirmed in several experimental conditions. Although present immediately after denervation, this effect becomes more complete after chronic denervation. As a matter of fact, with pharmacological or cold blockade the anti-arrhythmic effect is immediately evident. When ventricular tachyarrhythmias are induced by brief (<90 sec) coronary artery occlusions in the anesthetized dog, they are reproducibly prevented by reversible cold blockade of the left stellate ganglion [16]

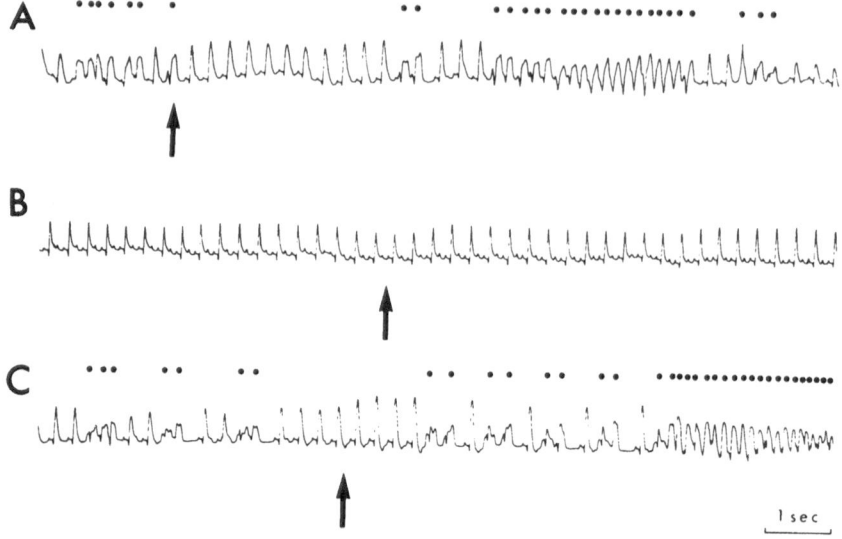

Fig. 2. Effect of a 90 sec occlusion of the circumflex coronary artery in a dog having the descending coronary artery ligated at the beginning of the experiment, in control condition and during left stellate ganglion blockade (SGB). A: coronary artery occlusion (CAO) in control condition. Episodes of VT before and after release of the occlusion. B: CAO during left SGB. No arrhythmias. C: CAO in control condition after restoration of the normal function of left SG. Several PVC's followed by VT which degenerates into ventricular fibrillation. A, B and C are consecutive trials. The arrows mark the release of occlusion. The dots indicate ectopic beats. (From Schwartz et al. [16].)

(Fig. 2). In these experiments major arrhythmias, such as ventricular tachycardia and fibrillation, required the presence of an intact stellate ganglion.

Left stellectomy modifies two electrophysiological parameters relevant to arrhythmogenesis: ventricular refractory period and ventricular fibrillation threshold. Left stellectomy shifts the strength-interval curve, commonly used as an index of ventricular excitability, later in diastole indicating an increased ventricular refractoriness [17]. The ventricular fibrillation threshold, measured by means of a train of stimuli scanning the entire vulnerable period, is increased, by either left stellectomy or cold blockade, by 72% when compared

Table 1. Effects of left stellectomy.

1. ↓ Arrhythmias associated with myocardial ischemia
2. ↑ Ventricular refractory period
3. ↑ Ventricular fibrillation threshold
4. ↑ Myocardial reactive hyperemia
5. ~ Cardiac performance during exercise
6. ↓ Incidence of spontaneous ventricular fibrillation

112

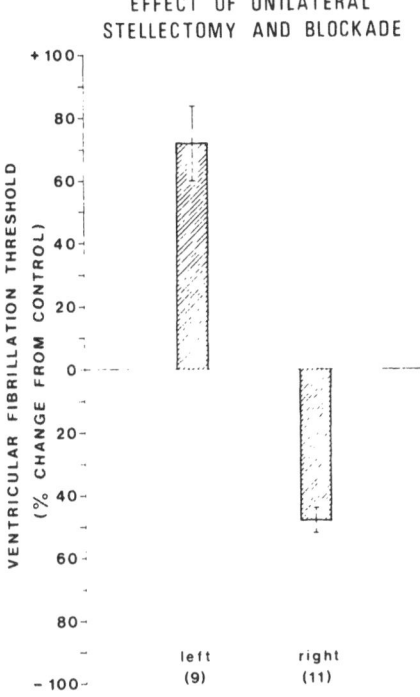

EFFECT OF UNILATERAL
STELLECTOMY AND BLOCKADE

Fig. 3. Effect of unilateral stellectomy and blockade on ventricular fibrillation threshold. Left stellectomy or blockade (9 animals) raised the ventricular fibrillation threshold by $72 \pm 12\%$ compared with control values ($p<0.001$). Right stellectomy or blockade (11 animals) lowered ventricular fibrillation threshold by $48 \pm 3\%$ (mean $\pm$ SE) compared with control values ($p<0.001$). (Modified from Schwartz et al. [18].)

to control conditions (Fig. 3) indicating a decrease in the propensity of the heart to fibrillate [18].

These studies suggest a tonic influence of the sympathetic nerves on cardiac function; later on, a tonic vasoconstrictor activity on coronary bed dependent on the sympathetic nerves was shown in conscious dogs [19]. Using the coronary flow response to a 10-second occlusion of the left circumflex coronary artery, it was found that left stellectomy greatly increased the myocardial reactive hyperemia, which is an index of the capability of the coronary bed to dilate. α-blockade produced qualitatively similar results while propranolol decreased the reactive hyperemia (Fig. 4). This indicates a dominance of an α-mediated vasoconstrictor tone, which may antagonize metabolic regulation. Furthermore this beneficial effect of left stellectomy on coronary flow could be demonstrated in dogs even when the metabolic demand is physiologically increased by exercise [20].

A protective effect of left sympathectomy on the degree and extent of

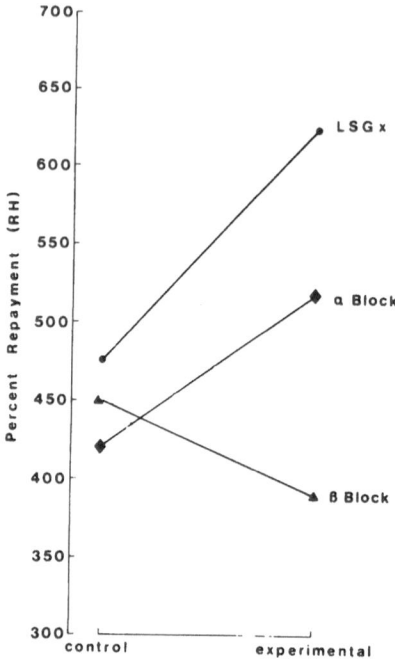

Fig. 4. Reactive hyperemia in conscious dogs before and after left stellectomy (LSGx), phentola-mine (α-block) and propranolol (β-block). The data points represent the mean of 130 trials in 16 dogs. They indicate that left stellectomy and α-adrenergic blockade increase reactive hyperemia, whereas β-adrenergic blockade has an opposite effect. The same kind of responses were found when heart rate was kept constant by pacing. (Modified from Schwartz et al. [19].)

ischemia induced by a coronary artery occlusion was observed in a collab-orative study with Janse. In anesthetized dogs 5-min coronary occlusions were performed in control conditions and after left or right stellectomy, while recording DC extracellular electrograms simultaneously from 60 left ventric-ular epicardial sites [21]. The degree of TQ segment depression, interpreted as a quantitative marker of ischemia, was reduced by left stellectomy. According-ly to these data left stellectomy reduced the infarct size, produced by an eight-hours occlusion of anterior descending coronary artery in anesthetized cats, by 23% of the total heart weight [22].

Through α-adrenergic mechanisms, left sided cardiac sympathetic nerves play an important role in the control of the coronary circulation. Under pathologic conditions (such as coronary occlusion) these effects may influence the extent of myocardium which will undergo irreversible damage. Left stel-lectomy is likely to reduce the extent of ischemia probably by allowing a better perfusion to the border zone through collateral vessels.

One of the limitations of these experiments is that the effects of sympathetic

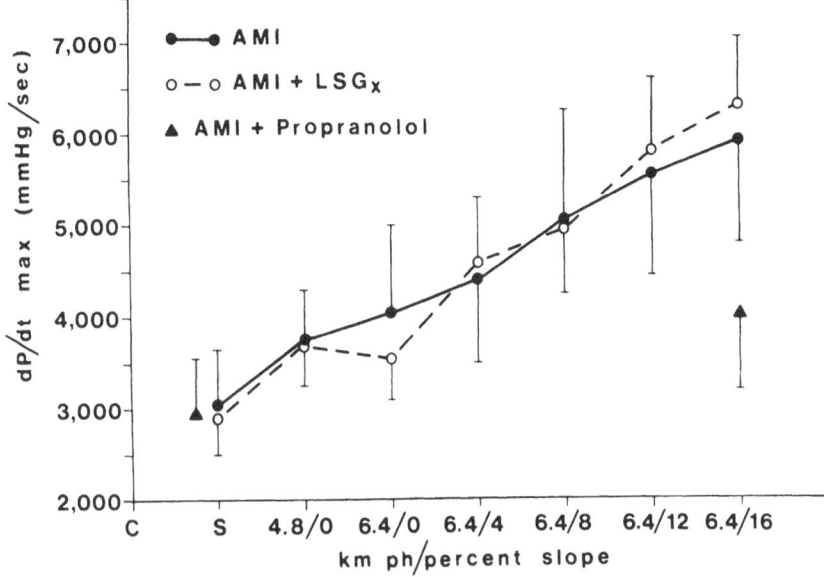

Fig. 5. The average maximal rate of rise of left ventricular pressure (dP/dt max) response to submaximal exercise in five dogs with a prior myocardial infarction in control condition and after left stellectomy (LSGx). In contrast with the effect of left stellectomy, propranolol (5 dogs), while leaving unmodified contractility at rest, severely reduced its increase during exercise. The bars through the points represent 1 standard error of the mean.

denervation were studied either in anesthetized animals or in hearts that were completely normal until the moment of the acute coronary occlusion. This is not comparable to the largely atherosclerotic and ischemic heart of most patients dying suddenly [23]. For this reason the anti-arrhythmic effect of left stellectomy was studied in an experimental model more similar to the clinical situation [24]. One month after the production of an anterior myocardial infarction dogs engage in an exercise stress test on a motor treadmill. At the beginning of the last minute of exercise a balloon occluder, previously positioned around the circumflex coronary artery, is inflated for 2 minutes to produce myocardial ischemia. This brief ischemic episode affects the last minute of exercise and the first minute after exercise. Ventricular fibrillation occurred in 23 of 35 (66%) control dogs, compared to none of 14 (0%) dogs with left stellectomy.

This study indicates that left sympathectomy exerts an important protective effect in reducing the incidence of ventricular fibrillation in an experimental situation that reminds of what may happen to a patient with a prior myocardial infarction who engages in exercise and has an increase in oxygen demand, myocardial ischemia, pain and stopping of exercise.

It is worth noting, for the implications concerning the use of left stellectomy in man, that left cardiac denervation is not accompanied by a negative inotropic effect. Myocardial contractility is not reduced either at rest or during exercise [20]. It is of clinical importance the fact that this lack of negative inotropic effects in the left ventricle is observed in dogs with prior myocardial infarction performing an exercise stress test [25] (Fig. 5).

Side effects of left stellectomy

While in the usual laboratory animals, cats and dogs, most of the sympathetic outflow pass through the stellate ganglia, a more extensive surgical procedure is needed in man to provide a sufficient denervation. The left sympathetic chain must be ablated down to the fourth-fifth thoracic ganglia while the cephalic pole of the stellate ganglion should be left intact in order to avoid the Bernard-Horner syndrome. The correct terminology would therefore be 'high thoracic left sympathectomy' (3), but we will use here the more familiar expression 'left stellectomy'.

Left stellectomy, performed extrapleurally, is a surgical procedure which practically has no risk, provided that manipulations of locally anesthetized nerves are carefully performed. The fact that, after unilateral sympathetic cardiac denervation, sweating stops on the ipsilateral hand and, at times, on the ipsilateral half forehead does not disturb the patient and constitutes a minor side effect. In about 5–8% of the patients paresthesias and even bursts of pain at the level of the left arm or shoulder may occur but usually subside within a few days.

We have already seen that in dogs left stellectomy does not decrease the ventricular pump function neither at rest nor during exercise, even after a myocardial infarction. Can these data be applied to man? Although quantitative data on ventricular hemodynamics are not available, an apparent positive answer comes from a non-invasive study of 70 patients affected by the Raynaud's syndrome who underwent, as a treatment, either right, or left, or bilateral stellectomy. Among patients of the same age group dyspnoea during an exercise stress test appeared in 30% of the patients with bilateral stellectomy but was never observed in the patients with left stellectomy [26]. This lack of detrimental effect on ventricular function is probably due to the fact that both right and left stellate ganglia contribute to myocardial contractility [27] and that unilateral stellectomy, while suppressing sympathetic activity in the ipsilateral side, may reflexly increase it in the contralateral side [9]. Also the possibility of denervation supersensitivity to catecholamines after left stellectomy has been excluded in a series of experiments in conscious dogs [28]. The left ventricular dP/dt max increases during intravenous injection of norepinephrine in conscious dogs and was identical before and two weeks after denervation. On the basis of these data left stellectomy can be reasonably considered a safe therapeutic intervention. On the other hand, with this surgical approach a protection against life-threatening arrhythmias is continuously provided, without the need of assuming drugs 1–3 times a day, thus avoiding the difficult problems related to the patient's compliance.

Clinical use of left stellectomy

Treatment of ventricular tachyarrhythmias could take advantage of left sympathetic cardiac denervation in subgroups of patients at high risk in whom a relationship between arrhythmias and increased or imbalanced sympathetic activity has been shown. The idiopathic long QT syndrome is a paradigmatic example of such a situation.

The idiopathic long QT syndrome

This disease probably represents the most interesting example of neurally mediated, noncoronary sudden cardiac death [6, 29, 30]. The affected patients have syncopal attacks in conditions associated with sudden increases in sympathetic activity, such as violent emotions or physical stresses. The syncopal episodes are due to 'torsades de pointe' which often degenerates to ventricular fibrillation. Frequently these episodes are self-terminating but each one could prove fatal. The only two evident abnormalities are in the electrocardiogram:
1. a marked prolongation of the QT interval usually due to a large, often bizarre, T wave which is sometimes notched;
2. the alternation of the T wave, in polarity or in amplitude, usually induced during emotional or physical stresses.

The acceptance of the pathogenetic hypothesis proposed in 1975 [30] of an imbalance in sympathetic cardiac innervation with left dominance probably due to a lower than normal right sympathetic activity pointed to left stellectomy as the most selective therapy for the long QT syndrome. The first surgical interventions were performed in 1970 by Moss and McDonald [31] and later on, in 1973, by Schwartz and Malliani [32].

Data available now on 763 patients, thanks to the cooperation of physicians around the world, show an extremely high mortality (71%) in untreated patients; with miscellaneous treatment, not including β-blockers, it remains high (35%) while with β-blockers it is markedly decreased (6%).

We have now data on 53 patients resistant (continuation of syncopal episodes) to full dose β-blockade, who have been treated with high thoracic left sympathectomy. In this group which clearly is at even higher risk, as indicated

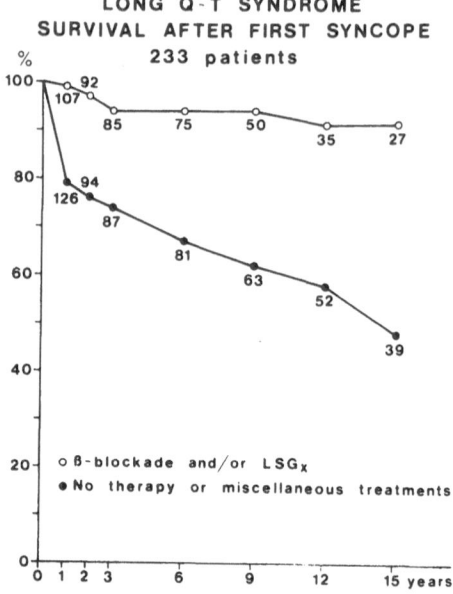

LONG Q-T SYNDROME
SURVIVAL AFTER FIRST SYNCOPE
233 patients

Fig. 6. Effect of therapy on the survival, after the first syncopal episode, of 233 patients affected by the idiopathic long QT syndrome. The protective effect of β-adrenergic blockade and of left stellectomy (LSGx) is dramatically evident. For example the mortality 3 years after the first syncope is 6% in the group treated with anti-adrenergic interventions and is 26% in the group treated differently or non-treated. Fifteen years after the first syncope the respective mortality is 9% and 53%.

by the failure of the β-blockers, there have been only three deaths (6%). The effect on survival of β-blockers and left stellectomy compared to no anti-adrenergic therapy in 233 patients for whom we have detailed information is shown in Fig. 6.

At present time it seems still rationale to begin the treatment with full-dose β-blockade. Should another syncopal episode occur, left stellectomy should be performed in a short time. Any other treatment (implantable defibrillator?) has to be considered 'experimental' and reserved only for those patients with ongoing syncopal episodes after left stellectomy.

Myocardial infarction

Patients with a prior myocardial infarction (M.I.) constitute a group at risk for death (8% to 12% during the first year and 5% in each subsequent year [33–35]). Up to 80% of these deaths are sudden cardiac deaths. It has been classically considered [36] that for patients with M.I. to have or not to have an episode of ventricular fibrillation does not modify the prognosis after discharge from hospital. Most studies supporting this concept have been made without taking into consideration the site of myocardial infarction. However it is well known [37] that sympathetic overactivity accompanies the early phase of anterior M.I.

According to these considerations, a retrospective case-control study on the survival after anterior and inferior myocardial infarction complicated or not by ventricular fibrillation has been performed in 250 male patients under 75 years of age [38]. For patients with an inferior myocardial infarction an episode of VF did not modify the prognosis (6% mortality in the first year in both groups) while in patients with anterior M.I. the mortality was importantly affected by the occurrence of ventricular fibrillation (in the first year 9% in the uncomplicated group, 32% in the VF group).

Why should the electrical cardiac instability be so high in patients after anterior myocardial infarction? A possible explanation comes from the experimental observation by Barber et al.: they found that a transmural infarction produces a sympathetic denervation even in non-infarcted areas below the infarct site probably due to destruction of the nerve fibers passing through the infarcted area [39, 40]. Myocardial infarction involving the anterior ventricular wall would result in a greater destruction of the right sided than left sided adrenergic terminals, thus producing a sympathetic imbalance with left dominance.

This observation may also partially explain the occurrence of QT prolongation in patients with myocardial infarction. It has been shown that QT prolongation has a strong association with lethal arrhythmias in the acute phase of myocardial infarction [41] and is an important predictor of subsequent sudden death [42]. These clinical data and the anti-arrhythmic effect of left stellectomy have led to a clinical trial, involving more than 40 hospitals in northern Italy, begun in 1979 and terminated at the end of 1983. A subgroup of patients at high risk for sudden death (anterior myocardial infarction complicated by primary ventricular fibrillation) was randomized between placebo, the β-blocker oxprenolol and high thoracic left sympathectomy. This trial independently from its results, indicates how tight may be the relationship between experimental and clinical cardiology.

Conclusions

There is a sufficient experimental and clinical background to provide a solid rationale for the use of left stellectomy in subgroups of patients at high risk of sudden death. In subjects affected by the idiopathic long QT syndrome the data available in 53 patients refractory to β-blockers leave no doubts. If a patient under full-dose β-blockade still has syncopal episodes, left stellectomy is mandatory. In post M.I. patients at high risk left stellectomy may be protective by limiting new ischemic episodes and by its direct anti-arrhythmic effect. This possibility is under evaluation through an ongoing multicenter clinical study in northern Italy.

References

1. Schwartz PJ, Brown AM, Malliani A, Zanchetti A: Neural Mechanisms in cardiac arrhythmias. Raven Press, New York, 1978.
2. Lown B: Sudden cardiac death: the major challenge confronting contemporary cardiology. Am J Cardiol 1979; 43: 313–328.
3. Malliani A, Schwartz PJ, Zanchetti A: Neural mechanisms in life-threatening arrhythmias. Am Heart J 1980; 100: 705–715.
4. Verrier RL, Lown B: Autonomic nervous system and malignant cardiac arrhythmias. In: Wiener H, Hofer MA, Stunkard AJ (eds) Brain, behavior and bodily disease. Raven Press, New York, 1981; 273–291.
5. Schwartz PJ, Stone HL: The role of the autonomic nervous system in sudden coronary death. Ann NY Acad Sci 1982; 382: 162–181.
6. Schwartz PJ: The long Q-T syndrome. In: Kulbertus HE, Wellens HJJ (eds) Sudden death. M. Nijhoff, Dordrecht, 1980; 358–378.
7. Hjalmarson A: Beta-blocking agents: current status in the prevention of sudden coronary death. Ann NY Acad Sci 1982; 382: 305–323.
8. Corr PB, Sharma AD: Alpha- versus beta-adrenergic influences on dysrhythmias induced by myocardial ischemia and reperfusion. In: Zanchetti A (ed) Advances in β-blocker therapy II. Excerpta Medica, Amsterdam, 1982; 163–180.
9. Schwartz PJ: Sympathetic imbalance and cardiac arrhythmias. In: Randall WC (ed) Nervous control of cardiovascular function. Oxford University Press, New York, 1984; 225–252.
10. Armour JA, Hageman GR, Randall WC: Arrhythmias induced by local cardiac nerve stimulation. Am J Physiol 1972; 223: 1068–1075.
11. Hageman GR, Goldberg JM, Armour JA, Randall WC: Cardiac dysrhythmias induced by autonomic nerve stimulation. Am J Cardiol 1973; 32: 823–830.
12. Kralios FA, Martin L, Burgess MJ, Millar CK: Local ventricular repolarization changes due to sympathetic nerve branch stimulation. Am J Physiol 1975; 228: 1621–1626.
13. Schwartz PJ, Vanoli E: Cardiac arrhythmias elicited by interaction between acute myocardial ischemia and sympathetic hyperactivity: a new experimental model for the study of anti-arrhythmic drugs. J Cardiovasc Pharmacol 1981; 3: 1251–1259.
14. Harris AS, Otero H, Bocage AJ: The induction of arrhythmias by sympathetic activity before and after occlusion of a coronary artery in the canine heart. J Electrocardiol 1971; 4: 34–43.
15. Vanoli E, Zaza A, Zuanetti G, Facchini M, Pappalettera M, Schwartz PJ: Pharmacologic prevention of malignant arrhythmias due to acute myocardial ischemia and sympathetic hyperactivity. Circulation 1982; 66: 27.
16. Schwartz PJ, Stone HL, Brown AM: Effects of unilateral stellate ganglion blockade on the arrhythmias associated with coronary occlusion. Am Heart J 1976; 92: 589–599.
17. Schwartz PJ, Verrier RL, Lown B: Effect of stellectomy and vagotomy on ventricular refractoriness in dogs. Circ Res 1977; 40: 536–540.
18. Schwartz PJ, Snebold NG, Brown AM: Effects of unilateral cardiac sympathetic denervation

on the ventricular fibrillation threshold. Am J Cardiol 1976; 37: 1034–1040.

19. Schwartz PJ, Stone HL: Tonic influence of the sympathetic nervous system on myocardial reactive hyperemia and on coronary blood flow distribution. Circ Res 1977; 41: 51–58.

20. Schwartz PJ, Stone HL: Effects of unilateral stellectomy upon cardiac performance during exercise in dogs. Circ Res 1979; 44: 637–645.

21. Janse MJ, Schwartz PJ: Effect of cardiac sympathetic nerves on electrophysiologic changes induced by acute myocardial ischemia in dogs. Eur Heart J 1983; 4 (Suppl E): 38.

22. Vanoli E, Zaza A, Zuanetti G, Pappalettera M, Schwartz PJ: Reduction in infarct size produced by left stellectomy. IX World Congr Cardiol. Moscow, 1982; 2: 1312.

23. Baroldi G, Falzi G, Mariani F: Sudden coronary death. A post-mortem examination in 208 selected cases compared to 97 'control' subjects. Am Heart J 1979; 98: 20–31.

24. Schwartz PJ, Billman GE, Stone HL: Autonomic mechanisms in ventricular fibrillation induced by myocardial ischemia during exercise in dogs with healed myocardial infarction. An experimental preparation for sudden cardiac death. Circulation 1984; 69: 790–800.

25. Schwartz PJ, Gwirtz PA, Stone HL: Cardiac performance before and after left stellectomy in dogs with an anterior myocardial infarction. Proc 8th Eur Congr Cardiol. Paris, 1980; 121.

26. Austoni P, Rosati R, Gregorini L, Bianchi E, Bortolani E, Fox U, Schwartz PJ: Effects of stellectomy on exercise induced QT changes in man. Circulation 1977; 56 (Suppl III): 184.

27. Randall WC, Rohse WG: The augmentor action of the sympathetic cardiac nerves. Circ Res 1956; 4: 470–475.

28. Schwartz PJ, Stone HL: Left stellectomy and denervation supersensitivity in conscious dogs. Am J Cardiol 1982; 49: 1185–1190.

29. Moss AJ, Schwartz PJ: Delayed repolarization (QT or QU prolongation) and malignant arrhythmias. Mod Conc Cardiovasc Med 1982; 51: 85–90.

30. Schwartz PJ, Periti M, Malliani A: The long Q-T syndrome. Am Heart J 1975; 89: 378–390.

31. Moss AJ, McDonald J: Unilateral cervicothoracic sympathetic ganglionectomy for the treatment of long QT syndrome. N Engl J Med 1971; 285: 903–904.

32. Schwartz PJ, Malliani A: Electrical alternation of the T wave: clinical and experimental evidence of its relationship with the sympathetic nervous system and with the long QT syndrome. Am Heart J 1975; 89: 45–50.

33. Moss AJ, DeCamilla J, Davis H: Cardiac death in the first 6 months after myocardial infarction: potential for mortality reduction in the early post-hospital period. Am J Cardiol 1977; 39: 816–820.

34. Kannel WB, Sorlie P, McNamara PM: Prognosis after initial myocardial infarction: the Framingham study. Am J Cardiol 1979; 44: 53–59.

35. Lawrie D: Long term survival after ventricular fibrillation complicating acute myocardial infarction. Lancet 1967; 2: 1085–1087.

36. Geddes JS, Adgey AAJ, Pantridge JF: Prognosis after recovery from ventricular fibrillation complicating ischemic heart disease. Lancet 1967; 2: 273–275.

37. Webb SW, Adgey A, Pantridge JF: Autonomic disturbance at onset of acute myocardial infarction. Br Med J 1972; 3: 89–92.

38. Schwartz PJ, Zaza A, Sbressa C, Lotto A, Grazi S, Lombardo M: Poor long term prognosis when ventricular fibrillation complicates an anterior myocardial infarction. Circulation 1982; 66 (Suppl II): 10.

39. Barber MJ, Mueller TM, Zipes DP: Evidence that transmural infarct ablates electrophysiologic responses to sympathetic nerve stimulation outside the infarct. Clin Res 1981; 29: 749A.

40. Barber MJ, Mueller TM, Phillips JP, Zipes DP: Chronic transmural infarction prevents refractory period shortening by sympathetic nerve stimulation in noninfarcted areas apical to infarct. Am J Cardiol 1982; 49: 899.

41. Taylor GJ, Crampton RS, Gibson RS, Stebbins PT, Waldman MTG, Beller GA: Prolonged Q-T interval at onset of acute myocardial infarction in predicting early phase ventricular tachycardia. Am Heart J 1981; 102: 16–24.
42. Schwartz PJ, Wolf S: QT interval prolongation as predictor of sudden death in patients with myocardial infarction. Circulation 1978; 57: 1074–1077.

3.3 Surgical Treatment of the Cardiac Arrythmias

J. MÁRQUEZ MONTES, J.J. RUFILANCHAS, J. ALZUETA,
J. UGARTE, C. HERNANDEZ, G. LINACERO, J.J. ESTEVE,
J. ARNAU and D. FIGUERA

**Endoepicardial mapping: techniques for the intraoperative
electrophysiological study**

Endoepicardial mapping of the heart is a technique for studying the sequence
of cardiac activation. The electrical signals obtained are evaluated as an
integrated function of time. It was first described in dogs by Lewis and
Rothschild [13] and later, in the adult human in the basic studies of Durrer et
al. [14] and in the fetus by Brusca and Rossetani [15].

In the course of the development of surgical mapping for the treatment of
Kent bundles, ventricular tachycardias or atrial arrhythmias, we must mention
the efforts of Frank and Fontaine [5] in Paris, Gallagher-Sealy and Josephson
in the United States and Durrer, Janse and Van Dam in Holland, among
others [10, 16].

Endoepicardial mapping can be performed in several ways, depending on
the arhythmia to be studied, the zone of the heart to be explored and the time
available. The results can be interpreted manually or by computer.

Endoepicardial mapping requires complex electronic instrumentation that
permits a large number of electrophysiologic signals to be recorded and
processed. As for recording, 32 to 64 simultaneous signals from bipolar electrodes may have to be received, requiring the same number of differential
amplifiers with their corresponding band filters. It is obvious that processing
must be oriented toward ascertaining the activation sequence in the different
endoepicardial zones, which can be done manually or instrumentally, with
evident advantages for the latter. The elaboration of isochronic line maps of
epicardial activation implies the use of a computer (16 bit – Word) and
considerable programming work. Gallagher and colleagues use a drawing with
the algorithm of Davidow and Brown [12, 17], and since the number of
epicardial points over which the delay in activation is measured is reduced,
interpolation techniques (Lagrange Spline, Coon) and definitively, 'smooth-
ing' techniques must logically be used.

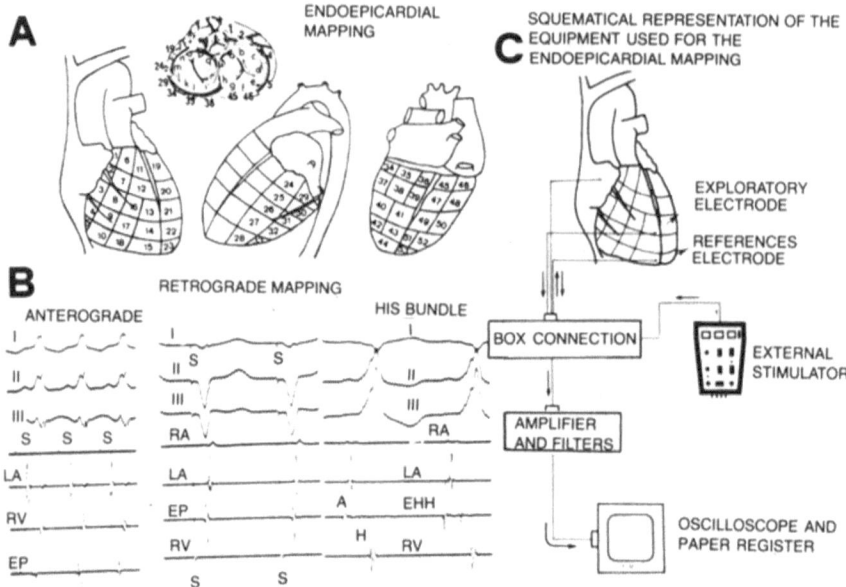

Fig. 1. Diagram of the old mapping system used by the authors. In A and B are old maps and examples of antegrade and retrograde ventricular mapping and bundle of His mapping. C shows the instrumentation used.

Considering strictly the operation, these maps often provide the surgical team with little information regarding the origin or pathways of the arrhythmia, because the origin is frequently not epicardial, but deeper in the endocardium. In these cases, epicardial mapping is insufficient and has to be complemented with other endocardial or intramyocardial signals, such as those obtained with the exploring electrode, Durrer's multielectrode needles, insertion of catheters, etc.

Our opinion is that the system design should be oriented toward achieving versatile multifunctional systems and improving the on-line processing algorithms.

Mapping can be done in sinus rhythm, after stimulation or with tachycardia. In each situation, the point to be mapped should be defined by an imaginary *graticule.* We use 53 points for the ventricular epicardium, 13 in the AV ring and 43 in the atrial epicardium. The number of points can be duplicated, at least, by realizing endocardial mapping or using multielectrode accessory plates [18] (Fig. 1).

Various types of *electrodes* are used:
a) Fixed electrodes (bipolar or pentapolar) that serve as references (REF. E.) in any chamber or the heart.
b) Exploratory electrodes (EXPL. E.), either tripolar or bipolar, of diverse

shapes to adapt to the surgical field (pencil, horseshoe, thimble), or plates of 8 to 24 pairs of electrodes of varying form and size according to function. Our group has designed an EXPL. E. in which the amplitude of the signal is unmodified by the incidence of the cardiac activation vector [11]. We have described [18] the use of bipolar and monopolar recordings and their utility.

c) Conventional ECG electrodes for recording 8 leads (generally I, II, III, and V_1 to V_6.

The system designed by our group to perform mapping techniques in patients with tachyarrhythmia functions in the following manner:

a) *recording* of data by electrodes placed in the heart (epicardial and endocardial) and the peripheral ECG;

b) *detection* of deflections;

c) *measurement* of delays (positive or negative) in the deflections observed with respect to a reference (origin of times);

d) *data processing* and interaction with the exterior by a series of E/S organs; and

e) *data storage* on a flexible disk for later studies.

These tasks should be realized in real time and near the operating theater. The system therefore has two different units situated in different places:

a) *Within the operating room* and beside the operating table, there is a box of connection for the endoepicardial electrodes, the peripheral ECG and the plates with 8 to 24 pairs of electrodes. The diversity of signals proceeding from the operating field requires four different types of preamplifiers: for the peripheral ECG, bipolar endoepicardial signals, monopolar signals, the tetrapolar EXPL. E. and those of plates designed to record postpotentials. This unit also contains a high persistance oscilloscope that the surgeon uses to visualize the type of mapping being realized, the most interesting electrograms obtained and the delay between the EXPL. E. and REF. E. in digits that appear automatically on the screen.

b) *The unit situated outside the operating room* functions as an input entry stage, conditioning the four types of signals received by the preamplifiers from the operating field and differentially filtering them according to their destination. All the amplifiers have an additional exit cable for a 12-channel polygraph, multiplexors, the surgeon's *display* screen, the A/D conversion stage, a system interface for the printer, plotter, flexible disk drive and a graphic screen that are grouped as a unit in a room adjacent to the operating theater.

The REF. E. is usually one of the four fixed pentapolar electrodes in the RA, LA, RV or LV, according to the section of the menu with we are working. Data collection (input) from diverse mapping points is done with the EXPL. E. placed over the heart at the site chosen (point by point method) or using plates of 8 to 24 pairs of electrodes of appropriate form and size for the task to

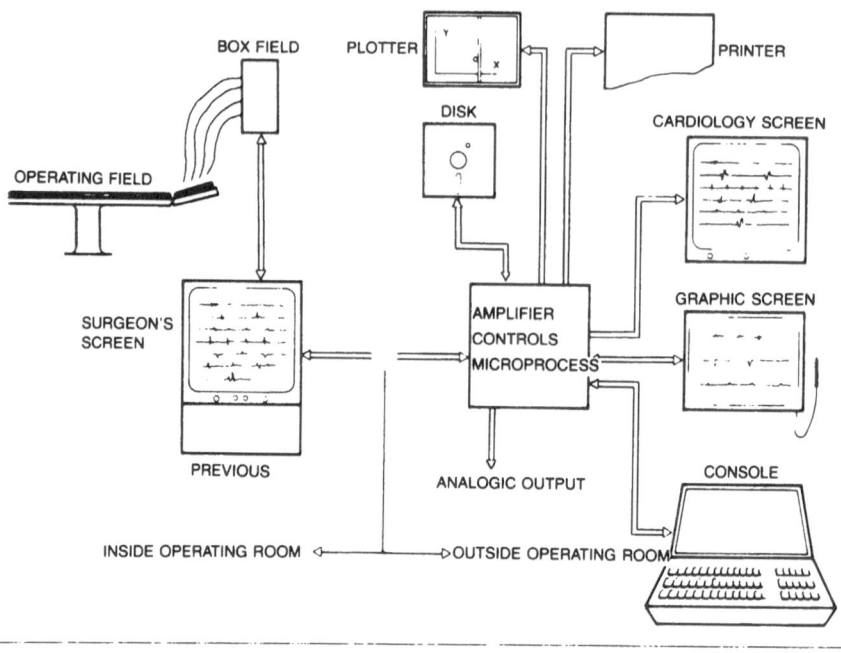

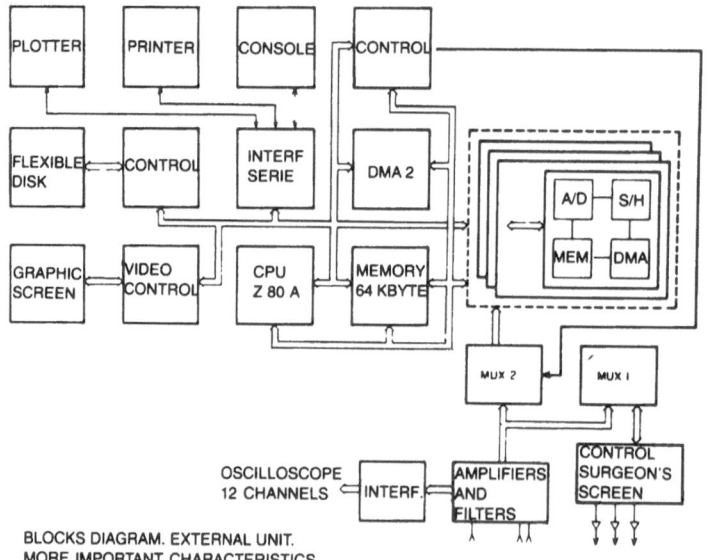

BLOCKS DIAGRAM. EXTERNAL UNIT.
MORE IMPORTANT CHARACTERISTICS.

1. 64 channels of simultaneous input
2. Buffer memory of 64 kbytes for each 32 channels
3. CPU Z80 A (4 MHz)
4. Three types of amplifiers and filters for
   a) Exploratory E, b) Bipolar E, c) Postpotentials E.
5. Transfer of samples from memory buffer to central memory

Fig. 2. Diagram of the new mapping system. *Above:* operating room unit. *Below:* diagram of external system.

be performed. If stimulation is used, data can be collected with any of the four pentapolar reference electrodes or the EXPL. E.

Aside from quantifying the EXPL. E.-REF. E. delay, for each measurement, the delay between other pairs of fixed electrodes (control delays) is determined to ensure that all are realized under similar conduction conditions. An appreciable variation between a measurement and the control delays would suggest the existence of conduction variations during data collection, which can be corrected by again measuring this point with appreciable variation in the control delays.

In each section of the mapping menu we use, the following operations can be realized: measure, validate, score, list, print, draw, erase, plate (which indicates to the system that a plate is being used instead of the exploratory electrode) and menu (when the work in the desired section is concluded, this operation is used to return to the main menu).

The main menu has 10 sections, in each of which the system offers prompts for the stimulation point, if there is one, reference point, number of points to be mapped, whether auxiliary catheters or plates will be used, and if the measurements will be made during tachycardia.

The sections of the menu are:

a) initial operational data;

b) endoepicardial atrial mappig;

c) retrograde AV atrial mapping;

d) retrograde mapping of the crux;

e) endocardial mapping of the atrial floor;

f) mapping of the bundle of His;

g) antegrade ventricular mapping;

h) antegrade ventricular mapping with atrial fibrillation;

i) ventricular mapping with ventricular tachycardia; and

j) endocardial ventricular mapping with ventricular tachycardia.

Each section of the menu will be described when we deal with the diverse types of arrhythmia surgery.

The experience of our group in arrhythmia surgery is shown in Table 1.

Table 1. Arrhythmia surgery (Clínica Puerta de Hierro, 1976–1983).

Surgical treatment of SVT	69 patients
1. Focal atrial tachycardia	2
2. Reentry atrial tachycardia	2
3. RTAV	1
4. Rapid atrial fibrillation (sinus disease)	2
5. WPW	62
Surgical treatment of Vt	12
1. Ischemic heart disease	10
2. Arrhythmogenic RV dysplasia	2

Arrhythmias originating proximal to the His bundle or bundle branches

In this group, we can differentiate three main groups of arrhythmias:
a) *Atrial tachycardia:*
– due to reentry (atrial flutter and other macroreentries),
– due to ectopic automaticity.
b) *AV junctional tachycardias;*
– tachycardia due to intranodal reentry or incorporating adjacent fibers or tracts; permanent tachycardia that incorporates fibers of accessory bundles with decremental conduction,
– due to an increase in AV junction automaticity.
c) *Tachycardias that incorporate Kent bundles (WPW).*
The tachycardias due to an increase in atrial ectopic automaticity are the result of abnormal atrial impulse formation and generally have clinical importance if they produce elevated ventricular rates, which occurs because the AV node does not evert a correct filtering function or this function is short-circuited. The reentry mechanism of the supraventricular tachycardias appears when there are two pathways with different conduction properties in the system[2] and an adequate mechanism for production.

In general, the supraventricular tachycardias (SVT) are maintained by a reentry mechanism, and can be produced and eliminated with an adequate stimulation program [19]. However, the arrhythmias caused by the atrial ectopic focus are difficult to provoke with stimulation and usually do not cease with electrical treatment. In this type of arrhythmia, the difficulty of reproducing the arrhythmia during surgery makes it impossible to localize it by mapping.

Two types of surgical measures are considered for SVT:
a) *Direct:* intervention at the origin of the arrhythmia or selectively in the reentry route. Ablation of the Kent bundle is one of the most well known [5, 17, 18], followed by ablation of the His bundle to create AV block [20–22]. Recently, since the experience of Coumel et al. [23] with elimination of a left atrial focal arrhythmia by excision of atrial tissue, other authors [24–26] have reported new cases of atrial focal tachycardia treated by surgical excision.

Resection of slow accessory bundles with decremental conduction to treat permanent forms of tachycardia [27] and interruption of the macroreentry circuit in patients with atrial flutter [28] complete the list of options for atrial procedures.
b) *Indirect:* this type of surgery does not attempt to eliminate the arrhythmia, but to prevent elevated ventricular rates by isolating the arrhythmia in the chamber/s where it is produced (surgical isolation of the LA or RA) [20, 29], in the atrial septum [30], or by producing AV block to isolate atrium

from ventricle, followed by pacemaker implantation [22]. Recently, the catheter fulguration techniques for producing AV block compete with the indirect techniques, and sometimes with the direct ones that act on the origin of the arrhythmia [31].

The *surgical techniques* used to treat the atrial arrhythmias can be summarized as follows:

a) *Section-ablation* used for Kent bundles, production of AV block or interruption of a macroreentry route.

b) *Ligature* is practically in disuse now, but was used mainly to produce AV block.

c) *Electrocauterization and injection of chemical substances* (formalin-alcohol) have precise indications and only exceptionally used at present.

d) *Selective longitudinal, V-shaped and circular atriotomy* is used for ablation or disconnection of part of the atrial muscular tissue [24, 32].

e) *Cryosurgery* is presently one of the most promising techniques, both to create an AV block [22, 23] and eliminate automatic foci [29]. In WPW, it is fundamentally indicated for superficial or ventricular epicardial Kent bundles [2, 17], for septal accessory routes [33] or in combination with surgical section [17]. One of the advantages of using cryotherapy is the possibility of practicing a reversible test by cooling to $0°C$ for 30 sec prior to destroying the muscular tissue, the effects of which disappear when the tissue temperature returns to normal. It is more effective for producing AV block than ligature, section or utilization of chemical substances and it is free of complications like tricuspid incompetence or production of VSD. The lesion produced by cryosurgery is less extensive, produces less vascular damage, is not arrhythmogenic *per se* and in the AV junction has less of a tendency to rupture or formation of aneurysm [21].

Surgical treatment of atrial tachycardias

The SVT with the greatest surgical interest are those produced in the sinus, predominantly symptomatic SVT with a tachycardiac phase, in atrial fibrillation or flutter with elevated ventricular rate and refractory to pharmacologic and electrical treatment, and for focal tachycardias or those due to increased automaticity refractory to medical treatment.

In *sinus node disease* with predominantly tachycardiac phase, pacemaker therapy only avoids the symptoms derived from bradycardia. On occasions, use of permanent atrial or sequential stimulation prevents, to a certain degree the tachycardic episodes by avoiding atrial bradyarrhythmia phases, but these patients usually continue to have tachycardias. In this case and in *atrial fibrillation* with poor response to pharmacologic treatment, there are two forms of alternative treatment:

a) catheter fulguration to produce AV block; and

b) creation of a surgical AV block that may be selective at various levels:

– section or ablation of the His bundle;

– proximal AV block,

– microsurgery of the AV node (experimental).

Section of the His bundle is not a well known technique, is more difficult to perform and has less satisfactory results than those obtained by sectioning parietal Kent fibers [34]. Our group uses a combination of *cryosurgery* and selective *section-atriotomy* of the atrial floor immediately below the AV junction. After a cryotest to 0° C, three points of about 1 cm in diameter are injured at −60° C for a minute and a half to two minutes in a proximal zone where the bundle of His mapping detects this structure's greatest amplitude electrogram with an atriogram of sufficient amplitude, generally near the fibrous right trigone and the membranous ventricular septum in the atrium. It is completed with a V-shaped atriotomy that has one limb in the inner part of the Todaro tendon and the vertex near the coronary sinus. For the technique, *bundle of His mapping* is important and is practiced during *bypass* surgery with moderate hypothermia, right atrial stimulation and determinations in 12 prefixed points at two levels (atrial and AV). The system automatically measures the AH and HV distances and the H amplitude in each point. The type of EXPL. E. is important, since bipolar electrodes are not valid because they can be placed perpendicular to the activation vector of the His bundle (isoelectric) and tripolar electrodes are inappropriate because the sum of the potentials of 1-2, 2-3, 3-1 produces small deflections. We prefer the tetrapolar electrode designed by our group, which has been previously described and does not have these disadvantages [11].

Probably, cryocauterization of the endocardial zone at the point where the largest hisian deflection is located affects the AV node and trunk of the His bundle, although it is later limited. For this reason, we prefer to do it more proximally, thus obtaining a good subsidiary pacemaker with fine QRS in the peripheral ECG and rates of 40 to 60 bpm that can be modified by isoproterenol, atropine and occasionally, exercise. This does not occur in more distal sections of the His trunk [21] (Fig. 3).

We have performed this intervention in five patients:

a) a young patient with AF and cardiomyopathy;

b) a 30-year-old patient with rapid atrial fibrillation in sinus disease with symptomatic bradycardiac and tachycardiac phases and refractory to medical treatment (Fig.3);

c) a coronary patient, in whom SVT induced symptomatic ventricular tachycardia;

d) a patient with SVT refractory to drug treatment; and

e) a patient with an intrahisian Kent bundle.

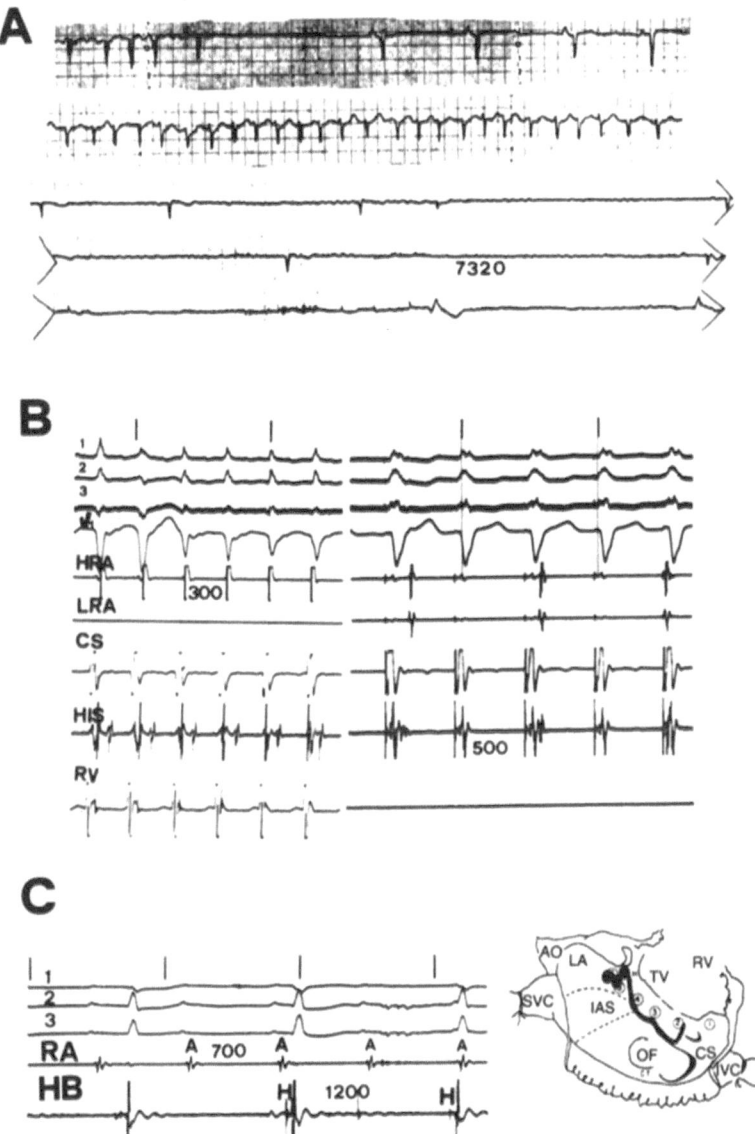

Fig. 3. Surgical treatment of rapid atrial fibrillation with sinus node disease. In panel A. Holter ECG strips where rapid and slow atrial fibrillation is shown with pauses of up to 7.320 msec. In B, electrophysiologic study that demonstrates 1 : 1 AV conduction with atrial stimulation at 300 msec and VA dissociation when the ventricle is stimulated with a 500 msec CL. In panel C, the atriotomy performed (thick black line) and the points of cryosurgery (black points). The final result was a suprahisian AV block with an escape rhythm at 1200 msec, which was modified by exercise, atropine and aleudrine. SVC/IVC = superior/inferior vena cava. TV = tricuspid valve. OF = oval foramen. CT = crista terminalis. HRA = high right atrium. LRA = low right atrium. CS = coronary sinus. RV = right ventricle.

In all of these, the AV block produced was stable, less so in coronary patients in whom it was done with an electrode needle and chemical infiltration guided by blind mapping of the His bundle and without cardiotomy or *bypass* procedures. However, the residual II degree AV block was sufficient to prevent appearance of VT due to the mechanism indicated above.

In surgery of the *paroxysmal focal atrial tachycardias,* our experience is limited to two patients: a 23-year-old women with atrial septal defect (ASD) and an automatic focus in the area of the coronary sinus, and a 12-year-old girl with no demonstrable heart disease and paroxysmal SVT (250 msec cycle), with and without aberrancy of the right bundle branch, originated in the posterosuperior part of the fossa ovalis (Fig. 4).

The refractoriness of these arrhythmias to pharmacologic treatment and the impossibility of electrical treatment made these patients candidates for surgery. Various methods have been used, some *indirect,* like ablation of the nodal-His area to create a permanent AV block followed by pacemaker implantation, and others *direct,* as in the case of Wyndham et al. [24], with resection of the right atrial appendage in a patient in whom the preoperative arrhythmia detected was reproduced in the tissue removed. Coumel [23] electrocoagulated the origin of an atrial arrhythmia, situated above the right pulmonary vein, but the method did not become popular because of the problems it produces. Anderson et al. [26] successfully treated another focus in a similar site by making a circular incision to exclude the origin of the arrhythmia. Josephson et al. [25] successfully treated a focal arrhythmia located in the posterior part of the limbus of the fossa ovalis by resecting a 1.5×2 cm piece of atrial tissue including the fossa ovalis. Sealy et al. [30], in an experimental study, realized three fundamental atrial resections to observe the subsidiary rhythms.

To perform these operations, the atrial epicardium and endocardium are mapped, which is difficult to do and, sometimes, to interpret, because of the anatomic complexity of the atrium. Our group uses a type of *endoepicardial atrial mapping* with an atrial stimulation point, or in tachycardia, reference electrodes in the RA or in the LA, and mapping at 58 predetermined endoepicardial points, which can be extended by using plates with 24 electrodes in diverse areas of interest in the atrium [11] (Fig. 4).

In some cases in which the origin of the arrhythmia cannot be detected or atriotomy is unadvisable, in zones like the pulmonary vein or superior vena cava (AVC), *an atrium can be electrically isolated.* Williams et al. [29] demonstrated the experimental possibility of electrically excluding the LA. Note that there is no conduction between the LA and the rest of the heart, AV conduction is conserved and the intervention seems to be well tolerated.

Our group has successfully used a new technique that produces a type of *RA disconnection* in a patient with chronic atrial flutter and operated atrial septal

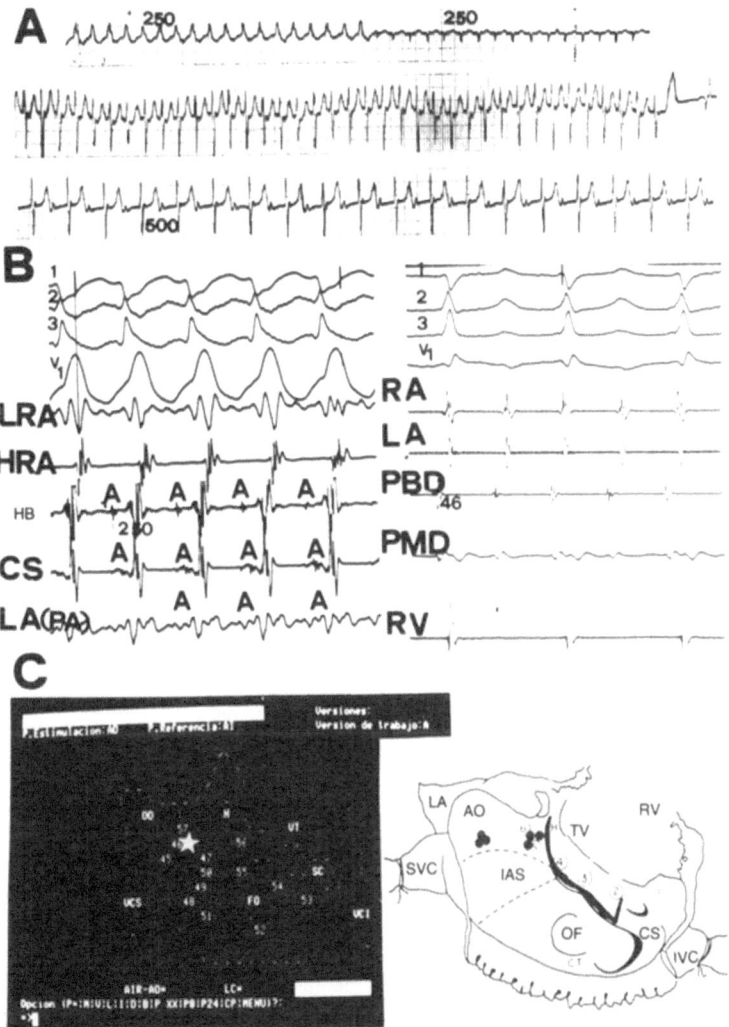

Fig. 4. Focal atrial tachycardia. Panel A shows a recording of tachycardia with a 250 ms cycle conducted with aberrancy and on other occasions, with narrow QRS. A later recording of the same tachycardia with 2 : 1 AB block. in B, atrial mapping in the operating room, with the earliest activation point near the right atrial appendage. In C, atriotomy practiced and point of cryo-surgery at the origin of the arrhythmia.

defect. The ECG and electrophysiologic study demonstrated common and uncommon atrial flutter that appeared and disappeared with a conveniently coupled extrastimulus, and transformation with a single extrastimulus from one type of flutter into another with the same 280 ms cycle, but the arrhythmia easily recurred with symptomatic 1 : 1 flutter refractory to pharmacologic treatment. Selective atriotomy was performed that involved the *crista termina-*

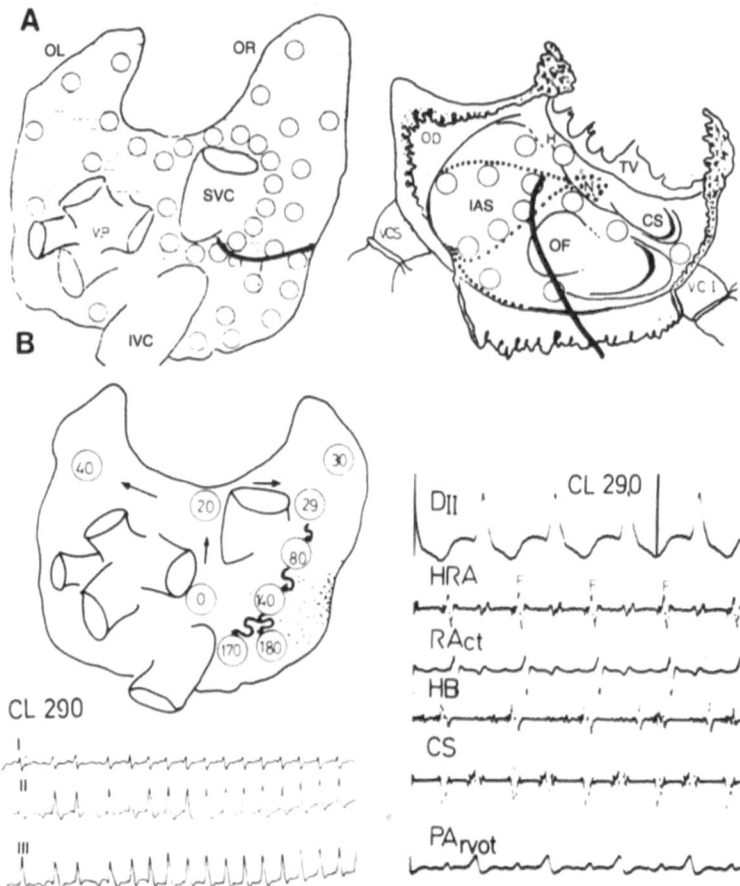

Fig. 5. In A common atrial flutter. In B, atrial mapping during surgery, where the origin is in the lower part of the right atrium and there is important conduction delay (curved line). In the upper section, right atrial atriotomy (black line) involving the *crista terminalis*, lateral wall of the right atrium and atrial septum. HRA = high right atrium. RAct = right atrium (crista terminalis). SVC/IVC = superior/inferior vena cava. CS = coronary sinus. OF = oval foramen. HB = His bundle. PArvot = Pulmonary artery (right ventricle outflow tract).

lis in its middle third, the lateral wall of the RA and the atrial septum divided the right atrium in two portions:

a) anterosuperior, including the upper part of the right atrium, the SVC and the anterosuperior part of the interatrial septum; and

b) posteroinferior, that included the IVC, the lower posterior part of the atrial septum and the RA near the floor of the AV union.

After a 2-year follow-up, the patient is free of arrhythmias, and atrial flutter has not been reproduced in the electrophysiologic study. The AV conduction remained intact and no postoperatory hemodynamic deterioration was observed (Fig. 5).

Surgical treament of atrioventricular junctional tachycardias

The surgical treatment most commonly used in the management of the AVRT is surgical section or cryoablation of the area of the AV node or His bundle followed by pacemaker implantation. Catheter fulguration in the area of the bundle of His after electrophysiologic detection of the area [33] using an antitachycardiac pacemaker or surgery are the three therapeutic options when pharmacologic treatment fails. Election of an adequate site for producing the AV block and elimination of the arrhythmia are, at present, subject to discussion. Various surgical possibilities are considered:

a) Section or cryosurgery of the bundle of His trunk, already commented on.

b) Incision at the nodal level (in the experimental phase). The difficulty of practicing microsurgery in this region and the appearance of postsurgidal arrhythmias that are induced by the method itself make the technique little recommendable.

c) Interruption of the tachycardia reentry circuit at the upper part of the AV union by selective atriotomy of the atrial floor, accompanied or not by cryosurgery.

Our group has been working mainly with the third option, on an experimental basis [32], and we have had the opportunity to perform this operation in a patient with Akthar type I symptomatic AVRT refractory to drug treatment, for whom a VAT pacemaker with simultaneous stimulation of the atrium and ventricle was the only possibility for permanent electrical treatment. The patient chose surgery for selective disconnection of the most proximal area of the AV junction. The underlying idea is that of Josephson et al. [33], who assume that the atrium, or part of it (atrial floor), is necessary to maintain many AVRT. It is important to make a specific atrial mapping in this situation, with reference electrodes at two levels:

a) Distant from the tachycardia circuit in the RA and LA.

b) Near the arrhythmia circuit situated in the interatrial septum and in the neighborhood of the coronary sinus – Todaro tendon – to record the activation wave that enters to or emerges from the AV area.

An exploring electrode and plates of 8 to 24 electrodes in multiple points of the atrial floor and the area of the His bundle complete the mapping (Fig. 6). The objective is to permanently interrupt the arrhythmia circuit while preserving the antegrade AV conduction. There are only two published cases in which these objectives have been achieved, one by Pritchett et al. [34] and another by our group [35] in the patient previously described. In our patient, after mapping the atrial floor, we performed a V-shaped atriotomy with its long limb parallel to the Todaro tendon and directed toward the membranous ventricular septum in the atrium and a short limb, with the inflection vertex, in the area of the coronary sinus (Fig. 6). In an earlier experimental study [32],

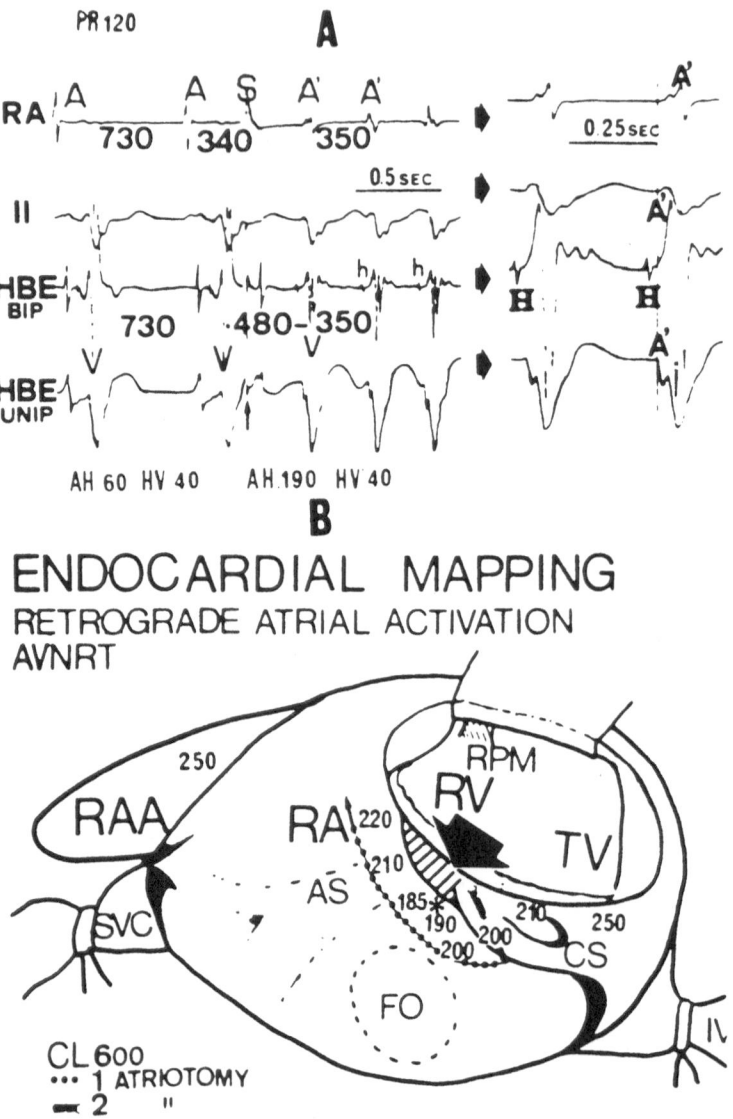

Fig. 6. Surgical treatment of AVRT in a patient with peroxysmal type I tachycardia. Panel A shows the beginning of the tachycardia with atrial extrastimulation. Note the lengthening of the PR interval at the expense of the AH and the situation of the retrograde atriogram (A') in the QRS complex. In B, atrial map of the floor of the atrium during surgery where earlier activation of the portions of the lower atrial septum near the crest of the AV node is shown. The atriotomy is shown by the dotted and black arrows. The atriotomy completely blocked retrograde VA fibers while only producing a conduction delay in the antegrade AV pathway. RAA = right atrial appendage. SVC = superior vena cava. AS = atrial septum. F° = foramen oval. RV = right ventricle. TV = tricuspid valve. CL = cycle length of ventricular stimulation. CS = coronary sinus.

complete AV block was produced in only 2/10 animals and transitory II degree block, in 2/10. The procedure therefore allowed AV conduction in 7/10 dogs, the conduction being dissociated in VA sense in 9/10 experiments. This coincides with our earlier experience and that of Pritchett in that the abolition of the AVRT is achieved while preserving AV conduction, which is an advantage over the His bundle ablation, which requires a permanent pacemaker.

Cases of incessant AV tachycardia involving a slow conduction accessory bundle (rapid-slow form) have been treated successfully by Ward et al. [27] with cryosurgery. The localization of the slow retrograde fibers by mapping at different points of the coronary sinus, and their surgical elimination not only confirm the electrophysiologic hypotheses concerning this type of arrhythmias, but open an interesting field for their surgical treatment.

Surgery for supraventricular tachycardias that incorporate Kent bundles

In the last decade, the WPW syndrome has undergone a profound revision [2–3]. Today it is included in the group of malformations of the fibrous skeleton of the heart or it is considered to be integrated in the larger group of the congenital heart disease [36]. After the first successful attempt to surgically section an AV accessory bundle, made by Sealy et al. [37] in 1968, surgery for this syndrome has progressed greatly with the development of new and more sophisticated mapping and surgical techniques, and the use of this type of therapeutic procedure has been extended to other groups [4, 17, 18].

Selection of candidates for surgical treatment is determined by the clinical features of the syndrome and its electrophysiologic characteristics. Classically [2, 4, 18], patients with tachycardia refractory to medical treatment, short refractory period or short RR in atrial fibrillation and risk of induction of ventricular tachycardia or fibrillation are considered to be possible candidates for surgery. Since the surgical results of each group have improved, young patients who have had pharmacologic treatment for years, who require cardiac surgery for other reasons, or have suffered a serious deterioration in their quality of life are at present also considered as candidates for surgery.

The experience of our group is shown in Tables 2 and 3, which list the global results obtained with this type of surgery during 1976–1983.

As to the *localization or classification* of the Kent bundles, various criteria are followed:
A) *General anatomic criteria:*
A1) Free wall Kent bundles (right and left).
A2) Septal Kent bundles (anterior and posterior).
A3) Combinations of the first two (bilateral or multiple bundles).
B) *Specific localization criteria:*
B1) Localization of the atrial insertion of the Kent bundle.

B2) Localization of the ventricular insertion of the Kent bundle.

B3) Is it a ring Kent bundle or does it pass through the fat of the furrow, avoiding the ring?

B4) Is the ventricular insertion endocardial or superficial epicardial?

These criteria are easily applicable to Kent bundles in the wall, although criterion B3 is difficult to study and B4 needs complementary utilization of Durrer needles or the monopolar lead morphology at the point of maximum preexcitation. The septal Kent bundles present different localization difficulties, whether they are anterior or posterior. The anterior Kent bundles (in front of the right fibrous trigone) are easily located, but the posterior ones are difficult to find because of the anatomic complexity of the pyramid of the crux of the heart and the problems inherent in performing successful mapping.

As to the *mapping techniques,* we have instrumentally developed three different types:

a) antegrade ventricular mapping to detect the ventricular Kent bundle insertion, with a variant for performing it in atrial fibrillation;

b) retrograde mapping of both AV rings to find the atrial insertion of the bundle; and

c) specific endoepicardial mapping of the cardiac crux for posterior or posterior septal fibers.

Table 2. Wolff-Parkinson-White syndrome (general table).

Free wall accessory bundles		35
Left	28	
Right	7	
Septal accessory bundles		22
Posterior	19	
Anterior	3	
Multiple accessory bundles		13
Kent bundles	11	
Atriohisian tracts	2	
Total		70

Table 3. Summary of WPW surgery (CPH, 1976–1983).

Results	
Kent bundles sectioned (curative)	51/62
Kent bundles injured	5/62
Injury or ablation of the His bundle	1/62
Early postoperative mortality	5/62
Asymptomatic patients	53/62

Antegrade ventricular mapping, in sinus rhythm or with atrial stimulation to obtain the maximum preexcitation, can be performed either point by point or by using plates of 8 to 24 pairs of electrodes, the shape and size of which vary according to the zone to be explored. The system provides security parameters for each point, such as the AV and RV-LV intervals and the basic cycle in case the mapping conditions change in the course of the study. For retrograde atrial mapping, we use 13 atrial epicardial points near the AV groove.

As security parameters, the ventricular St-RA intervals and the reference LA and reference Ra-LA are measured simultaneously and automatically in each point.

In septal bundles with preexcitation on each side of the posterior interventricular groove (right-left), two years ago we use to open both atria to make a retrograde endocardial mapping of the 18 points mentioned above with ventricular stimulation or in reciprocal tachycardia. Recently, in the same situation we do not open the LA, and instead we introduce a tetrapolar electrode through the coronary sinus into the RA and evaluating the deflections as a reference, along with the RA and LA readings, for those detected by the exploring electrode in the AV ring (Fig. 7). We only perform left atriotomy when the presence of an associated left bundle after correcting the right posterior septal bundle has been confirmed.

Experience has shown us that meticulous ocular inspection of the AV ring prior to mapping is important, since it occasionally reveals the presence of large or small anatomic defects in the ring where mapping will later show maximum preexcitation. We have seen small aneurysms or atrial sacs in the AV ring in the area of the crux in cases with an ECG morphology of right posterior septal Kent bundle and 'superficial fibers' mapping characteristics in the same site. In another patient, we found malformations in the posterior part of the right atrial appendage together with others in the AV ring.

Absence of preexcitation (due to the anesthetic, previous pharmacologic factors, especially amiodarone, surgical manipulation, etc.) is one of the *complications* encountered in WPW surgery, although we have only observed it on three occasions and it was only antegrade. The appearance of atrial fibrillation refractory to repeated electrical shock is another factor that complicates localization of the bundle; to overcome this difficulty we have developed an electronic instrument that only detects the beats with maximum preexcitation, selectively measuring them and ignoring the rest. We have observed on various occasions the appearance of low cardiac output due to tachycardia (atrial fibrillation or reentry tachycardia), or during stimulation, a circumstance that obliges us to shorten the mapping procedure. When there are multiple pathways, stimulation at various points as near as possible to the atrial or ventricular insertion of the bundles, is recommended. In this case, the ventricular reference electrodes are placed as near as possible to the respective

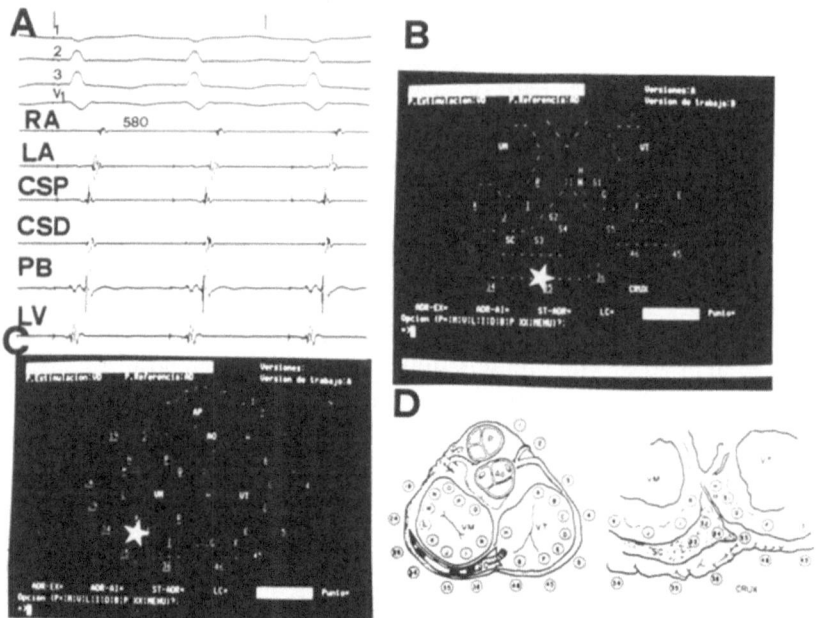

Fig. 7. Left posterior WPW syndrome. In A, map of the AV ring with ventricular stimulation, the earliest electrogram appearing in the proximal coronary sinus. In B and C, map of the AV ring and the crux, where the location of the Kent bundle is shown (white star). Observe in D the diagram of the tetrapolar catheter used for endocardial mapping of the AV ring. PA = pulmonary artery. AO = aorta. MV/TV = mitral/tricuspid valves. H = His bundle. BP = electrogram of the bipolar probe. PCS and DCS = proximal and distal coronary sinus.

AV ring to facilitate retrograde conduction. When there is discrepancy between the atrial and ventricular origin of the Kent bundle on each side of the AV groove, the existence of an oblique trajectory should be considered. In general, the number of points showing maximum preexcitation is usually greater on the ventricular side of the bundle, the proportion being 1 : 3. The meaning of this is still subject to discussion.

Accessory bundles can be *surgically interrupted* by sectioning or by cryo- or chemical (formaldehyde or alcohol) electrode ablation. Reiterated pressure on, or excessive handling of the Kent area under study should be avoided because of the possibility of being momentarily undetectable during surgery. Cryosurgery is especially interesting for the elimination of superficial fibers (not controllable with AV atriotomy) and septal fibers. In bundles located in other sites, cryosurgery is occasionally used as a complementary or backup technique for the procedure done.

Free wall bundles, once localized by endoepicardial mapping, are treated by making an internal atriotomy that slightly exceeds this area anteriorly and posteriorly, carefully dissecting the fat in the coronary groove and cryocauterizing points at $-60°$ C for two minutes. The adjacent ventricular epicardium can be optionally treated.

For anterior septal fibers, right atriotomy is performed in the usual site, the bundle of His is mapped and margins of security are marked to prevent AV block. Later, an internal atriotomy is made in the area of preexcitation, with or without cryosurgery. In the fibers adjacent to the bundle of His, we must act simultaneously on the His and Kent bundles, followed by implantation of a ventricular pacemaker.

Posterior septal fibers (Fig. 8) present more surgical problems because of the anatomic complexity of the region. The anterior boundary of the area is the fibrous trigone and posteriorly it forms a pyramid composed of the right and left atrial walls, the left ventricular epicardium and the septum. It contains, in the abundant fat of the region, sections of the coronary arteries, the coronary sinus and, in the anterior vertex, the conduction system. The posterior septal accessory fibers entail delicate dissection of these structures, since we have observed in some patients that the fibers responsible for the accessory pathway were those bordering the coronary sinus.

We *evaluate* the surgical results at three stages:

a) during surgery and after completing the intervention, requiring that VA and AV block appear after programmed stimulation;

b) a week after the operation, the RA, LA and ventricle are stimulated through steel wires temporarily left in the heart after surgery; these wires are removed after this study; and in the months after surgery, serial Holter recordings or an electrophysiologic study are made.

We consider appearance of preexcitation in the first 72 hours postoperatively as an indication for reoperation, for which we use an abbreviated technique. In the 5 patients in whom we have performed such a technique, there have been no complications and Kent bundle conduction was eliminated in all of them. Patients who have received elevated doses of antiarrhythmics for years, especially amiodarone, have required postoperative support with high doses of catecholamines due to cardiac pump failure. This was probably the main cause of death in two of our patients in the immediate postoperative period.

It can be anticipated that advances in drug treatment of the arrhythmias, technological progress, research into new and more sophisticated antitachycardiac pacemakers and the introduction of techniques like catheter fulguration will broaden the horizons of the treatment of patients with WPW syndrome and tachycardias, allowing separation of groups of patients who will benefit from one or another therapeutic method or combination of methods.

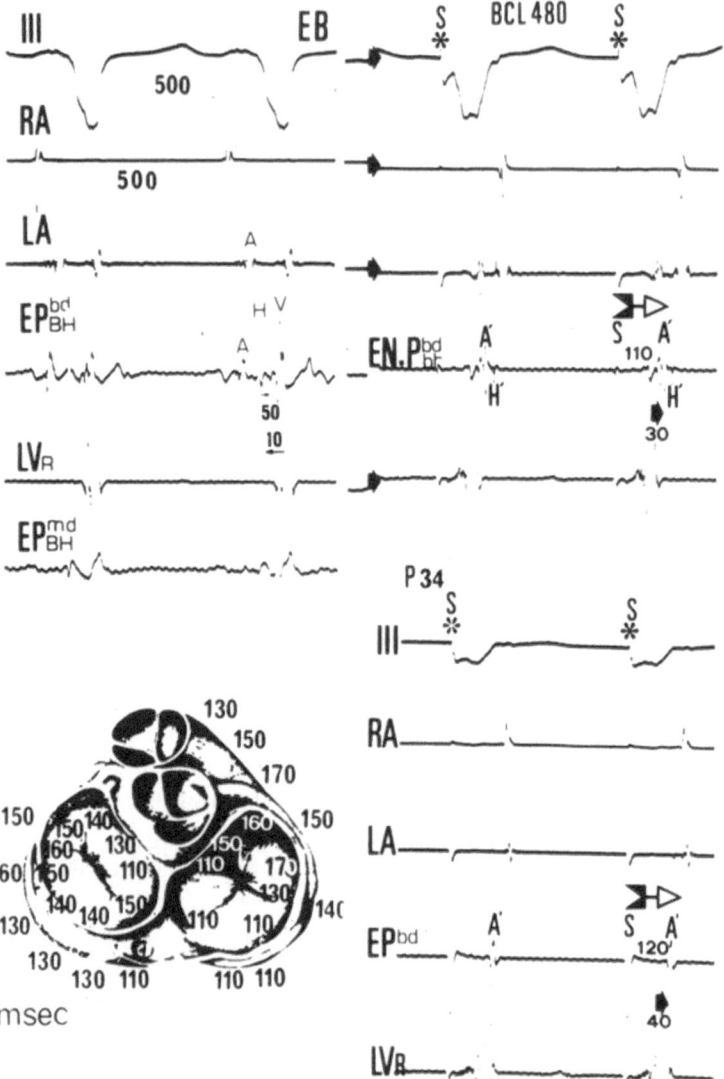

Fig. 8. Posterior septal Kent bundle. Recording obtained during intraoperative mapping of a septal WPW with AVRT. In the lower part of the figure the exploring electrode encounters a delay of 120 msec in the posterior atrial wall after the ventricular stimulus, being earlier than the right and left atriograms. In the upper part of the figure, mapping in sinus rhythm and with ventricular stimulation with the exploring electrode in the His zone; the atriogram of this zone precedes by 10 msec that of the atrial wall and bundle of His. S = ventricular stimulus artifact. LVr = Left ventricular reference electrogram. EPbd/bh = Bipolar endocardial electrogram in the bundle of His. EPmd/bh = Monopolar endocardial electrogram in the area of the His bundle.

Surgical treatment of the ventricular tachycardias

Certain types of ventricular tachycardias (VT) that are refractory to pharmacologic or electrical treatment, or both, can be successfully treated with surgery. Years ago, some authors observed that resection of a left ventricular
aneurysm in coronary patients with repetitive VT occasionally improved these
arrhythmias. Technological and electrophysiologic advances motivated the
Fontaine-Giraudon group in Paris and Waldo and colleagues in the United
States to present mapping techniques for use in the surgical treatment of VT,
fundamentally by ventriculotomy [38, 39]. From that time to the present,
important developments have taken place in both electrophysiology and the
speed and precision of the mapping techniques, and in the conception of new
surgical techniques.

Etiologically, there are three large groups of VT with respect to its interpretation and surgical treatment:
a) VT associated with ischemic heart disease;
b) VT occurring in arrhythmogenic RV dysplasia; and
c) others (idiopathic VT, cardiomyopathy, postventriculotomy, etc.).
The surgical indications for the VT are determined by the clinical consequences of the arrhythmia and a poor or insufficient response to pharmacologic
and/or electrical treatment. An additional and important factor is the experience of the surgical team and the option presently available of using catheter
fulguration techniques in a selected group of patients.

Three large groups an be made with respect to the electrophysiologic
mechanism of production on perpetuation of the VT:
a) reentry;
b) increased automaticity; and
c) *trigger* activity.
As regards the surgical treatment of the VT, our main interest has been
focused on those caused by a reentry mechanism that can be reproduced and
eliminated by means of a programmed stimulation (reproducibility). This
mechanism is equated with the presence of an anatomic circuit, as in the WPW
syndrome. The condition of being a sustained VT (time criterion) and the
reproducibility of the arrhythmia make the surgical indication possible.

Generally speaking, patients with chronic VT refractory to pharmacologic
treatment that is reproducible with programmed stimulation and sustained,
represent the most common indication for this type of surgery.

The use of *mapping techniques* to localize VT in the operating room is
subject to debate [39, 40] and research continues into both the mode of
collecting data (new types of electrodes, multielectrode plates, etc.) and data
analysis. The Fontaine-Frank [38] group uses epicardial mapping, which produces a complex expression in the form of isochronic lines. This method

presents problems for rapid interpretation, difficulties in repeating the technique when a patient has more than one tachycardia and provides no information on what occurs in the endocardium. Gallagher's group [12] uses a simple numeric system at each mapping point of the ventricular epicardium and a less complicated, more operative, system of isochronic lines. New, more sophisticated systems have been more recently developed, basically oriented toward saving time in the data collection phase (use of electrode net, multielectrode plates, etc.) and more rapid data processing. Using these systems, a single beat can be experimentally recorded in more than 100 different points, although in the surgery of arrhythmias, a maximum of 20–60 points are analyzed simultaneously [11]. Considering that to make an electrophysiologic analysis in the operating room, 53–80 points must be maped in sinus rhythm and in VT and that this must be done in a coronary patient undergoing not only surgery of the arrhythmia but coronary bypass and/or aneurysmectomy, the surgical time allotted to mapping should be minimal, making computarized sytems and the development of multielectrode plates necessary.

The main limitation of epicardial mapping is the endocardial origin of most VT. In these cases, the procedure would pick up the epicardial signal in one or more points of an endocardially originated VT that may be far from the epicardial point(s). For this reason to make intraoperative studies of the VT, we use epicardial and endocardial references that are compared with the electrogram of the exploring electrode (point by point mapping) or with those recorded by using plates of 8 to 24 electrodes [11]. The reference electrograms are arranged on paper using a special technique similar to that of the M mode echocardiogram (Figs 9 and 10). With this technique, in just a few VT beats an indication of te origin (right or left) and location of the VT is obtained.

The search for pre- and postpotentials and their location is also an indication for specific ventricular mapping.

Some authors [39] consider that mapping can be done in normothermia, but we prefer to use extracorporeal circulation and mild hypothermia to reproduce the VT by stimulating from the endocardial or epicardial reference electrodes with the most favorable stimulation program.

The surgical techniques are dinded into:

a) *Direct techniques*, such as the *subendocardial resection* proposed by Josephson [41], which is presently the least invasive surgical procedure to treat VT. This procedure requires a complete electrophysiologic support and maintenance of the VT in the operating room in a stable form, sometimes difficult to achieve in spite of the reproducibility of the arrhythmia in the presurgical EPS. This type of surgery may be associated with coronary bypass and occasionally with aneurysmectomy.

This technique is difficult to perform in certain areas of the heart, such as the anterior papillary muscle and the upper ventricular septum. Cryo-

144

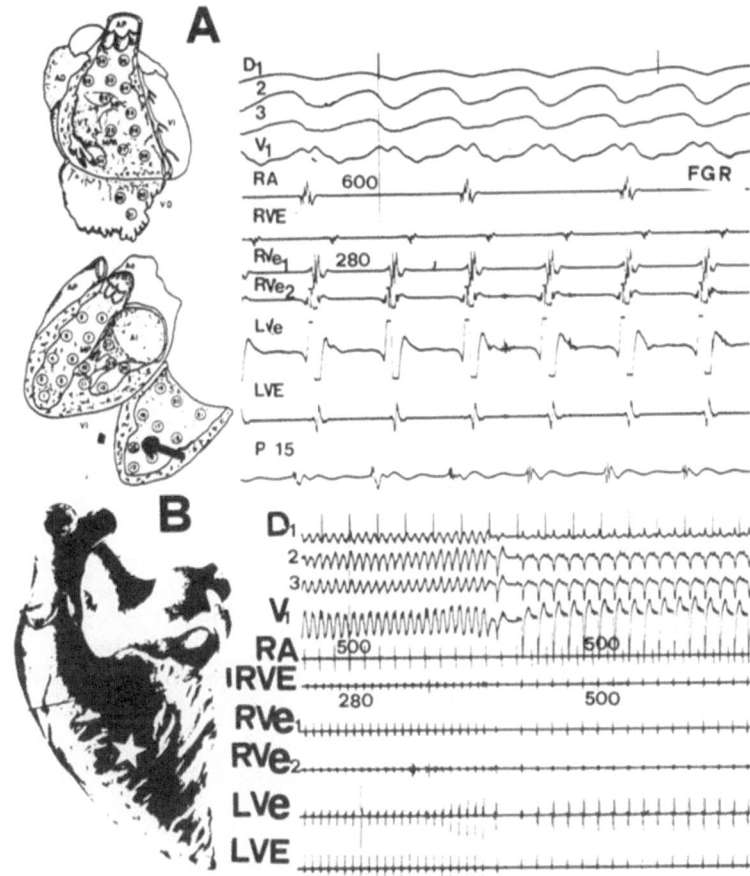

Fig. 9. Subendocardial resection of ventricular tachycardia. In A, endocardial mapping during VT. The exploring electrode is at the point of earliest activation, corresponding to point 15. In the lower panel (B), the tachycardia has been terminated after resecting the zone of origin. RA = right atrium. RVE = right ventricular epicardium. RVe₁ = proximal right ventricular endocardium. RVe₂ = distal right ventricular endocardium. LVe = left ventricular endocardium. LVE = left ventricular epicardium. P-15: electrogram of the bipolar exploring electrode at point 15.

surgery is presently used with success in these two locations. In some cases where the VT has a parietal location, cryosurgery has been used as a complement to subendocardial resection. Fig. 9 shows tracings from a patient with ischemic heart disease and refractory VT in whom elimination of the VT by resection of the subendocardial plaque over the zone of origin of the arrhythmia was accouplished.

b) *Indirect techniques:* previous studies reported a therapeutic success in VT of aneurysmectomy [1], and later of ventriculotomy with ventricular epicar-

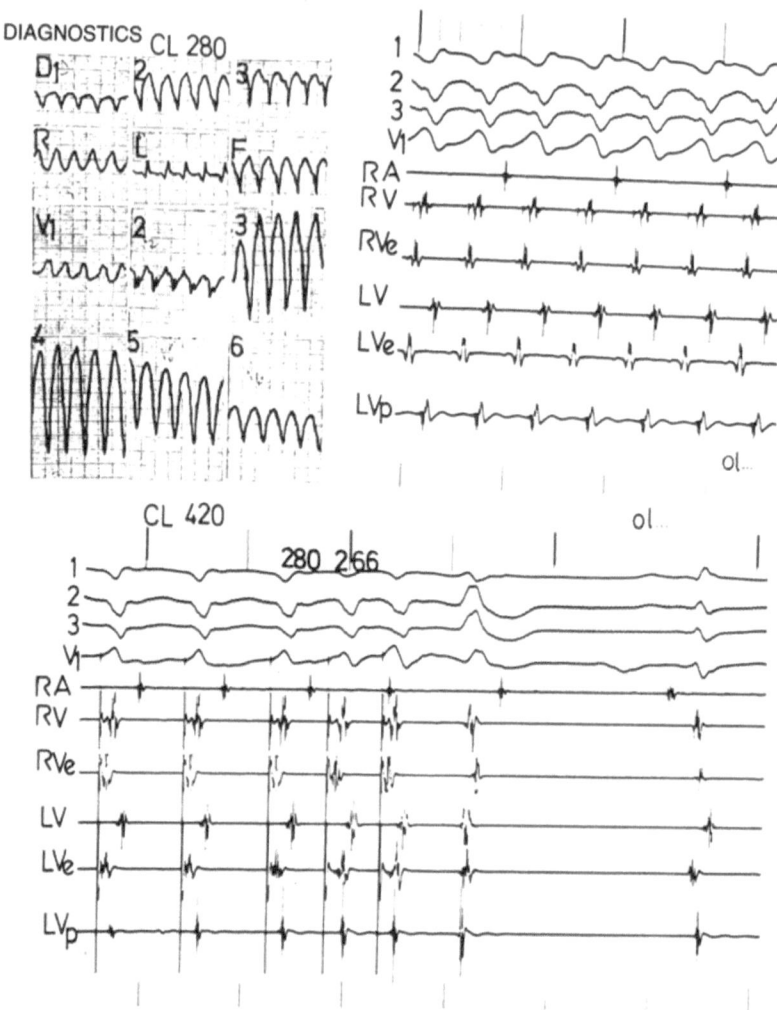

Fig. 10. Ventricular endocardial mapping. In the upper part of the figure, electrocardiographic recording of the VT and endocardial mapping during the tachycardia. In the lower panel, the same VT morphology is obtained with pacemapping. RA = right atrium. RV = right ventricular epicardium. RVe = right ventricular endocardium. LV = left ventricular epicardium. LVe = left ventricular endocardium. LVp = electrogram of the bipolar exploring electrode situated in the left ventricle.

dial mapping [5]. Based on these facts, the circular epicardial ventriculotomy described by Giraudon [42] is commonly used, consisting in an incision reaching the subepicardium in depth at the edge of the plaque and in healthy muscle. This technique does not require electrophysiological support. Among its disadvantages is a greater deterioration in left ventricular function in comparison with the direct techniques.

146

The *results are evaluated* in the operating room, after completing the surgical procedure in normothermia, with reference electrodes and the same programs that induced VT during mapping with stimulation. On the second or third postoperative day a limited electrophysiological study is made using steel wires that are temporarily left after surgery. Serial studies are later performed with Holter recordings and/or by electrophysiological study 2–3 months after surgery.

Our experience with this type of surgery involves 12 patients (Table 1), 10 of whom had refractory VT due to ischemic heart disease and 2 had arrhythmogenic RV dysplasia. In the immediate postoperative period there were 2 deaths, one corresponding to a patient with recurrent sustained VT refractory to medical treatment in whom surgery had to be performed in the acute phase of acute myocardial infarction, and the other to a cardiomyopathy of ischemic origin. The rest of the group remained asymptomatic without drug treatment, except for three cases; one with ischemic heart disease and two with types of VT demonstrated in the operating room, one of upper posterior septal origin. We could only act on the endocardial origin of one VT and at present the patient is on drug treatment and asymptomatic. In the other two cases, treatment was motivated by frequent ventricular extrasystolia shown in consecutive Holter ECGs, without VT having been demonstrated.

The progressive improvement in surgical techniques for patients with very high risk of sudden death, as well as the development of antitachycardiac pacemakers and implantable defibrillators, harbor some hope for this group of patients who have a poor prognosis.

Summary

The surgical treatment of cardiac arrhythmias has received an important impulse in the last decades. Beginning with the first cases of surgical section of Kent bundles, new techniques have been developed to treat other alterations in heart rate, mainly ventricular tachycardias. The development of electrophysiology and intraoperatory mapping techniques have served as an impulse and basis for progress in this type of surgery, making the indications for it progressively more precise and applicable to new groups of patients.

Together with these techniques, the introduction of new and more sophisticated antitachycardiac pacemakers and implantable defibrillators, the initiation of fulguration by catheter, and continuous research into new antiarrhythmic drugs, mean that new and more effective means of treating heart rate alterations are becoming available.

Surgery for cardiac arrhythmias is presently conceived as an alternative form of treatment when antiarrhythmic drugs or other therapeutic means prove ineffective for their control. Antitachycardiac pacemakers, implantable defibrillators and catheter fulguration techniques constitute the array of therapeutic possibilities that can be offered to a selected group of patients.

In 1913, Mines demonstrated that it was possible to interrupt an excitation wave maintained within a circle [1]. However, it was not until 1968 that Sealy and colleagues applied a technique for surgical section of a Kent bundle. Later, mapping techniques came into use for more precise localization of the Kent bundles in the WPW syndrome [2–4] and surgical ablation of the His bundle was developed [5, 6]. The groups of Giraudon-Fontaine-Frank in Paris and Sealy-Gallagher in the United States were responsible for promoting surgery for WPW and sustained ventricular tachycardias [7, 8]. The development of cryosurgery is an important advance, not only for ablation of the His bundle, but for use in the WPW syndrome, especially for epicardial fibers and some locations of ventricular tachycardia, such as those originated in the papillary muscle or upper ventricular septum [7].

At present, certain anesthetic techniques [9] and sophisticated endoepicardial mapping techniques [10–12], most of them still in the experimental stage, facilitate the precise detection of the origin and route of the arrhythmia.

The surgical procedures can be direct (resection of an arrhythmogenic area) or indirect (isolation of a chamber, bypass, aneurysmectomy, cardiac denervation, etc.).

Better knowledge of the electrophysiologic mechanisms of cardiac arrhythmias together with the use of new surgical techniques, such as those that act on ectopic atrial or ventricular foci, or selective disconnection of the left atrium (LA), right ventricle (RV) or right atrium (RA), make this field of therapy one that has progressed most in recent years and presents a promising future in the radical treatment of severe arrhythmias.

The cardiac arrhythmias can be classified by diverse anatomic (atrial or Kent bundle tachycardial), electrophysiologic, clinical (inducible or sustained reentry tachycardia, refractory to treatment, etc.), or etiologic criteria (idiopathic or ischemic tachycardia, association with heart disease) and different combinations of them. It is important that the type of arrhythmia and the clinical features of the patient be well defined when making a surgical decision. We use the following criteria:

a) anatomo-electrophysiologic criteria (inducible or sustained ventricular tachycardia, supraventricular tachycardia due to increased automaticity);
b) etiologic-clinical criteria (ischemic, absence of underlying heart disease, etc.); and
c) type of surgery (circular ventriculotomy, resection-cryosurgery).

The indications for this type of surgery are fundamentally determined by anatomo-clinical and electrophysiologic criteria. Some authors include important deterioration in the patient's quality or life produced by the arrhythmia as

148

a factor that decides the surgical indication. On the other hand, many arrhythmias should be considered as one of the many symptoms that accompany congenital malformation (accessory AV bundle due to a defect in the fibrous ring) [2] or acquired defects of the heart (lipoma or fibrous plaque of the atrial septum). The criteria for surgery in these cases should be different from those used for other diseases that involve the endocardium, myocardium or pericardium.

Other parameters to consider when establishing the surgical indication are the natural history of the disease, its clinial repercussions and the risk the intervention has in a certain surgical environment. Likewise, an arrhythmia associated with specific types of heart disease may have its own surgical indication, in which case it may be possible to treat it in the same operation. On the other hand some specific arrhythmias, not life-threatening but associated with a specific heart disease, can cause important hemodynamic deterioration. In summary to correctly treat an arrhythmia, a complete knowledge of the patient, the arrhythmia and the therapeutic options available is necessary. Once the intervention has been decided on, this can be divided into three operatory sections:

a) Diagnosis of location (ECG, precise endoepicardial mapping, and sometimes, imaging techniques like angiocardiography or echocardiography).

b) Elimination of the arrhythmia (section, resection, cryosurgery, chemical ablation, combined techniques).

c) Evaluation of results.

Acknowledgment

This study was partially financed by project no 385/81 of the 'Fondo de Investigaciones Sanitarias del INSALUD'

References

1. Gallagher JJ, Cox JL: Status of surgery for ventricular arrhythmias. Circulation 1979; 60: 1440–1442.
2. Gallagher JJ, Pritcher ELC, Sealy WC, Kasel J, Wallace AG: The preexcitation syndromes. Prog Cardiovasc Dis 1978; 20: 283–327.
3. Gallagher JJ, Gilbert M, Svenson RH, Sealy WC, Kasell J, Wallace AG: Wolff-Parkinson-White syndrome. The problem, evaluation and surgical correction. Circulation 1975; 51: 767–785.
4. Iwa T, Kawasuji M, Misaki T, Iwase T, Magara T: Localization and interruption of accessory conduction pathways in the Wolff-Parkinson-White syndrome. J Thorac Cardiovasc Surg 1980; 80: 271–279.
5. Fontaine G, Guiraudon G, Frank R, Vedel J, Grosgogeat Y, Carbol C, Facquet T: Stim-

ulation studies and epicardial mapping in ventricular tachycardia: study of mechanisms and selection for surgery. In: Kulbertus HE (ed) Reentrant arrhythmias. MTP Press, Lancaster, 1977; 334–350.

6. Hernandez C, Márquez J, Linacero G, Gonzalez MA, Cabo C, Castillo-Olivares JL: Modalidades de cartografía endoepicárdicas en cirugía de arritmias: sistema versátil basado en microprocesador. Rev Esp Cardiolog 1983; 36-I: 49–52.

7. Fontaine G, Guiraudon G, Frank R: Mechanism of ventricular tachycardia with and without associated chronic myocardial ischemia: Surgical management based on epicardial mapping. In: Narula OS (ed) Cardiac arrhythmias. Electrophysiology, diagnosis and management. Williams and Wilkins, Baltimore, 1979; 516–545.

8. Sealy WC, Wallace AG: The surgical treatment of the supraventricular tacyarrhythmias. J Thorac Cardiovasc Surg 1974; 68: 757–764.

9. Gomez Arnau J, Márquez Montes J, Avello F: Fentanyl and droperidol effects on the refractoriness of the accessory pathway in the Wolff-Parkinson-White syndrome. Anesthesiology 1983; 58: 307–313.

10. Bakker J, Janse M, van Capelle F, Durrer D: Intraoperative electrophysiologic mapping to guide the surgical treatment of life-threatening ventricular arrhythmias. In: Cats M (ed) Arrhythmias in myocardial ischemia. Amsterdam, 1983; 87–99.

11. Hernandez C, Marquez-Montes J, Linacero G, Rufilanchas JL, Gonzales MA, Cabo C, Castillo-Olivares JL: Versatile system for endoepicardial mapping in surgery of atrial, AV, and ventricular arrhythmias. 10th Annual Meeting Computers in Cardiology. Aachen, 1983.

12. Gallagher JJ, Kasell JH, Cox JL: The techniques of intraoperative electrophysiologic mapping. Am J Cardiol 1982; 49: 221–240.

13. Lewis T, Rothschild MA: The excitatory process in the dog's heart. II. The ventricles. In: Philosophical transactions of the Royal Society, London 1915: 81–206.

14. Durrer D, van Dam R, Freud GE, Janse MJ, Meuler FL, Arzbaecher RC: Total excitation of the isolated human heart. Circulation 1970; 41: 899–912.

15. Brusca A, Rossetani E: Activation of the human fetal heart. Am Heart J 1973; 86: 79–87.

16. Josephson ME, Horowitz LN, Farshidi A, Spear J, Kastor JA, Moore EN: Recurrent sustaied ventricular tachycardia. 2. Endocardial mapping. Circulation 1978; 57: 440–452.

17. Sallagher JJ, Sealy WC, Kasell JH: Intraoperative localization and division of accessory pathways associated with Wolff-Parkinson-White syndrome. In: Birchs W (ed) Medical and surgical of tachyarrhythmias. Springer-Verlag, Berlin Heidelberg New York, 1980; 114–137.

18. Márquez-Montes J, Rufilanchas JJ, Esteve Alderete JJ: Tratamiento quirúrgico en 24 pacientes con cíndrome de Wolff-Parkinson-White y taquiardias: diagnóstico toporáfico de los haces de Kent y evaluación de los resultados. Rev Esp Cardiol 1981; 34: 271–283.

19. Josephson ME, Kastor JA: Supraventricular tachycardia: mechanism and management. Ann Int Med 1977; 87: 346–357.

20. Rosen KM, Dhingra RC, Wyndham C: Trading arrhythmia for atrioventricular block. Circulation 1980; 61: 16–18.

21. Klein G, Sealy W, Prichett E, Harrison L, Hackel DB, Davis D, Kasell J, Wallace A, Gallagher JJ: Cryosurgical ablation of the atrioventricular node-His bundle: Long-term follow-up and properties of the junctional pacemaker. Circulation 1980; 61: 8–15.

22. Camm J, Ward DE, Spurrell R, Rees GM: Cryothermal mapping and cryoblation in the treatment of refractory cardiac arrhythmias. Circulation 1980; 62: 67–74.

23. Coumel PH, Aigueperse J, Perrault MA, Fantoni A, Slama R, Bouvrain Y: Réperage et tentative d'exeróse chirugical d'un foyer ectopique auriculaire gauche avec tachycardie rebelle. Evolution favorable. Ann Cardiol Aneiol 1973; 22: 189–193.

24. Wyndham CR, Arnsdorf MF, Levitsky S, Smith TC, Dhingra RC, Denes P, Rosen KM: Successful surgical excision of focal paroxysmal atrial tachycardia. Circulation 1980; 62: 1365–1372.

25. Josephson ME, Spear JF, Harken AH, Horowitz LN, Dorio RJ: Surgical excision of automatic atrial tachycardia: Anatomic and electrophysiologic correlates. Am Heart J 1982; 104: 1076–1085.
26. Anderson KP, Stinson EB, Mason JW: Surgical exclusion of focal paroxysmal atrial tachycardia. Am J Cardiol 1982; 49: 869–874.
27. Ward DE, Camm J, Pearce RC, Supurrell RA, Rees GM: Incessant atrioventricular tachycardia involving an accessory pathway: Preoperative and intraoperative electrophysiologic studies and surgical correction. Am J Cardiol 1979; 44: 428–433.
28. Márquez J, Alvarez Ayuso L, Escudero C, Mendez J, Hernandez C, Rufilanchas JJ, Castillo-Olivares JL: Partial surgical isolation of right atrium: As a surgical approach of macroreentry atrial flutter. An experimental study. Eur Surg Res 1984; 16-1: 153.
29. Williams JM, Underleider RM, Lofland GK, Cox JL: Left atrial isolation. New technique for the treatment of supraventricular arrhythmias. J Thorac Cardiovasc Surg 1980; 80: 373–380.
30. Sealy WC, Seaber AV: Surgical isolation of the atrial septum from the atria. Identification of an atrial septal pacemaker. J Thorac Cardiovasc Surg 1980; 80: 742–749.
31. Gallagher JJ, Svenson RH, Kasell JH, German LD, Bardy GH, Broughton A, Critelli G: Catheter technique for closed-chest ablation of the atrioventricular conduction system. N Engl J Med 1982; 306: 194–200.
32. Márquez-Montes J, Alvarez L, Esteve JJ, Benecet J, Hernandez C, Castillo-Olivares JL: New type of deep atrial mapping used for treatment of AV reentry tachycardia. Eur Surg Res 1982; 41-2: 85.
33. Josephson ME, Kastor JA: Paroxysmal supraventricular tachycardia. Is the atrium the necessary link? Circulation 1976; 54: 430–436.
34. Pritchett ELC, Anderson RW, Benditt DG, Kassell J, Harrison L, Wallace AG: Reentry within the atrioventricular node: Surgical cure with preservation of atrioventricular conduction. Circulation 1979; 60: 440–446.
35. Márquez-Montes J, Rufilanchas JJ, Esteve JJ, Alvarez J, Benezet J, Burgos R, Figuera D: Paroxysmal nodal reentrant tachycardia. Surgical cure with preservation to atrioventricular conduction. Chest 1983; 83: 690–693.
36. Lunel AVV: Significance of annulus fibrosis of heart in relation to AV conduction and ventricular activation in cases of Wolff-Parkinson-White. Br Heart J 1972; 34: 1263–1271.
37. Sealy WC, Hatler BG, Blumensdein SD, Cobb FR: Surgical treatment of Wolff-Parkinson-White syndrome. Ann Thorac Surg 1969; 8-1: 11–17.
38. Fontaine G, Frank R, Guiraudon G: Surgical treatment of resistant reentrant ventricular tachycardia by ventriculotomy. The new application of epicardial mapping. Circulation 1974; 50-III: 319–325.
39. Waldo AL, Arciniegas JG, Klein H: Surgical treatment of life-threatening ventricular arrhythmias: the role of intraoperative mapping and consideration of the presently available surgical techniques. Prog Cardiovasc Dis 1981; 23: 247–264.
40. Spielman SR, Michelson EL, Horowitz LN, Spear SF, Moore EN: The limitation of epicardial mapping as a guide to the surgical therapy of ventricular tachycardia. Circulation 1978; 57: 666–670.
41. Josephson ME, Harken AM, Horowitz LN: Endocardial excision: A new surgical technique for the treatment of recurrent ventricular tachycardia. Circulation 1979; 60: 1430–1439.
42. Guiraudon G, Fontaine G, Frank R, Eslade G, Etienent P, Carbol C: Encircling endocardial ventriculotomy: a new surgical treatment for life-threatening ventricular tachycardias resistant to medical treatment following myocardial infarction. Ann Thorac Surg 1978; 26: 438–442.

3.4 Early Experience in Endocardial Fulguration for the Treatment of Ventricular Tachycardia
Long-term Follow-up

R. FRANK, G. FONTAINE and J.L. TONET

We call fulguration the destruction of a small amount of myocardium by an electric shock delivered through an endocavitary catheter. This method was first applied on the His bundle for the creation of therapeutic AV block by Scheinman [1] and Gallagher [2] in 1982. It has been applied the first time in 1983 for the treatment of ventricular tachycardia by Hartzler [3] and Puech [4].

Our experience in the treatment of ventricular tachycardia by the endocardial fulguration technique started in March 1983. The aim of this paper is to present the first 22 cases who underwent the procedure until May 1984 and who have had a minimum of two years' follow-up.

Clinical series

This report concerns 18 men and 4 women aged between 14 and 74 years (mean 44 ± 19). Clinical data are reported in Tables 1 and 2.

There were 9 cases of right ventricular dysplasia (ARVD), 7 cases of VT occuring at least one month after a myocardial infarction, 3 cases of non-obstructive cardiomyopathy (one after surgery on the right ventricular outflow tract) and two were idiopathics, one right septal and the other of left ventricular origin. Tachycardias have been occurring in 9 cases for less than 6 months, and in 13 from one to 14 years. Fulguration was proposed after a thorough antiarrhythmic evaluation including the use of amiodarone and its association with Class IC drugs. Despite medical treatment, 7 patients had a permanent VT or daily relapses, 13 and at least one monthly relapse, and 3 had VT still inducible by programmed pacing.

Method

The procedure is done under general anesthesia, induced either at the begin-

Table 1.

	Age	SX	FE	IVT	NB	IC	IL	IF
Myocardial infarction								
1 CORM	60	M	12%	1	> 20	< D	I	Inces
2 BANT	29	M	42%	24	4	M	M	Parox
3 BEC	73	M	22%	1	> 20	< D	I	Inces
4 GALI	65	M	–	1	2	< D	W	IPP
5 HOUS	55	M	–	12	10	M	M	Parox
6 ZAIE	60	M	< 25%	24	10	M	M	Parox
7 FORT	67	M	< 25%	1	2	< D	M	IPP
Idiopathic non-obstructive cardiomyopathy								
8 POLC	18	M	< 30%	12	> 20	M	I	Inces
9 MANI	14	F	< 20%	168	> 20	I	I	Inces
10 LECA	56	M	20%	36	6	Y	M	Parox
Idiopathic left ventricular tachycardia								
11 DROU	22	M	–	60	> 20	M	W	Parox
Arrhythmogenic right ventricular dysplasia								
12 DUVA	35	M	–	> 20	> 20	M	–	Parox
13 CARO	62	F	–	36	> 20	M	W	Parox
14 GENS	74	M	52%	12	3	M	M	Parox
15 NAIT	37	M	58%	6	3	< D	M	Parox
16 MICH	27	M	25%	120	6	Y	I	Inces
17 MORA	40	F	59%	48	16	M	M	Parox
18 GELI	56	M	45%	84	> 20	Y	M	Parox
19 BARB	32	M	–	4	2	< D	W	Parox
20 CORA	30	M	28%	12	2	M	M	IPP
Infundibular surgery								
21 MOIR	21	M	61%	120	10	M	D	PVC
Idiopathic VT								
22 RAGA	53	F	59%	96	> 20	M	D	Inces

Legend of the tables

SX	: Sex
LOC	: Location of the arrhythmogenic area.
FE	: Ejection fraction (Echography, Angiography, Scintigraphy).
IVT	: Arrhythmia follow-up in months dating from first attack of VT.
NB	: Total number of VT prior to fulguration.
IC	: Shortest interval between two episodes of VT in Day Month Year.
IL	: Longest interval between two episodes of VT in D M Y Week.
Inces	: Permanent VT.
Parox	: Paroxysmal.
IPP	: Inducible by programmed pacing.
Nb S.	: Number of fulguration sessions.
Nb C.	: Number of shocks.
TRT	: Current antiarrhythmic treatment.

Table 2. (updated 01 aug 86).

	LOC	Nb S.	Nb C.	TRT	IND	10D	Follow
Myocardial infarction							
1 CORM ...	VG	2	2 + 1	AMI0	PR0	NI	37M
2 BANT ...	VG	2	7 + 7	A + Pr	TH	IN	26M
3 BEC ...	VG	2	4 + 1	AMI0	PR0	?	30M
4 GALI ...	VG	1	5	0	0	NI	28M
5 HOUS ...	VG	4	3 + 4 + 2 + 2	AMI0	TH	NI	23M
6 ZAIE ...	VG	1	2	?	?	?	DC4D
7 FORT ...	VG	1	2	AMI0	PR0	?	DC1M
Idiopathic non-obstructive cardiomyopathy							
8 POLC ...	VG	1	5	AMI0	TH	0	DC14M
9 MANI ...	VG	1	3	0	0	0	DC2M
10 LECA ...	VG	1	3	AMI0	PR0	NI	DC16M
Idiopathic left ventricular tachycardia							
11 DROU ...	VG	1	2	0	0	?	26M
Arrhythmogenic right ventricular dysplasia							
12 DUVA ...	VD	2	2 + 1	?	?	?	DC0D
13 CARO ...	VD	1	5	0	0	MC	32M
14 GENS ...	VD	1	1	AMI0	PR0	NI	31M
15 NAIT ...	VD	2	1 + 6	SOTAL	PR0	MC	28M
16 MICH ...	VD	1	17	0	0	MC	DC8D
17 MORA ...	VG	2	7 + 1	0	0	MC	22M
18 GELI ...	VD	2	1 + 4	A + Pr	TH	MC	19M
19 BARB ...	VD	1	4	AMI0	PR0	NI	25M
20 CORA ...	VD	1	6	A + Fl	TH	IN	25M
Infundibular surgery							
21 MOIR ...	VD	1	4	AMI0	PR0	NI	31M
Idiopathic VT							
22 RAGA ...	VD	2	1 + 2	0	0	NI	26M

IND	: Therapy indication.
FOLLOW	: Follow-up.
10D	: Results of provocative technique on the 10th day.
IN	: Inducible by programmed stimulation.
MC	: Morphological change.
PRO	: Low dosage antiarrhythmics for nonrelated arrhythmia.
TH	: High dosage antiarrhythmics after VT relapse.
?	: Result not available.
NP	: Provocative test not performed.
NI	: Noninducible.
J	: Day.
S	: Week.
M	: Month.
Y	: Year.

ning of the session or just before the first shock. Bipolar or multipolar catheters with 1 cm interelectrode distance are inserted transcutaneously in the subclavian and the femoral veins, and placed in different parts of the right atrium, coronary sinus, right ventricular apex, His bundle site and right ventricular outflow tract. These catheters serve as reference or as pacing electrodes. The other catheters already selected to withstand the fulguration shock [5] are moved into different parts of the ventricles to record bipolar endocardial potentials. A long sheath (Cordis femoral ventricular catheter/ sheath set) is inserted via the femoral artery, inside the left ventricle, to allow easier catheter positioning. Filters are set between 10 and 300 Hertz. Signals are amplified between 1000 and 10000 times. One millivolt calibration mark and time marks are automatically generated on the tracing. All the data are recorded on an analogue tape (EMI tape recorder). The position of the catheters is monitored on a bidirectional fluoroscope and stored on a video tape. Haemodynamic monitoring is performed using radial arterial pressure, pulmonary wedge pressure through a Swan-Ganz catheter, and serial cardiac output by thermodilution.

To minimize the time during which the patient remains in ventricular tachycardia and the risk of haemodynamic compromise, the study starts by pacemapping. This is done by pacing the ventricle at the tachycardia rate, at different endocardial sites. Twelve-lead ECG recordings are made, and compared with the spontaneous VT morphology. When a good match is obtained, VT is triggered by programmed pacing, and the endocardial potentials are analysed. Time measurements are made on the rapid portion of the signal, corresponding to the moment when the activation wave passes under the recording electrode, as suggested by previous simulation studies [6]. The catheter is slightly moved in the same region, and when the earliest occuring potential has been determined, fulguration is sent to that site.

Mapping may take any time between 30 minutes and several hours according to the ease with which the leads can be manipulated. VT has to be haemodynamically tolerated during long periods of time and, for this purpose, the patients are left under chronic amiodarone therapy (400 mg per day) to produce a slower tachycardia. All Class I antiarrhythmic drugs which have a more negative inotropic effect are stopped for 5 half-lives. Hemodynamic monitoring is continuous through the whole procedure and VT is interrupted in case of deterioration of heart function.

The fulguration shock of 160 of 240 joules is given by the distal electrode of the catheter, connected to the positive output of the defibrillator. Its negative output is connected with a large-surface back electrode. After a period of 10 minutes the programmed pacing protocol is reinitiated to induce the tachycardia again. The session is interrupted in the following circumstances: when a tachycardia is no longer inducible, when the induced VT is nonsustained (i.e.

when it is of less than 30 seconds duration), when the clinical VT cannot be reinitiated, and sometimes when the duration of the session is too long.

The left subclavian catheter electrode is left in the right ventricular apex for ulterior re-evaluation of the arrhythmia, with the same pacing protocol. The patient stays for 10 days under computerized rhythm monitoring without any antiarrhythmic therapy. If the patient has a spontaneous relapse during this period of time, a new session is indicated. On the tenth day, programmed pacing is performed in order to induce ventricular tachycardia again. If the clinical VT is triggered, a new trial with antiarrhythmic drugs is proposed and, if the patient has a relapse during ulterior follow-up, a new session is proposed.

Results (Table 2)

The patients underwent 1 to 3 sessions, and received 1 to 7 shocks per session.

CPK MB elevation was moderate from 0 to 105 units with a mean value of 34 ± 30 S.D. Peak CPK occurs 5 hours after the session.

Results were globally favourable since, after one or more sessions, with or without associated antiarrhythmic therapy, 17 patients had no relapse with a follow-up of 16 months to 3 years; recall that they had recurrent attacks before fulguration, and 3 were moribunds at the time of the procedure. Four are off drugs, 8 take a low dosage of antiarrhythmics against ventricular extrasystoles, 5 had postoperative relapses but previously ineffective medical therapy became effective and has not had to be changed since.

However, each case must be examined in respect of mortality, other complications, relapses, and criteria of success.

Mortality

Two patients died within the session. The cause of death was related to the protocol, but not to the shock itself.

The first (no 12) had a right ventricular dysplasia operated 7 years before, but a new type of VT had just occurred. VT was again triggerable 3 days after a first fulguration, and the patient was submitted to a second session. Endocardial mapping in VT was prolonged for 29 minutes, and the heart went into low output, with a progressive widening of the QRS. The low output could not be overcomed despite conventional therapy. Since that patient, we carefully monitor cardiac output during VT, which is interrupted as soon as any deterioration is observed.

The second patient (no 6) had syncopal attacks of VT due to an old myocardial infarction. That patient was not under anaesthesia at the beginning of the session, and when the first tachycardia was triggered, a depressant anaesthesic drug was given, resulting in electromechanical dissociation, and bronchospasm with anoxia. An endocardial shock was given to reverse the ventricular fibrillation and the hemodynamic status could be restored after 15 minutes. Unfortunately the patient stayed unconscious and died 4 days later without any relapse of VT.

Three other patients had a later death, unrelated to the procedure:

– One (no 16) had an ARVD with advanced heart failure. He was referred unconscious in permanent VT after multiple episodes of VT and VF, in low output, with a refractory hypoxemia. It took 17 shocks of low energy (160 joules) to slow the VT rate, which then stopped without antiarrhythmics. The patient died 8 days later, without arrhythmia, with a stable cardiac output, but with a refractory hypoxemia.

– Two other patients died of heart failure during the following months. One (no 7) already had a class III left ventricular dysfunction due to coronary artery disease, and was beyond any surgical therapy. The other (no 9) was a young girl with a dilated cardiomyopathy in an advanced stage. None of them had recurrence of VT, while the arrhythmia was paroxysmal in the first, and permanent in the second before fulguration.

Anatomical and histological studies could be carried out in 2 cases (nos 12 and 16). It showed localised and superficial lesions on the endocardium, comparable to the experimental data [7, 8].

Other complications

Two patients (nos 1 and 3) had a temporary third degree AV block after a left ventricular fulguration. In others, temporary intraventricular conduction disturbances occurred some minutes after fulguration. In 2 cases (nos 3 and 18) pulmonary oedema occurred after the session, and was treated in the conventional way.

After 20% of the shocks a ventricular flutter appeared, immediately reversed by an external countershock. However, no ulterior worsening of the arrhythmias was observed after the session.

Relapses after the first session

We call relapses a spontaneous occurrence of VT after fulguration. Nine patients had such relapses, 8 of them had a second session and 1 a third one.

Our first case (no 8) had a monomorphic permanent VT complicating a dilated cardiomyopathy despite a daily treatment with 400 mg amiodarone combined with 300 mg flecainide. These tachycardias totally disappeared after fulguration, and antiarrhythmic therapy has been interrupted. However tachycardias relapsed one month later, similar to the original one, but this time a previously ineffective dosage of 400 mg amiodarone alone allowed prevention of the arrhythmia, which recurred each time the antiarrhythmic was suspended. Fulguration seemed to have modified the arrythmogenic substrate which became sensitive to amiodarone. However, the hemodynamic status of this patient degenerated after 14 months, and he underwent a sudden death.

Two patients (nos 1 and 3) had recurrent VT which had started one month after a myocardial infarction, complicated by a left ventricular aneurysm. The relapses occurred some hours and some days after the first session, respectively. The failure has been related in the first patient to the lead's destruction by the shock, preventing the energy reaching the myocardium. In the other patient, moving inside the left ventricle was very difficult and did not allow us to find the earliest endocardial potential. However the series of shocks had been sent on the border zone of the aneurysm. In both cases, a new procedure with a different catheter allowed us to deliver the shock at the appropriate site, and these 2 patients had no relapse for 37 and 30 months, respectively.

Patient no 5 had an old septal myocardial infarction and underwent 4 sessions. During the first two, the programmed pacing technique could only trigger nonclinical tachycardias, most of them quickly degenerating into ventricular fibrillation. Fulguration was unsuccessfully performed in the left ventricle. During the third session, the clinical VT was induced, with a right ventricular origin. Two shocks of 240 joules prevented reinitiation. However the patient had a spontaneous relapse two weeks later, and needed a fourth session. Tachycardia was then no longer inducible but the patient was left on the amiodarone therapy. Two months later, he had a new spontaneous relapse, but tachycardia was slower and better tolerated. Since that time, he is still under amiodarone therapy, 200 mg/day and has had no relapse for a period of 23 months.

Patient no 18 had a right ventricular dysplasia with a dyskinetic zone in the left ventricular posteroseptal area where endocardial mapping localized the origin of VT. The arrhythmia recurred one month after the first session, and the endocardial mapping on the same zone localized an endocardial potential occurring earlier than during the previous study. Ten days after fulguration of that site, VT could again be triggered, but with a different morphology. The patient had a spontaneous relapse 4 months later, despite a treatment with 400 mg amiodarone combined with 300 mg flecainide. He had another relapse after a third session; however, a previously ineffective combination of amiodarone and propaphenone could then prevent the tachycardia with a follow-up now of 19 months, the VT relapsing when propaphenone is discontinued.

In patient no 2, VT mapping localized the earliest potentials in the inferior part of the left ventricle. These potentials were occuring in the mid diastole, in such timing that it was difficult to recognize whether they were premature potentials linked to the origin of the VT or late potentials. Continuous activity could be recorded in the vicinity of the zone. Fulguration was performed on that region. After VT relapse a second session was proposed, and the same recordings were found, but 7 shocks in that zone did not prevent VT recurrence. However, medical therapy with amiodarone combined with propafenone could then prevent tachycardia for 26 months.

Two patients (nos 15 and 22) had relapses shortly after the first session, while exercising. Mapping localized a new zone of early potential near the previously fulgurated site, with the same prematurity to the surface QRS, and after a new session there has been no relapse, with a follow-up of 26 and 28 months, respectively.

The last patient (no 17) had 2 morphologies of VT. One was treated during the first session, and the other relapsed after one month. A second session allowed total prevention with a 22 month follow-up.

Criteria for success

The results of programmed pacing during the early follow-up had a good prognostical value:
– In 2 cases (nos 13 and 17) the provocative technique could trigger before the session two different morphologies of VT, of which only one seemed clinical. In these 2 cases, fulguration was carried out on the site of origin of the clinical VT, the other tachycardia still being triggerable. Patient no 13 never had new relapse of arrhythmia with a follow-up of 32 months, while the other had a relapse one month later of the second morphology of VT, needing a new session which proved successful.
– In 5 cases (nos 2, 5, 12, 18, 20) VT was still triggerable one week to 10 days after the first session. Patient no 12 was one of our first patients who in fact had no relapse during that week. However, a new session was done and was complicated by the patient's death (vide supra). All the others had ulterior spontaneous relapses controlled either by new sessions or by medical treatment.

The effectiveness of antiarrhythmic therapy is assessed by comparing the rate of occurrence of VT before and after therapy, but it has also to take account of the spontaneous evolution of the arrhythmia. There is no question about the effectiveness of the therapy when VT is permanent or has daily relapses, and disappears immediately after fulguration. This applies to 7 cases (nos 1, 3, 8, 9, 16, 21, 22). The same applies to the patients in whom tachycardia relapsed every month, when there had been no relapses after more than 4 months, as in 7 of the patients (nos 10, 11, 13, 14, 15, 17, 19).

By contrast, when fulguration has been done on patients with rare ventricular tachycardia, still triggerable under antiarrhythmic therapies but with no spontaneous relapses (nos 4, 7, 20), only a prolonged follow-up can prove the effectiveness of therapy, as in 2 cases (nos 4 and 20) with two year follow-up. Case no 7 died after one month of heart failure pre-existant to the fulguration, but without relapse or antiarrhythmic therapy.

However, it is important to note that 5 of the 17 patients with long term follow-up are still under antiarrhythmic therapy. That subgroup of patients had early relapses of VT, but previously ineffective drugs had become effective after fulguration, which somehow modified the arrhythmogenic substrate. Therefore, an effective therapy resulted from the combination of fulguration and medical treatment.

Comments

Hartzler, in 1983, published the first cases of VT treatment by fulguration in one case of drug-resistant infundibular tachycardia, which also resisted surgery, and in two cases after myocardial infarction [3]. Puech in the same year also reported one case of VT originating from a right ventricular dysplasia [4]. Since that time our results, and others demonstrate that this technique is effective in the treatment of ventricular tachycardia resistant to medical antiarrhythmics, and for which until then only surgery was available, with a high risk for the patients with a bad haemodynamic status.

The risk of the procedure seems low, considering the fact that most of these patients had a compromised myocardium, especially those in whom the ejection fraction was inferior to 30%, and in which surgical mortality is particularly high.

Relapses can be explained in most of the cases. It may be the failure of the catheter which cannot withstand the energy sent by the defibrillator. This problem has since been overcome by the careful selection of the electrodes before the procedure. It can also be due to the impossibility of placing the electrode in the zone of origin of the tachycardia, defined as the one where the earliest potentials can be recorded. In some cases (nos 2 and 5) relapses are more difficult to explain, as they happened after fulguration in a zone activated 50 to 70 msec before the onset of the surface QRS in VT. In such cases, it may be supposed that the arrhythmogenic zone is wider than the one modified by the shock.

Many points are still under investigation in the use of fulguration for the treatment of ventricular tachycardia. The mechanism of action of fulguration is not simple. The local thermal effect seems to be without importance. A mechanical effect due to the barotraumatism provoked by the spark generated inside the heart, and an electrical effect due to the flow of current between the catheter and the neutral electrode may explain the results of fulguration [9]. The small elevation of the CPK MB shows that a small amount of myocardium is destroyed by the procedure, which is in the range of $1\,cm^2$ according to experimental studies and the two anatomical cases.

160

Endocardial mapping is limited by the difficulties of properly positioning the endocavitary lead, which cannot always enter all the areas of the ventricular endocardium. It is always difficult to acertain that there is not an earlier point of activation which has not been recorded by the catheter. The pacemapping technique also has some limitations and does not seem to be very accurate, distinct localisations of the pacing lead being capable of giving a similar electrocardiographic pattern. However, that technique has been very useful in one case (no 11) where the arrhythmia could not be triggered during the session, and for which two shocks were only directed by that method. That patient has been asymptomatic for two years, while his tachycardia was recurring once or twice a month before fulguration.

Conclusion

Fulguration methods for the treatment of ventricular tachycardia can be an alternative to surgery. The treatment has the advantage of being able to treat patients who cannot be operated, and of being easily repeated in case of failure. It has the disadvantage of needing a long session of endocardial catheterization while the patient has to stay in ventricular tachycardia, in a haemodynamic situation which can be ill-tolerated if too prolonged. However, the encouraging results of the actual short series are in favour of the technique.

Acknowledgment

This study was supported in part by grants from the 'Centre de Recherche sur les Maladies Cardiovasculaires de l'Association Claude Bernard'.

References

1. Gonzalez R, Scheinman MM, Marsaretten W, Rubinstein M: Closed chest electrode-catheter technique for His bundle ablation in doss. Am J Physiol 1981; 241: H283–H287.
2. Gallagher JJ, Svenson RH, Kasell JH, German LD, Bardy GH, Broushton A, Critelli G: Catheter technique for closed-chest ablation of the atrioventricular conduction system. N Ensl J Med 1982; 306: 194–200.
3. Hartzler GO: Electrode catheter ablation of refractory focal ventricular tachycardia. J Am Coll Cardiol 1983; 2: 1107–1113.
4. Puech P, Gallay P, Grolleau R, Koliopoulos N: Traitement par électrofulsuration endocav- itaire d'une tachycardie ventriculaire récidivante par dysplasie ventriculaire droite. Arch Mal Coeur 1984; 77: 826–835.
5. Fontaine G, Cansell A, Lechat Ph, Frank R, Grosgogeat Y: Method of selecting catheters for endocavitary fulguration. Stimucoeur 1984; 12: 285–289.

6. Frank R, Fontaine G, Pierfitte M, Grosgogeat Y: Simulation studies for the interpretation of delayed potentials. In: Schlepper M (ed) Proceedings of the rythmonorme symposium. Springer-Verlag, Heidelberg, 1983; 53–61.

7. Lechat Ph, Fontaine G, Cansell A, Grosgogeat Y: Epicardial and endocardial myocardial damage related to catheter ablation techniques (Abstract). Eur Heart J 1984; 5 (Suppl 1): 258.

8. Bardy GH, Kasell JH, Ideker RE, Worley SJ, Smith WM, German LD, Gallagher JJ: Transvenous catheter ablation of the atrioventricular conduction system for treatment of refractory supraventricular tachycardia. Electrophysiologic and Pathologic Observations in Dogs. Am J Cardiol 1982; 49: 1012.

9. Ward DE, Davies M: Transvenous high energy shock for ablatins atrioventricular conduction in man. Observations on the histological effects. Br Heart J 1984; 51: 175–178.

3.5 The Implantable Cardioverter-Defibrillator

M. MIROWSKI, PHILIP R. REID, MORTON M. MOWER, LEVI
WATKINS JR, EDWARD V. PLATIA, LAWRENCE S.C. GRIFFITH,
THOMAS GUARNIERI and JUAN M. JUANTEGUY

The automatic implantable defibrillator[1] is a self-contained diagnostic-therapeutic system designed to continuously monitor the heart, identify ventricular fibrillation and potentially lethal ventricular tachycardias, and then to deliver electrical discharges to restore normal rhythm [1–3]. The main objective of this device is to protect high-risk patients from sudden cardiac death whenever and wherever they are striken by the lethal arrhythmia. Because the device performs its functions promptly and automatically, the constraints of time and the need for trained personnel, the two major stumbling blocks in conventional out-of-hospital resuscitation, are largely eliminated.

The initial clinical model of the device (AID) was designed for treatment of ventricular fibrillation but its recent version, the automatic implantable cardioverterdefibrillator (AICD), has the additional capability of detecting and treating the broad spectrum of ventricular tachycardias (Fig. 1). The hermetically sealed device is encased in titanium and weighs 298 g. There are two defibrillating electrodes. One is located on the distal end of an intravascular catheter and is placed in the superior vena cava near the right atrial junction. The second electrode has the form of a flexible rectangular patch and is designed for placement over the apex of the heart. In addition, a third bipolar catheter electrode is wedged into the right ventricular apex and serves for reliable rate sensing and R-wave synchronization [4, 5]. In the near future it will be used for pacing as well.

The AICD is powered by special lithium batteries characterized by low resistance and high energy density; they have a discharge capability of over 100 shocks and a projected monitoring life of approximately three years. The sensing system monitors both the heart rate and a sampled probability density function of the ventricular electrical activity. This function defines the fraction of time spent by the differentiated input electrogram between two amplitude limits located near zero potential. For all practical purposes ventricular fibrillation is identified by the striking absence of isoelectric potential segments, while a ventricular tachycardia, in order to be treated, must be faster than a predetermined heart rate.

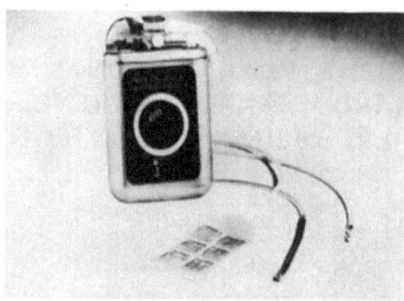

Fig. 1. The automatic implantable cardioverter-defibrillator with, left to right, the apical patch and superior vena cava electrodes, and the bipolar right ventricular electrode. For more details, see text.

When a suitable ventricular tachyarrhythmia is detected, the device delivers Schuder's truncated exponential pulse [6] of 25 joules some 20 seconds after onset of the arrhythmia; the pulse duration ranges between 3 and 8 msec as a function of the interelectrode resistance. In presence of ventricular tachycardia, the cardioverting discharge is R-wave synchronized. The device can recycle 3 times if the initial discharge is ineffective, with the strength of the 2nd, 3rd and 4th pulses being increased to 30 joules. After the 4th discharge, about 35 seconds of nonfibrillating rhythm is required to reset the counter and to allow a full series of pulses to be delivered again at the next episode.

Noninvasive testing of the automatic defibrillator before and periodically after implantation can be accomplished using an external analyzer.[2] Transient placement of a magnet over the device initiates the capacitor charging cycle, with the charge being delivered into a built-in test-load resistor rather than through the leads to the patient. An electromagnetic transducer measures the capacitor charging time. Progressive increases in this time denote battery depletion, while failure to initiate the charging cycle indicates abnormal operation of the device. The analyzer also stores and telemeters out the total number of defibrillating pulses received by the patient. The physician can thus easily determine the number of discharges, if any, which have occurred since the previous follow-up visit. The device can also be activated and deactivated at will by proper application of the magnet. The status of the device is indicated to the physician by coded audio signals emitted by a piezoelectric tone generator located within the pulse generator.

Clinical evaluation study of this new therapeutic modality began in February, 1980 [7]. The initial entry criteria into the study were stringent. Specifically, the candidates for implantation were required to have survived at least 2 episodes of cardiac arrest not associated with acute myocardial infarction, with the life-threatening arrhythmia documented at least once and occurring despite treatment with antiarrhythmic agents. Subsequently, their criteria have been relaxed to require only one episode of arrhythmic cardiac arrest outside the context of acute myocardial infarction, and evidence of incomplete protection as determined by continuing inducibility during electrophysiologic studies, stress testing, or on clinical grounds.

While the superior vena cava and the right ventricular electrodes are inserted percutaneously, a left thoracotomy and medial sternotomy are frequently used for implantation of the apical patch electrode. More recently, a subxiphoidal approach obviating a thoracotomy is also being performed [8]. This relatively simple procedure involves a small vertical incision made below the xiphoid process. The pericardium is then exposed and incised, the apical electrode introduced and its proximal edge sutured to the pericardium. The leads are then tunneled under the skin and connected to the pulse generator implanted in a left para-umbilical pocket.

As of March 1984, some 300 patients have undergone implantation of the device in 25 institutions in the United States and at several European centers that have recently joined the program. Over 2700 implant-months have so far been accumulated; the longest follow-up is 50 months and the average implant time is 9.75 months. The ongoing evaluation study of this new therapeutic modality has allowed a critical assessment of the device's functional performance, of the risks associated with its use, and of its impact on survival rates of the implantees.

In the series of 89 patients operated upon at The Johns Hopkins Hospital in Baltimore, the age of the implantees ranged between 16 and 75 years with a mean of 54. Coronary artery disease was the underlying disease process in 69 patients, various types of cardiomyopathies were present in 19, and one patient had a prolonged QT interval syndrome. The great majority of the implantees had markedly compromised left ventricular function, the mean ejection fraction being 33%. Prior to the implantation of the device, these patients had survived an average of 3.5 arrhythmic cardiopulmonary arrests requiring resuscitation and had failed an average of 4.5 antiarrhythmic drugs; 14 had undergone coronary artery bypass grafting, one a myectomy and 10 were being treated with permanent electronic pacemakers. At the time of implantation, 31 patients underwent concomitant cardiovascular surgery: 21 had endocardial resection which was combined with aneurysmectomy in 15 and coronary bypass grafting in 11. Ten patients had bypass grafting alone, and one case had grafting plus mitral valve replacement. Virtually all patients in this series were maintained on some type of antiarrhythmic medication following implantation of the device.

The functional performance of the AICD was assessed in a variety of settings [9]. Under the controlled conditions of the electrophysiology laboratory, the diagnostic accuracy of the AICD was 98% for both ventricular fibrillation and ventricular tachycardias. The rare instances of non-detection were due to such clearly identifiable and correctable causes as fracture or malposition of a lead, 60 cycle interference, or interaction with an implanted unipolar pacemaker.

Termination of the malignant rhythm is usually accomplished with a single internal discharge, although in some instances the device has to recycle once or even twice to achieve this goal. The time from the onset of the arrhythmia until its termination ranges between 11.5 seconds and 36 seconds, with a mean of 17 seconds. Ineffectiveness of the standard 25-joule discharge using the spring-patch lead configuration has been observed in 12% of patients, but routine determination of the defibrillation threshold during implantation has helped immensely to address the problem of high energy requirements. In a number of instances, it has been possible to reduce an excessive energy threshold by correcting the patients' metabolic disorders such as hypokalemia or by modifying their pharmacological regimens. Amiodarone, in particular, has been shown to increase the energy requirements for cardioversion/defibrillation. A patient whose threshold, despite all efforts to reduce it, exceeds the output of the device should not have the system implanted.

As far as the patient's subjective reaction is concerned, internal discharges cause momentary discomfort but are generally well tolerated even in a conscious state. The sensation most frequently described by implantees is that of a moderate blow to the chest. In contrast to the experience of the Stanford group [10], no serious emotional problems that could be related to the internal discharges were observed in the Hopkins series. This is probably so because this group is using 'rate-only' devices which not only have a higher incidence of false-positive discharges but also correct bona fide arrhythmias more rapidly, often before the patient can become symptomatic. Figures 2 and 3 exemplify the functional performance of the device.

A number of problems and complications related to the use of implanted defibrillators have been observed during the study period. While many of these problems were rapidly solved and are of only historical interest, others remain of clinical importance as they are inherent in techniques and technology employed.

Since implantation of the device at present still requires extensive surgery and general anesthesia, peri- and post-operative complications can be expected to occur in these very sick patients. In the Hopkins experience of 89 patients, for example, primary infectious complications occurred in 6 patients; in 4, the problem was traced to the pulse generator pocket, in one to an ante-cubital cut-down, while in another the origin was unknown. All patients responded well to antibiotics. There was one operative death due to perforation of the subclavian vein by a Swan-Ganz catheter. Post-operatively, transient pericardial rubs were the rule. There was one episode of superior vena

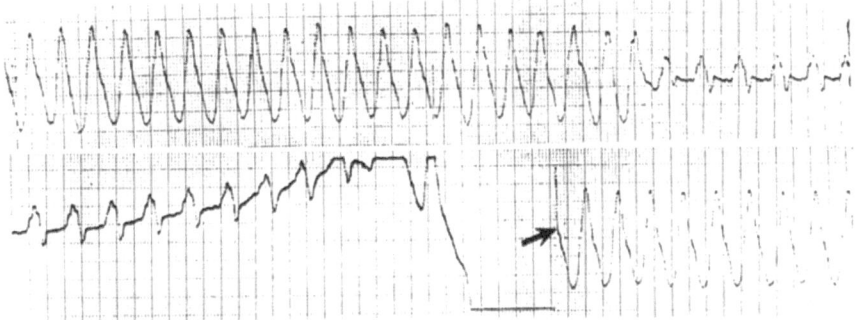

Fig. 2. Spontaneous ventricular tachycardia at a rate of 155 beats per minute is terminated automatically by the AICD within 11 seconds from its onset (arrow). Strips are continuous.

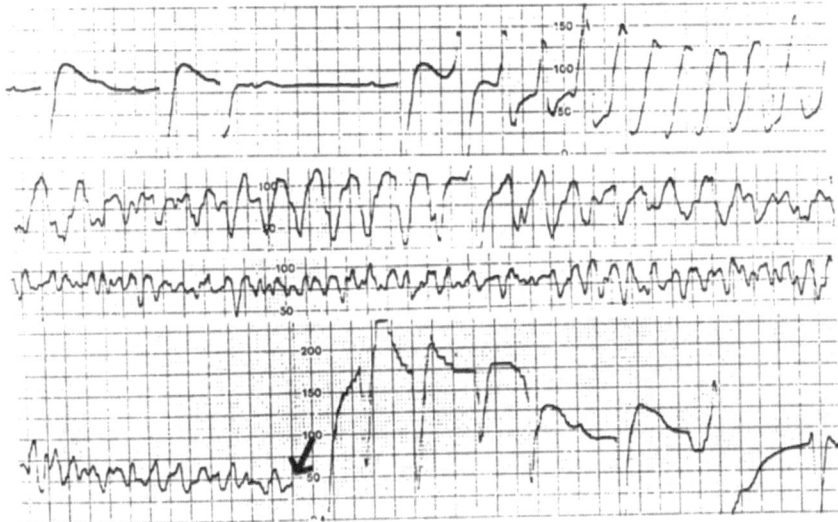

Fig. 3. Spontaneous ventricular tachycardia degenerating into ventricular fibrillation is automatically terminated with AICD within 36 seconds. This relatively long time is explained by the fact that the ventricular tachycardia was initially slower than 167 beats per minute, the cut off rate of the device. Strips are continuous.

cava thrombosis which was resolved with anticoagulants but no embolic phenomena were noted. Lead fractures were observed early in the study; this complication was virtually eliminated by replacing the silver tinsel wire with drawn braised strands. Lead dislodgement occurred in 7 patients requiring repositioning.

False-positive discharges occur whenever the input signal satisfies the sensing algorithm of the device. In the early stages of the study, the most frequent

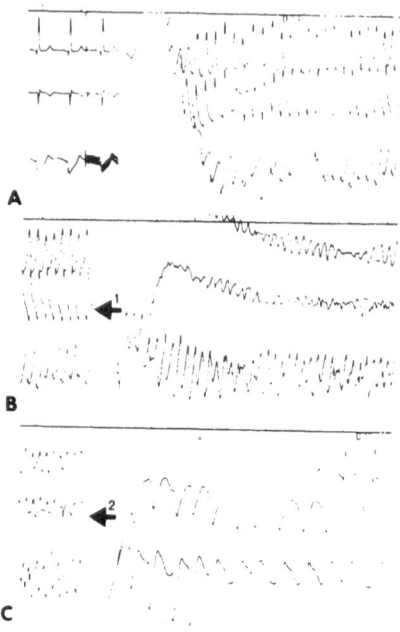

Fig. 4. Automatic correction of an accelerated arrhythmia. *Panel A:* ventricular tachycardia at a rate of 250 beats per minute is induced with low-level alternating current. *Panel B:* (Arrow 1) the initial internal shock accelerates the tachycardia into ventricular fibrillation. *Panel C:* (Arrow 2) a second automatic shock restores normal sinus rhythm. In each panel, the upper tracing is the surface lead II, the middle tracing is the right ventricular bipolar electrogram, and the lower tracing is the transcardiac electrogram. Strips are not continuous.

mechanism was miscounting of the heart rate as sensed by the transcardiac electrodes. However, with the addition of a separate rate channel, reliable determination of the heart rate became possible except for instances of interaction with an implanted unipolar cardiac pacemaker. In the past, interference signals due to lead discontinuity also resulted in unwanted discharges. At the present time, spurious discharges may still occur due to particularly rapid supraventricular rhythms which satisfy the morphology sensing criteria of the device. Although still a problem of concern, spurious shocks never resulted in serious arrhythmias or other untoward effects.

As it is true with an electronic device, one might expect some incidence of random component failures. The clinical experience to date, however, has been extremely good. The number of such component failures was a mere handful and no clinical harm resulted.

Acceleration of the ventricular tachycardia into a faster rhythm or even into ventricular fibrillation may occur with any type of electrical treatment of this arrhythmia. While R-wave synchronization theoretically minimizes the fre-

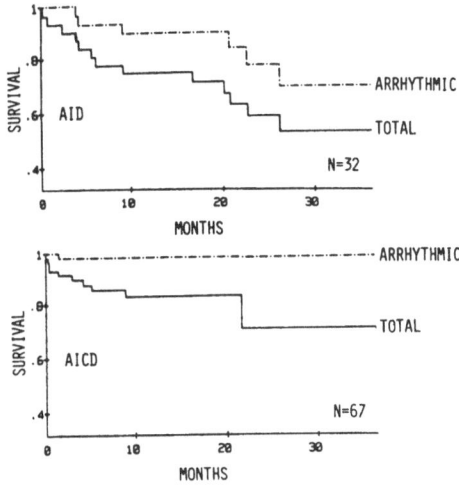

Fig. 5. Kaplan-Meier survival curves of patients with automatic implantable defibrillators. The upper two curves are from implantees who received the first generation device (AID) while the lower two curves are derived from patients with the AICD. The solid lines indicate the total survival experience, while the broken lines depict the observed mortality which was due to arrhythmias. For more details, see text.

quency of acceleration, it does not eliminate it completely; in fact, its occurrence is basically unpredictable and can be observed at all energy levels. Because of this complication, patients with implanted antiarrhythmic devices not having defibrillating back-up capabilities are at an unacceptable risk. The AICD is the only automatic system capable of dealing effectively with acceleration through recycling: the device recognizes the accelerated rhythm de novo and corrects it with a subsequent discharge. This unique function of the device was observed several times in our series and is exemplified in Fig. 4.

It has already been possible to determine what effect the automatic defibrillator has had on the survival rate of the implantees [9, 10]. Figure 5 depicts the respective effectiveness of the first and second generation devices used, as observed in the 89 Baltimore patients. These implantees were divided into 2 groups according to the model they had received. Patients whose early models were subsequently replaced with the AICD were withdrawn alive at that time from the AID group and entered anew into the AICD population. These Kaplan-Meier survival curves indicate that at one year, the mortality due to arrhythmias was 10.6% for the AID group and 2% for the AICD series, while the total one-year mortality was 26% and 16.6% respectively (p<0.01). These results are consistent with those recently reported by Echt and co-workers [10] who studied 70 patients treated with the AICD model at Stanford Medical Center; the arrhythmic one-year mortality in their group was 1.8%, a figure strikingly similar to ours.

The AICD has clearly proven its ability to diagnose and treat ventricular fibrillation and tachycardia, resulting in an impressive decrease in the implantees' arrhythmic mortality. The potential risks and dangers of this diagnostic-therapeutic system are quite similar to those observed with the use of implanted electronic pacemakers, particularly when the epicardial implantation approach is used. Further confirmation of the current clinical experience in much larger series will most probably lead to broadening of the patient population who could benefit from this therapeutic intervention.

Summary

The automatic implantable cardioverter-defibrillator is an electronic device designed to continuously monitor the heart, identify malignant ventricular tachyarrhythmias, and then to deliver effective countershock to restore normal rhythm. There are 2 defibrillating electrodes which are also used for waveform analysis; one is located in the superior vena cava, the other is placed over the cardiac apex. A third bipolar right ventricular electrode serves for rate counting and R-wave synchronization. When ventricular fibrillation occurs, a 25-joule pulse is delivered; when ventricular tachycardia faster than a preset rate is detected, the discharge is R-wave synchronized. The device can recycle 3 times if required. Special batteries can deliver over 100 shocks or provide a three-year monitoring life. Implantation of the device is made either through a thoracotomy, by a subxiphoid, or subcostal approach. Thus far, the device has been implanted in over 300 survivors of sudden arrhythmic death with a follow-up period up to 50 months. Acceleration of ventricular tachycardia to a faster rhythm or to ventricular fibrillation occurred only rarely and is dealt with most successfully through recycling. Actuarial analysis has indicated significant impact on the survival rate of the implantees; the one-year mortality rate attributed to arrhythmias was reduced to 2%. Thus, the automatic cardioverter-defibrillator can reliably identify and correct potentially lethal ventricular tachyarrhythmias, leading to a substantial increase in survival in properly selected high-risk patients.

Notes

1. Developed and manufactured by Intec Systems, Inc., Pittsburgh, Pennsylvania, U.S.A., under the trademark AID[R].
2. Developed and manufactured by Intec Systems, Inc., Pittsburgh, Pennsylvania, U.S.A., under the name AIDCHECK[R].

References

1. Mirowski M, Mower MM, Staewen WS, Tabatznik B, Mendeloff AI: Standby automatic defibrillator: an approach to prevention of sudden coronary death. Arch Intern Med 1970; 126: 158–161.
2. Mirowski M, Mower MM, Staewen WS, Denniston RH, Mendeloff AI: The development of the transvenous automatic defibrillator. Arch Intern Med 1972; 129: 773–779.
3. Mirowski M, Mower MM, Langer A, Heilman MS, Schreibman J: A chronically implanted system for automatic defibrillation in active conscious dogs: experimental model for treatment of sudden death from ventricular fibrillation. Circulation 1978; 58: 90–94.
4. Reid PR, Mirowski M, Mower MM, Platia EV, Griffith LSC, Watkins Jr L, Bach SM, Imran M, Thomas A: Clinical evaluation of the internal automatic cardioverter-defibrillator in survivors of sudden cardiac death. Am J Cardiol 1983; 51: 1608–1613.
5. Winkle RA, Bach Jr SM, Echt DS, Swerdlow CD, Imran M, Mason JW, Oyer PE, Stinson EB: The automatic implantable defibrillator: local ventricular bipolar sensing to detect ventricular tachycardia and fibrillation. Am J Cardiol 1983; 52: 265–270.
6. Schuder JC, Rahmoeller GA, Stoeckle H: Transthoracic ventricular defibrillation with triangular and trapezoidal waveforms. Circ Res 1966; 19: 689–694.
7. Mirowski M, Reid PR, Mower MM, Watkins L, Gott VL, Schauble JF, Langer A, Heilman MS, Kolenik SA, Fischell RE, Weisfeldt ML: Termination of malignant ventricular arrhythmias with an implanted automatic defibrillator in human beings. N Engl J Med 1980; 303: 322–324.
8. Watkins Jr L, Mirowski M, Mower MM, Reid PR, Freund P, Thomas A, Weisfeldt ML, Gott VL: Implantation of the automatic defibrillator: the subxiphoid approach. Ann Thorac Surg 1982; 34: 515–520.
9. Mirowski M, Reid PR, Mower MM, Watkins Jr L, Platia EV, Griffith LSC, Guarnieri T, Thomas A, Juanteguy JM: Clinical performance of the implantable cardioverter-defibrillator. PACE 1985; 10: 120–128.
10. Echt DS, Armstrong K, Caltagerone P, Oyer PE, Stinson EB, Winkle RA: Clinical experience, complications and survival in 50 patients with the automatic implantable defibrillator (AID) (Abstract). J Am Col Cardiol 1984; 3: 535.

3.6 Conclusions

E. PICCOLO

Until just a few years ago, treatment of the arrhythmias was conceived and realized only with drugs using empirical methods. As the mechanisms of arrhythmias have been understood and tested, new therapeutic approaches have been devised.

Invasive and specific treatment by means of surgery directed toward interrupting the electophysiologic mechanism of the arrhythmias has been developed recently. In the previous reports four techniques have been described that differ from each other technically, instrumentally and in the pathophysiologic mechanism they attempt to correct.

Left stellectomy, proposed by Schwartz and Facchini, now has a solid experimental and clinial basis to be applied to potentially malignant arrhythmias of the congenital long QT syndrome. Recently, the same authors have performed this technique in the postinfarction period, when dangerous arrhythmias can occur, but the results of such intervention are not yet available.

Various surgeons around the world, as Dr Márquez has reported, have developed a surgical approach to the therapy of arrhythmias by cutting the myocardial areas responsible for the reentry circuit. The first attempt was a resection of necrotic an fibrotic areas of the myocardium (postinfarctional ventricular aneurysms) without attending to specific electrophysiologic controls. The results were not satisfactory because the limiting zone, responsible for the reentry circuit, was preserved. The second technique is that of Guiraudon, who cuts the myocardium in the limiting zones around the infarct from endocardium to epicardium. In terms of the arrhythmia the results have been good, but they are clinically unsatisfactory because of the danger of producing important unpairment of left ventricular function. The technique of subendocardial resection of the necrotic zone guided by electrocardiographic endocardial mapping seems more adequate.

The Fontaine-Frank group is testing a fulguration technique by means of an intracardiac catheter. This method, which does not require open heart surgery, assumes that the reentry circuit can be precisely located by endocardial mapping, and that the circuit can be reached by the fulgurating catheter. It has the disadvantage of producing uncontrollable damage.

For several years Dr Mirowski of Baltimore has been working to develop an implantable defibrillator, similar to the pacemaker of everyday use, to be used in selected cases of dangerous arrhythmias (ventricular tachycardia or fibrillation). The results described have improved as the implanted devices have been perfected. There are still some technical problems (generator weight, surgical intervention, unnecessary defibrillation) and the selection of cases that may benefit from this measure has to be made. In any case, the line of research that Dr Mirowski is following will surely bear more fruit with further technological improvement.

4. Pacemakers

4.1 Introduction

J. COSÍN AGUILAR

For almost three centuries, mankind has had written testimony of the causal relationship between extreme bradycardia and convulsive crises, but it is has only been a little more than 30 years since the Stokes-Adams syndrome was first effectively treated by direct application of an electrical current to the chest wall with the intention of stimulating the heart. In this way Zoll (1952) demonstrated the possibility of substituting the cardiac pacemakers' function with an energy source other than that of the organism. However, the method resulted impractical in nonanesthetized patients.

Nonetheless, the conceptual advance produced and the existent technological possibilities enabled Ake Senning, six years later, to implant a pacemaker from the Elema-Schonander company equipped with a nickel-cadmium battery and an electrode-catheter terminating in a disk sutured to the ventricular epicardium, which supplied constant, longlasting and fixed (asynchronous) ambulatory stimulation. This introduced the first generation of cardiac stimulators, to the development of which Zoll, and especially Chardack's studies, contributed.

Furman, in the same year that Senning implanted the first pacemaker, used the trans-venous route to 'position' the stimulation chatheter in the right ventricular cavity without previous thoracotomy. This is the 'access' used today in more than 90% of implantations, thus transforming the procedure into minor surgery.

After a dozen years of using fixed rate stimulators (VOO), 'deaf' to the heart's own activity and therefore competitive with it and potentially arrhythmogenic, a second generation of pacemakers appeared that only discharge impulses capable of activating the heart when reguired ('on demand'), the rest of the time being inhibited (VVI) or discharged (VVT) by the spontaneous cardiac activity. These stimulators 'listen', conforming their activity to the needs of each moment. They avoid competitive arrhythmias and improve the hemodynamic output of the organ.

The third stage of the history of the cardiac stimulation is being written at present. The concept of development is oriented in different direction: physiologic or intelligent pacemakers, programmable pacemakers and antitachycardiac devices.

Since 1964, when Medtronic made the first programmable stimulator, one or several of the stimulation parameters can be externally noninvasively changed at will, the new parameters continuing until reprogramming.

Finally, among the most recent developments we must consider the antitachycardiac stimulators, with parameters adaptable to the previously studied electrophysiologic characteristics of each arrhythmia and capable of detecting the arrhythmia and producing a stimulation to interrupt it, or of being activated by the patient. Dr Phyllis M. Holt, assistant to Dr Sowton of Guy's Hospital, has dedicated her professional efforts to clinical research in the field of ventricular tachycardias and antitachycardiac pacemakers, and will speak to us on this type of 'pacemaker'.

These conceptual advances have been possible thanks to parallel technological developments in the field of energy sources (we have progressed from the classic mercury-zinc batteries to lithium batteries that last 4–5 times as long), resistance of the materials (catheters, unit covering, etc.) and especially electric circuits, which have advanced from those constituted by discrete elements to integrated circuits and build-in microprocessors.

Given the relative harmlessness and great efficiency of pacemakers in treating hypokinetic arrhythmias, the number of implantations in the western world is growing. In certain situations, the indication for pacemaker implantation is undeniable; in these cases, the clinial manifestations are supported by the cardiologic findings. On the contrary, there are groups of patients in whom evident clinical manifestations of cerebral ischemia, such as syncope, are not accompanied by signs indicative that the pacemaker implantation will resolve the disorder. In these cases a series of special studies are necessary; Dr García Civera, who is at present working in electrophysiology at the Department of Cardiology of the Hospital Clínico of Valencia, will describe his personal experience in this field.

Once a pacemaker has been implanted, both the patient and the device must undergo periodic controls to guarantee its correct function. In the first 6 weeks, these controls should be frequent (every 15 to 20 days) until stimulation thresholds stabilize. Late, controls can be performed (in lithium generators) every 6 months or less. Dr Botella Solana (pioneer in this field, who has directed for years one of the few Units in Spain dedicated to studying functional pacemaker alterations in vivo and in vitro), will describe in the last paper of this chapter the methods used in his laboratory of the Department of Cardiology of the Hospital Clínico of Valencia; his contribution will focus on the role of transthoracic stimulation in the diagnosis of anomalies of pacemaker function and in the study of the dependence of the patients.

4.2 Electrophysiological Studies in Patients with Syncope of Unknown Cause

R. GARCÍA CIVERA, R. SANJUAN, S. MORELL, S. BOTELLA,
E. GONZALEZ, E. BALDO, J. LLAVADOR and V. LOPEZ MERINO

Introduction

Syncope or minor equivalents of syncope are a relatively frequent cause for medical consultation [1–3]. The wide etiological spectrum of syncope and the transitory nature of its presentation make determination of its cause very difficult. However, diagnosis is of great prognostic and therapeutic importance because the causes of syncope range from banal to life threatening [3, 4].

Among the cardiac causes of syncope, the paroxysmal arrhythmias, either hyper or hypokinetic, occupy a preferential position. When the episodes are frequent, a clinical examination or a diagnostic electrocardiographic tracing (with conventional ECG or Holter) can be obtained during a crisis, but when the syncopal episodes are infrequent, documentation of the potential arrhythmias becomes practically impossible.

Not long ago it was suggested that the use of electrophysiologic studies (EPS) in patients with syncope of unknown cause could help in the diagnosis and therapy of these cases [5–7]. The present communication deals with the results of a prospective study in which 36 patients with syncope of unknown origin were submitted to EPS and followed during a mean of 19.75 months.

Material and methods

Selection of patients

The study was carried out in patients selected from those referred for evaluation of syncope by the Cardiology and Internal Medicine departments.

Prior to performing EPS all the patients were submitted to a study protocol that included the tests indicated in Table 1.

Criteria for inclusion in the study were the followings:

a) absence of clinical or laboratory data suggestive of an extracardiac origin of the syncope;

b) absence of significant arrhythmias both in the conventional ECG or in the electrocardiographic monitoring.

The following were considered to be significant arrhythmias: sinus pauses of 2 seconds or more; sinoatrial block; second and third degree AV block; and ventricular tachycardia (more than 5 consecutive beats at a rate of more than 100 bpm). Isolated sinus bradycardia and supraventricular tachyarrhythmias were only considered significant if a relation with the syncopal episode could be demonstrated.

In accordance with these criteria 36 patients, 27 males and 9 females, were included in the study. Their most relevant clinical data are summarized in Table 2.

Table 1. Initial patient evaluation.

Clinical history
Cardiovascular and neurologic examination
Determination of blood pressure, supine and erect
Electrocardiogram
Electroencephalogram
Continuous ECG monitoring: in 11 patients with 24-hour Holter and in the others by telemetry with the patient hospitalized
Echocardiogram, exercise test, hemodynamic studies and CAT of the skull, when it was considered clinically indicated

---

Table 2. García Civera.

Pat.	Age ES sex		Clinical diagnosis	ECG	EPS results	Treatment	Follow-up Mos	Symptoms
1	80 M	3	CMI	PR = 0.24 RBBB + AH Inf. necr.	HV = 150 Aj. test +	Pacemaker	12	SD
2	71 M	4	CMI HF	RBBB Inf. necr.	HV = 50 Aj. test +	Pacemaker	17	D by LVF
3	80 M	7	HF	PR = 0.28 LBBB	HV = 80 Aj. test +	Pacemaker	4	D by LVF
4	56 M	1	CMI	RBBB + AH Ant. necr.	HV = 85 Aj. test +	Pacemaker	6	Asymp.
5	74 M	1	HF	AF RBBB + AH	HV = 80 Aj. test +	Pacemaker	1	Asymp.
6	67 M	2		Normal	Intrahis. block	Pacemaker	6	Asymp.
7	59 M	2	CMI	RBBB + AH Ant. necr.	HV = 70 Aj. test +	Pacemaker	1	Asymp.
8	64 M	1		PR = 0.32 RBBB	HV = 50 Aj. test +	Pacemaker	1	Asymp.
9	57 F	2		LBBB	HV = 70 Aj. test +	Pacemaker	59	Asymp.

Table 2. (Continued).

Pat.	Age sex	ES	Clinical diagnosis	ECG	EPS results	Treatment	Mos	Symptoms
10	59 M	2	COPD	RBBB + AH	HV = 60 Aj. test +	Pacemaker	38	Asymp.
11	70 M	6	Angina	RBBB	HV = 60 Aj. test + Nonsust. VT	Pacemaker Amiodarone	33	Asymp.
12	71 M	4	CMI	Ant. necr.	Sust. VT (CL = 285)	Mexiletine	33	1 Symp. (29 mo.) D by S
13	59 F	2	Cong. CMP	RBBB	Sust. VT (CL = 240)	Amiodarone	6	SD
14	65 M	10	CMI + WPW	WPW	Sust. VT (CL = 290)	Propaphenone	1	D by LVF
15	57 M	1	CMI	Ant. necr.	Nonsust. VT (CL = 260)	Amiodarone	3	Asymp.
16	28 M	1	CMI + WPW	WPW	Sust. VT (CL = 200)	Mexiletine	12	Asymp.
17	55 M	3	OMI	RBBB + AH Ant. necr.	Sust. VT (CL = 280)	Amiodarone	3	Asymp.
18	85 M	6		Normal	SSS		36	Asymp.
19	73 F	3		AH	SSS		36	Asymp.
20	71 M	3		PR = 0.24 RBBB	SSS + SCH	Pacemaker	49	Asymp
21	65 M	2	Hip. Heart. id.	LVE	SSS		24	Asymp.
22	51 M	3	COPD	Normal	SSS + SCH	Pacemaker	2	Asymp.
23	67 M	6		Normal	SSS + SCH	Pacemaker	1	Asymp.
24	67 M	12	COPD	LBBB	SCH	Pacemaker	9	Asymp.
25	77 M	4		AH	SCH	Pacemaker Cortico steroids	8	Symp.
26	67 M	4	OMI	Inf. necr.	SCH	Pacemaker	6	LHF
27	66 M	6	OMI	Inf. necr.	Atrial flutter	Amiodarone	47	Asymp.
28	49 F	1		Normal	SVPT (CL = 240)	Propaphenone	15	Asymp.
29	27 M	6		Normal	Normal		55	Symp.
30	70 F	2		Normal	Normal		54	Asymp.
31	78 F	3		RBBB + AH	Normal		42	Asymp.
32	77 M	2	COPD	PR = 0.24 RBBB + AH	Normal		29	SD
33	44 F	3		PR = 0.22	Normal	Antihypert.	36	Symp.
34	38 F	8		Normal	Normal	drugs	4	Asymp.
35	34 M	11		Normal	Normal		4	Asymp.
36	70 F	3		RBBB	SVPT nodal (CL = 400)	Aprindine	6	Asymp.

OMI = old myocardial infarction.

Protocol for electrophysiological study

With the patient's prior consent, the studies were realized without sedation and in the postabsorptive state. Cardioactive drugs were previously discontinued for a period equivalent to at least five half lives.

Three to four catheters – bipolar, cuatripolar and hexapolar – with an interelectrode distance of one centimeter, were introduced percutaneously and the electrodes were positioned in the apex of the right ventricle (RV), over the tricuspid valve in the zone for recording the hisiogram, in the high right atrium and in the coronary sinus. The intracavitary electrograms were filtered between 50 and 500 Hz and simultaneously recorded with various surface ECG leads by a Mingograf 80 polygraph. In cases selected blood pressure readings were obtained at the same time with a percutaneously introduced catheter in the radial or femoral artery.

The tracings were made by flow-writer inscription at a paper speed of 100 mm/sec for electrophysiological measurements and at 10 to 100 nm/sec for hemodynamic measurements.

The heart was stimulated with a Medtronic 5325 or Biotronick As-20 stimulator at a stimulation intensity equivalent to twice the threshold value. The protocol for recording and stimulation was the following:
a) basal recording of the AV conduction intervals;
b) right and left carotid sinus massage, in sinus rhythm and with atrial stimulation at a slightly higher rate than the sinus rate;
c) atrial stimulation at progressively greater rates until intolerable symptoms appeared or a rate of 230 bpm was attained;
d) atrial extrastimulation test at sinus cycle (Strauss test);
e) atrial extrastimulation test at two base cycles (generally 600 and 500 ms) with introduction of 1 or 2 extrastimuli;
f) ventricular stimulation at progressively higher rates until ventricular arrhythmia was produced, intolerable symptoms appeared or a maximum rate of 230 bpm was reached;
g) introduction of 1 or 2 (in case arrhythmias were not induced with one) ventricular extrastimuli at 2 base stimulation cycles (generally 600 and 500 msec);
h) ventricular stimulation was always produced in the RV apex, and if no tachycardia was induced it was repeated in the RV outflow tract; and
i) introduction of short 'bursts' of ventricular stimulation at rates of 250–300 bpm.

Pharmacological tests

Thirty two patients underwent phamacological tests during the EPS. The tests were chosen on the basis of the results of the basal study and were of three types:

Ajmaline test. This test was performed in 18 cases following the method and criteria that have been described [8]. All the patients who presented ventricular conduction disorders were submitted to this test, as well as 2 patients with narrow QRS in whom the possibility of intrahisian conduction disorders was excluded.

Pharmacological autonomic blockade. This was done in 9 cases with basal EPS suggestive of sinus node dysfunction. The method proposed by Jordan et al. [9], was used based on techniques described by Jose et al. [10]. Propranolol and atropine were administered together in 3 minutes at doses of 0.2 mg/kg and 0.04 mg/kg, respectively. The intrinsic heart rate was obtained 5 minutes after the injection. The results were analyzed according to Jordan et al. [9].

Serial drug tests in patients with tachycardia. In 6 patients in whom sustained tachyardia was induced (5 ventricular and 1 supraventricular), serial drug tests were made on successive days following the methodology proposed by Horowitz et al. [11]. The drug probands were: mexiletine (5 occasions), propaphenone (4 occasions), oral amiodarone (on 2 occasions after 2 weeks of treatment), lidocaine and procainammide (one occasion each).

Follow-up

Patient follow-up was done by periodic visits to the outpatient clinic of the hospital and by telephone communication with patients or family members. The follow-up ranged from 1 to 59 months (mean $\pm$ SD of 19.75 ± 18.33 months).

Results

The most relevant data of the EPS, treatment and follow-up of the patients are summarized in Table 2. The cases were divided into 6 groups according to the most sinificant EPS data.

Group I: study results suggestive of paroxysmal AVB

This group was composed of 10 cases. In 9 patients the basal ECG showed intraventricular conduction disorders, and one had a normal QRS. Three patients had chronic myocardial infarction, two had heart failure and one was diagnosed as having chronic *cor pulmonale.*

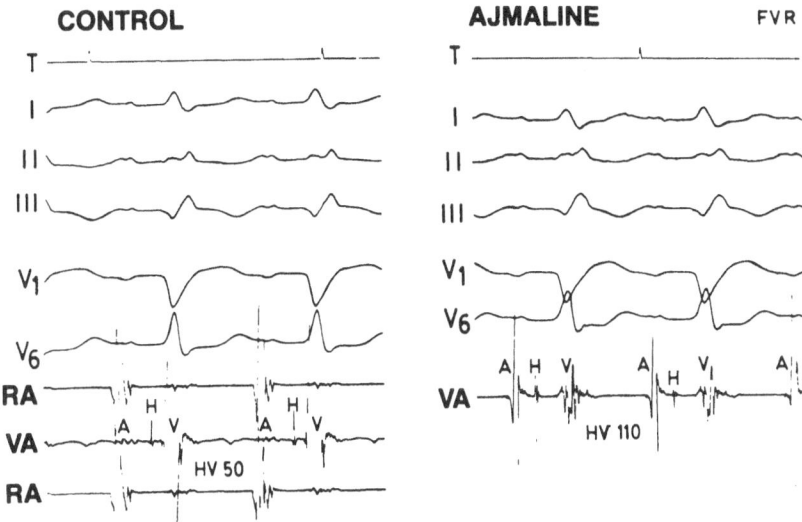

Fig. 1. Effect of the ajmaline test on a patient with syncope and left bundle branch block in the ECG. In the control study the HV interval was 50 msec. After ajmaline, the HV increased to 110 msec. T: time in seconds; I, II, III, V_1 and V_6: surface ECG leads; RA: intracavitary bipolar recording of the right atrium; VA: bipolar intracavitary recording of the zone of the hisiogram recording.

In the only patient with normal QRS, the EPS revealed the presence of truncal AV block (splitting of the hisian potential) with production of a high degree intrahisian block with atrial stimulation and paroxysmal intrahisian AV block after ventricular stimulation; a pacemaker (PM) was implanted, and the patient is asymptomatic 6 months later.

In the other 9 patients with intraventricular conduction disorders, the HV interval was superior to 65 msec in 6 patients and inferior to 65 msec in 3. In all 9 patients the ajmaline test response was abnormal, in 3 cases showing HV lengthening of more than 100% and high degree infrahisian AV block in the rest (Figs 1 and 2). PM were implanted in all these patients: 6 remain asymptomatic, 1 died suddenly at 12 months and 2 died as a consequence of refractory ventricular failure 4 and 7 months after implantation.

Group II: ventricular tachycardia

During basal EPS, sustained ventricular tachycardia was induced in 5 patients (Fig. 3); in 3 of them (cases 12, 13, 16) the tachycardia rapidly produced a syncopal episode and had to be terminated by synchronized electrical cardioversion. In the others, tachycardia was stopped by programmed electrical stimulation.

POST AJMALINE

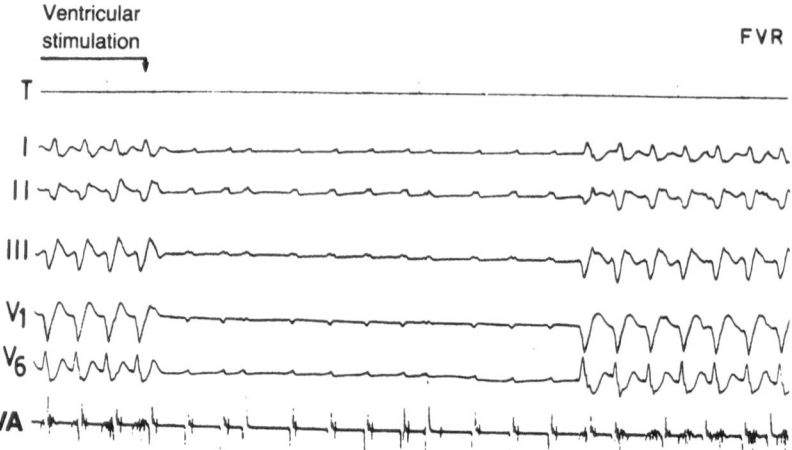

Fig. 2. The same case as in Fig. 1. After ajmaline, the abrupt suppression of ventricular stimulation leads to appearance of a paroxysmal infrahisian block that makes renewal of ventricular stimulation necesary. Abbreviations as in Fig. 1.

In the 5 cases, the mean cycle length of the tachyardia was 253 ± 33 msec. Nonsustained ventricular tachycardia (spontaneous reversion before 30 sec) was induced in 2 cases; in both of them repeat attacks of more than 15 beats of monomorphic tachycardia were induced, with cycle lengths of 285 and 240 msec respectively; in one of the cases (11) with a basal intraventricular conduction disorder tachycardia was induced by ventricular stimulation after only 50 mg ajmaline, which also produced a lengthening of the HV interval of more than 100%.

The 2 cases with nonsustained tachycardia were treated with amiodarone, and PM implantation in one case, and are still asymptomatic at 15 and 33 months. In the 5 cases with sustained tachycardia, an average of 2.6 tests per case were made with different drug dosages. Three patients were treated with drugs that impeded tachycardia induction during the study and 2 were treated with amiodarone when no other effective drug was found. Of the 3 patients treated on the basis of study results, one experieced an early hospital death (in the first month) from refractory heart failure; another died in hospital from a stroke at 33 months of follow-up, during which the patient had been asymptomatic except for a syncope at 29 months; the third patient, treated with a drug proven to be effective remains asymptomatic at 12 months. Of the 2 patients for whom no effective regime was found during the study and who were treated with amiodarone one died suddenly at 6 months of follow-up and the other is asymptomatic at 3 months.

184

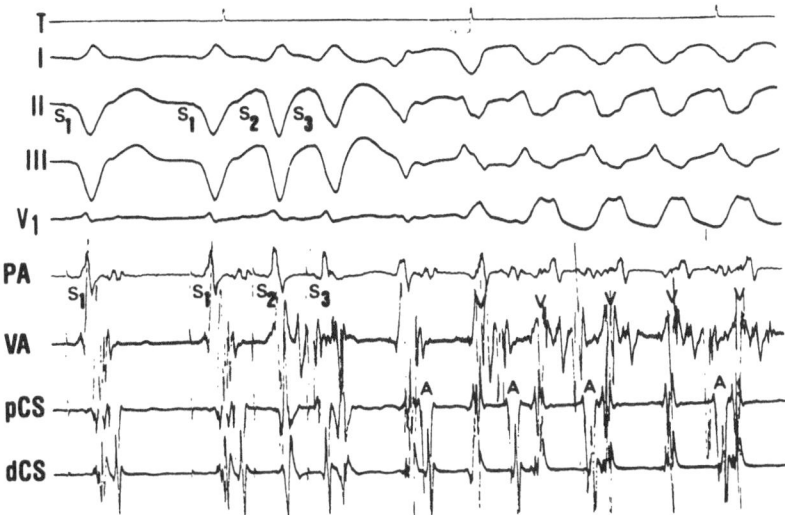

Fig. 3. Patient in group II. Induction of a monomorphic ventricular tachycardia with two ventricular extrastimuli (S_2, S_3) introduced in a 500 msec base cycle of ventricular stimulation (S_1, S_2). PA: bipolar recording of the pulmonary artery; pCS and dCS: bipolar recordings in the proximal and distal coronary sinus, respectively. Other abbreviations as in preceding figures.

Group III: sinus node dysfunction

Six patients showed evidence of sinus node dysfunction during EPS. In 4, the corrected basal sinus recovery time (CSRT) exceeded 525 msec. Two had a normal basal CRST, but the intrinsic heart rate after autonomic blockade was abnormal. On the basis of these findings, 3 cases were considered to have intrinsic sinus node dysfunction and 3 extrinsic sinus node dysfunction. In 3 cases, carotid sinus hypersensitivity was an associated finding. In 3 patients permanent PM were implanted and the other 3 received pharmacological treatment (vasodilators, vagolytic drugs, etc.). In an average follow-up of 24 months, the 3 cases with PM remained asymptomatic, and of the 3 without PM 2 remained asymptomatic and one died at 36 months as a result of a bronchial neoplasm.

Grade IV: carotid sinus hypersensitivity

Three patients were diagnosed as having hypersensitivity of the carotid sinus undetected prior to the EPS. This diagnosis was based on the following criteria:
1. Normality of the results of electophysiological tests for sinus node function (CSRT, ASRT) in the 3 cases.

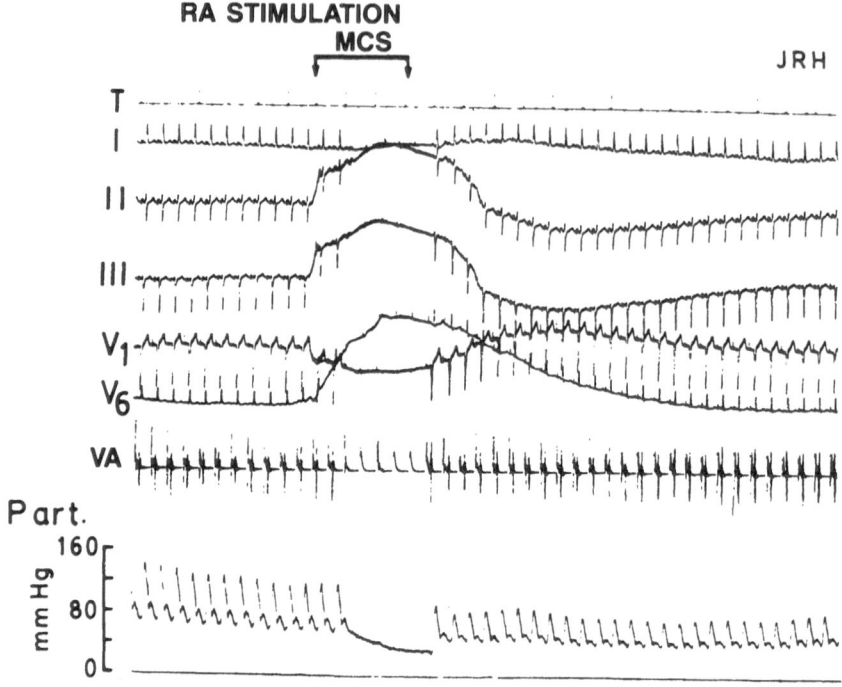

Fig. 4. Patient with hypersensitivity of the carotid sinus of mixed type. When the right carotid sinus is massaged (MCS) while stimulating the right atrium is made at fixed rhythm, loss of atrial capture that produces a pause of 3 sec is seen. Note the fall of more than 50 mm Hg in the arterial blood pressure that persists in spite of atrial rate recovery.

2. Abnormal response to carotid massage characterized by:
a) sinus pause of more than 3 seconds (cases 25 and 26);
b) high degree AV nodal block (cases 24 and 26) and
c) a fall in systolic blood pressure of more than 50 mm Hg unrelated to brady-cardia (Fig. 4).

Two of the 3 cases were diagnosed as carotid sinus hypersensitivity of the cardio-inhibitor type and treated with PM, remaining asymptomatic at 6 and 9 months of follow-up. The third case (25) corresponded to a mixed hypersensitivity with vasodepressor predominance and was treated by implantation of a sequential PM (DDD type) and corticoids, the patient's symptoms persisting, although with less frequency.

Group V: supraventricular tachyarrhythmias

In 2 cases EPS induced supraventricular arrhythmias that were considered responsible for the syncope. One case was treated for AV reentry tachycardia

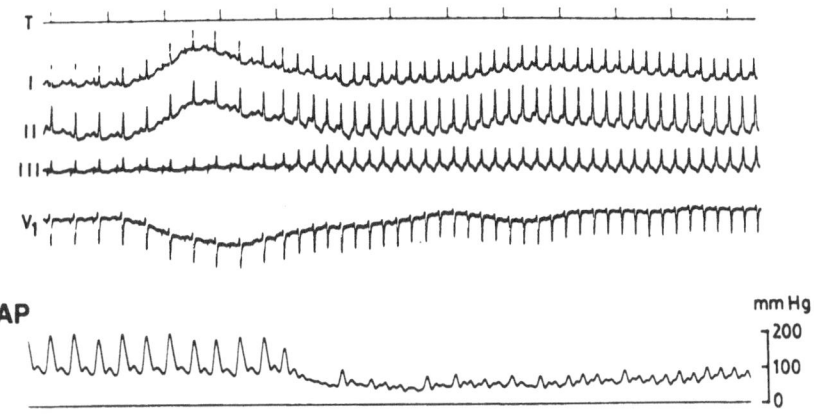

Fig. 5. Patient with syncope in whom the EPS demonstrated the presence of supraventricular paroxysmal tachycardia through an occult accessory AV bundle. The tachycardia rate was 250 bpm and its initiation was accompanied by an abrupt fall in blood pressure.

with a concealed left AV accessory bundle; induction of this tachycardia at a rate of 250 bpm in the supine patient led to an abrupt fall in blood pressure (Fig. 5) and appearance of presyncopal symptoms (dizziness, blurred vision). This case was treated with propaphenone and the patient is asymptomatic at 15 month follow-up. In another case, episodes of atrial flutter with 2 : 1 AV conduction could be reproducibly induced and interrupted by programmed atrial stimulation. During the induced arrhythmia the patient presented symptoms (dizziness, sweating) that were recognized as preceding the syncopal episodes. This patient was treated with amiodarone and is asymptomatic at 47 months.

Group VI: inconclusive studies

In 8 patients (22.2%) (cases 29 to 36) the EPS was considered inconclusive as to the cause of syncope. In 5 cases, the EPS was strictly normal. In the remaining 3, in one case atrial fibrillation was produced with a ventricular response of about 100 bpm. In another, tachycardia due to nodal reentry with a cycle length of 400 msec (corresponding to a heart rate of 150 bpm) was induced but did not correspond to the patient's symptoms. The last case had a long PR and an AH of 120 msec with a point of nodal Wenckebach at 160 bpm. These patients were treated empirically as detailed in Table 2. In the follow-up (average of 25 months), 5 remained asymptomatic. One case with right bundle branch block and anterior hemiblock and normal study results remained asymptomatic for 48 months, then died suddenly after presenting precordial pain. Another case with fine QRS and long PR, in which only AV node dysfunction was detected and that was not considered significant, had a syncope at 30 months of follow-up. Finally, a patient without heart disease (case 29) with a normal ECG and EPS underwent PM implantation at 32 months due to persistent syncopal episodes in spite of the fact that numerous ECG and Holter recordings failed to detect significant arrhythmias. After PM implantation, the patient continues to complain of the same clinical picture.

Discussion

Given the wide variety of causes of syncope, the sensitivity of EPS for detecting its etiology largely depends on the selection of the study group.

Our study group was made of patients mainly referred for electrophysiological evaluation by the Internal Medicine and Cardiology Services of two hospitals. All the possible candidates for study were submitted to a careful clinical investigation and noninvasive laboratory tests. Patients whose preliminary evaluation suggested extracardiac cause of the syncope as well as those in whom 'significant arrhythmias' (see Material and methods) were detected were excluded. Heart disease or ECG abnormalities were present in 27 cases (75%) in the series. Given the selection method, the group was composed of patients in whom the syncope was suspected of having an arrhythmic origin, but this had not been demonstrated by noninvasive methods.

The protocol of the EPS was designed to detect the arrhythmias most often implicated in the syncope: ventricular arrhythmia, paroxysmal AV block, and sinus node dysfunction. Addition of the ajmaline test [8] and autonomic pharmacological blockade [9, 10] should improve the sensitivity of EPS to detect the later two causes. Likewise, certain causes of supraventricular arrhythmias (presence of occult accessory bundles, intranodal reentry, etc.) should be easily identified with this protocol.

A general problem of this type of studies is the eventual lack of correlation between the electrophysiological findings and the clinical symptoms. Indeed, the arrhythmias induced in the laboratory often do not reproduce the syncope, and on the other hand some severe arrhythmias that are induced on EPS may not appear spontaneously. The solution to this problem is difficult since spontaneous arrhythmias are often undocumented. Nonetheless, some general principles should aid in the interpretation of results:
a) Only arrhythmias or electrophysiological abnormalities capable of producing clinical symptoms should be considered.
b) In the evaluation of the electrophysiological abnormalities, its relation to the spontaneous production of arrhythmias observed in clinico-electrocardiographic series should be taken into consideration.
c) For ethical reasons the natural course of these patients cannot be studied.

Thus, once the treatment indicated on the basis of the EPS is prescribed the clinical cause constitutes the most adequate guide for interpreting the EPS results.

Paroxysmal AV block is a frequent cause of syncope in Stokes-Adams crisis. In these cases the block is almost always located in the His-Purkinje system. It is generally conceded that detection of conduction disorders at this level, such as truncal block or prolongation of the HV interval, in patients with syncope is an indication for PM implantation [12]. However, in an earlier study 73 patients with intraventricular conduction disorders (IVCD) and documented intermittent AV block we found that in 37% there were HV intervals of 55 ms or less between crises, while only 46% presented HV intervals of more than 60 msec [13, 14]. In accordanc with previous studies [8], the ajmaline test increases the sensitivity of EPS for detecting intermittent AV block, with second or third degree infrahisian block or HV interval lengthening of 100% being the most valuable criteria for positivity. In the present study, a case of truncal block was detected and a PM was implanted, the patient remaining asymptomatic. Of the 16 patients with IVCD an HV interval of more than 65 msec was detected in 6 (all of whom had a positive ajmaline test), and an HV under 65 msec was found in 10, in 4 of them with a positive ajmaline test (in one of these cases ventricular tachycardia was detected and included in the group). PM was implanted in every patient with a basal HV over 65 msec and a positive ajmaline test. In the follow-up of this group one patient with associated ischemic heart disease died suddenly and two died of left ventricular failure.

Induction of sustained or nonstained monomorphic ventricular tachycardia (always superior to 15 beats in our cases) was considered significant. With protocols that use single or double ventricular extrastimuli, like that of our study, this type of arrhythmia generally is not induced in patients who do not present them spontaneously [15–17]. Although it cannot be categoricaly stated that these arrhythmias are the cause of syncope, in the absence of other anomalies they seem to be the most probable cause and provide an indication for treatment. The evolution observed in this group supports this hypothesis. Syncope was abolished with antiarrhythmic treatment (in one case associated with PM implantation) in 5 of the 7 cases (although one died early because of irreversible left ventricular failure). Of the other two, one presented a syncopal episode at 29 months in spite of the fact that antiarrhythmic treatment indicated to be effective by the study had been given. The other patient, for whom an effective drug could not be found, died suddenly at 6 months.

In our study, 9 patients were diagnosed as having sinus node dysfunction due to carotid sinus hypersensitivity. In 3 cases the hypersensitivity was 'pure' and in 3 it was associated with sinus node dysfunction. Pharmacologic autonomic blockade tests allowed detection of 2 cases of sinus node dysfunction with normal basal EPS. In cases of sinus node dysfunction, there is not always a direct relation between the electrophysiological anomalies detected and the importance of the symptoms. The variability in sinus node response to diverse situations that modify the vegetative tone can partially explain these discrepancies. In any case, electrophysiological diagnosis of sinus node dysfunction even in the absence of other anomalies strongly suggests it as the cause of the syncope. In 6 of our cases of sinus node dysfunction 3 were treated with PM implantation and 3 with medication, and no syncopal episodes have appeared during follow-up. Of the 3 cases with 'pure' carotid sinus hypersensitivity treated with PM implantation only one still presents symptoms.

Supraventricular tachyarrhythmias are less frequently a cause of syncope than ventricular tachyarrhythmias. In this study, only the cases in which induction of the arrhythmia produced syncope or minor equivalents were considered diagnostic. In the 2 cases in this group treatment suppressed the symptoms. Nonetheless, another case with tachycardia due to nodal reentry that was considered nonsignificant because of its low rate and good tolerance is also asymptomatic with antiarrhythmic treatment.

In our series EPS was considered to be diagnostic of the cause of syncope in 77% of the cases. In previous studies (Table 3), the sensitivity of these studies has been estimated from 17% to 68% [5–7, 18]. The lowest sensitivity (17%) was observed in the series of Gulamhussein et al. [18], who studied patients with syncope or presyncope and excluded cases with heart disease or with some electrocardiographic anomaly. Given these premises, a large number of cases of syncope of extracardiac origin must have been included which accounts for the low sensitivity of the EPS. In other reports [5–7] the sensitivity of the diagnostic studies ranged between 56% and 68% lower to that obtained in our study. These series also differ from ours in the distribution of the possible causes of syncope. Indeed, in these studies, cases with ventricular arrhythmia predominate and those suggestive of paroxysmal AV block are scarce. These differences could be due to:

Table 3. Results of EPS in patients with syncope of unknown origin.

Series	No of cases	VT	Diagnoses (% of cases)				Est. + (%)
			SVT	ND	pAVB	Others	
DiMarco et al. [5]	25	36	–	4	16	16	68
Hess et al. [6]	32	34	–	15	3	3	56
Gulamhussein et al. [18]	34	–	9	9	–	–	17
Akthar et al. [7]	30	36	–	13	3	–	53
Present study	36	19	5	16	27	8	77

VT: ventricular tachycardia; SVT: supraventricular tachyccardia; ND: nodal disease; pAVB: paroxysmal AV block.

a) Differences in the study protocol. As such, utilization of the ajmaline and autonomic block tests in our study should increase the diagnostic capability for cases of paroxysmal AV block and sinus node dysfunction, respectively. In a study like that of Hess et al. [6], the use of three ventricular extrastimuli should increase the incidence of induction of ventricular tachycardia.

b) Differences in the composition of the different series. Of the 28 patients in whom the EPS were considered diagnostic 23 (8%) had some type of heart disease or anomalies in the basal ECG whereas of the 8 patients with negative study results only 4 presented this type of anomaly.

Altogether, it can be concluded that

a) EPS are useful in the diagnosis and therapy of patients with syncope of unknown origin, particularly in those with heart disease or basal ECG changes; and

b) the use of pharmacological provocation tests (ajmaline test, autonomic blockade) increases the sensitivity of the EPS.

Summary

Electrophysiological studies (EPS) were performed in 36 patients with syncope of unknown cause despite a careful clinical investigation. EPS led to a presumptive diagnosis in 28 patients (77%). Paroxysmal AV block was suspected in 10 patients (27%) because there was a prolonged HV interval, splitting of the hisian potential or a positive ajmaline test. In 7 patients (19%), paroxysmal monomorphous ventricular tachycardia was produced that was sustained in 5 cases and nonsustained in 2. Six cases (16%) had sinus node dysfunction and 3 (8%) had a hypersensitive carotid sinus. Finally, in 2 cases (5%) supraventricular tachycardia associated with presyncopal symptoms was induced.

In all these cases therapy was based on EPS results, and the clinical follow-up (mean of 19 ± 18 months) suggested that in every case the presumptive EPS diagnosis was correct.

Of the 28 cases with diagnostic EPS, 23 had some type of heart disease or anomalies in the basal ECG. In contrast, of 8 patients with negative studies, only 4 presented anomalies. We conclude that:

a) EPS are useful in the diagnosis and therapy of syncope of unknown cause, particularly in patients with heart disease;

b) the addition of pharmacologic provocation tests (ajmaline, autonomic blockade) increases the diagnostic sensitvity of the EPS.

References

1. Wright KE, McIntosh HD: Syncope: a review of pathophysiological mechanisms. Prog Cardiovasc Dis 1971; 13: 580–594.
2. Friedberg CK: Syncope: pathological physiology: differential diagnosis and treatment. Mod Concepts Cardiovasc Dis 1971; 40: 55–63.
3. Kapoor WN, Karpf M, Wieand S, Paterson JR, Levey GS: A prospective evaluation and follow-up of patients with syncope. H Engl J Med 1983; 309: 197–204.
4. Lown B: Cardiovascular collapse and sudden cardiac death. In: E Braunwald (ed) Heart disease. A textbook of cardiovascular medicine. WB Saunders, Philadelpohia, 1980; 778–817.
5. DiMarco SP, Garau H, Hartorne W, Ruskin SN: Intracardiac electrophysiologic techniques in recurrent syncope of unknown cause. Ann Intern Med 1981; 95: 542–548.
6. Hess DS, Morady F, Schieman MM: Electrophysiologic testing in the evaluation of patients with syncope of undetermined origin. Am J Cardiol 1982; 50: 1309–1315.
7. Akhtar M, Shenasa M, Denker S, Gilbert CJ, Riswi N: Role of cardiac electrophysiologic studies in patients with unexplained recurrent syncope. Pace 1983; 6: 192–201.
8. Sanjuan R, García Civera R, Morell S et al.: Valor del test de ajmalina en la detección del bloqueo AV intermitente. Rev Esp Cardiolog 1982; 35: 259–264.
9. Jordan JL, Yamaguchi I, Mandel WJ: Studies of the mechanism of sinus node dysfunction in the sick sinus syndrome. Circulation 1978; 57: 217–223.
10. Jose AD: Effect of combined sympathetic and parasympathetic blockade on heart rate and cardiac function in man. Am J Cardiol 1966; 18: 476–478.
11. Horowitz LN, Josephson ME, Farshidei A, Spielman SR, Michelson EL, Greenspan AH: Recurrent sustained ventricular tachycardia. 3. Role of the electrophysiologic study in selection of antiarrhythmic regimens. Circulation 1978; 58: 986–997.
12. Scheinman MM, Peters RW, Suac MJ et al.: Value of the HQ interval in patient with bundle branch block and the role of prophylactic permanent pacing. Am J Cardiol 1982; 50: 1316–1324.
13. Cabades A, Sanjuan R, García Civera R, Ferrando C, Ruano M, Segui J: Valor del intervalo HV en la detección del bloqueo AV intermitente. Rev Latina de Cardiolog 1981; 2: 123–130.
14. Sanjuan R, García Civera R, Cabades A, Ferrando C, Segui J, Ruano M: Intraventricular conduction time (HV interval) in the detection of intermittent AV block. In: Feruglio GA (ed) Cardiac pacing: electrophysiology and pacemaker technology. Piccin Medical Books, 1982.
15. Vandelpol CL, Farshidi A, Spielman et al.: Incidence and clinical significance of induced ventricular tachycardia. Am J Cardiol 1980; 45: 725–731.
16. Livelli FD, Bigger JTh, Reiffel JA et al.: Response to programmed ventricular stimulation: sensitively, specificity and relation to heart disease. Am J Cardiol 1982; 50: 452–458.
17. Brugada P, Green M, Abdollah H, Wellens HJJ: Significance of ventricular arrhythmias initiated by programmed ventricular stimulation: the importance of type of ventricular arrhythmia induced and the number of premature stimuli required. Circulation 1984; 69: 87–92.
18. Gulamhussein S, Nacarelli GV, Ko PT et al.: Value and limitations of clinical electrophysiologic study in assessment of patients with unexplained syncope. Am J Med 1982; 73: 700–705.

4.3 Tachylog P43 in the Control of Tachyarrhythmias

E. SOWTON, P.M. HOLT and J.C.P. CRICK

Introduction

In patients with paroxysmal tachycardias, drug treatment may be ineffective or produce unacceptable side effects. In this situation an implantable pacemaker capable of rapidly terminating tachyarrhythmias is an attractive therapeutic alternative.

The Tachylog P43 unit (Siemens Elema AB, Stockholm, Sweden) is an implantable single chamber multiprogrammable pulse generator designed for the elective termination of tachycardias as well as bradycardias. It can be used with either atrial or ventricular electrodes, and may be fully automatic or patient-activated. Early units were unipolar but more recent generators can be programmed to unipolar or bipolar modes.

On distinguishing a pathological from a physiological tachycardia, one of four anti-tachycardia programmes are available for its termination:

1. *Critical fixed time stimulation or burst stimulation.* This delivers a sequence of a fixed programmable number of stimuli. The first 16 intervals are programmable independently of each other.
2. *Self-searching.* From 1–5 pulses are emitted. If unsuccessful, the interval(s) of the next attempt will be adjusted. If the unsuccessful attempt resulted in a reset of the tachycardia the interval(s) are decreased next time. Otherwise the interval(s) are increased within programmable limits. The sequence of stimuli that prove successful are used first with the next tachycardia.
3. *Adaptive table scanning.* Up to five sets of timing for stimuli can be programmed. When a tachycardia is detected impulses from the first set of the table are delivered. If unsuccessful the second set are used, and so on down the table. If the final timings fail to terminate the tachycardia then a searh will be initiated until successful timings are found. These intervals are then entered at the top of the table and the bottom set erased.
4. *Centrifugal scanning.* This utilises a table of impulses, the timing of which is based upon the tachycardia cycle length. If the first attempt fails, the beat

stimuli are taken from the row above the first in the table, and then from the row below, and so on. If unsuccessful the search may be continued with single, double or triple extra stimuli.

In all programmes the total number of searches to be made ranges from 0–256 (infinite) attempts. Having terminated the tachycardia the memory function of the Tachylog records the tachycardia rate, whether the attempt was successful or not and the total number of attempts made. This memory function is an excellent objective method of assessing the efficiency of the chosen programme. Additionally, the generator has an interactive mode (AAT/VVT) which allows non-invasive electrophysiology studies to be performed at any time after implanting the unit.

Programming is carried out with an HP 85 computer and a Siemens interface. This is also used to interrogate the memory.

Patients

Tachylog generators have been implanted in 17 patients since December, 1982. There are nine males and eight females whose ages ranged from 17–66 years (mean 40 years). Twelve had Wolf-Parkinson-White syndrome with L-sided accessory pathways, three patients had ventricular tachycardia and two patients had dual AV nodal pathways.

One patient had had aortic valve disease and required aortic valve replacement, one had undergone complete repair of Fallot's tetralogy and a third patient had a mild dilated cardiomyopathy.

All patients had a history of frequent palpitation, requiring multiple hospital admissions. Eight had had syncopal attacks. Drug therapy (includig amiodarone) had been ineffective or produced severe side effects. Extensive electrophysiological investigation was performed in all patients prior to implantation.

Results

Fourteen unipolar and thre bipolar units have been implanted in the 17 patients. Ten patients have electrodes positioned in the right ventricle (RV), (two with epicardial leads), one has a left ventricular epicardial electrode, and in one patient the electrode originally positioned in the coronary sinus displaced to the RV. The remaining five patients have right atrial electrodes. Positioning of the pacing wire was critical in this latter group, requiring a site producing a suitably large atrial electrogram for reliable sensing, and from which tachycardias could be repeatedly and efficiently terminated using the minimum number of stimuli.

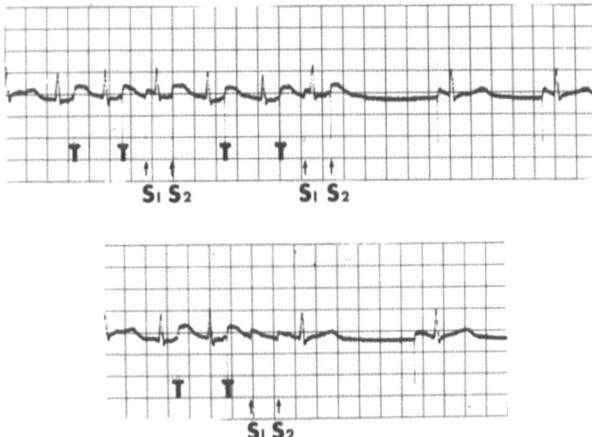

Fig. 1. The top tracing illustrates the first attempt to terminate this patient's orthodromic reentry tachycardia, using the self-searching mode. The successful intervals are memorised and the second tachycardia is stopped first time. T = atrial tracking signal; S_1, S_2 = the two extra stimuli.

Termination programmes

As previously described [1] the termination 'window' of a tachycardia varies greatly with posture and exercise. In 14 patients tachycardia termination was reliably achieved by two extra stimuli, and in one patient, by three stimuli, in one four stimuli, and in one man burst overdrive was used because of a very narrow termination zone on exercise. Fourteen patients were programmed to self-searching mode (Fig. 1), two had the adaptive table scanning programma and one had burst overdrive, as described above.

The time to termination ranged from a few seconds at rest in most patients, to 1–2 minutes on exercise in some.

Long-term outcome

Follow-up time ranges from 2–17 months (mean approximately eight months). Two patients with WPW syndrome developed atrial fibrillation with ventricular rates over 300/minute and have required surgical division of their accessory pathway. Eleven patients are controlled by the Tachylog alone and four require additional drug therapy for complete control.

In all patients the Tachylog generator rapidly terminates most episodes of tachycardia, with considerable symptomatic benefit. There is high patient acceptance

Complications

The most common complication has been myopotential sensing. In two patients, both young and very active, this has produced an increase in the frequency of their tachycardias due to the generation of inappropriate stimuli. These tachycardias are correctly terminated by the generator but nevertheless mean that these patients curtail their physical activity. Both these men are awaiting implantation of bipolar units.

Myopotential sensing has been a slight problem in a further six patients with unipolar units.

Four bipolar units have been implanted, three in patiens with atrial electrodes. In two of these the sensing characteristics are insufficient for reliable identification of the trial electrogram, and these units have required programming to the unipolar mode.

There has been no infection, perforation or other complication in patients with implanted Tachylogs.

Discussion

Moe et al. [2] in 1963, laid the foundation for the modern clinical use of the cardiac pacemaker with their experimental work on dogs. Subsequently electrophysiology studies have firmly established the role of re-entry in SVT [3] and VT [4] and the vulnerability of such arrhythmias to appropriately timed electrical stimuli [5].

Implantable pacemakers capable of delivering critically timed stimuli have recently been developed, followed by units that were capable of changing the intervals of their stimuli, depending upon the tachycardia response [6].

The Tachylog is a sophisticated generator with four tachycardia termination modes. It has proved successful in the management of re-entry tachycardias in 17 patients. Only four required additional drug therapy. In all patients most tachycardias are rapidly terminated, resulting in considerable symptomatic benefit. Most of our patients have been freed from the necessity to take drugs, and none need carry a magnet to activate their system.

Patients are extremely pleased with their generators which in nearly all cases have allowed them to lead normal lives.

Sensing problems have been encountered with unipolar and bipolar systems, but further modifications should produce significant improvements in the near future.

Summary

The Tachylog P43 generator is an implantable single chamber, multiprogrammable pacemaker capable of functioning as an anti-tachyardia unit or VVI bradycardia pacemaker.

It has been implanted in 17 patients, nine males and eight females whose ages ranged from 17–66 years, for control of their paroxysmal tachycardias. Twelve had Wolf-Parkinson-White syndrome with orthodromic tachycardias, two had dual AV nodal pathways and three had ventricular tachycardia. Unipolar units have been implanted in 14 and bipolar units in three patients.

Programmes of two extra stimuli were employed in 14 patients, three extra stimuli in one patient, four in extra stimuli in one, while the remaining patient is now controlled by burst overdrive.

The tachycardias of 11 patients are completely controlled by the pacemaker alone, while four patients are controlled by the P43 plus drug therapy. Self-searching mode is employed in 12 of these patients, adaptive table scanning in two, and burst overdrive in one. Two patients with WPW syndrome developed AF with ventricular rates over 300/minute and required surgical division of their accessory pathway.

Myopotential sensing is a significant problem in two patients with unipolar units, while atrial sensing has been unreliable in two patients with bipolar units.

However tachycardias in all patients with the Tachylog generator are rapidly controlled, and patient acceptance is high.

References

1. Crick JCP, Way B, Kappenberger L, Sowton E: Variation in tachycardia termination window with posture and exercise. Proceedings of the 2nd European Symposium on Cardiac Pacing. In: Feruglio GA (ed) Cardiac pacing: electrophysiology and pacemaker technology. Piccin Medical Books, 1982; 273–276.
2. Moe GK, Cohen W, Vick RL: Experimentally induced paroxysmal AV nodal tachycardia in the dog. Am Heart J 1963; 65: 87.
3. Wit AL, Goldreyr BN, Damato AN: An in-vitro model of paroxysmal supraventricular tachyardia. Circulation 1971; 43: 862.
4. Wellens HJJ, Schuilenberg RM, Durrer D: Electrical stimulation of the heart in the study of ventricular tachycardias. Circulationn 1972; 46: 216.
5. Kappenberger L, Sowton E: Programmed stimulation for long term treatment and non-invasive investigation of recurrent tachycardia. Lancet 1981; 1: 909–914.
6. Sowton E: A self-searching tachycardia pacemaker. Proc Br Card Soc Autumn Meeting. Br Hear J 1981; 45: 340–341.

4.4 Control of the Pacemaker Patient

S. BOTELLASOLANA, J. OLAGUE DE ROS, L. INSA PEREZ,
J. AGUILAR BOTELLA, R. GARCÍA CIVERA and
V. LOPEZ MERINO

From the moment that a permanent pacemaker is implanted in a patient, three types of periodic reviews should be initiated:
a) primary level, under the care of the family physician;
b) secondary level, under supervision of the cardiologist; and
c) third level, in a hospital unit for pacemaker control.
Attention to the pacemaker carrier should be oriented towards:
a) confirmation of correct pacemaker function with verification of the different analyzable parameters:
b) detection of the first signs of failure of the power source;
c) evaluation of the state of the heart; and
d) reintegration of the patient into normal life.
The rhythm of the pacemaker control should be greater during the first 6 weeks of postimplantation, since this is the time it usually takes to stablize stimulation thresholds. After the sixth week, controls are more spaced until the first indications of failure are detected, thus requiring a closer monitoring until the decision to replace the generator has been taken. Nonetheless, our criterion is that the maximum time between two successive controls be no more than 6 months and in no case should it exceed a year.

In each pacemaker control a predetermined routine must be followed (Fig. 1) to allow the necessary tests to reach a correct diagnosis of possible pacemaker dysfunction and for detection of latent failure.

Diagnostic analysis of pacemaker malfunction leading to arrhythmia can be based on *alterations in spike emission, stimulation defects or sensing failures*. These three functional defects may be isolated or in association, although because of their importance separate consideration will be given to each of them.

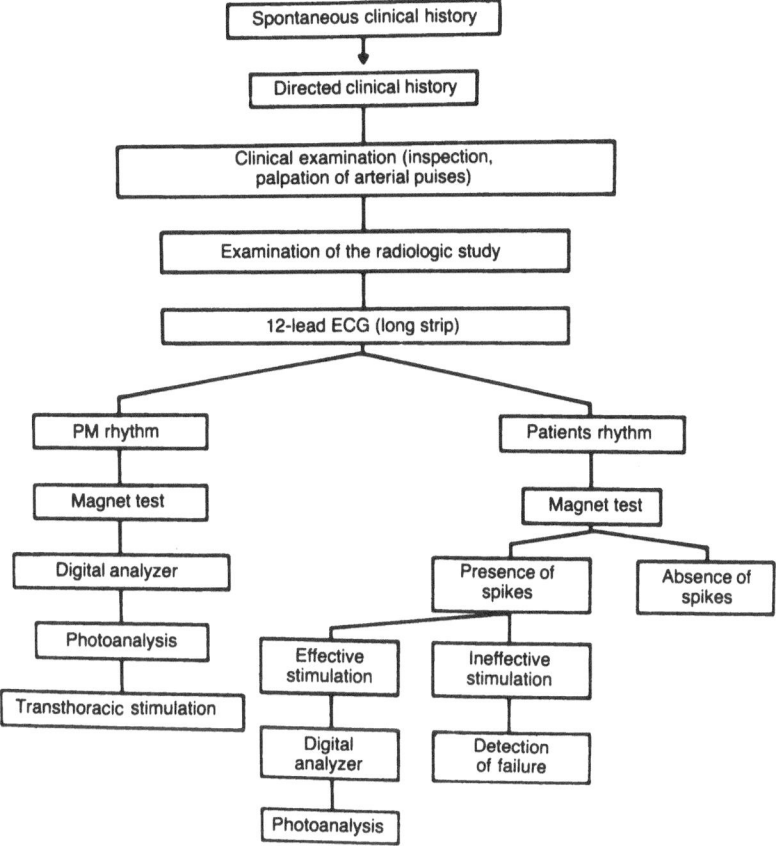

Fig. 1. Control routine for the pacemaker carrier.

Alterations in spike emission under the effects of the magnet test

Total absence of spikes

If this appears during the magnet test, it means that there is a failure in the power source or in the generator-cathether-patient electrical circuit. The solution for either of these situations is surgical; in the former case by substitution of the generator, and in the later by checking the electrical connections or substituting the electrode catheter.

Irregularities in spike emission

Under the effects of the magnet test, irregularities in spike emission suggest the existence of a malfunction in some circuit component or intermittent loss

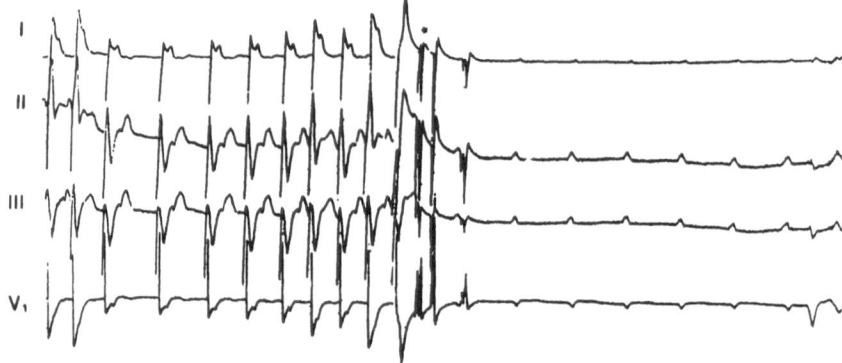

Fig. 2. Acceleration of pacemaker rate or 'runaway'.

of continuity in the stimulation system. Here, it is also important to know the variations in behavior of different demand generators in response to the magnet test to avoid a false diagnosis of malfunction.

Change in spike frequency

This may consist of acceleration or slowing. Slowing is always related to progressive power source failure. *Runaway* frequency acceleration [1–2] may be due to depletion of the power source or alteration in the timing circuit and is easy to diagnose because the stimulation rhythm exceeds the maximum threshold imposed by the refractory period of the device (Fig. 2). The clinical situation can be serious and may require sectioning the catheter to halt stimulation [3]; an external pacemaker should be implanted before doing this.

Spikes that do not induce myocardial depolarization (stimulation failure)

The causes of stimulation failure will be discussed in the following.

Increase in the stimulation threshold

If the stimulation failure appears soon after pacemaker implantation it may be due to an acute local reaction (maturation of the stimulation point), and if it is late to perielectrode fibrosis. In cases such as acute myocardial infarction, metabolic or water-electrolyte disorders, correction of the underlying cause usually suffices to restore stimulation effectiveness [4]. In the other situations, if the generator is not energy programmable, the catheter should be implanted in another point or the generator substituted by a higher voltage one.

Displacement of the electrode catheter

This originates inefficient stimulation and depends on the greater or lesser flexibility of the electrode catheter. Displacement at the level of the right ventricle usually takes place in the first month after implantation, although instances of late displacement at sixteen months have been reported [5].

Electrocardiographically this situation usually presents as a permanent or intermittent stimulation failure. If the right ventricular wall is perforated the stimulation failure is usually associated with diaphragmatic contractions simultaneous with the pacemaker discharge. If the electrode slips into the left ventricle there will be an electrocardiographical morphology of right bundle branch block. In every case the treatment is reimplantation of the catheter. The diagnosis of displacement can be confirmed by a radiologic study.

Detection failure (sensing failure)

Incorporation of an electronic sensing circuit to interrupt stimulation under certain conditions is accompanied by the risk of provoking untimely apparatus recycling. The causes for this are diverse, for example, external interferences, such as electromagnetic fields, or may proceed from the stimulation system itself.

The sensing circuit's design means that it is sensitive to determined signals, specifically to autonomic cardiac depolarization, both atrial and ventricular. In general, the conditions necessary for sensing a signal are the following [6]:
a) an amplitude greater than the nominal amplitude of the sensor circuit;
b) a slope that can be sensed, and
c) occurrence outside the refractory period.

Detection defects (undersensing)

This occurs when a pacemaker is incapable of detecting autonomic cardiac complexes. This may happen in *battery failure* because the sensor circuit does not receive sufficient voltage to be activated by spontaneous ventricular complexes.

Another sensing malfunction may result from a *permanent or intermittent block of the plate interruptor*. The electrocardiographical recording of this malfunction translates into the appearance of a shorter cycle than would correspond to basal pacemaker frequency and coincides with the value of the magnetic cycle (Fig. 3). The cause of this phenomenon is spontaneous and sporadic approximation of the magnetic interruptor plates, which situates the

Paper speed 50 mm/sec

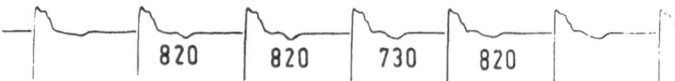

820   820   730   820

Fig. 3. Intermittent block of the plate interruptor. Observe the reduction in the 4th cycle (730 msec), corresponding to the magnetic frequency of this device, in relation to the nominal interval (820 msec).

pacemaker in asynchronic mode. The diagnosis is easy when the magnetic frequency is superior to the basal frequency, but if this is not the case it can be diagnosed by the presence of a competitive rhythm between autonomous contractions and electroinductive complexes.

However, the sensing defects most often observed in clinical practice are those due to *autonomic complexes with insufficient amplitude and/or slope to activate the sensor circuit of the pacemaker* (Fig. 4).

Diagnosis will be confirmed by an electrogram recording of the chamber where the electrode catheter is placed and by studying the characteristics of the sensitivity curve of the implanted generator. Treatment consists in changing the device or placing the catheter at another point where there is a greater difference of potential and/or autonomic complex inscription slope. Finally, another cause of sensing failure due to malfunction is an *abnormally long generator refractory period.* Only if the pacemaker is multiprogrammable for

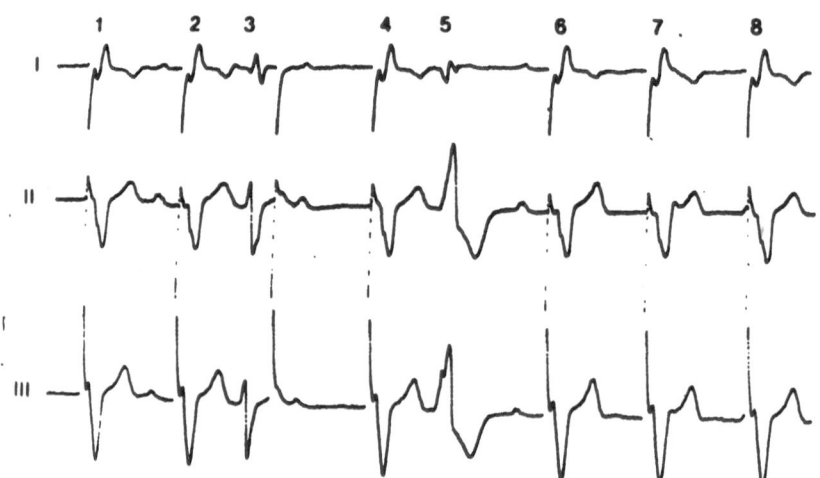

Fig. 4. The third beat with right bundle branch block and left anterior hemiblock morphology is not detected by the pacemaker, in contrast with the fifth beat with right deviation of the electrical axis that is sensed by the generator because it has sufficient amplitude and/or slope.

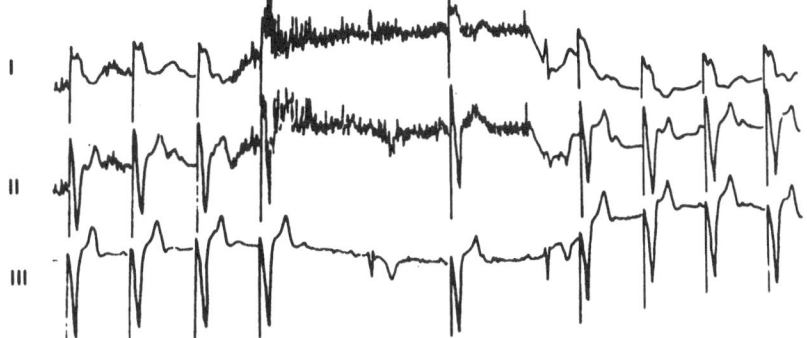

Fig. 5. Temporary inhibition of the pacemaker due to myopotentials.

this parameter can the problem be resolved by external programming; otherwise, treatment consists in changing the generator.

Excessive detection (oversensing)

This malfunction practically only occurs in monopolar pacemakers and consists in the abnormal detection of signals other than those of the QRS complex. The diagnoses is based on the presence of abnormally long cycles of variable duration that disappear under the effects of the magnet. The most frequent causes are described below.

Detection of myopotentials

Described by various authors [7–8], it has been found that its incidence can reach 69% in Holter system studies [9]. It is produced after muscular contraction, generally of the pectorals covering the generator. If these contractions attain higher potentials than the nominal value of the sensing circuit, they are sensed by it and a more or less long pacemaker recycling is produced (Fig. 5). The diagnosis is easily made by electrocardiographic control while the patient isometrically contracts the pectoral covering the generator. Treatment depends on the type of pacemaker. If it is multiprogrammable sensitivity should be reduced or the stimulation mode changed to VVT. If it is not, the generator should be changed.

Detection of the T wave

This is another cause of VVI demand pacemaker recycling. It is due to excessive sensing circuit sensitivity to slow signals together with a short refractory period.

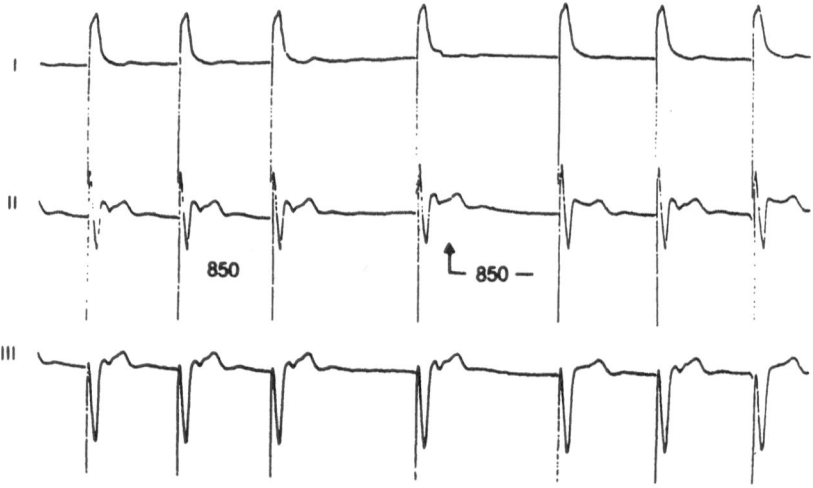

Fig. 6. Recycling on the T wave. Observe that the escape interval from the T wave is identical to the automatic one (850 msec).

The diagnosis is confirmed if the initiation of the escape interval coincides with that of the T wave (Fig. 6). This disorder does not usually produce syncopal symptomatology, but a slowing of the heart rate. Treatment involves changing the generator or, if it is programmable for refractory period and sensitivity, to increase the refractory period and decrease the sensitivity. Sometimes both parameters will have to be adjusted.

Detection of postpotentials

This is an infrequent malfunction produced by generator discharge that produces a high continuous current potential in the electromyocardial interphase which, when dissipated in the form of voltage, receives the name of 'postpotential phenomenon'. If the postpotentials surpass the refractory period in duration and the stimulation threshold in voltage, recycling will occur.

Detection of abnormal phenomena

Incomplete fracture of the conducting wire

This is characterized by intermittent contacts between the fractured terminals that produce abrupt changes in resistance at this level and changes in voltage between the pacemaker anode and cathode. This generates false signals that are detected by the sensor circuit and cause unneeded pacemaker recycling

[10, 11]. The electrocardiogram shows an irregular spike duration, equal to or greater than the sum of the base cycle and the value of the refractory period of the pacemaker.

The radiologic diagnosis is not easy, and the magnet test should always be performed [11], as well as an oscilloscopic study which will reveal by photoanalysis the variability of spike morphology in each successive cycle. The catheter should be changed.

Electrical leak syndrome

This concept was introduced by Fontaine [12], and consists in the sporadic detection and stimulation failures with variations in spike amplitude and changes in the electrical axis. These express electricity loss at some point of the conducting wire (erosion of the catheter sheath or loss of isolation at the level of the connector system) (Fig. 7).

Treatment always requires a surgical review of the stimulation system followed by a therapeutic decision that can range from changing the catheter to a simple repair of the leak with silicone.

Special problems in pacemaker control

Pacemaker dependence

There is general awareness of the depression produced after stimulation of subsidiary autonomic cardiac foci and its relation with the frequency of the stimulation used [13]. The emission of weak external stimuli applied to the chest wall of patients carrying demand pacemakers, known as the transthorac-

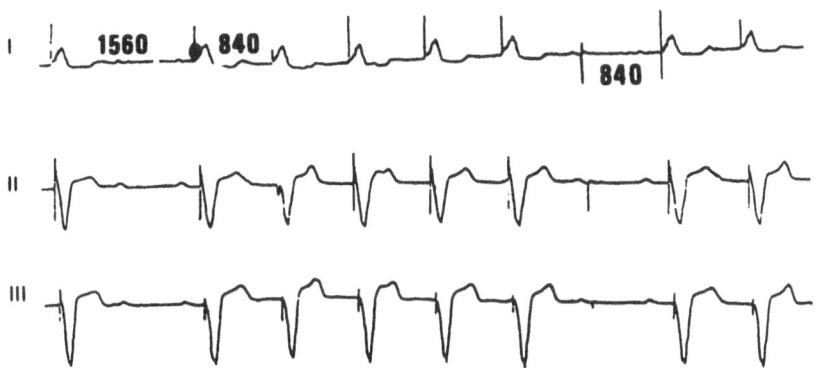

Fig. 7. ECG tracing that presents intermittent variations of the electrical axis of spikes with occasional stimulation and sensing failure. These alterations point out to an electrical leak.

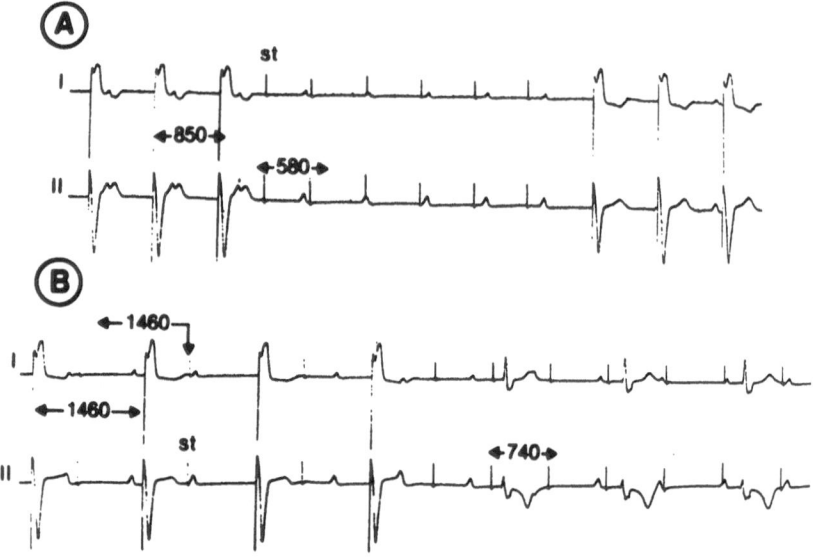

Fig. 8. Panel A: transthoracic inhibition of a demand pacemaker at 850 msec interval (70 bpm) producing ventricular asystolia and requiring cessation of external stimulation. *Panel B:* reduction of the stimulation rate of the pacemaker by means of transthoracic stimulation at 1460 msec (41 bpm) and the abrupt passage of the external stimulation to a rate greater than the nominal one (which will inhibit it permanently) induces the appearance of an escape rhythm.

ic external stimulation phenomenon, allows identification or not of a protective escape rhythm (Fig. 8A). Its absence requires careful observation of the patient, especially in the control sessions that reveal battery failure. In frequency-programmable pacemakers, frequency should be set as low as possible, since the appearance of the first spontaneous cycles is inversely related to stimulation frequency. In standard, or nonprogrammable, pacemakers, slow frequencies can be obtained by external stimulation at equally slow frequencies (cycles longer than the sum of the automatic interval and the duration of the stimulation refractory period). After 2–3 minutes of slowed pacemaker frequency, a sudden change in the external frequency to one greater than the nominal pacemaker frequency will inhibit it permanently (Fig. 8B).

Pacemaker-induced arrhythmia

The VOO or fixed rhythm pacemakers generally produce competition between the rhythm of the patient and the rhythm generated by the pacemaker. On rare occasions ventricular tachycardia or fibrillation can be induced as a result of the pacemaker stimulus falling in vulnerable ventricular period, that

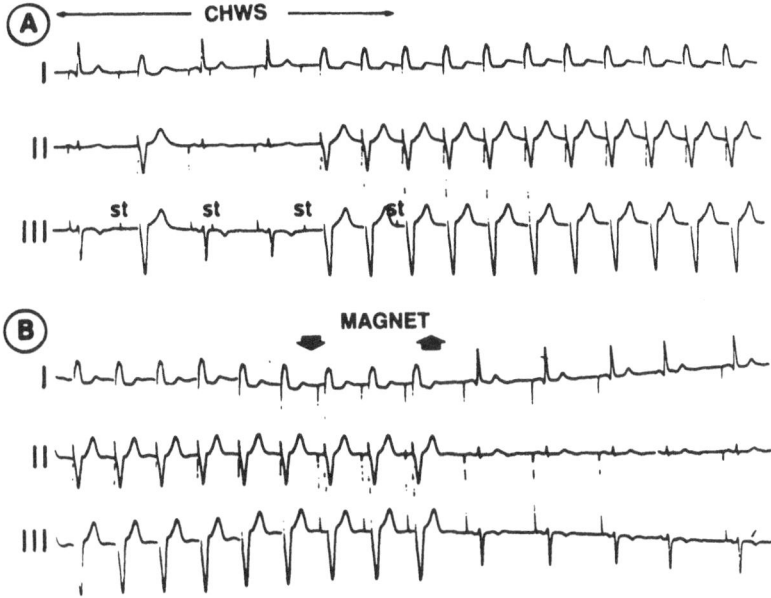

Fig. 9. Transthoracic stimulation provocation of closed loop tachycardia in a DDD generator. Use of the magnet produces an AV stimulation at a fixed rhythm which induces cessation of the tachycardia.

is, on the T wave of the cardiac cycle [14]. This possibility has disappeared with the introduction of demand stimulation.

With the availability of double chamber stimulation the production of a new type of pacemaker induced arrhythmia ('closed loop tachycardias') has been facilitated [15].

Clinically, closed loop tachycardia can be induced by:
a) premature ventricular contractions;
b) loss of atrial capture;
c) detection of myopotentials; and
d) unconducted premature atrial beats.

The tachycardia is easily interrupted by placing the magnet over the generator and producing a synchronic AV stimulation (Fig. 9). The incidence of these tachycardias has decreased with the new DDD pacemakers, which have longer post ventricular stimulation atrial refractory periods (235 msec) and an anti-bigeminy protection system that disables the timed AV circuit for 342 msec after sensing a second ventricular beat.

Pacemaker syndrome

This term is applied to the appearance of clinical symptoms secondary to ventricular stimulation [16]. Pathophysiologically this is due to the loss of the atrial contribution to cardiac output or to the absence of atrioventricular synchronization. The left atrial contraction contributes to 25–30% of the cardiac output; its absence, as in patients with severe myocardial disease, valvular lesions, acute myocardial infarction or arterial hypertension, can lead to the pacemaker syndrome which is clinically characterized by fatigue, dizziness or vertigo, or even syncope. The treatment in these cases is to restore the physiologic atrioventricular sequence. Ventricular stimulation should be converted into atrial or sequential stimulation, according to the state of the patient's conduction system.

References

1. Odabashian HC, Brown DF: Runaway in a modern generation pacemaker. Pace 1979; 2: 152–155.
2. Santini M, Messina G, Masini V: Intermittent and arrhythmic 'runaway' pacemaker. Pace 1980; 3: 730–732.
3. Bosch R, Fiz LN, Rivas LE, Granena J, Senador G, Paravisini J: Taquicardia paroxística ventricular inducida por marcapaso 'desbocado'. Rev Esp Cardiolog 1975; 28: 601–603.
4. Rubio Alvarez J, Fuster Siebert M, Sierra Quiroga J, Carrera-Carbo F, Garcia Bengoechea JB: Variaciones temporales de los umbrales de estimulación en un paciente en programa de hemodiálisis. Estimulación cardiaca 1980; 1: 9–11.
5. Rubio Alvarez J, Fuster Siebert M, Sierra Quiroga J, Garcia-Bengoechea JB: Desanclaje tardío de electrodo endocárdico: presentación de un caso. Estimulación cardiaca 1981; 2: 247–249.
6. Dodinot B, Buffet J, Meunier JF, Dodinot JL: Defectos de detección. Parte I. Estimulación cardiaca 1980; 1: 38–56.
7. Godin JF, Guiheneuc P, Neumann JL, Dodinot B: Blocage des stimulateurs sentinelles par les potentiels musculaires. Arch Mal Coeur 1974; 11: 1317–1326.
8. Candel JM, Sabatel F, Guerrero JA, Gonzalez R, Galvan J, Rodriguez JJ, Megias M, Marti JL: Inhibición e interferencia de un marcapasos de demanda en un enfermo con hemiparesia espástica. Estimulación cardiaca 1982; 3: 221–227.
9. Breivik K, Ohm OJ: Myopotential inhibition of unipolar QRS-inhibited pacemaker assessed by ambulatory Holter monitoring of the electrocardiogram. Pace 1980; 3: 470–478.
10. Mugica J, Dubois M, Duconge R, Ricordeau G: Inhibition d'un stimulateur à la demande par courant de rupture dans un cas particuliérement typique de fracture d'electrode. Coeur 1977; 8: 875–881.
11. Coumel PH, Mugica J, Barold SS: Demand pacemaker arrhythmias caused by intermittent incomplete electrode fracture. Am J Carciol 1975; 36: 105–109.
12. Fontaine G, Sautel JM, Bonner M, Stoltz J, Grosgogeat Y, Welti JJ: Le syndrome de fuit electrique chez les porteurs de pacemaker. Arch Mal Coeur 1972; 65: 190–196.
13. Cosín J, Gimeno JV, Martin G, Garcia del Jalon P, Lastra L, Baguena J: Respuesta de los marcapasos cardiacos primarios y subsidiarios ante la sobreestimulación. Parte I. Estimulación cardiaca 1980; 1: 40–50.
14. Zoll PM, Weintraub MJ: Safety of competition from fixed rate pacemakers. In: Watanabe Y (ed) Cardiac pacing. Excerpta Medica, Amsterdam 1976; 325–327.

208

15. Furman S, Fisher JD: Endless loop tachycardia in an AV universal (DDD) pacemaker. Pace 1982; 5: 486–489.
16. Otero JE, Bognolo DA, Pollicina F: Síndrome del marcapaso ventricular: fisiopatología, diagnóstico y tratamiento. Estimulación cardiaca 1981; 2: 229–235.

4.5 Conclusions

F. FURLANELLO

At present, pacemaker implantation frequently represents a complex decision-making process to select the specific stimulator type: programmable; single or double-chamber; regulated by biosensors. In an attempt to prevent or interrupt a tachy-arrhythmia, particularly if it is ventricular, the semiautomatic or orthorhythmic system is now available.

The main problem is still clinical, because many ventricular and some supraventricular arrhythmias (such as cardiac preexcitation that threatens to produce atrial desynchronization) can behave unpredictably in time as the electrophysiological properties of the diseased heart change. This is often seen in recurrent sustained postinfarctional ventricular tachycardia and dilated cardiomyopathy.

A new aspect of the problem of electrostimulation is related to one discussed in the preceding round table on the clinical use of implantable defibrillators of the 'catheter cardioverter' or Mirowski type. This makes the decision making process more complex in a given patient.

5. Arterial Hypertension

5.1 Introduction

G. HERGUETA GARCIA DE FUADIANA

Essential arterial hypertension (AH) is one of the main cardiovascular risk factors, along with hypercholesterolemia and tobacco use.

The prevalence of AH varies from one country to another as a result of the influence of diverse factors, since it is considered to be a multifactorial disease with a chronic, almost asymptomatic, evolution. On the basis of numerous epidemiological studies, it has been concluded that the incidence of AH reaches a figure of approximately 18–20% of the world population. It is alarming to think that it is calculated that there are 5 or 6 million hypertensives in Spain and that in relation with age, one fourth of the individuals over 50 years of age in the world are hypertensive, as well as one of every six persons over 30 years and one of every eight over 16. The disease is a modern scourge and must be considered a true community health problem. We agree with Balaguer in stating that any increase in blood pressure, including borderline values, whether systolic or diastolic, and those that are only occasionally raised, bears a risk and that after 50, AH is catalogued as the prime factor: 'AH is the main individual cardiovascular risk factor in the community'.

AH reduces the life expectancy by 10 years, while life expectancy of a hypertensive who is correctly treated is identical to that of the normotensive. Aside from detecting the disease, it now seems that the concept and philosophy of the management of hypertension has changed enormously in the last ten years. This is especially so at the educational level, in view of the fact that treatment should be permanent and lifelong. However, at the 10th Congress of the International Hypertension Society in Interlaken (Switzerland), for the first time mention was made of the possibility of witholding pharmacological treatment in certain hypertensive patients after prolonged control with various drugs. In a randomized study, it was found that 55% of such patients can discontinue their medication.

In the United States, only 16% of hypertensives were controlled in 1962, while in 1982, this figure raised to 70%, as an evidence of the effects of the campaigns developed and the results that can be achieved.

214

The main objective of treating the hypertensive patient is to keep normal blood pressure levels. For this purpose a committee of WHO experts has established pertinent clinical diagnostic and therapeutic criteria.

Two problems presently occupy the forefront with regard to antihypertensive therapy: one is the treatment of mild or moderate hypertension; the other is the treatment of the elderly hypertensive patient. In general there is sufficient justification for treating both, after general non-pharmacological measures have failed and a clinical and functional evaluation of the patient (control of obesity, reduction in salt and alcohol intake, rest, etc.) has been made. With respect to mild hypertension, a joint meeting on the subject celebrated in 1980 (WHO/International Hypertension Society) favored the policy of making new pressure measurements (two more times in a month) and to decide afterwards; medical treatment is only recommended to patients whose diastolic blood pressure remains higher than 180 mm Hg.

One of the reasons for therapy, perhaps the most important, is that, except for coronary heart disease, it prevents cardiovascular complications.

The other problem is treatment of hypertension in the elderly. The arguments center on dosages and selection of drugs without adverse effects, especially orthostatic hypotension and reduction of cardiac output. In the patients systolic pressure should not be lowered to less than 140 since undesirable effects, like cerebral hypoperfusion, can appear.

Guidelines and indications of AH therapy will be reviewed in this meeting, which should be eventually modified in accordance with the new therapeutic arsenal available. In this context, the calcium antagonists, inhibitors of the renin-angiotensin-aldosterone system and the new generation of diuretics must be included.

Generally speaking, the objective in treating AH is an inexpensive monotherapy free of adverse effects.

References

Guidelines for the treatment of mild hypertension: memorandum from a WHO/ISH Meeting. Lancet 1983; 1: 457–458.

The Pooling Project Research Group: Relationship of blood pressure, serum cholesterol, smoking habit, relative weight and ECG abnormalities, incidence of major coronary events. Final report of the Pooling Project. J Chron Dis 1978; 31: 272–302.

Trafford AP, Horn CR, O'Neal H, McGonicle R, Halford L, Evans R: Five years follow-up of effects of treatment of mild and moderate hypertension. Br Med 1981; 282: 1111–1113.

Veterans Administration Cooperative Study Group on Antihypertensive Agents: Effects of treatment on morbidity in hypertension I: Results in patients with diastolic blood pressures averaging 115 through 129 mm Hg. JAMA 1967; 202: 1028–1034.

Veterans Administration Cooperative Study Group on Antihypertensive Agents: Effects of treatment on morbidity in hypertension II: Results in patients with diastolic blood pressure averaging 90 through 114 mm. JAMA 1970; 213: 1143–1152.

5.2 The Value of Treatment in the Prevention of Hypertension Complications

L. THOMÁS ABADAL

Introduction

Arterial hypertension (AH) constitutes the main problem in primary medical practice in most industrialized countries. In England, in 1974, it generated five times more visits to the general practitioner than problems related to diabetes control.

Assuming that 110 mm Hg diastolic pressure (DP) is the lower limit for prescription of treatment and that 90 mm Hg is the lower limit for effecting annual check-ups, it was calculated that in the British population in 1981, at least 4% of males and 5.5% of females between 35 and 64 years could probably prolong their life expectancy and drastically reduce the danger of being handicapped by stroke. Thirty per cent of the individuals in this age group would also require organized care over the years to detect changes in blood pressure that might require the initiation of pharmacological treatment. The complications AH can produce justify an intervention at a primary level.

The growing interest in the direction and control of hypertensive patients in the community is due to both the elevated prevalence of AH in the adult population of most developed countries and to the fact that the majority of epidemiological studies confirm a direct relationship between high blood pressure (BP) and overall mortality, as well as cardiovascular mortality and morbidity (Fig. 1).

The studies carried out by American Insurance companies as well as the cooperative program of detection and followup of hypertension by the American National Heart Lung and Blood Institute [1] and others [2] demonstrate the risk involved with borderline or moderately elevated blood pressure.

Prospective epidemiogical studies have shown the predictive value of both systolic and diastolic BP and even the value of a simple routine determination as indicator of cardiovascular risk. The correlation is direct and significantly increases with age.

216

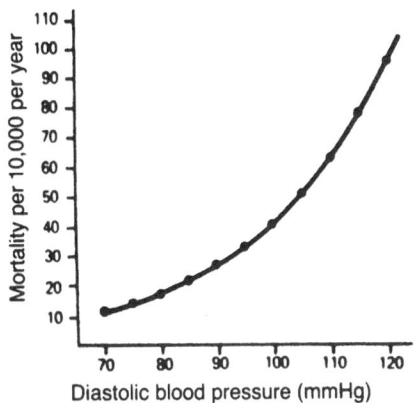

Fig. 1. Function of the risk of mortality and diastolic blood pressure in males of 35–44 years (Framingham Study).

Cardiovascular complications of AH

These may be:
a) Directly related to the BP level.
– Accelerated or malignant form of AH due to fibrinoid necrosis of the renal arteries as a consequence of severe sustained diastolic hypertension.
– Left ventricular failure due to systolic overload.
– Chronic renal insufficiency. Cerebral hemorrhage due to rupture of microaneurysms of the cerebral arterioles.
– Formation and rupture of dissecting aneurysms of the aorta.
b) Indirect: due to acceleration of the arteriosclerotic process.
– Acute myocardial infarction (AMI) and other syndromes of coronary heart disease.
– Aterothrombotic cerebral vascular stroke.
– Intermittent claudication due to trunk involvement and obliteration of the arteries of the lower extremities.
The acceleration of the arterio sclerotic process is probably due to a mechanical factor, adding other factors of coronary risk, mainly hypercholesterolemia and tobacco. The predictive risk of hypertension increases with age, while it decreases with the other factors.

For cerebral arteriosclerotic processes and stroke AH is undoubtedly the most important risk factor of any age.

Epidemiology of the complications of AH

The prospective studies on the complications of different blood pressure levels are based on three types of information:
a) Actuarial data from American insurance companies. These studies involve a large number of individuals for long follow-up periods.

Lew [3] has combined the results of six of these studies, a total of one million persons. These subjects were healthy at the onset of the study and were followed for 10 to 20 years. Those who had a BP of 140/90 mm Hg at the onset were found to have a 50% higher mortality than the average for the whole group. Those with a pressure of 145/95 mm Hg had twice the mortality and those with 160/100 mm Hg had a total mortality that was three times greater than the average rate of all the individuals in the study.

One of the disadvantages of this type of study is that the individuals are selected by socio-economic status, as determined by the fact that they can pay for life insurance. This is important in the case of stroke because the rate of this disease is higher in the poor. In addition, the pressures recorded are underestimated by the fact that the individual interested in being accepted can take drugs to correct hypertension before the examination.
b) Hospital data. Selection criteria vary and the population at risk is rarely defined. The results are very difficult to extrapolate to the general population.
c) Prospective epidemiological data. These are the most reliable data and those most easily applicable to the primary assistance level.

In all these studies the role of hypertension as a risk factor for coronary disease and sudden death is evident. The data obtained in the Framingham study after 10 years follow-up of males between 30 and 39 years demonstrates, using discriminatory function analysis, that hypertension is the third factor in importance after age and tobacco use in the prediction of coronary disease. Coronary artery disease and sudden death constitute a third of all the causes of death for middle-aged males in almost every industrialized society and hypertension contributes greatly to this phenomenon. Since death from coronary causes is more common than death from stroke or injury to other organs, the most frequent fatal complication of hypertension is naturally coronary artery disease. Coronary episodes usually occur 10 years earlier than stroke [4] in the hypertensive population.

These studies also demonstrate that elevation of blood pressure is a much more exact predictive factor for stroke or acute or chronic left ventricular failure than it is for coronary or peripheral arterial disease. In a 14-year follow-up of 387 males and females in the Framingham study, a positive association between systolic hypertension and development of cardiovascular disease was twice as frequent as that of stroke, more than double that of left

218

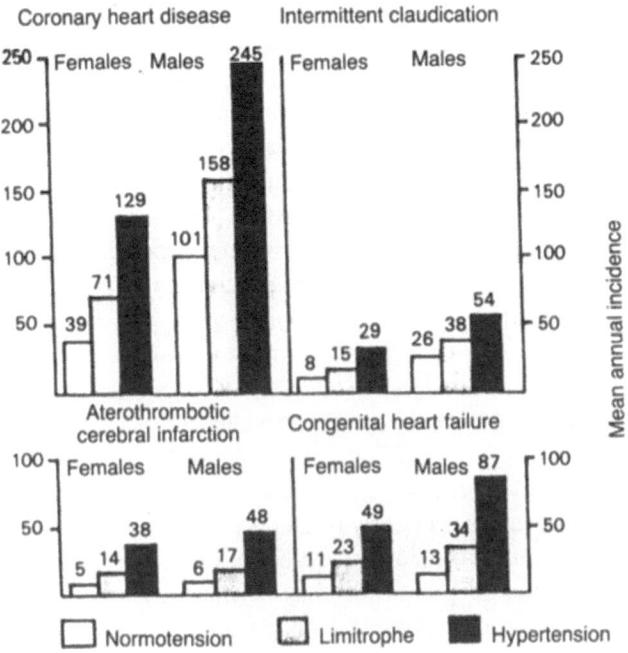

Fig. 2. Risk of morbidity for cardiovascular diseases, adjusted for age, according to the degree of hypertension in each biannual examination. Males and females of 45–74 years. (Framingham Study: 18 years' follow-up.) Statistical significance: p = 0.01.

ventricular failure and one-and-a-half times that of intermittent claudication. This association was much less marked in coronary artery disease [5] (Fig. 2).

Coronary artery disease, the most frequent cause of death in hypertensive patients is less dependent on AH. Other complications such as stroke, although less frequent, are more clearly determined by it. For this reason alone, any strategy for AH control will have a much greater impact on the incidence of stroke and heart failure than on the incidence of coronary disease.

Differences in mortality between males and females

The differences in the mortality rates of male and female hypertensives are so large that Lew, after analyzing the data of the Society of Actuaries in 1967, concluded that females seemed to be 'another species'. After 5-year follow-up of 439 untreated hypertensives, most of them in their forties, the mortality of the males was double than that of the females for each hypertension level group: 250+/130+, 200−/110− and 150−/90 mm Hg [6]. Here again, the panorama changes when coronary artery disease, stroke and heart failure are considered separately. At equivalent hypertension levels, the cerebrovascular mortality in men and women is almost the same at all ages. As such, under 50 years there is a slight predominance of hypertension in men and a slightly greater rate of death from cerebrovascular causes. Over 50, the prevalence of hypertension and stroke in women increases disproportionately. On the other hand, for coronary artery disease, although the relative risk increased equally in both sexes with increases in blood pressure [7], the absolute risk in premenopausic women for equivalent BP levels is almost half that of males [8]. Coronary artery disease in the hypertensive population affects females almost 20 years later than males.

Does any feature of BP have a predictive value?

The association between blood pressure and disease is quantitative, not qualitative. Each AH levels is linearly related to the complications of the disease. The predictive value of a single determination is less than that of multiple readings. A quality of pressure behavior that has been observed to have predictive value is the response to the cold test of Hines and Brown [9]. A follow-up of 279 men, mean age of 47 years, without coronary artery disease at the onset showed that those who responded to the cold test with an increase of 20 mm Hg or more in the basal BP had a coronary risk in 20 years double than that of the rest of the individuals. This effect was independent of BP level at the onset.

Another feature that seems to have predictive value is the rate of increase in systolic BP with age. Rabkin, Mathewson and Tate [10] demonstrated that the individuals who suffered stroke in a 26-year observation period had an increment over the initial BP figure of 40% with time, whereas those who did not have strokes only had a 15% increment. This was valid for all the BP levels observed at the beginning of the study. The association between the rate of BP increment with age and cardiovascular complications is much less marked for coronary artery disease than for stroke.

Reversibility of hypertension and prevention of complications

For unknown reasons but probably due to differences in the natural history, the diverse hypertensive complications can be prevented to a large degree by reducing blood pressure levels in the middle-age patient.

An observation consistently made in all the controlled epidemiological studies is that reduction in BP is very effective in preventing left ventricular failure, hypertensive retinopathy and stroke, but not coronary heart disease.

220

Such studies involve persons over 50 years of age. It could be anticipated that the beneficial preventive effect would be greater if hypertension control were begun earlier. However, it could also be expected that the iatrogenic affects of the medications would be compounded by use for a longer time. There are great hopes that the recent AH treatment with β-blocking agents may be more beneficial in preventing all cardiovascular complications without unfavorable side effects.

Controlled randomized studies of BP reduction

The study of the Veterans Administration group [11, 12], undertaken in the United States and initiated in 1964, constitutes the most complete source of information on different AH complications and on the effectiveness of treatment as regard to the probability of its prevention (Table 1). The study was carried out in 523 hypertensive males from 30 to 73 years of age randomly distributed into two groups: control and treatment. Treatment consisted of reserpine, thiazide and/or hydralazine. On the basis of DE these groups were divided into two subgroups:
a) 90–114 mm Hg, and
b) 115–129 mm Hg.
In the DP subgroup of 90–114 mm Hg (380 individuals), treatment produced a decline in DP to 79 mm Hg. In the control group DP continued at 106 mm Hg. In the second subgroup (DP 115–129 mm Hg), treatment reduced DP to 93 mm Hg, while in the controls it remained at 119 mm Hg (Table 2). In the first three years of follow-up, there was no death in the treated group and there was only one stroke. There were four deaths in the control group: three due to rupture of an aortic aneurysm and one sudden death. There were also 199 cardiovascular accidents: 9 grade IV retinopathies, 3 strokes, 1 transient ischemic attack (TIA), 2 myocardial infarcts, 2 episodes of left ventricular failure and 2 of renal failure (Tables 3 and 4).

After 3 years, treatment was also initiated in the control group because of the evidence of the benefits obtained in preventing complications.

Similar randomized studies have been carried out on treated hypertensives

Table 1. Veterans Administration Study.

Randomization: control – treatment
523 males
Age: 30–73 years
Onset: 1964
Treatment with: reserpine – thiazide and/or hydralazine

and controls with the same DP levels: see Wolff and Lindeman, 1966 [13], Hamilton, Thomson and Wisniewski, 1964 [14]. One of the most recent studies is that of the cooperative group of the U.S. Public Health Services Hospitals [15], which includes 389 men and women randomized into control and treatment groups and followed up for 7 years. This study confirms the results of the Veterans Study and those of Hamilton's group: control of arterial hypertension effectively prevents stroke, left ventricular failure and renal failure, but its value in preventing coronary heart disease is not so clear.

Various studies [2, 12] indicate the effectiveness of treatment of AH with DP levels of 90–114 mm Hg. In the Veterans Study (II), 380 randomized hyperten-

Table 2. Veterans Administration Study. Effectiveness of treatment: DP level (mm Hg) 4 years after onset.

Subgroup*	N	Treatment	Control
90–114	380	79	106
115–129	125	93	119

*Subgroups according to DP at (mm Hg)onset.

Table 3. Veterans Administration Study. Effect of treatment on complications after 3 years of follow-up.

Group	Deaths		Major cardiovascular accidents	
Treated	0		1 Stroke	
Control	4	3: Ao rupture 1: Sudden death	17	9: Grade IV retinopathy 3: Stroke 1: Transient ischemic attack 2: Myocardial infarct 2: LV failure 2: Renal failure

Table 4. Veterans Administration II (380 individuals; 90–114 mm Hg DP).

	Control	Treatment
Cardiovascular death	19	8
Sudden death – Myocardial infarct	11	6
Nonfatal cases	37	13
Nonfatal infarct	2	5

sive patients were followed for 15 years. There were 19 cardiovascular deaths in the control group and 8 in the treated group; 37 nonfatal cardiovascular accidents were observed in the control group and 13 in the treated group. Analyzing the causes of death in both groups it was found that in the control group 11 were due to myocardial infarct or sudden death while 6 were recorded in the treated group. Considering all cardiovascular events, fatal or not, the differences for left ventricular failure, retinopathy and kidney failure were significant. As for stroke, the differences between the two groups were very significant, but for coronary heart disease, 11 patients in each group, the difference did not reach statistical significance. Fatal myocardial infarct and sudden death, 11 and 6 patients in the control and treated groups, respectively, showed differences, but nonfatal infarcts did not since there were 5 in the treated group and only 2 in the control group.

Considering all the controlled studies that compare treatment *versus* nontreatment in hypertension, it can be deduced that treatment has a slight advantage over nontreatment in the prevention of coronary heart disease. This advantage is neither definite nor conclusive for moderate diastolic hypertension levels (90–114 mm Hg) but at higher levels there are clear benefits from treatment, both in overall prevention of cardiovascular complications and for coronary heart disease in particular. Fewer benefits are seen in subjects under 50 years and in subgroups without coronary heart disease or renal failure at onset [16]. In the Veterans Administration study, the authors concluded that patients with diastolic pressure between 90–104 mm Hg profit relatively little from treatment unless they have some kind of renal or cardiovascular anomaly at the onset or are older than 50 years.

If we consider two subgroups in the treated group, *a)* those that consistently maintain diastolic pressures under 90 mm Hg, and *b)* those that do not, show a reduction in total cases proportional to the degree of control.

The Veterans Study also indicated that the benefits of decreasing BP appear soon and are cumulative in time (Fig. 3), reaching the greatest effectiveness after 3 years in approximately 50% of patients. This suggests that the benefits of long-term treatment may be greater than what the reference studies indicate. Likewise, early initiation of treatment (before 51 years) has still more advantages, particularly for reducing death from coronary heart disease. In practice, there are two interpretations of the results of the Veterans Study; one that considers that it is necessary and beneficial to treat all hypertensives with more or less sustained DP values over 90 mm Hg, and another, more conservative, view that only considers as candidates for treatment subjects with DP of 105 mm Hg or higher, middle-aged and without organic lesion. The higher the DP level was before randomization at the onset of the study, the more effective was the treatment.

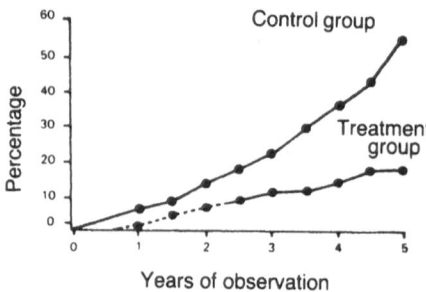

Fig. 3. Estimated accumulated incidence of all events in a period of 5 years occurring in the control and treatment groups (Veterans Study II, 1970).

Effect of treatment on specific complications

The greatest difference in the effectiveness of hypertension treatment is the prevention of stroke, retinopathy, and renal or cardiac failure in comparison with prevention of coronary heart disease. This difference depends clearly on variations in the natural history of these diseases and on their degree of reversibility at different stages of development.

Hypertension has always been considered the most important coronary risk factor; effective treatment of hypertension has reinforced this relationship.

In the controlled series BP reduction decreases the number of deaths from stroke by about 75%, while renal and cardiac failure almost disappear as causes of death. However, survivors are exposed to a greater risk of myocardial infarction. In 1952, in a study on life expectancy and cause of death in 1.294 patients attended in the hypertension clinic of the Hammersmith Hospital in London it was confirmed that treatment reduced mortality from all causes to 19% when only the efficacy of treatment with ganglionar blockers was evaluated. Mortality decreased to 3% in 1977, when neuronal adrenergic blockers and diuretics were introduced in hypertension treatment. Until 1952 myocardial infarction represented only 7% of the causes of death; in 1967 the proportion of mortal infarctions was 27% [17].

Can the risk of myocardial infarction be decreased by blood pressure reduction?

In studying the relationship between hypertension and ischemic heart disease two fundamental questions are relevant:
a) Can the risk of myocardial infarct be decreased by reducing BP?
b) Is the remedy worse than the disease? That is, do the pharmacological

effects of long-term treatment with hypotensive drugs increase coronary risk?

More attention and effort have been dedicated to resolving the first question than to clarifying the second one. The value of the treatment of hypertension in the prevention of ischemic heart disease has been discussed previously. It is clear that medical control of AH reduces both the incidence of myocardial infarct and its mortality. With the appearance of the βblocking agents in 1960, it has been demonstrated in numerous studies that while secondary prevention with these drugs is effective, two contradictory situations can occur with respect to postinfarction mortality in patients treated with β-blocking agents: postinfarction mortality increases due to heart failure or it decreases due to the preventive effect of these drugs against arrhythmias. However, less postinfarction deaths are caused by heart failure than by arrhythmias. For this reason, β-blocking agents are used in the postinfarction period.

The first evidence that β-blocking agents could reduce mortality from coronary disease does not come from experience with the treatment of hypertension but from the treatment of patients with angina. Amsterdam, Wolfson and Gorlin in 1968 [18] showed that mortality in patients with angina treated with β-blockers is lower than that of the patients treated only with nitrites.

The most notable evidence that treatment of hypertension has a preventive effect on coronary artery disease comes from the Goteborg study [19]. Initiated in 1970 and designed to be a longitudinal study of primary prevention of coronary heart disease, it included 1026 males from 47–57 years randomly selected from the general population. In this population 635 individuals were found to have BP values of 175/115 mm Hg in two or more determinations. These subjects were submitted to treatment with hypotensive drugs, were followed-up for an average of 4.3 years and results were compared with a control group of 391 individuals from the same population who had BP values of 175/115 mm Hg in single determination and were left untreated. In the treated group total mortality and cardiovascular mortality were half the control group values. In this study treatment was stepped, using thiazides, hydralazine and β-blocking agents, in contrast with the Veterans Study in which β-blocking agents were not used. It may be that the inclusion of these drugs in the treatment was responsible for the difference in mortality.

As a counterpoint to this consideration the disadvantages and possible danger of a long-term treatment with β-blocking agents must be kept in mind. If treatment of hypertension is begun early it can be assumed that some persons will be taking these drugs for 30 to 40 years. In this respect, Williams and Raine [20, 21] have shown a loss of 19% of the muscular mass in rabbits treated with propranolol for long periods, as well as changes in the cellular structure of the myocardium.

Likewise, the metabolic modifications that other antihypertensive treatments can produce and the fact that it may increase coronary risk by other means should be considered. Diuretics (thiazides and furosemide) can induce clinical diabetes or pathologically modify the glucose tolerance test. Lewis [22] demonstrated that in 137 hypertensive patients treated with diuretics, there was no change in the glucose tolerance after 14 months, but in 22% of 51 patients followed for 6 years a 13% increase in basal glycemia was observed. Intolerance to the glucose load test developed earlier and more rapidly in the elderly.

The study by Ames and Hill in 1976 and other studies published [23, 24] have demonstrated an increase in total cholesterol in hypertensive patients treated with thiazides.

The relative effectiveness and benefits of arterial treatment of hypertension with different drugs may be clarified by a study the Medical Research Council initiated in 1977 which includes 36,000 moderate hypertensive patients (DP = 90–110 mm Hg) given long-term treatment with thiazides and/or β-blockers. The results will not be published until 1985. In the meantime perhaps we should limit ourselves to acting on the basis of what has been well established: treatment of severe hypertension (DO of 105–110 mm Hg or more) produces sure benefits and prevents against stroke. Coronary heart disease has a more complex and less direct relationship with arterial hypertension, and the effects of elevated blood pressure may be already irreversible relatively early in life. Atheroma plaques were found in 20-year-old soldiers who died in Korea. It has also been observed that coronary atheromas appear earlier and are more developed in hypertensive patients. If treatment of hypertension is to be effective it should begin at early ages, although the dangers related to long-term treatment must be considered.

An alternative that would avoid the adverse effects of hypertension treatment and obtain all the advantages would be the use of general health-dietetic measures; these can greatly reduce blood pressure. Control of excess weight, salt restricted or salt-free diet, and avoiding the use of alcohol and tobacco, aside from controlling hypertension, constitute a multifactorial approach to the prevention of coronary heart disease.

Mortality due to coronary heart disease has decreased by 27% in the United States since 1970 for men between 35 and 44 years [25]. This phenomenon is undoubtedly due to changes in the habits of the population.

The present philosophy behind the prevention of coronary heart disease tends to consider that cardiovascular risk should be modified by hygienic-dietetic measures, avoiding drug prescription as much as possible.

The most recent studies on prevention of coronary heart disease show that modifications in one risk factor have substantial and unexpected repercussions on the others. Coronary risk factors act synergistically. Thus, a man with 250 mg/ml or more of serum cholesterol, or a systolic BP of 160 mm Hg or more, or a cigarrette habit of 20 or more a day has twice the average risk of the general population of suffering a myocardial infarct in the next 10 years. If the man has two of these three factors, the risk is multiplied by 3.5 and if he has all three, his risk is multiplied by 10 [26].

The most rational strategy in the prevention of coronary heart disease would be to make a concerted attack at an early age on the main risk factors in the population at the highest risk.

Summary

The risk of stroke and heart failure can be substantially reduced by treatment and control of severe arterial hypertension. By contrast, the risk of fatal or nonfatal myocardial infarction decreases only a little. Moreover, other coronary risk factors should also be controlled. In persons of advanced age, treatment with diuretics may even increase this risk. β-Blocking agents probably reduce the risk of myocardial infarction and postinfarctional cardiovascular death although the results of the prospective studies so far undertaken are inconclusive.

The advantages of the pharmacological treatment of moderate hypertension (diastolic pressure 90–104 mm Hg) in the prevention of cardiovascular complications in individuals without other organ lesions have not been convincingly demonstrated. In this population, general health and dietetic measures should be recommended before resorting to drugs.

All hypertensive patients, whether treated or not, are at high coronary risk. The effects of drugs on glucose and lipid metabolism should always be kept in mind since they may produce interference with other coronary risk factors in the form of increased cholesterol and glycemia levels.

Treatment of hypertension to prevent coronary heart disease should definitely be initiated as soon as possible in severe hypertensive patients, using drugs free of effects that potentiate other coronary risk factors.

References

1. Hypertension Detection and Follow-up Program Cooperative Group: The effect of treatment on mortality in 'mild' hypertension. N Engl J Med 1982; 307: 976–980.
2. Stamler R, Stamler J: 'Mild' hypertension: risks and strategy for control. Primary Cardiol 1983; 9: 150–166.
3. Lew EA: Blood pressure and mortality-life insurance experience. In: Stamler J, Stamler R, Pullman TN (eds) The epidemiology of hypertension. Grune and Stratton, New York, 1976.
4. Kannel WB, Gordon T: The Framingham study: an epidemiological investigation of cardiovascular disease. Section 26, Government Printing Office, Washington DC, 1970.

5. Kanner WB: Results of the epidemiologic investigation of ischaemic heart disease: illustrated by the Framingham Study. In: Hass JH, Hemker HC, Snellen HA (eds) Ischaemic heart disease. Leiden University Press, Leiden, 1970.

6. Sokolou M, Perloff D: The prognosis of essential hypertension treated conservatively. Circulation 1961; 23: 697.

7. Dauwer, TR, Kannel WB, Revostkie N, Kagan A: The epidemiology of coronary heart disease – The Framingham enquiry. Proc Royal Soc Med 1962; 55: 265.

8. Kannel WB: Assessment of hypertension as a predictor of cardiovascular disease: the Framingham Study. In: Burley DM, Birdwood GFB, Frya JH, Taylor SH (eds) Hypertension, its nature and treatment. CIBA Laboratories, Horscham, England, 1975.

9. Hines EA, Brown GE: A standard test for measuring the variability of the blood pressure: its significance as an index of the prehypertension state. Ann Intern Med, 1933; 7: 209.

10. Rabkin SW, Mathewson FAL, Tate RB: Long-term changes in blood pressure and risk of cerebrovascular disease. Stroke, 1978; 9: 319.

11. Taguchi J, Freis ED: Partial reduction of blood pressure and prevention of complications in hypertension. N Engl J Med, 1974; 291: 329.

12. Veterans Administration Cooperative Study Group on Antihypertensive Agents: Effects of treatment on morbidity in hypertension. JAMA, 1970; 213: 1143–1152.

13. Wolf IW, Lindeman RD: Effects of treatment on hypertension results of a controlled study. Chron Dis, 1966; 19: 227.

14. Hamilton M, Thompson EN, Wisniewski TKM: The role of blood pressure control in preventing complications of hypertension. Lancet, 1964; 1: 235.

15. Smith WMcF: Intervention trial in mild hypertension. Cooperative Study Group. Public Health Service Hospitals. Circulation, 1976; 95 (Suppl II): 95.

16. Veterans Administration Cooperative Study Group on Antihypertensive Agents: Effects of treatment on morbidity in hypertension III. Influence of age, diastolic pressure, and prior cardiovascular disease. Further analysis of side effects. Circulation, 1972; 45: 991–1004.

17. Breckenridge A, Dollery CT, Parry EH: Prognosis of treated hypertension. Changes in life expectancy and causes of death between 1952 and 1967. A J Med 1970; 39: 411.

18. Amsterdam EA, Wolfson S, Gorlin R: Effect of therapy on survival in angina pectoris. Ann Intern Med, 1968; 68: 1151.

19. Berglund G, Wilhelmsen L, Sannerstedt R, Hansson L, Anderson O, Sivertsson R, Wedel H, Wikstrand J: Coronary heart disease after treatment of hypertension. Lancet, 1978; 1: 1.

20. Williams EMVM, Raine AEG: Effect of prolonged β-receptor blockade on dry weight and electrophysiological responses of rapid heart. Lancet, 1974; 2: 1048.

21. Williams EM, Tasgal J, Raine AEG: Morphometric changes in rabbit ventricular myocardium produced by long-term β-adrenoreceptor blockade. Lancet, 1977; 2: 850.

22. Lewis PJ, Kohner EM, Petrie A, Dollery CT: Deterioration of glucose tolerance in hypertensive patients on prolonged diuretic treatment. Lancet, 1976; 1: 564.

23. Ames R, Hill P: Increase in serum lipids during treatment of hypertension with chlorothalidone. Lancet, 1976; 1: 721.

24. Schander H, Fitz A, Frohlich E, Goldman A, Perry HM, Steele B: Chlorthalidone and serum cholesterol. Lancet, 1977; 2: 295.

25. Walker WJ: Changing United life-style and declining vascular mortality: cause or co-incidence? N Engl J Med, 1977; 297: 163.

26. Dawber TR, Kannel WB, McNamara PM: The prediction of coronary heart disease. Transactions of the Association of Life Insurance Medical Divisions of America, 1964; 47: 70.

5.3 Use of β-Adrenergic Blocking Agents in Arterial Hypertension

E. ALEGRÍA EZQUERRA, J.A. ARRIETA, R. HUGUET, J. BARBA and D. MARTINEZ-CARO

Introduction

At present, antihypertensive treatment usually constitutes a preventive measure rather than a true therapeutic necessity. This is obviously due to the fact that arterial hypertension (AH) is one of the main risk factors for ischemic heart disease.

β-adrenergic blocking agents (BB) and diuretics are the drugs of first choice in the treatment of AH [1]. This is probably due not only to their effectiveness and favorable risk/benefit ratio [2], but to their efficacy in preventing complications. Indeed, BB are the only drugs with which significant reductions in coronary morbidity [3, 4] and vascular complications [5, 6] have been demonstrated in AH patients in whom blood pressure has decreased. The importance BB continue to have in AH treatment derives from these findings.

The present study deals briefly with some aspects of interest in relation to the pharmacokinetics and pharmacodynamics of the BB, as well as certain other practical aspects. Labetolol has been excluded from this discussion, although it is a useful antihypertensive medication, because its properties differ markedly from those of classic BB. For further details, more extensive papers can be consulted [2, 7–10].

Pharmacokinetic aspects

The BB are a structurally homogeneous group, but there are marked differences in the pharmacokinetics of the compounds in this group. Table 1 summarizes the most important pharmacokinetic properties of the principal BB.

Of these properties, the one with the greatest clinical importance is the degree of *liposolubility* [11] of the drug. Highly liposoluble drugs have a predominantly hepatic metabolism, suffer the so-called 'first pass effect', cross the blood-brain barrier and have a shorter half life (2–6 hours). Water soluble drugs are eliminated fundamentally by the kidney, cross the blood-brain barrier in much lower ratio and have a longer half life (7–20 hours).

More details on BB pharmacokinetics can be found in other studies [12–15].

Pharmacodynamic aspects

In spite of the fact that the twenty-fifth anniversary of the introduction of the first BB [16] has recently occurred, the mechanism of their antihypertensive effect is still not completely clear. The studies of Scriabine [7] and George [14] contain critical reviews of the diverse hypotheses that have been formulated.

β-blocking agents compete with the endogenous catecholamines for the β-adrenergic receptors, shifting the dose-response curve of the agonist to the right. For this reason, prior to studying the effects of these drugs, a brief physiological review seems in order.

In β-adrenergic receptors are subdivided into β_1 (cardiac) and β_2 subtypes [17]. In Table 2 the responses produced by stimulation of these receptors are summarized. In Fig. 1, modified from Opie [8] the biochemical mechanism of response to β-adrenergic stimulation is illustrated.

The blockade of the β-receptors produced by the BB is competitive, that is, the intensity of the β response depends on the respective concentrations of agonists (catecholamines) and their competitive antagonists (the β-blockers). Nonetheless, some compounds in this group also possess what is known as *intrinsic activity,* that is, a certain capacity for activating the β-receptor in certain circumstances and in relation with the preexistent β-adrenergic tone. This allows the preservation of a certain β-adrenergic response, always less than that obtained by catecholaminic stimulation.

Table 1. Pharmacokinetic properties of the principal β-blocking agents.

Drug	Intestinal absorption (% p.o. dose)	First pass effect	Bioavail- ability (% p.o. dose)	Plasma half-life (hours)	Elimination route	Nonmetabo- lized RE (% p.o. dose)	Lipo- solubility
Acebutolol	50		50	3–4	MH + RE	35	High
Atenolol	50	15	40	6–9	RE	40	Low
Metoprolol	95	50	50	3–4	HM	3	High
Nadolol	30		20–30	16–17	RE	90	Low
Oxprenolol	85	40	25–50	1–2	HM	2–5	High
Pindolol	95	13	90	3–4	HM + RE	40	High
Propranolol	90	60	30	3–6	HM	1	Very high
Sotalol	75	15	60	6–14	RE	60	Low
Timolol	90			4–5	HM + RE	20	High

Abbreviations: p.o.: per os; HM: hepatic metabolization; RE: renal excretion.

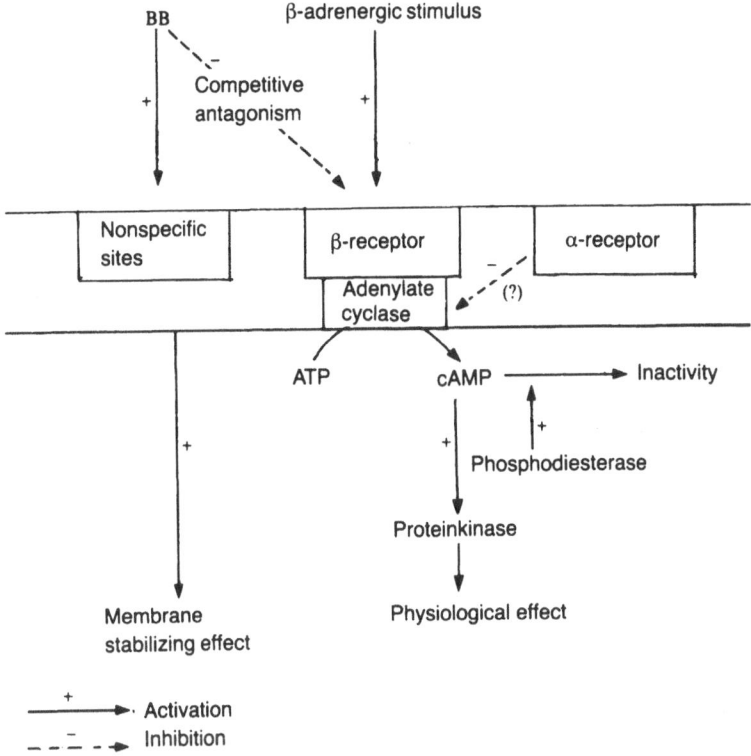

Fig. 1. Diagram of the adrenoceptor.

All the known BB are selective, blocking only the β-receptors. Neither α- or glucagon receptors nor the cardiostimulator effects of digitalis or calcium are related to BB activity. However, some BB preferentially or selectively block β_1-receptors, sparing the interaction of the agonist with the β_2-receptor. This property, which has been termed *cardioselectivity,* is relatively dose-dependent, progressively declining with an increase in the drug dosis.

Finally, numerous compounds in this group possess *membrane stabilizing* properties similar to those of quinidine, consisting in non-specific depression of the conductance of the biological membranes for certain ions. This property is manifested at higher doses than those required to produce β-blockade and its clinical repercussions seem to be scarce.

At present, it is believed that the principal mechanism involved in the antihypertensive effect of the BB is not, as was believed, a reduction of cardiac output produced by bradycardia and the decrease in inotropism. This mechanism would be the main one responsible for reducing blood pressure during effort or stress. The main antihypertensive mechanism of the BB would be to lower systemic vascular resistance, with presynaptic inhibition of transmission in the sympathetic nerve ends [18] and a central effect of reducing efferent sympathetic tone [19]. The decrease in renin secretion seems to exercise a secondary role.

Table 3 shows the most important β-blocking agents and their pharmacodynamic properties.

Table 2. Locations of the β-adrenergic receptors and pharmacologic effects derived from their stimulation.

Receptors	Location	Pharmacologic effect
β_1	Heart	Increase in sinus rate
		Increase in ectopic excitability
		Acceleration of A-V conduction
		Increase in contractility
	Adipose tissue	Lipolysis
β_2	Bronchi	Dilation
	Blood vessels	Dilation
	Uterus	Relaxation
	Digestive tract	Reduction in motility
	Pancreas	Insulin release
	Bladder	Relaxation of detrusor muscle
	Skeletal muscle	Contraction
		Glucogenolysis
	Kidney	Renin release
	Liver	Glyconeogenesis

Table 3. Pharmacodynamic properties of the principal β-blocking agents.

Drug	Intrinsic activity	Cardioselectivity	Membrane stabilization
Acebutolol	+	Yes	+
Atenolol	No	Yes	No
Metoprolol	No	Yes	±
Nadolol	No	No	No
Oxprenolol	++	No	+
Pindolol	+++	No	+
Propranolol	No	No	++
Sotalol	No	No	No
Timolol	±	No	+

Abbreviations: +: intensity of the effect; ±: doubtful or weak effect.

Practical aspects

Table 4 lists the BB available in Spain, their commercial presentation, and recommended *dosages* for AH treatment.

With respect to the *adverse reactions* of BB, these generally have less clinical relevance than might at first be expected. The most notable effects are listed in

Table 4. Presentation and dosages of the β-blocking agents available in Spain.

Drug	Commercial preparation	Presentation (mg/tabl.)	Usual dosage (mg/day	Doses/day
Acebutolol	Sectral	200 or 400	200–800	1–2
Atenolol	Tenormín, Blokium	100	50–200	1
Metoprolol	Lopresor, Selokén	100	150–300	2
Oxprenolol	Trasicor	80	80–320	2–3
	Trasicor Retard	160	160	1
Pindolol	Viskén	5	10–30	3–4
Propranolol	Sumial	10 or 40	100–320	2–3
	Sumial Retard	160	160	1
Timolol	Blocadrén	5 or 10	20–60	2–4

Table 5. Adverse reactions to β-blocking agents.

Due to β_1 blockade
Bradycardia
Atrioventricular block
Heart failure
Hyperlipoproteinemia

Due to β_2-blockade
Bronchial obstruction
Vascular effects (cold extremities, worsening of chronic arterial insufficiency, induction of Raynaud phenomenon)
Constipation
Fatigue
Potentiation of insulin hypoglycemia

Due to pharmacokinetics
Nervousness (insomnia, hallucinations, impotence, nightmares)
Rebound effect after abrupt withdrawal

Toxic effects
Practolol syndrome
Retroperitoneal fibrosis
Cutaneous lesions (psoriasiform or lichenoid)
Carcinogenesis

Table 5. Cruickshank's study [20] contains a complete review of this subject.

Obviously, the most frequent adverse effects are those directly related to the mechanism of action of these drugs. Bradycardia is rarely symptomatic and only dangerous if it is very marked or is associated with severe cardiac failure or advanced coronary insufficiency. Atrioventricular block is rare. There is little likelihood of aggravating heart failure if patients are carefully selected. It has not been demonstrated that there is less risk with drugs that possess intrinsic activity. With respect to hyperlipoproteinemia, slight elevations in the low density lipoproteins have been described, particularly with the non-cardioselective drugs. However, the clinical significance of this finding is still unclear. These adverse reactions, common to all β-blocking agents, are not necessarily dose-dependent. The possibility of their appearance should therefore be looked for when initiating treatment.

Bronchial obstruction is perhaps the most important adverse effect of these drugs, but it only constitutes a clinical problem in patients who have obstructive pulmonary disease. If these patients must be treated low doses of cardioselective drugs are preferable and an inhalatory β_2-stimulator can be associated, if necessary.

Cold extremities is not a problem except in patients with peripheral arterial insufficiency in whom noncardioselective drugs can worsen the disease. These same drugs can produce Raynaud phenomena. Muscular fatigue is a frequent problem, but it decreases progressively in the course of a few weeks of treatment, as does constipation. Finally, the β-blocking agents are generally well tolerated in diabetes, but cardioselective drugs should be used in insulin-dependent patients because they produce less insulin hypoglycemia, which is easier to treat.

CNS effects are varied but not very frequent. Among them are nightmares, migraine, hallucinations, insomnia, paresthesias and impotence. Depression has been described with propranolol and oxprenolol. The effects on the nervous system are much less frequent with water soluble drugs, such as atenolol and sotalol. The rebound effect that appears after abrupt suspension of BB can be a problem in angina pectoris but not in AH.

Finally, direct toxic effects have only been described in exceptional cases

Table 6. Absolute contraindications of the β-blocking agents.

Severe bradycardia
Overt cardiac failure
Advanced atrioventricular block
Severe asthma
Advanced peripheral arterial insufficiency
Severe depression

with practolol, and for this reason the product has been withdrawn. The so-called practolol syndrome consists in a psoriasiform hyperkeratosis, keratoconjunctivitis, sclerosing peritonitis, effusive middle otitis, pleuritis and pericarditis. These effects have not been observed with any of the drugs actually in use.

Finally mention will be made of the *contraindications* of BB. Except for those shown in Table 6, which are absolute contraindications, the rest are relative, conditioned by two facts: the need of BB treatment and the pharmacokinetic properties of the drugs used. An interesting study in this respect is that of Breckenridge [21].

Thus, BB can be used in AH complicated with compensated heart failure. It has not been demonstrated that medications with a partial agonist activity in this sense are safer.

As we have already mentioned, the cardioselective drugs are preferable in patients with AH and chronic obstructive pulmonary disease, combined if necessary with inhaled β_2-stimulants. In patients with depression, hallucinations or other psychiatric diseases, β-blocking agents should be avoided, or only BB with little liposolubility should be used. In peripheral arteriopathy, cardioselective or intrinsic activity drugs can be used with caution.

In patients with kidney failure, β-blocking agents can be used with a corresponding reduction in dose. Finally, in diabetics, cardioselective BB should be used and the insulin dose should be adjusted.

An important problem is hypertension during pregnancy. Although the BB have been traditionally considered to be contraindicated, it has recently been found that the cardioselective BB or those with intrinsic activity are effective and safe in this case [22, 23].

Summary

After having analyzed briefly the value of β-blocking agents in preventing the cardiovascular complications of hypertension, we have discussed the pharmacodynamic, pharmacokinetic and practical aspects related to these drugs.

References

1. World Health Organization: Arterial hypertension. Report of an expert committee. WHO Technical Report Series No 628, 1978; 1–57.
2. Meier M, Orwin J, Rogg H, Brunner H: β-adrenoceptor antagonists in hypertension. In: Scriabine A (ed) Pharmacology of antihypertensive drugs. Raven Press, New York, 1980; 179–194.
3. Berglund G, Wilhelmsen L, Sannerstedt R, Hansson L, Andersson O, Sivertsson R, Wedel

H, Wikstrand J: Coronary heart disease after treatment of hypertension. Lancet 1978; 1: 1–5.

4. Steward IMG: β-adrenoceptor blockade and the incidence of myocardial infarction during treatment of severe hypertension. Br Clin Pharmacol 1982; 13: 91–93.

5. Trafford JAP, Horn CR, O'Neal H, McGonigle R, Halford-Maw L, Evans R: Five years follow-up of effects of treatment of mild and moderate hypertension. Br Med J 1981; 282: 1111–1113.

6. Beevers DG, Johnston JG, Larkin H, Davies P: Clinical evidence that β-adrenoceptor blockers prevent more cardiovascular complications than other antihypertensive drugs. Drugs, 1983; 25 (Suppl 2): 326–330.

7. Scriabine A: β-adrenoceptor blocking drugs in hypertension. Ann Rev Pharmacol Toxicol 1979; 19: 269–284.

8. Opie LH: Drugs and the heart. I β-blocking agents. Lancet 1980; 1: 693–698.

9. Frishman WH: β-adrenoceptor antagonists: New drugs and new indications. N Engl J Med 1981; 305: 500–506.

10. Robertson JIS: State of the art review: β-blockade and the treatment of hypertension. Drugs, 1983; 25 (Suppl 2): 5–11.

11. Woods PB, Robinson ML: An investigation of the comparative liposolubilities of β-adrenoceptor blocking agents. J Pharm Pharmacol 1981; 33: 172–173.

12. Johnson G, Regards CG: Clinical pharmacokinetics of β-adrenoceptor blocking drugs. Clin Pharmacol 1976; 1: 233–263.

13. Frishman W: Clinical pharmacology of the new β-adrenergic blocking drugs. Part 1. Pharmacodynamic and pharmacokinetic properties. Am Heart J 1979; 97: 663–670.

14. George GF: Pharmacodynamics and pharmacokinetics of cardiovascular drugs. In: Coltart J, Jewitt D (eds) Recent developments in cardiovascular drugs. Churchill Livingstone, Edinburgh, 1982; 16$27.

15. Shand DG: State of the art: comparative pharmacology of the β-adrenoceptor blocking drugs. Drugs 1983; 25 (Suppl 2): 92–99.

16. Powel CE, Slater IH: Blocking of inhibitory adrenergic receptors by a dichloro analog of isoproterenol. J Pharmacol Exp Ther 1958; 122: 480–488.

17. Kaumann AJ: Herz β-Rezeptoren. Experimentelle Standpunkte. Z Kardiol 1983; 72: 63–82.

18. Langer SZ, Cavero I, Massingham B: Recent developments in noradrenergic neurotransmission and its relevance to the mechanism of action of certain antihypertensive agents. Hypertension 1980; 2: 373–382.

19. Tackett RL, Webb IG, Privitera PJ: Cerebroventricular propanolol elevates cerebrospinal fluid norepinephrine and lowers arterial pressure. Science 1981; 213: 911–913.

20. Cruickshank JM: How safe are the β-blockers? Drugs 1983; 25 (Suppl 2): 331–340.

21. Breckenridge A: Which β-blocker? Br Med J 1983; 286: 1085–1088.

22. Gallery EDM, Saunders DM, Hunyor SN, Gyory AZ: Randomized comparison of methyldopa and oxprenolol for treatment of hypertension in pregnancy. Br Med J 1979; 1: 1591–1594.

23. Rubin PC, Butters L, Clark DM et al.: Placebo-controlled trial of atenolol in treatment of pregnancy-associated hypertension. Lancet 1983; 1: 431–434.

5.4 Other Antihypertensive Drugs

J. TAMARGO MENÉNDEZ

Arterial hypertension (AH) is an important cardiovascular risk factor, and treatment reduces morbidity and mortality secondary to its complications [1, 2]. However, AH is a multifactorial disease of chronic evolution, and treatment usually requires association of various drugs which can induce important adverse effects in the long term. This has prompted a search for new antihypertensive drugs (AHD) as an alternative to those already available that could improve the risk-efficacy ratio of long-term treatment. Theoretically, blood pressure (BP) can be controlled by reducing peripheral vascular resistance (PVR) or decreasing cardiac output, although a reduction in cardiac output without modifications in the PVR can impair renal, cerebral or coronary perfusion. Therefore, most AHD reduce PVR because the increment in PVR constitutes the principal factor responsible for elevated BP in the hypertensive patient. Of the multiple AHD available (Table 1), in this chapter we will only refer briefly to those that have most recently been introduced. The main pharmacokinetic characteristics of these drugs, administration and dosage are shown in Tables 2 and 3, respectively.

α-Adrenoceptor agonists and antagonists

The α_1/α_2-adrenoceptors play an important role in the control of vascular tone and PVR [3, 4]. The α_1-adrenoceptors are located in the postsynaptic membranes of the smooth arteriovenous muscle and its blockade produces vasodilation and lowers BP. Peripherally, the α_2-receptors are located at the presynaptic level, where stimulation reduces norepinephrine release from the sympathetic nerve ends, and at the postsynaptic level. In the CNS, the α_2-receptors are located mainly at the postsynaptic level and stimulation produces a reduction in peripheral cardiovascular sympathetic tone and reflexly increases parasympathetic tone. We will now review the principal characteristics of prazosin (α_1-receptor antagonist), clonidine and guanfacine (central α_2-receptor agonists).

Table 1. General mechanisms of the antihypertensive effect.

Drugs that inhibit sympathetic nervous system activity
Selective α-1-adrenoceptor blockers: prazosin, trimazosin, labetalol, indoramine, medroxalol, doxazosin, tetrazosin, thiodazosin, E-643, bucindolol
Nonselective α-1-adrenoceptor blockers: phentolamine, phenoxybenzamine, timoxamine
Central α-2-adrenoceptor stimulants: clonidine, guanfacine, guanabenz, azepexole, alphamethyl-dopa, thiamenidine, lofexidine, B-Ht 920, FLA-136
α-2-blocker, α-1-adrenoceptor stimulant: urapidil
Norepinephrine release blockers: guanethidine, bethanidine
Drugs that modify catecholamine storage: reserpine, U-54
Ganglionar blockers: trimethaphan

Drugs that interfere with the renin-angiotensin-aldosterone system
Renin inhibitors: pepstatines, URI-73A, PE-104
Angiotensin II receptor blockers: saralasin
Converting enzyme inhibitors: captopril, enalapril, pivalopril, teprotide, phentiapril, lysinopril

Vasodilators
Hydralazine, nitroprusside, diazoxide, minoxidil, nitrates
Calcium antagonists: nifedipine, nimodipine, nicardipine, verapamil, diltiazem, felodipine
β-2-adrenoceptor stimulants: salbutamol, pirbuterol, terbutaline

Table 2. Principal pharmacokinetic characteristics and undesirable effects.

Drugs	Bioavail-lability (%)	C_{man} (hrs)	$t_{1/2}$ (hrs)	Protein binding (%)	Renal elimination (%)	Adverse effects
Prazosin	60	1–3	2–4	95	10	First dose effect Sedation Dryness of mouth
Clonidine	65–95	2–4	6–24	30	68	Sedation Headache Rebound AH
Guanfacine	95	1–3	17–21	20–30	80	Rebound AH Drowsiness Dryness of mouth
Captopril	68	1	4	30	60	Skin eruption Taste alterations Proteinuria
Nifedipine	65	1–2	4–5	90	80	Rubor Headache Tachycardia Pretibial edema
Verapamil	10–25	1–2	3–7	90	80	Constipation Headache Rubor Nausea Bradycardia AV block

Prazosin [5–18]

This substance is a quinazoline derivative that has arterio-venous vasodilator properties. The mechanism behind its vasodilator effect seems to be the capacity to selectively and competitively block the postsynaptic vasoconstrictor α-adrenoceptors [5]. Two more mechanisms that may help to explain its vasodilator effect are:

a) blockade of phosphodiesterase, increasing vascular AMPc levels, and
b) interference with norepinephrine synthesis by inhibiting dopamine-β-hydroxylase.

Nonetheless, these two effects appear at much higher drug concentrations than those habitually obtained in clinical practice. Participation of this mechanism in the hypotensive effect of prazosin is therefore doubtful [6, 7].

Pharmacologic effects [8–10]. Because of its arteriovenous vasodilator effect, prazosin decreases PVR and BP and increases cardiac output [17]. It also reduces venous return, which explains why its hypotensive effect is more marked when the patient is standing up than when lying down. Prazosin does not block the α_2-adrenoceptors, which when stimulated produce inhibition of norepinephrine release by sympathetic nerve ends: as a consequence, and in contrast with other vasodilators (minoxidil, diazoxide, hydralazine), its hypotensive effect is accompanied by a slight or null increase in heart rate, plasma renin activity, and circulating catecholamine levels [10]. In prolonged treatments it has been demonstrated that prazosin does not modify cerebral or renal blood flow or glomerular filtration rate (GFR), and that it decreases

Table 3. Preparations, routes of administration and dosages.

Drug	Commercial name	Presentation	Dosis	Effect (hrs)		
				Initial	Maximum	Total
Prazosin	Minipres	1, 2, 5 mg tablets	2–5 mg/6 hr	0.5	2–3	6
Clonidine	Catapresán	0.150 mg tablets	0.150 mg/6–8 hr	0.5	1	3–6
Guanfacine	Estulic	1, 2 mg tablets	1–3 mg/day	2	6	24
Captropril	Capotén	25, 50, 100 mg tablets				
	Cesplon	25, 50 mg tablets	25 mg/8 hr	0.5	2	6–8
Nifedipine	Adalat	10 mg capsules		0.5	1–2	6–8[a]
	Cordilan	10 mg capsules	5–20 mg/4–8 hr	5'	0.5–1	4–6[b]
	Dilcor	10 mg capsules				
Verapamil	Manidon	10, 80, 120 mg tablets	80–160 mg/8 hr	0.3	1–2	6–8

[a] Per os.

[b] Sublingual.

serum cholesterol or triglycerides while it increases the high density lipoproteins and cholesterol index [11]. Since prazosin does not alter heart rate and has no positive inotropic effects, but reduces filling pressure and BP, it reduces myocardial O_2 demand [6, 7].

Pharmacokinetics [8, 12, 13, 17]. Oral absorption of prazosin is good and effects appear in 30 minutes. Ninety five per cent is bound by plasma proteins, and the drug is widely distributed throughout the organism, reaching the maximum plasma concentration in 1–3 hours. Eighty-five per cent is biotransformed in the liver by O-dealkylation and glucuronoconjugation, forming 6-0-dimethylprazosin, with only 10% of the potency of prazosin. It is mainly eliminated in bile, 90% of the dosis given being excreted in feces; the rest is eliminated in urine. The pharmacokinetics of prazosin in the elderly patient do not differ, and plasma levels are not altered by hemodialysis.

Adverse effects. In hypertensive patients, the main adverse effect is postural hypotension, which is generally much more marked with the first dose; this first-dose phenomenon [8, 10, 16, 17] is characterized by dizziness, palpitations, vertigo, fainting and occasionally syncope in the 30–120 min immediately after giving the first dose of prazosin. This disorder appears most often in patients treated with β-blocking agents, in patients with a previous diuretic Na-depletion treatment or in those with kidney problems. This phenomenon may be due to inadequate venous return and is preceded by an abrupt descent in heart rate. The complication can be avoided by initiating treatment with low doses (0.5 mg), with the patient lying down and after interrupting diuretic treatment the day before and the first day of prazosin treatment.

Other mild adverse effects that appear during treatment include [8]: dizziness, headache, nausea, somnolence, confusion, lassitude, nervousness, hallucinations, cutaneous exanthema, dryness of the mouth, nasal congestion, diarrhea, tachycardia and frequent micturition. Prazosin also produces urinary retention and weight gain that can be controlled with diuretics, which in turn potentiate the antihypertensive effect of this substance. Postural hypotension and somnolence are two effects that limit the use of this drug in patients with cerebrovascular insufficiency. In some patients prazosin can increase heart rate and aggravate a prior angina. It should therefore be administered cautiously in patients with ischemic heart disease. In contrast with other antihypertensive drugs sexual alterations are not frequent in patients treated with prazosin.

Clinical uses. Prazosin is useful for the treatment of mild or moderate AH, in association with diuretics and/or β-blocking agents. This reduces the hydrosaline retention that prazosin produces, and potentiates its antihypertensive effects. Moreover, prazosin is a useful alternative for patients in whom diuretics are not indicated (gout, diabetes) or β-blocking agents (asthmatics, congestive heart failure [CHF]) [19]. Treatment should begin with 0.5 mg, and the dosis increased every 2–3 days until the effective dosis is reached, which may be as much as 20 mg daily. Prazosin is effective in patients with low plasma renin activity [15], AH associated with kidney failure [9] or congestive heart failure, in preoperative treatment of pheochromocytoma and in patients on chronic hemodialysis [18].

Clonidine [20–26]

This drug stimulates the central α_2-adrenoceptors located in the pontomedullary region (solitary tract nucleus, vasomotor center and vagus nucleus) [20]. The result of stimulation of the receptors depends on whether their location is pre- or postsynaptic. Postsynaptic receptor stimulation leads to activation of a medullospinal inhibitory neuron, while α_2-presynaptic receptor stimulation reduces norepinephrine release by depressing the activity of a facilitating neuron. In either case, the result is the same: reduction in peripheral sympathetic tone [21]. Favoring this hypothesis of clonidine's central effect are the findings that:
a) the hypotensive effect appears when concentrations that do not produce any hypotensive effect when administered intravenously are injected into the vertebral artery;
b) the effect is inhibited after pretreatment with yohimbine (a selective α_2-receptor blocker); and
c) the effect disappears in tetraplegics with brainstem system section [22].

Pharmacologic effects. Clonidine decreases PVR and BP, which is accompanied by a reduction in cardiac output and heart rate [23]. The bradycardia not only results from α_2-receptor stimulation, but from a reflex increase in vagal tone of central origin [3] and presynaptic cardiac α_2-receptor stimulation, which decreases norepinephrine release in the sinus node [24]. The hypotensive effect of clonidine does not modify renal flow or GFR, but it reduces plasma catecholamine levels and plasma renin activity. Given intravenously the hypotensive effect characteristic of clonidine is preceded by a brief hypertensive response possibly due to stimulation of the peripheral α_1-adrenoceptors [25]. This stimulation is more marked in venous capacitance vessels than in resistance vessels, which would explain why orthostatic hypotension phenomena are so infrequent during clonidine treatment [23, 26].

Pharmacokinetics [23, 26]. Oral absorption of clonidine is good, the bioavailability being 75%. The substance is widely distributed and undergoes biotransformation in the liver. Sixty per cent of the drug is eliminated in urine without biotransformation. The half-life increases from 4 hrs to more than 10 hrs in hypertensive patients.

Adverse effects. The main adverse effect is sedation (depression, somnolence) as a consequence of this drug's effect on the central α_2-receptors, which appears in 45–80% of patients. It is recommended that the drug be administered before retiring to lessen these effects. Somnolence is potentiated by use of hypnotics, tranquilizers, antiepileptics or alcohol [21]. Clonidine also produces: dryness of the mouth, bradycardia, hydrosaline retention, impotence, constipation, nausea, anorexia, fatigue, postural hypotension and skin eruptions. Moreover, abrupt suppression of treatment produces 'rebound AH' in the 15 hours after the last dosis [25, 26], accompanied by tachycardia, vomiting, nervousness, headache, sweating and increase in urinary catecholamines. These manifestations can be controlled by administering clonidine or an α-blocker (phentolamine) and a β-adrenergic blocker (propranolol).

Clonidine should be given with caution in patients with bradycardia, hepatorenal insufficiency, Raynaud's disease, thromboangiitis obliterans or clinical history of depressive psychosis, ischemic heart disease or cerebrovascular disease. Tricyclic antidepressants and phenothiazines competitively antagonize the hypotensive effects of clonidine, and their association with this substance in the hypertensive patient should be avoided.

Clinical uses [23, 26]. Clonidine is used to treat mild or moderate AH, although its adverse effects (in particular, the risk of rebound AH) limit its utility as a first choice drug or as a single option. It is recommended that it be used in association with diuretics, β-blocking agents or vasodilators. Treatment is initiated with 0.1 mg/12 hours and the dosis is increased until 0.8 mg/6–8 hours is reached. However, clonidine and guanfacine present some advantages over other AH drugs since they can be given safely to asthmatics, diabetics or patients with congestive heart failure. The incidence of orthostatic hypotension and sexual alterations is scarce during treatment [26].

Transdermic administration of clonidine is at an experimental stage (*Catapresán-TTS^R*). A 3.5 cm patch [27] applied to the skin releases 0.1 mg/day of clonidine for a week. After placement, plasma clonidine levels and the hypotensive effect increase progressively over 72 hours, followed by stabilization of plasma levels (0.4–0.6 ng/ml) and hypotensive effect. When the patch is removed, plasma levels remain stable for 8 hours, then decline during the following 72 hours, accompanied by a return to pre-treatment BP. This reduction in systolic and diastolic BP is similar to that observed when clonidine is administered orally, although the plasma levels of clonidine (1.6 ng/ml) are much higher in this case than those obtained transdermically. Preliminary findings [27] indicate that four or five days after affixing the patch, somnolence, dry mouth and skin alterations (erythema) can appear, effects that disappear rapidly after its removal.

Guanfacine [28–32]

This drug stimulates the central α_2-adrenoceptors and has properties similar to those described for clonidine. Like clonidine, it reduces PVR and BP, but hardly modifies cardiac output. In long-term treatment its hypotensive effect is accompanied by a reduction in plasma catecholamine, renin and prolactin levels [29, 30].

Pharmacokinetics [28]. Orally, guanafacine is absorbed well (95%), attaining maximum plasma levels in 60–90 min. Twenty per cent is carried by plasma proteins and widely distributed, crossing the hematoencephalic and placental barriers. It is biotransformed in the liver by hydroxylation and conjugation and eliminated mainly in the kidney, although a small portion is excreted in maternal milk. The elimination half-life is superior to 17 hours and together with the elevated tissular affinity of the drug, is responsible for its prolonged hypotensive effect.

Adverse effects [31]. Guanfacine produces somnolence, dryness of the mouth, constipation, orthostatic hypotension, asthenia, vertigo and headache. The appearance of rebound AH has also been described, although it is less dramatic than that induced by clonidine, appearing 2–7 days after suspending treatment [32]. Dryness of the mouth and sedation appear at the onset of treatment, with elevated doses and when associated with diuretics. As for clonidine, the sedative effect of the drug can be reduced by giving it at bedtime; hypnotics, tranquilizers and alcohol potentiate the sedative effect of guanfacine. β-blocking agents enhance the bradycardic effect of guanfacine, and tricyclic antidepressants increase its hypotensive effects. Guanfacine is contraindicated in patients with advanced AV block or with severe renal failure not on dialysis and should be used cautiously in patients with cerebrovascular insufficiency.

Clinical uses. The uses are similar to those of clonidine, guanfacine being of value in mild or moderate AH, generally associated with diuretics and/or β-blocking agents [28–30]. Treatment begins with 0.5 mg/day and the dose is increased weekly until 2 mg daily is reached.

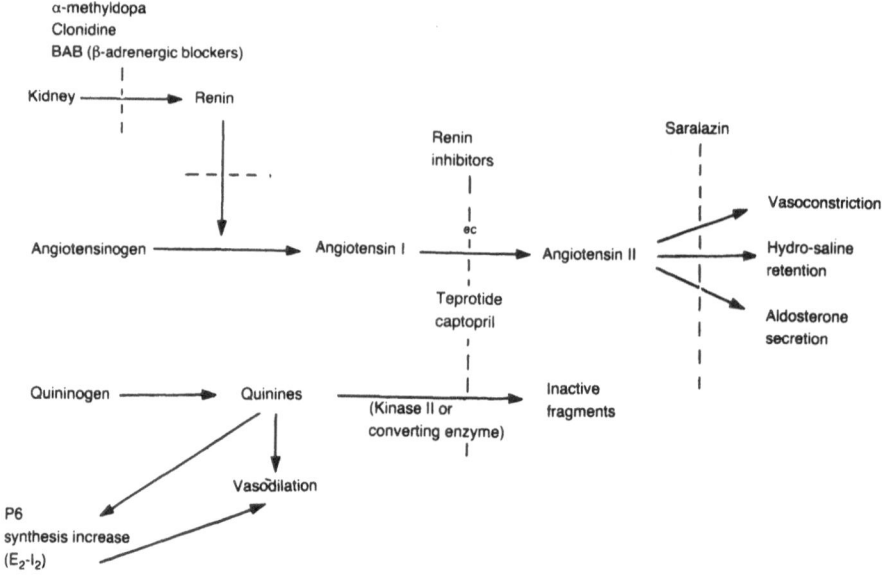

Fig. 1. Diagram of the renin-angiotensin-aldosterone system and the sites of action of the principal drugs that inhibit it. BAB: β-adrenergic blockers. CE: converting enzyme. α-MD: α-methyldopa. PGs: prostaglandins.

Inhibitors of the renin-angiotensin-aldosterone system [6, 33–43]

This system controls BP, fluid-electrolyte balance and PVR [33]. It thus seems logical that some types of BP are accompanied by alterations in this system. Fig. 1 shows the site of action of drugs that inhibit it.

Captopril

This drug acts by competitively blocking the converting enzyme (peptidyldipeptidase) [33–35] that transforms angiotensin I into angiotensin II (Fig. 1). As a result:

a) Captopril decreases plasma angiotensin II concentrations and its corresponding vasoconstrictive effect, and angiotensin III levels, reducing plasma and urine aldosterone levels and the Na and H_2O retention this substance produces [37].

b) It blocks kinase II, inhibiting enzymatic degradation of bradykinin, a vasodilator per se, and increasing prostaglandin E_2 and F_2 synthesis, also vasodilators. At present, there is no conclusive proof that the increase in kinins plays an important role in the long-term antihypertensive effects of captopril, although it may participate in the acute response.

c) It is possible that captopril exercises a direct venodilator effect, that may be exceptionally intense at the pulmonary level.

Pharmacologic effects. Captopril produces arteriovenous vasodilation, decreasing BP in both normo and hypertensive patients [37–43]. At the onset of treatment the hypotensive effect is related to plasma angiotensin II levels and plasma renin activity, but this relation disappears after a few weeks of treatment. Captopril also reduces plasma aldosterone and catecholamine concentrations and increases plasma renin activity (especially in patients with vasculorenal AH), possibly by impeding the negative feedback that angiotensin II exercises over renin release and by a reflex increase in SNS tone. The hypotensive effect of captopril is accompanied by a reduction in PVR without significant changes in cardiac output, pulmonary capillary pressure or right atrial pressure. However, in hypertensive patients with congestive heart failure, captopril increases cardiac output, reduces pulmonary capillary pressure and, by decreasing venous return, right atrial pressure. Heart rate remains unchanged or slightly decreases (10%). This finding suggests that captopril may reduce baroreceptor sensitivity.

Coronary and splanchnic blood flow increase; renal blood flow is also enhanced as a consequence of lower angiotensin II and higher bradykinin levels. An elevation in renal Na excretion is also observed perhaps due to reduction in the angiotensin II and aldosterone concentrations, a direct tubular effect, or to the inhibition of the sympathetic tone of the renal vessels [39]. Captopril does not affect, or may reduce, skin, muscle and hepatomesenteric circulation. The increased blood supply observed in other territories could be the result of a circulatory redistribution.

In hypertensive patients treated for 5–9 months with captopril, no changes were observed in left ventricular diameter, but there was a reduction in the thickness of the posterior left ventricular wall and ventricular septum, suggesting that the drug may decrease cardiac hypertrophy.

Pharmacokinetics. The pharmacokinetics of the drug are still not well known [7, 43]. Given orally, 70% is absorbed, but if given with food this percentage decreases to 30%. Thirty per cent is carried by the plasma proteins and is widely distributed, although it does not cross the blood-brain barrier and is not excreted in maternal milk. Thirty eight per cent is biotransformed at the hepatic level and is rapidly eliminated by urine, where 60% appears after 4 hours. There is a correlation between the rate of renal elimination and the creatinine clearance, and the dosis should be reduced in patients with renal failure.

Adverse effects [38–43]. These effects are relatively frequent (5–10% of patients). The following have been described:

a) hematologic alterations: neutropenia (after 3–12 weeks of treatment), leukopenia and agranulocytosis;

b) cutaneous alterations: maculopapular exanthema (a dose-dependent phenomenon that appears in 14% of patients in the first two weeks of treatment, associated with fever, pruritus and eosinophilia, and attributed to an increase in plasma kinins), and pemphigoid and aphthous ulcers that disappear after withdrawing treatment;

c) transitory loss of taste is seen in 6% of patients;

d) gastrointestinal disorders: nausea, vomiting and abdominal pain;

e) cardiovascular alterations: postural hypotension and tachycardia;

f) renal alterations: proteinuria appears in 2% of patients after 8 months of treatment, and nephrotic syndrome and membranous glomerulonephritis are rarely present [40]. These manifestations are accompanied by hyperpotassemia, and potassium should be monitored during treatment. It is unclear if these alterations are due to a nephrotoxic effect or to the reduction in renal blood supply produced by hypotension. In any case, these disorders improve when treatment is discontinued. For these reasons, periodic analyses are required, including blood cell count, differential leukocyte count and detection of proteins in urine.

The incidence of severe adverse effects (hematological and renal) increases with the dosis, in renal failure, previous proteinuria, autoimmune disease (LE) or under treatment with cytostatics or immunosuppressors. In hypertensive patients with high plasma renin activity due to Na^+ restriction or treatment with diuretics, or in patients with stenotis of the renal artery, there may be an intense hypotensive response to the first dosis of captopril. This can be avoided by giving small doses (5–12.5 mg) and having the patient lie down. In spite of these adverse effects, captopril represents an advance in the treatment of AH because it does not produce postural hypotension, depression, sleep or sexual disorders, glucose intolerance or tachycardia, nor does rebound AH appear on discontinuation of the drug.

Clinical uses [38–44]. Captopril is effective in the therapy of any type of AH. The initial dosis is 25 mg/8 hours, to be increased after 2–3 weeks until 150 mg/8 hours is reached. In patients with impaired renal function the dosis should be reduced and the administration intervals prolonged. Following these guidelines, 80% of the patients with essential AH respond to treatment with captopril, alone or in association with thiazides or furosemide. Since captopril increases kalemia by reducing aldosterone production, it should not be associated with K^+ saving diuretics; this effect accounts for the fact that when this drug is associated with thiazides or furosemide there is no risk of hypokalemia and potassium supplements are unnecessary. It is also effective in patients with severe AH resistant to other drugs [43], pulmonary AH or AH associated with Buttler syndrome, hemolytic uremic syndrome or scleroderma. As can be deduced from its mechanism of action, patients with AH and high plasma renin activity (vasculorenal AH and certain forms of malignant AH) respond very well to captopril [42]. However, it is not effective in patients with primary hyperaldosteronism. Associated with propanolol, captopril produces an additive effect in patients with normal or high plasma renin activity [44]. In patients with low renin concentration, captopril should be associated with diuretics; this combination can also be useful in hypertensive women in whom minoxidil produces hirsutism.

Enalapril

Since part of the undesirable effects of captopril have been attributed to the sulfhydryl group of the molecule, in recent years diverse converting enzyme inhibitors lacking this reactive group have been synthesized. Of these, the most promising is enalapril (Mk-421). Enalapril is a prodrug that does not have the converting enzyme inhibitory effect, but when given orally it is intestinally absorbed and biotransformed in the liver into a diazine that is converting enzyme inhibitor 6 to 10 times more potent than captopril. After oral administration of enalapril the hypotensive effect appears in 1–3 hours, reaching its maximum in 4–8 hours and lasting 24 hours. The incidence of adverse effects of enalapril seems to be lower than that of captopril.

Calcium antagonists [45–60]

The calcium antagonists constitute a heterogeneous group of drugs that have the pharmacologic property of blocking Ca inflow in cardiac muscular fibers and in vascular smooth muscle fibers. At present, they are interesting in AH treatment because they correct the anomalous vasoconstrictor response of the hypertensive patient.

In practically all cases of essential AH, the increase in BP is the consequence of an elevation in PVR, which is ultimately related to an increment in $[Ca]_i$ in the vascular smooth muscle. This increase in $[Ca]_i$ has been considered to be responsible for the abnormal vasomotor tone in the hypertensive patient [45]: an increased membrane Na gradient would lead to an increment in $[Ca]_i$ and to higher vascular wall tension and PVR. Diverse experimental findings support this hypothesis:

a) In resistance vessels, in contrast with what occurs in capacitance vessels, the vasoconstriction induced by catecholamines or sympathetic stimulation depends fundamentally on Ca inflow [46, 47].

b) The more intense vasoconstrictive response to norepinephrine observed in hypertensive animals is related to a greater Ca inflow in the vascular smooth fibers [46].
c) There is an increase in [Ca] in the vascular walls of the hypertensive patient that increments with age [60].

Pharmacologic effects [48, 60]. Nifedipine and verapamil produce both arterial and venous vasodilation, reducing PVR and BP. The hypotensive effect is related to the previous pressure level [49] and the age of the patient, but not to plasma renin activity. Thus, the hypotensive effect of nifedipine is minimal in normotensive patients, and its effect increases with BP, RVP and age [58].

The hypotensive effect of nifedipine is accompanied by an increase in sinus rate, cardiac index and output. Tachycardia disappears in a few hours, although the hypotensive effect persists for 6–8 hours; moreover, tachycardia progressively reduces its rate in the first 2–4 weeks of treatment. In any case, the higher the blood pressure of the patient, the lower the tachycardia. The hypotensive effect of nifedipine is accompanied by an increase in plasma renin activity and plasma catecholamine levels [50, 52], but aldosterone levels are unchanged. The increase in plasma renin activity is the result of a reflex increase in sympathetic tone and disappears at 3–4 weeks of treatment. In contrast with other vasodilators, nifedipine produces a natriuretic effect that may contribute to its hypotensive effect.

Verapamil reduces PVR and BP, but in contrast with nifedipine, does not modify or discretely increases heart rate and cardiac output during treatment [51, 53, 54]. The hypotensive response to verapamil is not accompanied by variations in plasma renin activity or in plasma catecholamine or aldosterone levels, although there is a positive correlation between basal catecholamine levels and the magnitude of the hypotensive response. Neither verapamil nor nifedipine modify or increase renal blood flow. After suppressing treatment with these drugs, BP gradually recovers to pre-treatment levels in 48 hours without rebound AH.

In the heart, Ca antagonists depress cardiac contractility, heart rate, and slow AV conduction (this effect is much more intense with verapamil). However, these effects do not appear at the usual doses due to the strong vasodilator effect these substances have. These drugs stimulate baroreceptors and increase sympathetic cardiac tone, manifested as an increase in cardiac contractility and rate. The result of these opposite effects is that at the usual dosage of nifedipine, a potent vasodilator, the reflex effects predominate and heart rate and dp/dt_{max} increase. Verapamil, a less powerful vasodilator, induces less reflex compensation and hardly modifies cardiac contractility or rate, although it increases the refractory period of the AV node. In patients with ischemic heart disease, the Ca antagonists exert antianginal and cardioprotective effects [6]. This antianginal effect is a consequence of the capacity to decrease myocardial O_2 requirements while increasing coronary blood flow and suppressing vasospastic phenomena.

In contrast with other vasodilators, verapamil and nifedipine do not produce hydrosaline retention, bronchoconstriction (they are bronchodilators), alterations in glucose tolerance or increased plasma lipids. Moreover, they increase cardiac output (which reduces the risk of hypotension secondary to a sharp decrease in PRV) and have antianginal effects. Their hypotensive effect does not decline in the course of treatment and there is no risk of rebound hypertension, all of which justify the interest in the Ca antagonists as first line drugs in the therapy of the hypertensive patient.

Pharmacokinetics [6, 48]. Although oral absorption of nifedipine is good, its bioavailability is 65% and maximum plasma concentrations are attained 1–2 hours after per os administration [48]. Ninety per cent is transported by plasma proteins and biotransformation into inactive metabolites takes place in the liver. Sixty per cent is excreted in the bile and part of the compound is eliminated in the feces. Metabolites are recycled enterohepatically and eliminated by the kidney.

Verapamil is absorbed very well orally, although its bioavailability is poor (10–25%) because it suffers an important first pass effect in the liver; bioavailability increases in liver diseases with the portocaval short-circuit. Orally, the maximum plasma levels are reached in 1–2 hours, while intravenously the effects are immediate. Ninety per cent is bound to plasma proteins, but it can be displaced by certain drugs (lidocaine, diazepam) that potentiate in this way its effects. The substance suffers a notable hepatic biotransformation and its demethylated metabolite (norverapamil) shows mild antihypertensive properties; the half-life of the drug increases from 4 hours to 14 hours in patients with liver cirrhosis or failure.

Adverse effects [6, 48]. During nifedipine treatment, the most frequent are those that originate from its vasodilator effect: reddening of the skin, headache, dizziness, shortness of breath, nausea and hypotension. These effects tend to ameliorate in the course of 2–3 weeks of treatment. Digital dysesthesias and malleolar edema can also appear; these effects are seen in up to 20% of patients, mainly women, and do not respond to diuretic treatment. In spite of the fact that the risk of depressing contractility is minimal at the usual doses, the drug should be given with care in patients with CHF.

Verapamil produces the following effects:
a) cardiovascular effects: bradycardia, AV block and depression of contractility; vasodilator effects: hypotension, headache, dizziness, skin reddening;
b) gastrointestinal alterations: nausea, vomiting, pyrosis, epigastric pain, constipation.

Its administration is contraindicated in patients with sinus node disease, sinoatrial or AV block, recent infarct, bradycardia, depression of contractility, WPW or atrial fibrillation.

Although association of β-blocking agents with Ca antagonists does not usually produce serious cardiovascular effects in the hypertensive patient, due care should be taken; Ca antagonists attenuate the vasoconstrictor effects of β-blocking agents and these diminish the reflex increase in heart rate produced by the Ca antagonists. The Ca antagonists potentiate the hypotensive effect of prazosin and when these drugs are associated, dosages should be reduced to avoid postural hypotension.

Clinical uses. Although there is still not enough clinical experience to reach definite conclusions the Ca antagonists have assumed an important role in recent years in the treatment of mild or moderate AH, especially in patients who do not respond to diuretics or β-blocking agents [51, 54]. Moreover, they may substitute diuretics as first line drugs in the elderly hypertensive patient.

Nifedipine is administered sublingually or orally at a dosage of 5–20 mg/6–8 hours [51–54, 59, 60]. Sublingually its effects appear in 5 min, reaching their maximum intensity in 15–20 min and disappearing in 6–8 hours. Orally, the hypotensive effect appears in 30 min, reaches its maximum in 1–2 hours and lasts 6–8 hours. Associated with β-blocking agents or alphamethyldopa, oral nifedipine is useful in the therapy of severe AH, especially in patients with high PVR, impaired renal function or in those in whom other treatments have failed. Alphamethyldopa not only potentiates the effects of nifedipine, but suppresses the tachycardia this substance produces. Sublingual nifedipine is a useful drug for the treatment of hypertensive emergencies (hypertensive encephalopathy, pheochromocytoma, AH associated with pulmonary edema or ischemic heart disease): its rapid and powerful hypotensive effect, easy administration (monitoring is not required) and limited adverse effects explain why traditional vasodilators of similar efficacy in the treatment of these patients are being replaced by nifedipine [59, 60]. Nonetheless, nifedipine is not indicated for AH associated with increased cardiac output.

Verapamil is given orally (60–160 mg/8 hours) or i.v. (5–10 mg). The intravenous route is reserved for severe AH or hypertensive emergencies; by this route its effect is immediate and persists for 15–20 min [55–60]. Orally, its effects are similar to those of the β-blocking agents and verapamil can substitute these drugs in patients in whom they are contraindicated or produce adverse effects. Verapamil seems to be very effective in elderly hypertensive patients with low PRA.

References

1. Veteran's Administration Cooperative Study Group on Antihypertensive Agents: Effects of treatment on morbility in hypertension. I. Results in patients with pressures averaging 115 through 129 mm Hg. JAMA 1967; 202: 1028–1034.
2. Veteran's Administration Cooperative Study Group on Antihypertensive Agents: Effects of treatment on mobility in hypertension. II. Results in patients with diastolic blood pressures averaging 90 to 114 mm Hg. JAMA 1967; 202: 1143–1152.
3. Kobinger W: Central α-adrenergic systems as targets for hypotensive drugs. Rev Physiol Biochem Pharmacol 1978; 81: 39–75.
4. Langer S: Presynaptic regulation of the release of catecholamines. Pharmac Rev 1981; 32: 337–362.
5. Cambridge D, Davey H, Massingham R: Prazosin, a selective antagonist for postsynaptic α-adrenoreceptors. Br J Pharmacol 1977; 59: 514–520.
6. Tamargo J, Lombrera F, Lopez Sendon J: Tratamiento con vasodilatores en la insuficiencia cardiaca y angina de pecho. Clin Cardiovasc 1982; 1: 89–107.
7. Lopez Sendon J, Tamargo J: Vasodilatores en la insuficiencia cardiaca. In: Avances en cardiología. Edited by the Sociedad Española de Cardiologia. Científico-Médica, Barcelona, 1983; 337–360.
8. Rawinds M, Geyer G, Beeued E (eds): European prazosin symposium. Excerpta Medica, Amsterdam, 1979.
9. Graham R, Murvihill-Wilson J: Clinical pharmacology of prazosin used alone or in combination in the therapy of hypertension. J Cardiovasc Pharmacol 1980; 2 (Suppl 3): S387–S398.
10. Graham R, Pettinger W: Prazosin. N Engl J Med 1979; 300: 232–236.
11. Lowenstein J: Effects of prazosin on serum lipids in patients with essential hypertension: a review of the findings presented at the satellite symposium on coronary heart disease, hypertension and other risk factors. Am J Cardiol 1984; 53: 21A–23A.
12. Hobbs D, Twomey T, Palmer R: Pharmacokinetics of prazosin in man. J Clin Pharmacol 1978; 18: 402–410.
13. Jahion P: Clinical pharmacokinetics of prazosin. Clin Pharmacokinet 1980; 5: 365–376.
14. Graham R, Thornell I, Gain J, Bagnolli C, Oates H, Stokes G: Prazosin: the first-dose phenomenon. Br Med J 1976; 2: 1293–1294.
15. Bolli P, Amann F, Buhler F: Antihypertensive response to postsynaptic α-blockade with prazosin in low – and normal – renin hypertension. J Cardiovasc Pharmacol 1980; 2 (Suppl 3): S399–S405.
16. Bendall N, Baloch K, Wilson P: Side effects due to treatment of hypertension with prazosin. Br Med J 1975; 2: 727–728.
17. Rubin P, Braschke T: Clinical pharmacology of prazosin. Br J Clin Pharmacol 1980; 10: 23–32.
18. Harter H, Delmez J: Effects of prazosin in the control of blood pressure in hypertensive dialysis patients. J Cardiovasc Pharmacol 1979; 1 (Suppl 6): 543–555.
19. Okun R: Effectiveness of prazosin as initial antihypertensive therapy. Am J Cardiol 1983; 51: 644–650.
20. Chalmers J: Brain amines and models of experimental hypertension. Circ Res 1975; 36: 469–480.
21. Van Zweiten P, Thoolen M, Timmermans P: The pharmacology of centrally acting antihypertensive drugs. Br J Clin Pharmacol 1983; 15: 455S–462S.
22. Reid J, Wing L, Mathias C: The central hypotensive effect of clonidine. Studies in tetraplegic subjects. Clin Pharmacol Ther 1977; 21: 375–382.
23. Pettinger W: Clonidine, a new antihypertensive drug. N Engl J Med 1975; 293: 1179–1180.

24. DeJonge A, Timmermans P, Van Zweiten P: Participation of cardiac presynaptic α_2-adreno-ceptors in the bradycardic effects of clonidine and analogues. Naunyn-Schmiedeberg 1981; 317: 8–12.

25. Hansson L: Clinical aspects of blood pressure crisis due to withdrawal of centrally acting antihypertensive drugs. Br J Clin Pharmacol 1983; 15: 485S–489S.

26. Dollery C, Davies D, Draffan G et al.: Clinical pharmacology and pharmacokinetics of clonidine. Clin Pharmacol Ther 1976; 19: 11–19.

27. Symposium: Transdermal delivery of cardiovascular drugs. Am Heart J 1984; 108: 195.

28. Scholtysick G: Pharmacology of guanfacine. Br J Clin Pharmacol 1980; 10: 21S–25S.

29. Fariello R, Agabitti-Rosei E, Alicandri C et al.: Clinical study of guanfacine in essential hypertensive patients: effects of therapy and withdrawal on blood pressure, heart rate, plasma catecholamines and plasma renin activity. Curr Ther Res 1981; 29: 968–975.

30. Jerie P: Clinical experience with guanfacine in long-term treatment of hypertension. Part I: efficacy and dosage. Br J Clin Pharmacol 1980; 10: 37S–47S.

31. Jerie P: Clinical experience with guanfacine in long-term treatment of hypertension. Part II: adverse reactions to guanfacine. Br J Clin Pharmacol 1980; 10: 157S–164S.

32. Zamboulis C, Reid J: Withdrawal of guanfacine after long-term treatment in essential hypertension. Observations on blood pressure and plasma urinary noradrenaline. Eur J Clin Pharmacol 1981; 1: 19–24.

33. Laragh J: The renin system in essential, renovascular and adrenocortical hypertension. An overview. Adv Nephrol 1978; 7: 157–165.

34. Antonaccio M, Cushman D: Drugs inhibiting the renin-angiotensin system. Federation Proc 1981; 40: 2275–2284.

35. Ferguson R, Brunner H, Turini G, Gavras H: Specific orally active inhibitor of angiotensin converting enzyme in man. Lancet 1977; 1: 775–778.

36. Nakkano J: Effects of bradykinin on cardiovascular dynamics. In: Sicuteri J, Rocha e Silva E, Back N (eds): Bradykinin and related kinins. Plenum Press, New York, 1970; 157–164.

37. Williams G, Hollemberg N: Accentuated vascular and endocrine response to SQ 20881 in hypertension. N Engl J Med 1977; 297: 184–188.

38. Bravo E, Tarazi R: Converting enzyme inhibition with an orally active compound in hypertensive man. Hypertension 1979; 1: 39–46.

39. Faxon D, Creager R, Halperin J: Regional circulatory response to converting enzyme inhibition in congestive heart failure. Br J Clin Pharmacol 1982; 14: 179S–186S.

40. Hoorntje S, Weening J, The T, Kallenberg C, Donker A, Hoedemaeker P: Immune complex glomerulopathy in patients treated with captopril. Lancet 1980; 1: 1212–1214.

41. Atkinson A, Robertson J: Captopril in the treatment of clinical hypertension and cardiac failure. Lancet 1979; 2: 836–839.

42. Gavras H, Brunner H, Turine G: Antihypertensive effect of the oral angiotensin converting-enzyme-inhibitor SQ 14225 in man. N Engl J Med 1978; 298: 991–995.

43. Captopril: Worldwide clinical experience. Br J Clin Pharmacol 1982; 14 (Suppl 2): 69S–209S.

44. Pickering T, Case D, Sullivan P, Laragh J: Comparison of antihypertensive and hormonal effects of captopril and propanolol at rest and during exercise. Am J Cardiol 1982; 49: 1566–1568.

45. Blaustein M: Sodium ions, calcium ions, blood pressure regulation and hypertension: a reassessment and a hypothesis. Am J Physiol 1977; 232: C165–176.

46. Cauvin C, Saida K, Van Breemen C: Effects of Ca antagonists on Ca fluxes in resistance vessels. J Cardiovasc Pharmacol 1982; 4 (Suppl 3): S287–S290.

47. Folkow B, Hallback M, Jones J, Sutter M: Dependence on external Ca for the noradrenaline contratility of the resistance in spontaneously hypertensive and renal hypertensive rats, as compared with normotensive controls. Acta Physiol Scand 1977; 101: 84–97.

48. Stone H, Antman E (eds): Calcium channel blocking agents in the treatment of cardiovascular disorders. Futura Publishing Co, New York, 1983.

49. McGreggor G, Markandu N, Bayliss J, Brown M, Roulston J: Circumstantial evidence that an abnormality of calcium transport may be important in essential hypertension. Clin Sci 1981; 60: 6–10.

50. Aoki K, Kondo S, Mochizuki A: Antihypertensive effects of cardiovascular Ca antagonist in hypertensive patients in the absence and presence of β-adrenergic blockade. Am Heart J 1978; 96: 218–224.

51. Guazzi M, Olivari M, Polese A, Fiorentini C, Magrini F, Moruzzi P: Nifedipine, a new antihypertensive with rapid action. Clin Pharmacol Ther 1977; 22: 528–534.

52. Corea L, Miele N, Bentivoglio M, Boschetti E, Agabiti-Rosei E, Muiesan G: Acute and chronic effects or nifedipine on plasma renin activity and plasma adrenaline and noradrenaline in controls and hypertensive patients. Clin Sci 1979; 57 (Suppl 1): 115S–117S.

53. Olivari M, Bartorelli C, Polese A, Fiorentini C, Moruzzi P, Guazi M: Treatment of hypertension with nifedipine, a calcium antagonistic agent. Circulation 1979; 59: 1056–1062.

54. Guazzi M, Fiorentini C, Olivari M, Bartorelli A, Necchi G, Polese A: Short- and long-term efficacy or a calcium-antagonistic agent (nifedipine) combined with methlydopa in the treatment of severe hypertension. Circulation 1980; 61: 913–919.

55. Vicenzi M, Allegri P, Gabaldo S, Maiolo P, Ometto R: Hemodynamic effects caused by i.v. administration of verapamil in healthy subjects. Drug Res 1976; 26: 1221–1228.

56. Midtbo K, Hals O: Verapamil in the treatment of hypertension. Curr Ther Res 1980; 27: 830–838.

57. Leonetti G, Sala C, Bianchini C, Terzoli L, Zanchetti A: Antihypertensive and renal effects of orally administered verapamil. Eur J Clin Pharmacol 1980; 18: 375–382.

58. Buhler F, Lennart U, Kiowski W, Muller F, Bolli P: The place of the calcium antagonist verapamil in antihypertensive therapy. J Cardiovasc Pharmacol 1982; 4: S350–S357.

59. Hulthen U, Bolli P, Buhler F: Calcium influx blockers in the treatment of essential hypertension. Acta Md Scand 1983; (Suppl 681): 101–108.

60. Symposium on calcium antagonists. Rev Esp Cardiolog 1983; 36: 459–483.

5.5 Problems in the Treatment of Chronic Primary Arterial Hypertension

V. LÓPEZ MERINO

Changes in the public health problems posed by hypertensives

Until a decade ago, statistics [1–3] indicated that in the United States in 1960 and 1967, 41% and 57%, respectively, of the persons surveyed were unaware of being hypertensive. The resulting figures gave rise to a public health aphorism of halves: 'Half the hypertensives don't know they have hypertension; of those that do know it, half don't treat it; of those who are treated, half don't follow the correct regimen'. The main problems were lack of knowledge of the disease and the side-effects of treatment.

Since then this situation has changed thanks to the efforts of the League Against Hypertension and the corresponding public health campaigns. In the United States 10 years later only 25–30% of the hypertensives were unaware of their disease [4, 5]. On the basis of figures taken from a study in Alameda County [5] (Fig. 1), the public health aphorism mentioned could be substituted by: 'More than two thirds of the hypertensive population knows they have hypertension; of these, two thirds are treated but less than a third attain therapeutic control of hypertension'.

The main problem now is that of *relative therapeutic failure,* and the study of its causes and the most opportune sanitary measures to take are the protagonists in the fight against hypertension.

In Table 1 the most frequent causes of therapeutic failure are summarized.

The absence of patient compliance continues to be one of the most important reasons for failure of therapy. This is conditioned by the fact that hypertension is a frequently asymptomatic process but its treatment obliges patients to take drugs for the rest of their lives – drugs which often produce side effects.

Better health education, with a health team 'constantly reinforcing' the patient's motivations, could palliate this situation, as well as a therapeutic regimen of single daily doses of drugs that do not produce side effects.

Patient behavior is characterized by the 'health model' we have and from which the factors related to noncompliance derive. The model suggests that

254

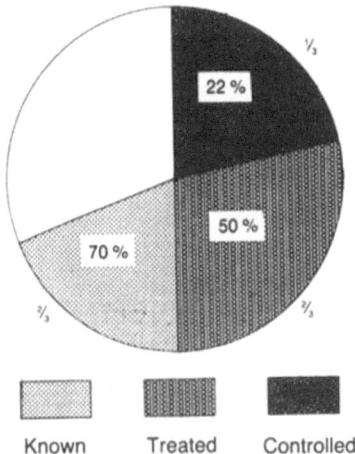

Fig. 1. Results of the Alameda County Study.

patients would adopt preventive measures and be more likely to follow the physician's recommendations:
a) if they felt sick or were aware of the importance of the disease;
b) if they believed they would become ill if they did not follow therapeutic norms;
c) if they were convinced of the effectiveness of treatment; and
d) if therapy were not a nuisance.

These conditions are not often encountered among hypertensive patients, as shown by Harris' trial [6], in which only 60% of the subjects were conscious of the seriousness of AH, young people being more skeptical (48%). Among asymptomatic patients, who were the majority, only 60% were cooperative [7]. Of the patients following treatment, 69% experienced side effects, most of which were not very important but still annoying [8].

The longer the patient has been treated, the less reliable patient compliance is [9], due to: ignorance or conceptual errors about the disease, insufficient motivation, lack of confidence in the physician or a complex therapeutic regimen. For this reason, we should attempt to resolve *the patient's problems by:*
a) facilitating patient information on the aim of the treatment and the need that it be permanent.
b) informing the patient of possible side effects of the drugs;
c) encouraging the patient to undergo periodic control, continue treatment and cooperate with the physician; and
d) informing the patient of the existence of other cardiovascular disease risk factors that should be eliminated.

To achieve this, well-trained family practitioners should be available or the periodic controls should be arranged in free access clinics that the patient can visit outside working hours and in which the control will be carried out by trained personnel.

The physician's problems are summarized in Table 2.

A good patient-doctor relationship is indispensable and the patient must be

Table 1. Causes of failure of a therapeutic regimen.

Discontinuation of treatment (the most frequent)
Ineffective dosage
Drug-linked factors (25–35%)
  Low blood level
  Refractoriness (renal failure, hypercalcemia)
Incorrect or insufficient regimen
Interference with treatment
  Water and salt intake
  Alcohol or other drug abuse
Uncontrolled drugs
  Contraceptives
  Amphetamines
  Cyclic antidepressants, IMAO
Inadequate BP control
  Emotional factors in the visit to the physician
  Psychiatric problems

Table 2. AH treatment. Physician's problems.

The patient should be completely informed about:
AH
  That it lasts a long time or forever
  That it is an important cause of stroke, heart failure or kidney failure
  That it can be controlled, but not cured
  That its risks can be reduced
The prescription
  Discuss the therapeutic plan with the patient (regimen, drugs)
  Clear and simple prescription
  Provide informative pamphlets
  Insist on life style and prophylaxis of other risk factors
  Explain actions and side effects of drugs

The patient should be motivated
  For adequate self-control
  To follow the prescription and accept trials variations in it

AH and treatment should be controlled
Prophylaxis and early detection should be made
Iatrogenesis should be avoided

---

convinced that mutual cooperation is fundamental to the success of the preliminary therapeutic trail-and-error period that will lead to final control. If this fails, Syme proposes an *alternative model* [5], based on experience in a program to stop smoking [10] designed for individuals at high risk of coronary artery disease: the patient-doctor relationship should not be allowed to become a paternal relationship; the patient should be responsible for taking decisions. Should the relationship become paternal, other alternatives should be sought, such as having other individuals assume the role of the patient's helper, in pairs or as support groups, as is done in associations for drug addiction or similar.

Which hypertensive patients should be treated?

There are two main problems at present: treatment of mild hypertension and treatment of systolic hypertension in the elderly patient.

Treatment of mild hypertension

Several studies [11–14] have made it clear that AH with a diastolic pressure of 105 mm Hg or more has to be treated and stepped guidelines for therapy have been given by the North American Joint National Committee [13] and the WHO [15].

Studies by the Hypertension Detection and Follow-up Program [16, 17] have attempted to clarify the effect of reducing blood pressure on the in-

Table 3. Reduction of mortality (%) in individuals according to patient characteristics at admittance to the Hypertension Detection and Follow-up Program.

Characteristics at admission	Stepped care (SC)		Referred care (RC)		
	No deaths	Incidence per 1000 pat./yr	No deaths	Incidence per 1000 pat./yr	Reduction in mortality (%)
Without organic alterations or antihypertensive treatment* Diastolic BP at admission					
90–94 mm Hg	36	7.0	54	10.6	34.0
95–99 mm Hg	39	8.4	53	11.6	27.6
100–104 mm Hg	31	9.3	44	11.6	19.8

*Organic alterations include: left ventricular hypertrophy in ECG; history of anterior myocardial infarction; history of stroke; history of intermittent claudication; serum creatinine 1.7 mg/dl.

cidence of acute myocardial infarction and death due to coronary disease in patients with mild AH. In a multicenter study with 10,940 participants, two groups of about 5,000 individuals were randomly assigned: one group to special centers where patients were rigorously treated using stepped care until blood pressure was reduced (SC group), while the other group (referred care group) (RC) continued with the usual medical care. At the end of the fifth year, BP had descended in both groups but was proportionally lower in patients in the SC group. Results and therapeutic benefits are listed in Tables 3 and 4.

An important finding was that complications clearly correlated to AH – specifically, left ventricular enlargement and cerebral stroke – decreased significantly in the SC group. Global mortality at 5 years in this group was 1.3% lower. However, patients under 50 years and Caucasian women obtained no benefits.

Various criticisms have been made of this study, which we will discuss below, the most important of them being the absence of a placebo control group and the fact that what is really demonstrated is that individualized and supervised treatment reduces global mortality.

In an Australian study [19], a reduction in cardiovascular mortality in patients with mild AH (diastolic pressure between 95 and 109 mm Hg) who were treated was shown as compared with a placebo group, although this decline was only observed in patients with diastolic pressure exceeding 100 mm Hg and not in those with diastolic pressure of 95–99 mm Hg. The earliest significant difference was obtained at the end of the fourth year. Therefore, this study does not demonstrate that treatment of AH in the case of diastolic pressures lower than 100 mm Hg is useful. Two important conclusions can be drawn: in half of the patients with a diastolic pressure of 95-109 mm Hg BP can be reduced to 95 mm Hg or lower without treatment; secondly, anti-hypertensive therapy reduces cardiovascular risk in patients with diastolic pressure over 100 mm Hg.

Table 4. Mild hypertension. Results of the Hypertension Detection and Follow-up Program (HDFP) (1979).

Cause of death	SC (n = 5485)	RC (n = 5455)	SC:RC (%) (Reduction)
Stroke	29	52	45
Myocardial infarct	51	69	26
All coronary deaths	131	148	20
All cardiovascular deaths	195	240	26
All noncardiac deaths	154	179	13

SC: stepped care group. RC: Referred care group.

258

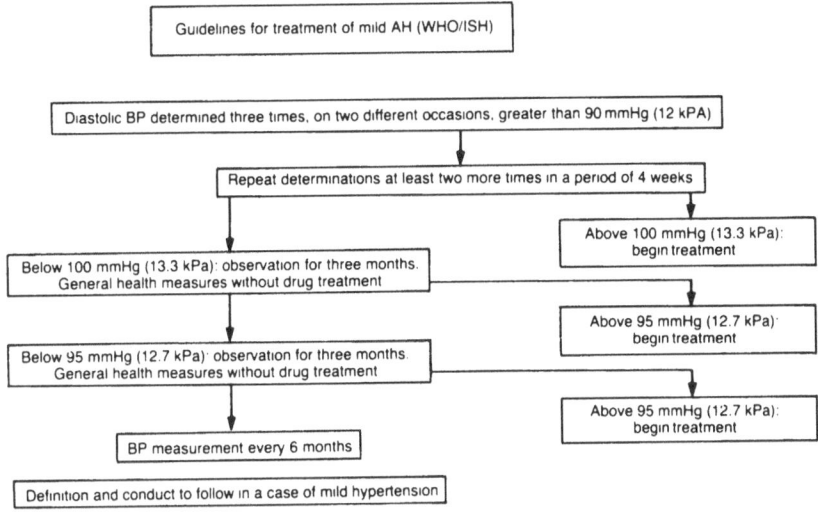

Fig. 2. Therapeutic guidelines for mild arterial hypertension (WHO/IHS) [22].

Nonetheless, other studies, such as the Oslo Study [20] or the Public Health Study on Mild Hypertension [12], seem to demonstrate that there is no benefit in treating mild AH. Both involve relatively small numbers of patients, and the data obtained should not be overestimated.

The Multiple Risk Factor Intervention Trial, designed to study the effects of modifications of the three major risk factors (AH, hypercholesterolemia, cigarrette smoking), concluded with the surprising result that patients with diastolic BP of 90–94 mm Hg who received antihypertensive treatment had a greater mortality and morbility than those not treated.

With this background, in 1982 the Mild Hypertension Liaison Committee of the WHO/ISH [21] analyzed the existing trials relative to treatment of mild AH and concluded that it was not justifiable to recommend drug treatment in patients with diastolic BP between 90 and 104 mm Hg, although they emphasized that individual considerations were important. One year later, although there had apparently been no new findings, the same group, enlarged to 31 members (instead of 7), decided to establish norms for the treatment of mild AH [22]. These guidelines are summarized in the diagram in Fig. 2. Any definitive attitude with respect to these patients is important because 70% of the total hypertensive population has a diastolic pressure between 90 and 105 mm Hg.

These recent guidelines and criteria of the WHO/ISH (1983) [22] have received numerous criticisms based on the following points:

1. These norms are premature since only one year earlier the WHO did not recommend drug treatment in these cases and no additional results had been produced in the interim [21].

2. The objective of obtaining a diastolic blood pressure of 90 mm Hg or less is questioned.

3. These results affect a large proportion of hypertensive patients (70%) and the psychological repercussions and the influence on the patient's personal awareness of health should be evaluated [23], as well as possible side effects and sociological costs [25–27]. Drug treatment, even with diuretics, is not harmless [28] especially when serious doubts have arisen from the negative results of the Multiple Risk Factor Intervention Trial.

Moreover, it is debatable if the BP taken in the clinical situation really corresponds to the patient's usual pressure [29]; patients can be shown to be falsely hypertensive when carefully monitored [30, 31].

4. The uncertainty of the positive results of some studies, the apparently negative results of other studies and the discordant contributions of many of them induce doubts. As such:

a) The Hypertension Detection and Follow-up Program results [6, 17] are dubious, because the study included no placebo group and did not test generic antihypertensive treatment but the favorable effects of special assistance, which were confirmed by the 14% reduction in deaths due to noncardiac disorders [32]. No significant effect was observed in patients under 50 years or in Caucasian women. In addition, both the accuracy of the sources of the diagnoses of death (death certificates) and the adequacy of the statistical analysis are questioned [32, 37]. In any case, according to this study, only 1.3% of the patients would benefit in 5 years. Given these results, it could be questioned how many physicians would apply the treatment and how many patients would accept it, considering the possible adverse effects of the medication.

b) The Australian Study [19] demonstrates that in 48% of patients, BP can decline to 95 mm Hg or less with a placebo.

c) Both the Oslo Study [20] and the Public Health Study on Mild Hypertension [12], although corresponding to small series, do not prove that treatment is useful.

d) The Multiple Risk Factor Intervention Trial contributes the finding that there is greater cardiovascular mortality and morbidity in treated than in untreated AH with diastolic BP between 90 and 94 mm Hg.

5. It would be prudent to await the results of the only study in course (British Medical Research Council Trial [34] that can clarify this situation.

As a consequence of these considerations and pending additional data, the following alternative proposals have been made in response to the WHO/ISH 1983 norms:

1. General norms should not be given for treatment of AH with diastolic BP under 100 mm Hg; therapy should be individualized.

2. If the patient presents no other risk factors, it is not clear if he should be

treated. In these cases or when there are very few risk factors, non-pharmacologic alternatives, such as the following could be used:

a) General health measures [35]: salt restriction; limitation or elimination of alcohol consumption; cessation of smoking; weight control (for each 1% of weight loss, diastolic BP declines by 1 mm Hg and systolic BP by 2 mm Hg [36]; regular physical exercise; avoidance of chronic stress, and use of relaxation techniques, meditation or similar measures [37, 38].
b) Blood pressure should be taken by the patient, if possible, to control the evolution of pressure levels and to encourage patient participation [35].
c) Health education of the patient.

Treatment of systolic AH in elderly patients

There is no consensus with respect to this group. The definition of AH in these subjects is debated and it is argued whether it has the same predictive value for cardiovascular risk as in younger persons. From the Framingham study results there is no doubt that AH is harmful to the elderly. Whether systolic or diastolic, and independently of sex, AH triples cardiovascular risk with respect to normotensives of the same age. The 1983 WHO/ISH publication maintains the criterion that treatment should be initiated in these patients from 170/100 mm Hg. However, there is no agreement for exclusive systolic elevation; since the origin of this increase in the loss of distensibility of the large vessels, any maneuver that decreases BP may compromise irrigation of vital zones. If systolic blood pressure is only moderate there is no proof that treatment is beneficial.

The question of how to treat these patients is even more debated. While some suggest the use of small doses of diuretics, others prefer β-blocking agents. It is evident that in the pathophysiologic circumstances mentioned, use of the peripheral vasodilators would be more logical, compensated by small doses of β-blocking agents if tachycardia is produced.

The European Working Party of High Blood Pressure in the Elderly [39] is studying a population of patients over 60, divided into two groups: half of them (group A) receive thiazide and triamterene and if BP does not decrease, methyldopa is added; the other half (group B) receives placebo. The results may provide conclusive guidelines to this problem.

How should arterial hypertension be treated?

Stepped or pathophysiologic care?

The Joint National Committee defined the concept of *stepped care* in 1977 [13]

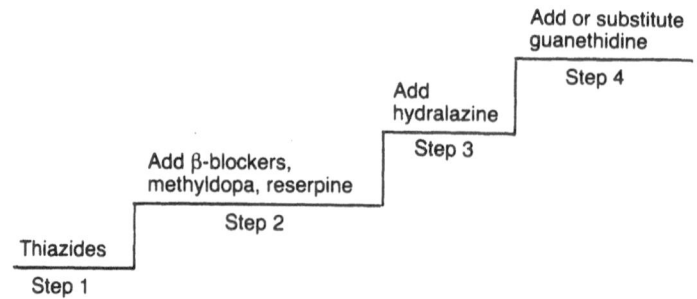

Fig. 3. Stepped care for arterial hypertension, according to the Joint National Committee [13].

and redefined it three years later [14]. This concept was also proposed in 1978 by the WHO [15] (Figs 3 and 4 and Table 5).

In all the norms, the diuretics are considered to be drugs of choice for initiating treatment.

The WHO shifted the β-blocking agents to the first step and they are presently used in this way in many cases.

The Rauwolfia alkaloids were already being used in many countries as initial treatment before these norms were established, and in recent years methyldopa was progressively become the drug of first choice. The same situation is now occurring with some calcium antagonists (verapamil or nifedipine) and even with captopril in small doses.

Most drugs have been commercially launched as definitive solutions for antihypertensive therapy and years later are being used in combination with

Table 5. Norms for stepped care of the Joint National Committee [14] (1980).

Step	Drugs
1	Diuretics (a)
2	Adrenergic inhibiting agents (b)
	Clonidine
	Methyldopa
	Metoprolol
	Nadolol
	Prazosin (c)
	Propranolol
	Rauwolfia alkaloids
3	Vasodilators (d)
	Hydralazine
4	Additional adrenergic inhibitors
	Guanethidine (e)

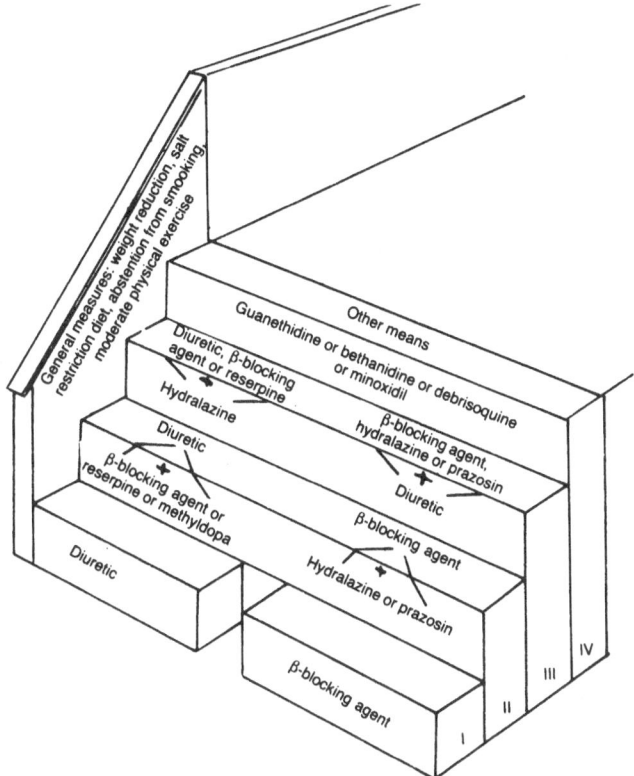

Fig. 4. Stepped care for arterial hypertension, according to the WHO [15].

diuretics. The diuretics thus appear to be a frequently necessary component of AH treatment, and they continue to constitute the first choice therapy. However, in practice first and second choice drugs are not clearly distinguished from each other and either of them may be used as a first choice.

At present, it would be more realistic to speak of *first choice drugs,* which are those listed in steps 1 and 2 of Table 5, *second line drugs* (step 3) and *third line drugs* (step 4). In first line therapy, the use of a *single drug* must be differentiated from *combined therapy.*

The questions to ask when selecting an antihypertensive agent are the following:

1. Does it directly correct a basic hypertensive mechanism?
2. Does it produce responses that might impede its efficacy?
3. Does it produce adverse effects?
4. Does it act synergistically with other antihypertensives?
5. Does disease of any organ (heart, cerebrovascular or renal failure) limit its use or contraindicate it?

The antihypertensive drugs have been stepped attending to the third question and for this reason steps 1 and 2 (first line drugs) are clearly separated from steps 3 and 4 (second and third line drugs).

Individual and physiopathologic approach to AH treatment

Individuals with AH do not form a homogeneous group as regards the physiopathologic mechanisms involved. In each patient, the following factors play different roles [40]:
a) cardiac output;
b) peripheral vascular resistance;
c) intravascular volume;
d) functional state of the sympathetic nervous system; and
e) functional state of the renin-angiotensin-aldosterone axis [41].
While we do not know all the factors implicated in every case, identification of the principal or most evident ones facilitates election of the drug or combination of drugs that best complies with the first criterion. It is generally not necessary to make complex analyses, as a detailed clinical examination will suffice (especially for (e)). Signs of cardiac hyperkinesia (a), skin appearance and temperature, diastolic arterial pressure and severity of AH (b), signs of plethora (c), intensity of the nervous component and regulation, signs of sympatheticotonia (d), and renal status and renin levels (e) should be considered, as well as the predisposition to secondary effects of each medication.

According to the relative weight of each of these components, a choice should be made between β-blocking agents (a), vasodilators (b), diuretics (c), sympatheticolytics or β-blocking agents (d), or if plasma renin is high, captopril and, if it is suppressed, high doses of spironolactone (e) or others.

The most constant factor in hypertensive patients is elevation of peripheral arterial resistance [42]. For this reason, effective vasodilators are acquiring a greater role in AH treatment. However, since the vasodilators usually induce or exacerbate cardiac hyperkinesia, their effectiveness is notably improved by associating small doses of selective β-blocking agents.

In spite of the fact that, theoretically, captopril would be most effective in cases with hyperreninemia, in reality its efficacy is restricted because its effect is not limited to the renin mechanism.

Twenty to thirty per cent of patients with AH have suppressed plasma renin activity probably because of overproduction or excessive activity of mineralcorticoid substances [43]. This group is characterized by its excellent response to high doses (200–400 mg) of spironolactone or, alternatively, to normal doses of any diuretic combined with other hypotensors if necessary [41].

Calcium antagonists, especially nifedipine and its analogues, and vasodilators will probably complete the first line of the pharmacologic spectrum. Combined physiopathologic therapies with small drug doses will allow reestablishing the hemodynamic equilibrium that in mild and moderate hypertensives.

References

1. National Health Survey: Blood pressure of adults by age and sex, United States, 1960–1962. National Health Survey, National Center for Health Statistics Series II no. 4. U.S. Department of Health, Education and Welfare. Public Health Service, 1964.
2. Wilver JA: Detection and control of hypertensive disease in Georgia, USA. In: Stamler J, Stamler R, Pullman RN (eds): The epidemiology of hypertension. Grune & Stratton, New York, 1967.
3. Schoenberger JA, Stamler J, Shekelle RB, et al.: Current status of hypertension control in an industrial population. JAMA 1972; 222: 559–562.
4. Hypertension Detection and Follow-up Program Cooperative Group: Blood pressure studies in 14 communities: A two-stage screen for hypertension. JAMA, 1977; 237: 2385–2391.
5. Syme SL: Implicaciones psicológicas y fisiológicas del tratamiento a largo plazo de la hipertensión. CVR&R, 1982; 3(7): 366–351.
6. Harris L, et al.: The public and high blood pressure: A survey conducted for the National Heart and Lung Institute. N & (NIH) 74: 356. U.S. Department of Health, Education and Welfare, 1973.
7. Sackett DL: The magnitude of compliance and noncompliance. In: Sackett, DL, Haynes RB (eds): Compliance with therapeutic regimens. Johns Hopkins University Press, Baltimore, 1976; 9–25.
8. Smith WM: Mild essential hypertension: Benefit of treatment. In: Perry HM, Smith WM (eds): Mild hypertension: to treat or not to treat. NY Acad Sci, New York, 1978; 74–80.
9. Veter W, Meyer E, Wursten D, Siegenthaler: Problemas del tratamiento prolongado de la hipertensión. Sandorana, 1983; II: 19–20.
10. Syme SL, Jacobs MJ: Smoking cessation activities in the Multiple Risk Factor Intervention Trial: A preliminary report. In: Smoking and Health. Proc 3rd World Conf, Vol. 2. National Cancer Institute. US Department of Health, Education and Welfare, 1975.
11. Freis E, et al.: Veteran's Administration Cooperative Study Group on Antihypertensive Agents. Effects of treatment on morbidity in hypertension. II. Results in patients with diastolic blood pressures averaging 90 through 114 mm Hg. JAMA, 1970; 213–1143.
12. Smith McFW, Edlavitch SC, Krushat WM: Public Health Service Hospitals Intervention Trial in Mild Hypertension. In: Onesti G, Klimt CR (eds): Hypertension determinants, complications and intervention. Grune & Stratton, New York, 1979.
13. Moser M, Finnerty F, Guyther JR: Report of the Joint National Committee on Detection, Evaluation and Treatment of High Blood Pressure. JAMA 1977; 237: 255.
14. Krishan I, Moser M, Curry C, et al.: Report of the Joint National Committee on Detection, Evaluation and Treatment of High Blood Pressure. Arch Intern Med 1980; 140: 1280.
15. WHO: Hipertensión arterial. Informe de un comité de expertos de la OMS. Serie de Informes Técnicos 628. WHO, Genève, 1978.
16. Five-year findings of the Hypertension Detection and Follow-up Program (1). Reduction in mortality of persons with high blood pressure, including mild hypertension. JAMA 1979; 242: 2562.
17. Hypertension Detection and Follow-up Program Cooperative Group: Five-year findings of

the hypertension detections and follow-up program. Mortality by race, sex, and age. JAMA 1979; 242: 2572–2577.

18. Hypertension Detection and Follow-up Program Cooperative Group: The effect of treatment on mortality in 'mild' hypertension. N Engl J Med, 1982; 307: 976–980.

19. Australian National Blood Pressure Study Management Committee: The Australian therapeutic trial in mild hypertension. Lancet 1980; 1: 1261–1267.

20. Helgeland A: Treatment of mild hypertension: A five-year controlled drug trial. The Oslo Study. Am J Med 1980; 69: 725–732.

21. WHO/ISH Mild Hypertension Liaison Committee: Trials of the treatment of mild hypertension: an interim analysis. Lancet 1982; 1: 149–156.

22. Normas para el tratamiento de la hipertension arterial ligera: Memorandum de una reunión de la OMS/SIH. Rev Esp Cardiolog 1983; 36(6): 497–500. (Also published in Bull WHO 1983; 61: 53–56. Lancet, 1983; 2: 48–50. Boletin de la OMS, 1983; 61: 67–71.)

23. McCormick JS: Pautas terapéuticas en la hipertensión ligera. (Cartas al Director). Lancet (Spanish ed), 1983; 3: 135.

24. Medical Research Council Working Party on Mild to Moderate Hypertension: Adverse reactions to bendroflumethiazide and propanolol for the treatment of mild hypertension. Lancet, 1981; 2: 539–543.

25. Gutzwiller F: Should mild hypertension be treated? (Letters to the editor.) N Engl J Med 1982; 307: 1524.

26. Schweizerisches nationales Forschungsprogramm 1, Autorengruppe: Epidemiologie des Blutdrucks in vier Schweizer Städten. Schweiz Med Woschenschr (Suppl) 1981; 12: 40–46.

27. Gutzwiller F, Shucan C, Junod B: Epidemiologische und Soziookonomische Aspekte der grenzwertigen Hypertonie. Praxis 1982; 71: 5–10.

28. Holland OB, Nixon JV, Kuhnert L: Diuretic-induced ventricular ectopic activity. Am J Med 1981; 70: 762–768.

29. Wadden TA, Stunkard AJ: Should mild hypertension be treated? (Letters to the Editor.) N Engl J Med 1982; 307: 1523.

30. Pickering TG, Hershfield GA, Kleinert HD, Laragh JH: Ambulatory monitoring in the evaluation of blood pressure with borderline hypertension and the role of the defense reflex. J Clin Exp Hypertens 1982; 675: 693.

31. Hershfield GA, Pickering TG, Kleinert HD, Blank S, Laragh JH: Situational variations of blood pressure in ambulatory hypertensive patients. Psychosom Med 1982; 44: 237–245.

32. Freis ED: Should mild hypertension be treated? (Letters to the Editor.) N Engl J Med 1982; 307: 1524–1525.

33. Freis ED: Should mild hypertension be treated? N Engl J Med 1982; 307: 306–309.

34. MRC Working Party on Mild to Moderate Hypertension: Randomised controlled trial of treatment of mild hypertension: Design and pilot trial. Br Med J 1977; 11: 48.

35. Mulcahy R: Tratamiento de la hipertensión ligera (Cartas al Director), Lancet (Spanish ed) 1983; 3: 219.

36. Eliahou HE, Iaina A, Gaon T, Shochat J, Modan M: Body weight reduction necessary to attain normotension in the overweight hypertensive patient. Int J Obesity 1980; 5: 157–163.

37. Benson H: Systemic hypertension and the relaxation response. N Engl J Med 1977; 296: 1152–1156.

38. Wadden TA, De la Torre C: Relaxation therapy as an adjunct treatment for essential hypertension. J Fam Pract 1980; 11: 901–908.

39. Amery A, Berthaux P, Birkenhager W et al.: European Working Party on High Blood Pressure in Elderly. Antihypertensive therapy in patients above age 60. Acta Cardiol 1978; 33: 113–134.

40. Dustan HP, Tarazi RC, Bravo EI: Physiologic characteristics of hypertension. Am J Med 1972; 52: 610.

266

41. Koch-Weser J: Correlation of pathophysiology and pharmacotherapy in primary hypertension. Am J Cardiol 1973; 32: 499.
42. Frohlich ED, Tarazi RC, Dustan HP: Reexamination of the hemodynamics of hypertension. Am J Med Sci 1969; 257: 9.
43. Crane MG, Harris JJ, Johns VJ Jr: Hyporeninemic hypertension. Am J Med 1972; 52: 457.

5.6 Conclusions

A. BISTENI

The participants in this symposium have provided evidence that arterial hypertension is an important problem because of its high incidence, the complications it produces in different areas of the human economy, its chronicity, and its effects on the cardiovascular system. The study of arterial hypertension, including its mechanisms, etiological factors, complications, risks, etc., has captured the attention of numerous researchers throughout the world.

Dr L. Tomás has referred to the value of treatment with preventing cardiovascular complications. One of the main objectives of treating arterial hypertension is to avoid complications that threaten life or function. There is an elevated frequency of systemic arterial hypertension in patients who suffer myocardial infarction, whether due to an increase in myocardial oxygen consumption, increase in intramyocardial pressure with the resulting reduction in subendocardial coronary blood flow, or because it favors atherosclerosis, etc.

Dr E. Alegría spoke on the utility of the β-adrenergic receptor blocking agents. His presentation emphasized the importance of these drugs used alone or in association with other drugs. β-adrenergic blocking agents have been shown to be useful in the prevention of sudden death due to ventricular arrhythmias, which are relatively common in anxious patients with tachycardia and mild or moderate hypertension. In these cases (catecholamine-dependent patients), β-blocking agents are indicated.

The introduction of new antihypertensive drugs has acquired an accelerated rate. Dr J. Tamargo has referred to several of these drugs, among which certain substances merit special mention because of their extensive application: diuretics, systemic vasodilators, slow calcium channel inhibitors and a wide variety of drugs, including alphamethyldopa. Pharmacologic research attempts to discover highly effective drugs with the least possible iatrogenic problems; at present what is being offered hardly satisfies these requirements. Unfortunately, modern antihypertensive medications are very aggressive, and in some cases the remedy might be worse than the disease.

Dr V. López Merino referred to the therapeutic regimen, which changes according to the nature of the disease and should consist in an intelligent association of hypertensive drugs, considering synergisms and antagonisms, with the double objective of controlling arterial hypertension and preventing its complications. There are numerous and widely varied regimens; one must judge which are the best of them by experience.

Finally, I would like to call attention to some important points:

1. Arterial hypertension is a disease that has a high incidence and an elevated morbidity and mortality in every country.
2. Whether mild, moderate or severe, it deserves consideration.
3. It is a source of diverse complications, some of them life-threatening and others that permanently alter function.
4. An important function of the treating physician is to convince the patient to follow the prescription carefully, even in asymptomatic cases.
5. Finally, we should not forget that the most important option, which should never be lacking, is a low-salt diet, either alone or with medication.

6. Heart failure

6.1 Introduction

M. CERQUEIRA GOMES

In recent years, important advances have been made in the treatment of heart failure. The role of the traditional drugs is being reevaluated, and various new pharmacologic approaches have been introduced. However, many unanswered questions persist with regard to these advances, such as those mentioned below.

1. With respect to digitalis, opinions on its long-term efficacy in patients with chronic heart failure in sinus rhythm are divided. Moreover, a growing number of drugs have been found to interfere with its clinical effectiveness, especially certain antiarrhythmic agents and calcium antagonists. On the other part, use of digitalis in acute myocardial infarction continues to be debated. Dr Johnson will review the limitations of digitalis utilization and will consider some of these important questions.

2. A great deal remains to be learned about the role of vasodilators in the treatment of congestive heart failure. Are they only effective in advanced phases of this syndrome or can they also be used for mild forms? Do they slow the progress of left ventricular failure as in mitral incompetence or aortic insufficiency? Should the main factors considered in the choice of a vasodilator be the relative efficacy of the drug for arterial or venous vasodilation and their administration route? Or on the contrary, are there other clinically important factors that should be weighted, for example, the influence of the drug on the sympathetic nervous system or on renin-angiotensin activity? What effect do the different vasodilators have in situations in which coronary artery perfusion pressure is of maximum importance, as in ischemic heart disease? If these drugs improve symptoms and the quality of life, do these effects prolong the patients' life expectancy? In other words: Do these drugs really change the natural history of chronic heart failure? Are there sufficiently extensive studies on this natural history in the literature? Dr Coma Canella will summarize the role of vasodilators in heart failure and will also analyze some of these questions.

3. A growing number of new and effective inotropic drugs are being in-

troduced. What is the clinical significance of the vasodilator effect some of them have? And what is the net effect of these powerful drugs on the balance between myocardial oxygen supply and demand? As a result, what is the true role these drugs play in the treatment of the congestive heart failure that complicates ischemic heart disease? What do we know about the influence of these new and powerful inotropic agents on life expectancy and the natural history of patients with heart failure? Dr Lejemtel will speak of the application of the new inotropic drugs and will comment on some of these crucial questions.

4. The role of right ventricular function on global cardiac pump function is a new and interesting subject that has only recently begun to receive the attention of the researchers. The influence of this factor in some situations has special significance, especially in myocardial infarction and other states of severe ischemia propagated to the right ventricle. In this field, Spanish authors have recently made notable contributions. Right ventricular failure in ischemic heart disease will be discussed by Dr Froufe.

6.2 Patients with Heart Failure and Normal Sinus Rhythm: Who Should Receive Digitalis?

ROBERT ARNOLD JOHNSON

In the spring of 1982 my colleagues and I published the results of a randomized, crossover trial of digitalis versus placebo in outpatients who suffered from heart failure but whose cardiac rhythm was a normal sinus mechanism [1]. This study, which showed that digitalis (digoxin) produces improvement in some patients and does not in others (and that some relatively simple observations help distinguish those patients who will benefit from those who will not), excited immediate and intense interest in journalists for newspapers, television, and radio. (I shall add that the interest sprang from the journalists themselves; we had not announced the publication beforehand.) Many reporters asked the same question: 'Why had such a study, simple in concept, only just been performed for a drug so long in use?'

To some extent the question overemphasizes the priority of the study, and I shall later discuss the history of studies that led up to it. Part of the answer to the question is matter-of-fact: the randomized, crossover, double-blind features of the study, which give it its power, are relatively new in comparison with the tenure of digitalis, and perhaps their application to new drugs before their application to old ones is not so surprising; and although the study is simple in concept it is not at all simple in execution. Even so, I found myself both embarrassed and amused by the question because I knew the reporters were on to something: they had glimpsed the peculiar susceptibility of clinical thinking and practice to authority, unproved assertion, and imaginative stalemate. My own memories of discussions anent the proper employment of digitalis proved them correct. I had had teachers who declaimed with evangelical fervor that digitalis was the first and best drug for heart failure. I had had teachers who declaimed with equal fervor that digitalis, however beneficial, was dangerous and should never be employed before diuretic. Neither seemed to know of or care about the existence of the other. An application for partial funding of this very study to the Massachusetts Heart Association had been rebuffed with the comment 'Clinicians believe they know who should be treated with digitalis and who should not'. (Fortunately, the National Institutes of Health took a broader view, and funded the whole of the study.) I knew too that part of the answer lay in a mistaken idea about the nature of heart failure, an idea that by then seemed unbearably naive: for decades clinicians and physiologists had held the view that heart failure resulted from a unitary pathway of contractile insufficiency which could be triggered by a large number of cardiac insults. True, the application of valvular operations, the study of idiopathic hypertrophic subaortic stenosis, and a flurry of publications about ventricular compliance abnormalities were making inroads on this view, but no systematic revision in the meaning of the term 'heart failure' had yet occurred in the minds of most clinicians or investigators. And still papers are published in which some problem of heart failure is examined as if heart failure had a unitary mechanism. My point is this: if heart failure is imagined as having a unitary mechanism, neither clinician nor investigator is likely to ask 'Who is helped by digitalis and who isn't?'.

Studies of the clinical employment of digitalis, a review

Studies to 1968

Dr William Withering was an ingenious and objective observer, but a busy practitioner; his brief case reports, 163 in all, describing the application of digitalis are neither complete nor systematic [2]. Often the heart rate is not described, and he could not make blood pressure recordings. The notes make clear that most of the patients were less than age 60. They suggest that bisided heart failure (constantaneous pulmonary and systemic venous congestion) accounted for many but by no means all of his patients, most of whom suffered from dropsy but some from dyspnea alone. He recognized alcoholism in some, and preceding streptococcal infection (scarlet fever) in others. That some of the patients improved after taking digitalis is incontestable, but whether each of the improved had atrial fibrillation, had some particular cause for heart failure, or had heart failure at all we cannot tell.

By the end of the nineteenth century, prevailing opinion, that of Mackenzie, for example, held that digitalis produced improvement only if heart failure coexisted with atrial fibrillation [3]. But in 1919 Henry Christian published an account of three patients with normal sinus rhythm whose heart failure improved after digitalis was administered [4]. At least two and possibly all three patients had uncontrolled hypertension. During the next decade, several more studies with oral digitalis confirmed Christian's findings [5–8]. Within another decade patients with heart failure and normal sinus rhythm could be investigated by right-heart catheterization: such studies showed that a parenteral preparation of a digitalis glycoside could produce a rise in cardiac output and a fall in the appropriate atrial pressure, whether heart failure was left-sided only or bisided [9–13]. With some exceptions, the authors of these studies do not seem to have been concerned that the cause of heart failure might have conditioned the response to digitalis [7]. The patients they studied most commonly suffered from uncontrolled hypertension, since their investigations preceded the advent of effective antihypertensive treatment.

By 1968, however, some special causes of heart failure had been selected out for study. Patients whose heart failure resulted from cor pulmonale were shown to experience a fall in right atrial pressure and a rise in cardiac output after parenteral administration of a digitalis glycoside [14]. Similarly, the left atrial pressure falls and the cardiac output rises in patients whose heart failure results from aortic-valve stenosis [15, 16]. By contrast, if heart failure results from mitral stenosis (accompanied by sinus rhythm), digitalis does not effect improvement [17]. And in patients whose heart failure results from hypertrophic cardiomyopathy with dynamic outflow-tract obstruction (IHSS), digitalis may produce more heart failure by advancing the degree of obstruction [16].

The mechanism by which digitalis affects improvement, when improvement occurs, was a popular subject of controversy during this era. Several investigators had noted that digitalis glycoside does not affect the cardiac output or atrial pressures when heart failure is absent [11, 18, 19]. This observation prompts the suspicion that digitalis may act through a diuretic effect rather than through direct stimulation of the heart. Withering seems to have considered digitalis as a diuretic, hence believing any cause of edema an appropriate subject for the study of its effectiveness. But he noticed that ascites owing to an intra-abdominal disorder (which in women he often referred to as 'ovarian edeme') was not responsive to the drug, nor was shortness of breath owing to tuberculosis. Observations in the 1960s, utilizing measurements of the contractile state of the heart that are more sensitive than those provided by hemodynamic assessment alone, proved that digitalis has an inotropic effect on the human heart even when heart failure is absent [20, 21]. These observations, in addition to those wherein a rise in cardiac output was recorded in heart-failure patients, mostly dispelled the argument that digitalis acts principally through a diuretic action. Some investigators still harbor misgivings about this conclusion, however [22].

Studies between 1968 and 1982

During the period a number of papers were published in which the chronic effect of oral digitalis in ambulatory patients with heart failure was reported. Each found either that the drug seemed to have no beneficial long-term consequence or that the number of patients receiving benefit was relatively small in comparison to the total [23–28]. Several explanations are possible for these results, which appear contradictory to earlier observations. A simple explanation would be that digitalis loses its action during chronic administration. An elegant study by Arnold and coworkers, however, proved this explanation untenable [29]. If the drug has an effect, the effect is maintained during long-term prescription.

In most of the earlier, short-term clinical studies, the degree of heart failure was quite pronounced or heart failure was proved to exist by hemodynamic measurements. In the later ambulatory studies, many of the patients seem to have had milder symptoms and less pronounced signs; an erroneous diagnosis of heart failure could easily have confounded their selection. My colleagues and I have found (unpublished observations) that one-third of outpatients who are taking digitalis are unlikely to be suffering from heart failure even though this diagnosis is the reason for its administration.

None of the earlier studies had been conducted in a double-blind fashion. This reservation seems unlikely to account for the results of the short-term studies, in which the effect of digitalis seemed dramatic, but it might have applied to the often-cited ambulatory study in 1931 of Harrison and coworkers; perhaps the seemingly beneficial effect of chronic digitalis prescription in their patients was an illusion [5]. Four of the six later studies were not blinded either. The absence of blinding could also act to reduce the likelihood of detecting an effect of digitalis. If the effect were subtle, it might be revealed by a double-blind, crossover technique but be unrevealed by casual clinical observations. A hemodynamic study during this later era showed that the effect of digitalis was slight in some instances [30].

The effect of diuretic prescription is another possible explanation. At the time of many of the earlier investigations, powerful diuretic drugs did not yet exist. By the time of the later investigations, the administration of a diuretic drug concurrently with digitalis was a common practice. By 1982 some studies had shown that the administration of diuretic modified the degree of improvement ensuing after subsequent administration of digitalis [12, 31].

In addition, in the time that lapsed between the earlier and later investigations, the distribution of causes of heart failure had shifted enormously. Effective medicines for the control of hypertension had been discovered, and were shown to be especially important for reducing the frequency of hypertension-associated heart failure [32–34]. Although hypertension remained a strong predisposing factor for the eventual development of heart failure in the population at large [35, 36], uncontrolled hypertension in itself was now a rare cause of heart failure. The application of operations for relieving the effects of valvular heart disease had greatly reduced the proportion of outpatients whose heart failure could be attributed to this cause. The very patients who had figured most prominently in the earlier studies of digitalis were now uncommon among patients undergoing long-term followup for chronic heart failure.

The controlled trial of digitalis versus placebo conducted at the Massachusetts General Hospital

In this study, which I have mentioned in my introductory comments, my colleagues and I hoped to answer two questions. First, does oral digitalis produce, when chronically administered, a clinically detectable degree of improvement in heart failure? Second, if some patients are improved and others are not (which seemed likely, see above), what factors help predict who will benefit from its administration and who will not? We chose digoxin as the glycoside for our study, because digoxin is by far the most commonly pre-scribed form of digitalis.

We studied only patients whose clinical records showed no history of atrial fibrillation or other arrhythmia for which digitalis might be a preferred treat-ment. The patients were chosen from the outpatient practices of internists and house officers on our staff. Once the selection began, the patients (25 in all) were taken consecutively provided that the diagnosis of heart failure seemed definite (both clinically and radiologically on at least one occasion in the past when no acute event, such as myocardial infarction, could explain the occur-rence) and that the patient and his or her physician gave consent.

The causes of heart failure were:
- multiple infarctions, 10 (left ventricular ejection fraction at rest, LVEF, 0.14–0.43);
- idiopathic dilated cardiomyopathy, 6 (LVEF 0.13–0.35);
- left ventricular aneurysm, 3 (LVEF 0.07–0.24);
- recurrent ischemia, 2 (LVEF 0.61–0.67); and
- hypertrophic cardiomyopathy, 4 (LVEF 0.52–0.64).

None of the patients with hypertrophic cardiomyopathy had outflow-tract obstruction, as judged clinically or echocardiographically; we applied this appellation if left ventricular hypertrophy, concentric or asymmetric, was the only cause of heart failure, whether or not a history of hypertension existed. No patient had uncontrolled hypertension or severe valvular heart disease. LVEF was measured by the radionuclide technique.

The protocol for the study is outlined in Fig. 1. A number of noninvasive measurements, including interviews and physical examinations, were made repetitively. During the lead-in period, the dose of diuretic (used in 22 pa-tients), vasodilator drug (used in 6 patients), or both were adjusted until the signs and symptoms were stable, and the daily number of 0.125 mg tablets of digoxin required to produce a target serum level of 1.2 ng/ml was determined. This was the number of study-drug (digoxin or placebo) tablets taken during the ensuing study periods. We planned for the study periods to be nine weeks in duration, but if heart failure appeared to be worsening the study period was terminated and a recovery period ensued during which known digoxin was

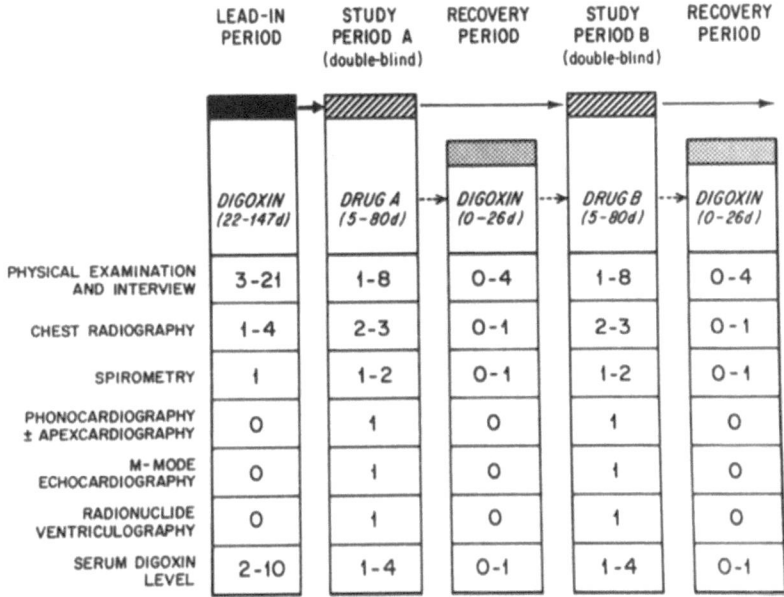

	LEAD-IN PERIOD	STUDY PERIOD A (double-blind)	RECOVERY PERIOD	STUDY PERIOD B (double-blind)	RECOVERY PERIOD
	DIGOXIN (22-147d)	DRUG A (5-80d)	DIGOXIN (0-26d)	DRUG B (5-80d)	DIGOXIN (0-26d)
PHYSICAL EXAMINATION AND INTERVIEW	3-21	1-8	0-4	1-8	0-4
CHEST RADIOGRAPHY	1-4	2-3	0-1	2-3	0-1
SPIROMETRY	1	1-2	0-1	1-2	0-1
PHONOCARDIOGRAPHY ± APEXCARDIOGRAPHY	0	1	0	1	0
M-MODE ECHOCARDIOGRAPHY	0	1	0	1	0
RADIONUCLIDE VENTRICULOGRAPHY	0	1	0	1	0
SERUM DIGOXIN LEVEL	2-10	1-4	0-1	1-4	0-1

Fig. 1. Design of the study protocol. Each period of the study is shown with duration in parentheses. Each value denotes the number of observations per category of observation during each period.

administered (but the study code, known neither to patient nor investigator, was not broken); when the status of the late lead-in period was approximated, the next study period commenced, or if both had been completed, the study ended. If the degree of heart failure appeared to have been worse in one study period compared with the other, we asked the patient to repeat the entire protocol (although we reduced the target length of the study periods to four weeks); six patients were willing to do this, some of whom subsequently iteratively completed the protocol a third time. The study code was not broken for any patient until all of the trials for each patient had been completed, as well as all of the scoring for the clinical and noninvasive data. Right-heart catheterization was performed during each study period for six patients. The degree of clinical heart failure was scored by combining observations from the interview, physical examination, and chest film, as shown in Table 1. The score so generated, HF, was found to correlate well with the pulmonary capillary wedge pressure (PCWP) in the twelve instances in which a direct comparison was possible (PCWP = 3.92 HF + 6.09, r = 0.85, P = 0.0004).

The average daily digoxin dose was 0.435 mg (range, 0.125–1.0 mg), and the average serum level of digoxin during the study period on digoxin was 1.125 ng/ml (range 0.2–2.1 ng/ml). All patients considered together, HF was 3.6 ± 0.7

Table 1. Criteria for determining heart-failure score.*

Point value	Criterion				
	Dyspnea	Crackles	Abnormal heart rate	Right-heart failure	Chest-film abnormality
1	Mild to moderate exertional dyspnea	At base(s) only	91–110 beats/min	Jugular venous pressure >6cm H_2O	Upper-zone flow redistribution
2	Paroxysmal nocturnal or increasing exertional dyspnea	More than at base(s)	>110 beats/min	Jugular venous pressure >6cm H_2O plus edema or hepatomegaly	Interstitial edema
3	Orthopnea or nocturnal cough				Alveolar edema, or interstitial edema with pleural effusions
4	Dyspnea at rest				
Maximum points/ category	4	2	2	2	3

* A composite clinical score is the sum of the highest number of points for each criterion. The maximum possible score, corresponding to the worst heart failure, is 13 points.

during the placebo period compared with 2.0 ± 0.4 during the digoxin period (P<0.05). A comparison of some other measurements, including those determined by echocardiography and radionuclide ventriculography, is shown in Table 2. The reductions in cardiothoracic ratio and left ventricular internal dimension during the digoxin period are significant. We did not detect an increase in LVEF during the digoxin period. Even so, a rise in LVEF, probably too small for detection by the radionuclide method but of hemodynamic significance, is the most likely mechanism for the changes that we could detect.

Considered individually, 14 patients improved during the digoxin period and 11 did not (Fig. 2: a positive value for $\triangle HF$, $HF_{placebo} - HF_{digoxin}$, is defined as improvement). Of the 14 patients who improved during digoxin administration, improvement was pronounced in 5 ($\triangle HF = 6$ or more) and mild in 9. Digoxin-induced improvement could be reproduced: 5 patients who were tested iteratively showed improvement during each digoxin period (Fig. 3). One patient who was unimproved showed no consistent response on iterative trials (Fig. 3). Of the six patients who underwent right-heart catheterization during both study periods, 4 were from the group showing clinical improvement on digoxin; these 4 patients showed hemodynamic changes consistent

Table 2. Comparison of effects of digoxin and placebo.

Variable	No of patients	Placebo[a]	Digoxin[a]	P Value[b]
Heart rate (beats/min)	23[c]	86 ± 3	81 ± 3	0.017
Mean blood pressure (mm Hg)	25	98 ± 3	99 ± 3	0.75
Body weight (kg)	25	78 ± 3	77 ± 3	0.012
Vital capacity (liters)	25	2.4 ± 0.1	2.5 ± 0.1	0.24
Cardiothoracic ratio[d]	25	0.53 ± 0.01	0.51 ± 0.01	0.00027
Left ventricular internal diastolic dimension (mm/m^2)[e]	21[f]	33 ± 1	31 ± 1	0.0026
Left atrial diameter (mm/m^2)[e]	22[f]	22 ± 0.8	22 ± 0.6	0.49
Preejection period/left ventricular ejection time[g]	24[f]	0.54 ± 0.05	0.52 ± 0.04	0.25
Left ventricular ejection fraction[h]	25	0.29 ± 0.04	0.30 ± 0.04	0.49

[a] Means $\pm$ S.E.M.
[b] Determined by paired t-test; P<0.005 considered significant according to the Bonferoni inequality.
[c] Two patients with continuous pacing were excluded.
[d] Measured by posteroanterior chest radiography.
[e] Measured by M-mode echocardiography.
[f] Patients in whom adequate data could not be obtained were excluded.
[g] Measured by phonocardiography in 23 patients and by eachocardiography in one patient.
[h] Measured by resting radionuclide ventriculography.

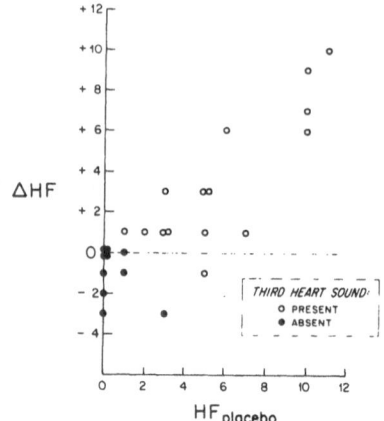

Fig. 2. Change in heart failure score ($\triangle$HF [i.e., $HF_{placebo} - HF_{digoxin}$]) plotted against heart-failure score during placebo administration. Patients whose $\triangle$HF was positive were considered to have responded clinically to digoxin and had an associated third heart sound.

with an improvement in left ventricular function (Fig. 4). The other 2 patients, clinically unimproved, were also unimproved as judged by hemodynamic measurements (Fig. 4).

We tested a large number of clinical variables, as well as the physiological variables that are listed in Table 2, for correlation with $\triangle$HF. Considering the correlations one-by-one, the following were related to digoxin-induced improvement: $HF_{placebo}$, chronic (contrasted with episodic) heart failure, a large

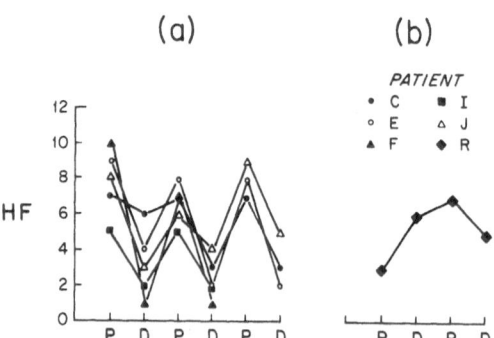

Fig. 3. Heart-failure scores of six patients during repetitive trials of placebo (P) versus digoxin (D). Panel a shows scores in five patients whose initial $\triangle$HF was positive, and Panel b shows those in one patient whose initial $\triangle$HF was negative. When chest-radiography data for all repetitions were not available, a modified score that omitted the point in the radiographic category was used. The order of study periods shown is not the actual order of drug administration, which was randomly determined for each trial.

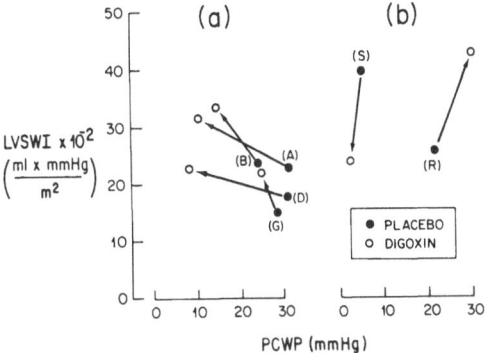

Fig. 4. Left ventricular stroke work index (LVSWI) plotted against resting pulmonary capillary wedge pressure (PCWP). The four patients shown in Panel a responded clinically to digoxin, and the two shown in Panel b did not. LVSWI = (stroke volume in milliliters × [mean arterial pressure − right atrial mean pressure]) body-surface area in square meters.

left ventricular internal dimension, a low value of LVEF, and the presence of a third heart sound. Using a multivariate technique, we found the third heart sound was the strongest correlate; once its presence or absence was taken into account, none of the other variables added more predictive information. All 14 of the patients who improved during the digoxin period had exhibited a third heart sound, whereas only one of the 11 patients who was not improved had exhibited this sign (Fig. 2) (the existence of an audible third heart sound was verified by phonocardiography or apexcardiography in all but one instance).

This data can be interpreted in two ways. The simplest interpretation is to conclude that digoxin provides benefit if heart failure is severe. A second interpretation, and the one that we favor, is that digoxin responsiveness depends not only on the severity of heart failure but also on its mechanism. Two observations suggest that truth more likely resides in the latter. First, the third heart sound was the only predictive variable in a multivariate comparison; the severity of heart failure, as expressed by $HF_{placebo}$, added nothing more. Second, in at least one individual patient we could demonstrate that severe heart failure (high resting PCWP) was unresponsive to digoxin (this patient, R in Fig. 4, did not have a third heart sound). In most instances, the genesis of a third heart sound appears to require that the left ventricle is dilated enough to strike the chest wall during protodiastole and that the left atrial pressure is high enough to produce an especially rapid inflow of blood in protodiastole [37]. If we are correct in our interpretation of this data, the third heart sound is the best predictor of digitalis responsiveness because it integrates information both about severity of heart failure and about its mechanism. If the cause of heart failure does not depend on ventricular dilation, such as in hypertrophic cardiomyopathy, amyloid heart disease, or recurrent ischemia, neither a third heart sound nor digitalis responsiveness exist. If heart failure results from ventricular dilation (in our study ventricular dilation had been produced by a substantial reduction in LVEF in each case), the existence of a third heart sound (and digoxin responsiveness) depends on whether other forms of treatment have mitigated the elevation of PCWP. If diuretic drugs, for example, have produced enough reduction in PCWP, the third heart sound is absent, heart failure is relatively mild or eliminated, and digitalis produces no further benefit. If the PCWP remains enough elevated, a third heart sound exists, and digitalis administration will produce improvement.

Since our study, two more investigations of chronic digitalis prescription for patients in normal sinus rhythm have been published [38, 39]. Neither found that benefit resulted from digitalis, but patients with a third heart sound were rare or absent in both.

A summary of the present indications for prescribing digitalis for patients suffering from chronic heart failure

Digitalis is still the best drug for controlling the ventricular response to atrial fibrillation in most instances, especially if heart failure coexists. In patients who have normal sinus rhythm and whose heart failure persists despite treatment with diuretic drugs, digitalis may be expected to produce improvement if

Table 3. Digitalis in patients whose heart failure is associated with normal sinus rhythm.*

Condition causing heart failure	Left ventricular dilation (rest)	LVEF (rest)	Third heart sound	Improvement expected from digitalis
Dilated cardiomyopathy	Yes	< 0.40	Yes	Yes
Remote infarction (CM-CAD or LV aneurysm)	Yes	< 0.40	Yes	Yes
Uncontrolled hypertension	Yes	Probably < 0.40	Yes	Yes
Aortic stenosis	Often	Often < 0.40	Often	Often
Hypertrophic cardiomyopathy	No	> 0.40	No	No
Amyloid heart disease	No	Often > 0.40	No	No
Recurrent ischemia	No	> 0.40	Not when ischemia is absent	No
Ventricular volume overload	Yes	> 0.40	Yes	Unestablished

*The statements in the table are based on the assumption that heart failure actually exists or is recurring, that is, that it has not been eliminated by other treatment. CM-CAD = cardiomyopathic syndrome owing to coronary artery disease. LV = left ventricular.

a third heart sound is present. I doubt that digitalis will effect improvement if a third heart sound is absent even if the heart failure is severe and persistent, but I should admit that this issue bears further study. In Table 3, I have listed several causes of heart failure and grouped them according to certain easily measured aspects of the mechanisms through which they produce heart failure and whether or not they are commonly associated with a third heart sound. If the LVEF is substantially depressed from a disorder of the left ventricular muscle (dilated cardiomyopathy or extensive remote infarction) or from excessive afteroad (aortic-valve stenosis or uncontrolled hypertension), the left ventricle is dilated and a third heart sound is common if heart failure (defined here as elevation of the PCWP) is severe. If the LVEF is not substantially depressed and ventricular dilation is absent, heart failure results from diminished ventricular compliance (hypertrophic cardiomyopathy, amyloid heart disease) or is abrupt and transient (acute ischemia); a third heart sound is uncommon even if heart failure is severe. Patients from this latter category of disorders are common. We have found, in a study which is not yet published, that one-half of outpatients with heart failure in the practices of general internists do not have ventricular dilation or substantial reduction of the LVEF, do not have a third heart sound, and are usually elderly women with a previous history of hypertension. We presume that heart failure results from an hypertrophy-induced diminution of left ventricular compliance in most of these patients, a disorder to which we apply the term hypertrophic cardiomyopathy (although it is probably not the genetic variant of hypertrophic cardiomyopathy, and the hypertrophy is often of the concentric form).

Neither we nor others have carefully studied digitalis responsiveness in patients whose heart failure results from ventricular volume overload, such as severe aortic or mitral regurgitation. The left ventricle is dilated and a third heart sound exists in such patients, but the LVEF is not substantially reduced (Table 3). For the present we should consider digitalis of unestablished efficacy for their treatment. A recent paper reported little or variable benefit of digitalis in infants with a left-to-right shunt, but I am unable to interpret the data in this paper because not all of the patients appear to have had heart failure [40]. In most patients with ventricular volume overload, of course, digitalis would find only temporary employment until a corrective operation is undertaken, even if the drug were known to cause improvement. The same is true of patients who suffer from aortic-valve stenosis, a condition for which digitalis produces short-term improvement if heart failure exists.

Many questions of practical importance for the wisest use of digitalis are still unanswerable. Although the clinician may now select patients who are likely to benefit from the drug, little precise information exists for selecting the best dose. This fact is hardly surprising when one realizes that the proof of efficacy in the modern era is so recent. We conducted our study by doing our best, given the confines of a double-blind protocol, to ensure a serum level of 1.0–1.5 ng/ml, a value that seemed likely to be adequate and yet unlikely to produce toxicity. My use of the words 'seemed likely to be adequate' is revealing because it exposes an appeal to intiution rather than to knowledge. It is true that a serum level of 2.0 ng/ml or less bears a small (small, not zero) probability of association with toxicity. But whether increments of serum concentration up to this level produce increments of clinical response is unknown. In an individual instance we found clinical benefit in a patient whose serum level was only 0.2 ng/ml. At the moment, the method of dose titration that we employed may be used as a guide to clinical practice, but careful studies of dose-response would be most welcome. Perhaps smaller doses are enough.

How should the clinician decide whether to use digitalis or diuretic drugs if either alone would be sufficient treatment? No studies of relative benefit in comparison with relative risk exist. My present practice is to use digitalis alone for patients with aortic-valve stenosis who are being readied for aortic-valve replacement (providing digitalis prompts enough relief from heart failure). Conversely, for patients with dilated cardiomyopathy or CM-CAD (multiple infarctions) I use diuretic first, and if a small or modest dose relieves the symptoms and signs of heart failure (including the third heart sound) I do not add digitalis. At best these practices are intuitively reasonable; at worst they are highly arbitrary. I shall dare even less advice for using digitalis in relation to vasodilator drugs except to say that I avoid the latter in patients in whom I suspect severe aortic stenosis and that in patients with delated cardiomyopathy or CM-CAD I employ vasodilator drugs when heart failure is relatively severe; I do not discontinue the digitalis prescription which has by then almost always commenced. The availability of amrinone, a non-glycoside cardiac stimulant, is about to prompt a new series of questions anent the treatment of heart failure. Relatives of amrinone, perhaps with less toxicity, may soon follow. Perhaps an enlivened spirit of inquiry among clinicians will provoke immediate investigation pertinent to the prescription of these drugs in relation to digitalis.

Summary

Several studies published between 1968 and 1982 reported that few or no ambulatory patients with heart failure and sinus rhythm receive benefit from chronic oral digitalis administration. I analyze several aspects of these studies in comparision with earlier (1919 to 1968) short-term clinical or hemodynamic studies with which they seem to conflict, emphasizing that the most common causes of heart failure have changed. My colleagues and I have recently shown

286

in a double-blind, crossover study of oral digoxin versus placebo, which I review, that digitalis does produce improved heart failure in a subset of patients with sinus rhythm, namely those whose left ventricular ejection fraction is greatly reduced, who exhibit left ventricular dilation, and whose heart failure is chronic and relatively severe despite diuretic treatment. Multivariate analysis showed that the third heart sound was the strongest correlate of a positive response to digitalis. I argue that the third heart sound reflects not only the severity but one of several mechanisms (left ventricular dilation) of heart failure, and that forms of heart failure for which a third heart sound is not typical are now relatively common in the practices of general internists and primary-care physicians.

Acknowledgment

This study was supported in part by grants (HL-22750 and HL-05769) from the National Heart, Lung and Blood Institute, USA.

References

1. Lee DC-S, Johnson RA, Bingham JB, Leahy M, Dinsmore RE, Goroll AH, Newell JB, Strauss HW, Haber E: Heart failure in outpatients. A randomized trial of digoxin versus placebo. N Engl J Med 1982; 306: 699–705.
2. Withering W: An account of the foxglove and some of its medical uses. Classics of Medicine Library, Burmingham, Ala, 1979 (an edition of the book first published in 1789).
3. MacKenzie J: Digitalis. Heart 1911; 2: 273–386.
4. Christian HA: Digitalis therapy. Satisfactory effect in cardiac cases with regular-pulse rate. Am J Med Sci 1919; 157: 593–602.
5. Harrison TR, Calhoun A, Turley FC: Congestive heart failure. The effect of digitalis on the dyspnea and on the ventilation of ambulatory patients with regular cardiac rhythm. Arch Intern Med 1968; 38: 1203–1216.
6. Luten K: Clinical studies of digitalis. I. Effect produced by the administration of massive doses to patients with normal mechanism. Arch Intern Med 1924; 33: 251–278.
7. Marvin HM: Digitalis and diuretics in heart failure with regular rhythm, with especial reference to the importance of etiologic classification of heart disease. J Clin Invest 1927; 3: 521–539.
8. Stewart HJ, Cohn AE: Studies on the effect of the action of digitalis on the output of blood from the heart. J Clin Invest 1932; 11: 917–944.
9. Ferrer IM, Conroy RJ, Harvey RM: Some effects of digoxin on the heart and circulation in man. Digoxin in combined (left and right) ventricular failure. Circulation 1960; 21: 372–385.
10. Harvey RM, Ferrer IM, Cathcart RT, Richards DW Jr, Cournand A: Some effects of the digoxin on the heart and circulation in man. Digoxin in left ventricular failure. Am J Med 1949; 7: 439–453.
11. Lagerlof H, Werko L: Studies on the circulation of man. The effect of cedilanid (lanatoside C) on cardiac output and blood pressure in the pulmonary circulation in patients with compensated and decompensated heart disease. Acta Cardiol 1949; 4: 1–21.

12. Rader, Smith WW, Berger AR, Eichna LW: Comparison of the hemodynamic effects of mercurial diuretics and digitalis in congestive heart failure. Circulation 1964; 29: 328–345.

13. Weissler AM, Schoenfeld CD: Effect of digitalis on systolic time interval in heart failure. Am J Med Sci 1970; 259: 4–20.

14. Ferrer IM, Harvey RM, Cathcart RT, Webster CA, Richards DW Jr, Cournand A: Some effects of digoxin upon the heart and circulation in man. Digoxin in chronic cor pulmonale. Circulation 1950; 1: 161–186.

15. Yankopoulos NA, Dawai C, Frederici EE, Adler LN, Abelmann WH: The hemodynamic effects of ouabain upon the diseased left ventricle. Am Heart J 1968; 76: 466–480.

16. Braunwald E, Brockenbrough EC, Frye RL: Studies on digitalis. IV. Comparison of the effects of ouabain on left ventricular dynamics in valvular aortic stenosis and hypertrophic subaortic stenosis. Circulation 1962; 26: 166–173.

17. Beiser GD, Epstein SE, Stampfer M, Robinson B, Braunwald E: Studies on digitalis. XVII. Effects of ouabain on the hemodynamic response to exercise in patients with mitral stenosis in normal sinus rhythm. N Engl J Med 1968; 278: 131–137.

18. Harvey RM, Ferrer IM, Cathcart RT, Alexander JK: Some effects of digoxin on the heart and circulation in man. Digoxin in enlarged hearts not in clinical congestive failure. Circulation 1951; 4: 366–377.

19. Selzer A, Hultgren HN, Ebnother CL, Bradley HW, Stone AO: Effect of digoxin on the circulation in normal man. Br Heart J 1959; 21: 335–342.

20. Mason DT, Braunwald E: Studies on digitalis. IX. Effects of ouabain on the nonfailing human heart. J Clin Invest 1963; 42: 1105–1111.

21. Sonnenblick EH, Williams JF Jr, Glick G, Mason DT, Braunwald E: Studies on digitalis. XV. Effects of cardiac glycosides on myocardial force-velocity relations in the nonfailing human heart. Circulation 1966; 34: 532–539.

22. Guz A: Value of digitalis in heart failure (Letter). N Engl J Med 1982; 306: 626.

23. Starr I, Luchi RJ: Blind study of the action of digitoxin in elderly women. Am Heart J 1969; 78: 740–752.

24. Dall JLC: Maintenance digoxin in elderly patients. Br Med J 1970; 2: 705–706.

25. Dobbs SN, Kenyon WI, Dobbs RJ: Maintenance digoxin after an episode of heart failure: Placebo-controlled trial in outpatients. Br Med J 1977; 1: 749–752.

26. Fonrose HA, Ahlbaum N, Bugatch E, Cohen M, Genovese C, Kelly J: The efficacy of digitalis withdrawal in an institutional aged population. J Am Geriatr Soc 1974; 22: 208–211.

27. Hull SM, Mackintosh A: Discontinuation of maintenance digoxin therapy in general practice. Lancet 1977; 2: 1054–1055.

28. Johnston GD, McDevitt DG: Is maintenance digoxin necessary in patients with sinus rhythm? Lancet 1979; 1: 567–570.

29. Arnold SB, Byrd RC, Meister W, Melmon K, Cheitlin MD, Bristow JD, Parmley WW, Chatterjee K: Long-term digitalis therapy improves left ventricular function in heart failure. N Engl J Med 1980; 303: 1443–1448.

30. Cohn K, Selzer A, Kersh ES, Karpman LS, Goldschlager N: Variability of hemodynamic responses to acute digitalization in chronic cardiac failure due to cardiomyopathy and coronary artery disease. Am J Cardiol 1975; 35: 461–468.

31. McHaffie D, Purcell H, Mitchell-Heggs P, Guz A: The clinical value of digoxin in patients with heart failure and sinus rhythm. Q J Med 1978; 47: 401–419.

32. Hodge JY, Smirk FH: The effect of drug treatment of hypertension on the distribution of deaths from various causes. Am Heart J 1967; 73: 441–452.

33. Veterans Administration Cooperative Study Group on Antihypertensive Agents. Effects of treatment on morbidity in hypertension. II. Results in patients with diastolic blood pressure averaging 90–114mm Hg. JAMA 1970; 213: 1143–1152.

34. Wolff FW, Lindeman RD: Effects of treatment in hypertension. Results of a controlled study. J Chronic Dis 1966; 19: 227–240.

35. Kannel WB, Castelli WP, McNamara PM, McKee PA, Feinleib N: Role of blood pressure in the development of congestive heart failure. The Framingham study. N Engl J Med 1972; 287: 781–787.

36. McKee PA, Castelli WP, McNamara PM, Kannel WB: The natural history of congestive heart failure. The Framingham study. N Engl Med 1971; 285: 1441–1446.

37. Reddy PS, Meno F, Curtiss EI, O'Toole JD: The genesis of gallop sounds: Investigation by quantitative phonocardiography and apexcardiography. Circulation 1981; 63: 922–932.

38. Fleg JL, Gottlieb SH, Lakatta EG: Is digoxin really important in the treatment of compensated heart failure? A placebo-controlled crossover study in patients with sinus rhythm. Am J Med 1982; 73: 244–250.

39. Gheorghiade M, Beller GA: Effects of discontinuing maintenance digoxin therapy in patients with ischemic heart disease and congestive heart failure in sinus rhythm. Am J Cardiol 1983; 51: 1243–1250.

40. Berman W Jr, Yabek SM, Dillon T, Niland C, Corlew S, Christensen D: Effects of digoxin in infants with a congestive circulatory state due to a ventricular septal defect. N Engl J Med 1983; 308: 363–366.

6.3 Vasodilators in the Treatment of Congestive Heart Failure

I. COMA CANELLA and J. LÓPEZ SENDÓN

Introduction

The use of vasodilators has been an authentic innovation with respect to the classic treatment of heart failure with digitalis and diuretics. In the last decade the use of vasodilators has extended in such a way that in many cases they are not only given to potentiate digitalis but to substitute it in the treatment of patients with CHF.

The vasodilators presently available are numerous and every year new drugs are synthesized and added to the list of those already being offered. In a short review it is impossible to exhaustively study each of these drugs, the different groups will be studied according to their predominant effect, with special attention to those most used. Other problems of interest, such as the effect on myocardial oxygen balance and exercise capacity, neuroendocrine effects, long-term response and tolerance will also be dealt with.

A brief summary of the pathophysiology of CHF will be made, which is essential for understanding the effects of vasodilators and for selecting the most appropriate drug.

Pathophysiology of congestive heart failure

Heart failure has been classically defined as a condition in which the heart is incapable of moving a sufficient blood supply in relation to venous return and metabolic tissue needs in a certain period. According to this definition any heart can be insufficient if metabolic demand is excessive. However, CHF usually results from dysfunction or myocardial disease, whether of primary or secondary origin or due to overload.

Independently of the cause of CHF, the result is that cardiac output and blood pressure decline and the compensatory mechanisms for ensuring sufficient blood flow immediately operate [1].

PATHOPHYSIOLOGY OF CONGESTIVE HEART FAILURE

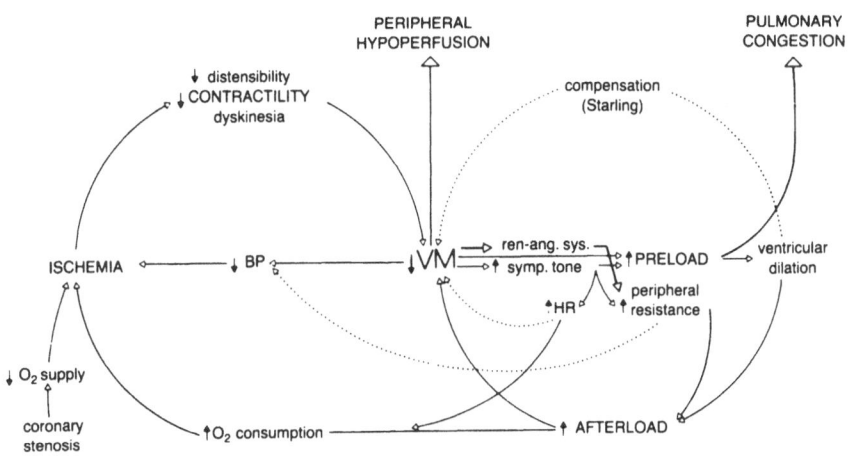

Fig. 1. Pathophysiology of congestive heart failure. The activation of the compensatory mechanisms for cardiac output reduction (CO) can overcome a slight deficit in contractility but may produce clinical symptomatology or even aggravate congestive heart failure [1]. BP: blood pressure; HR: heart rate.

First, the Frank-Starling mechanism is activated. This consists in an increase in ventricular diastolic volume and results from the heart's incapacity to eject the blood volume corresponding to a determined filling volume. Within certain limits the longer the myocardial fiber length the more powerful the cardiac contraction [2]. Another relatively rapid compensatory mechanism is hypertrophy, which increases the size and number the myocardial fibers, that generally improve contractility [3]. Aside from the cardiac mechanisms, there are extracardiac ones, such as vasoconstriction, increased tissular oxygen extraction and, in the most extreme cases, anaerobic metabolism.

Vasoconstriction is mediated by different systems:

a) reflex elevation of sympathetic tone and an increment in neuronal norepinephrine release;

b) increased release of norepinephrine produced by the adrenal medulla;

c) increased renin secretion when renal perfusion pressure decreases; renin reacts with a plasma globulin to produce angiotensin I, which in turn is converted into angiotensin II by the mediation of converting enzyme [4];

d) it has been confirmed that in CHF, vascular smooth muscle responds poorly to intrinsic or extrinsic vasodilator stimuli [5] producing a predominance in the vasoconstrictive response.

Norepinephrine and angiotensin II are powerful vasoconstrictors that act at the arterial level; norepinephrine also acts at the venous level. At the arterial level, vasodilation occurs mainly in skeletal muscle, the splanchnic territory,

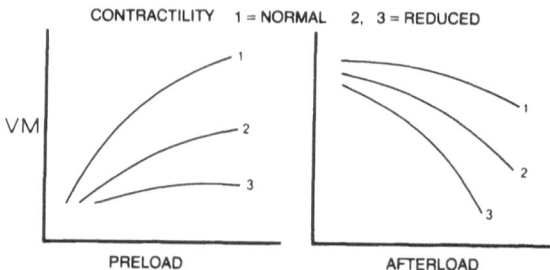

Fig. 2. Preload-cardiac output (CO) relationship. For the same increase in preload, the better contractility the greater the CO. The contrary occurs with afterload, which is inversely related to CO. The influence of preload is maximum in congestive heart failure [1].

skin and kidneys. When systemic vascular resistances increase blood pressure is maintained in spite of the reduction in cardiac output ($BP = CO \times R$). Moreover, selective vasoconstriction redistributes the blood volume to preserve an adequate blood flow in organs of vital importance like the heart and brain at the expense of producing a various degrees of ischemia in organs of secondary interest. The generalized vasoconstriction increases the blood return to the heart. Moreover, angiotensin II stimulates aldosterone secretion by the adrenal cortex, which increases volemia by retaining water and sodium. These two mechanisms help to increase the preload, or diastolic volume, and therefore favor the Frank-Starling mechanism (Fig. 1).

Unfortunately, the compensatory mechanisms generally do not improve heart failure but worsen it. Although the sympathetic nervous system manages to maintain an adequate blood supply to vital organs by vasoconstriction, it increases systemic vascular resistance. This has hardly any effect on the cardiac output in the normal heart but reduces it still more in the failing heart. On the other hand, an increase in diastolic ventricular volume in the normal heart raises the cardiac output, but in the failing heart, which has a flattened ventricular function curve, cardiac output is barely modified [6] (Fig. 2).

Oxygen balance

Myocardial oxygen consumption depends directly on heart rate, contractility and wall tension. Wall tension is calculated as left ventricular pressure × radius/2 × wall thickness; for systolic tension all variables are measured immediately after the aortic sigmoid cusps open, and for diastolic tension, they are measured at the end of the diastole.

The oxygen supply to the myocardium depends directly on aortic pressure and the patency of the coronary arteries, and inversely on vascular and

292

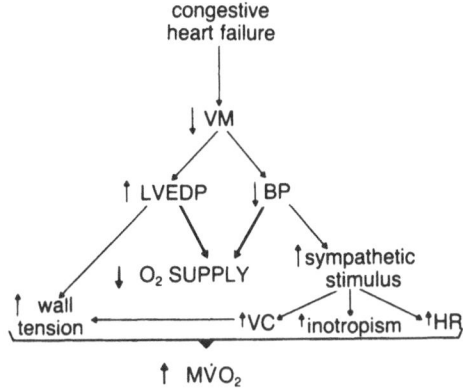

Fig. 3. Mechanisms of reduction of O_2 supply and increase in consumption in congestive heart failure: the increase in wall tension, heart rate (HR) and inotropism contribute to raising O_2 consumption, while the reduction in blood pressure (BP) and left ventricular end diastolic pressure (LVEDP) diminish O_2 supply [15]. CO: cardiac output; VC: vasoconstriction.

extravascular coronary resistance or intramural pressure. Since intramural pressure is very high during the systole there is only coronary blood flow during the diastole. Extravascular coronary resistance is represented by the passive transmission of ventricular cavity pressure to the myocardium. The myocardial perfusion gradient (MPG) can thus be calculated with the formula: MPG = diastolic aortic pressure − diastolic left ventricular pressure [7].

In CHF, sympathetic hyperstimulation produces vasoconstriction and a secondary increase in wall tension, as well as an increase in heart rate and contractility, which increases oxygen consumption. Oxygen supply varies in accordance with the relation between diastolic aortic pressure and diastolic left ventricular pressure (Fig. 3).

Parameters of ventricular function

Global ventricular function, represented by the cardiac output, depends directly on preload, or end-diastolic ventricular volume, contractility and heart rate, and inversely on afterload, or wall tension. Nonetheless, it has been seen that in CHF, increased preload hardly changes the cardiac output and mainly produces pulmonary congestion. The possibility of acting on the afterload is much more interesting because an afterload reduction in these patients can notably raise the cardiac output. Using vasodilators, heart failure can be improved by lowering preload and afterload, which are markedly elevated. The vasodilators act on preload by reducing venous return and consequently decreasing end-diastolic ventricular pressure and volume, which in turn alleviates pulmonary congestion. They act on the afterload by reducing systemic vascular resistances, which increases the cardiac output. When preload and afterload decline, oxygen consumption decreases. These substances do not directly affect heart rate and contractility, although contractility may be bettered as a result of the improvement in the oxygen balance.

Classification of the vasodilators

In Table 1, the vasodilators are classified by their predominant site of action. No drug is exclusively an arterial or venous dilator, but in some instances, the effect is more marked in the arterial territory or the venous territory, while the mixed drugs have a balanced effect on both vascular beds.

Mechanism of action

Numerous vasodilators produce nonspecific relaxation of the smooth muscle of the vascular wall. This is the case of the nitrates, molsidomine, nitroprusside, hydralazine, endralazine, diazoxide and minoxidil. Other vasodilators block the α-receptors; for instance, prazosin acts on the postsynaptic α_1-receptors [8] and phentolamine and phenoxybenzamine are nonspecific α-blockers. Phentolamine also has a direct smooth muscle relaxation effect and a β-adrenergic stimulation effect [9]. The structure of trimazosin is similar to that of prazosin [10] and its mechanism of action is probably the same. Captopril, teprotide and enalapril [11] inhibit the enzyme that mediates the conversion of angiotensin I into angiotensin II, while saralasin is a competitive angiotensin II antagonist [12]. The vasodilator mechanism of the prostaglandins depends on their effect on cyclic AMP [13], which increases adenylcyclase. Finally, nifedipine is a calcium antagonist [14].

Table 1. Classification of vasodilators according to predominant site of action.

Venous	Mixed	Arterial
Nitroglycerin	Nitroprusside	Hydralazine
Isosorbide dinitrate	Prazosin	Endralazine
Molsidomine	Trimazosin	Minoxidil
	Captopril	Phentolamine
	Enalapril	Nifedipine
	Saralasin	Diazoxide
	Teprotide	Phenoxybenzamine
	Prostacyclin	
	Prostaglandin E_1	

VASODILATORS IN AMI WITH CHF

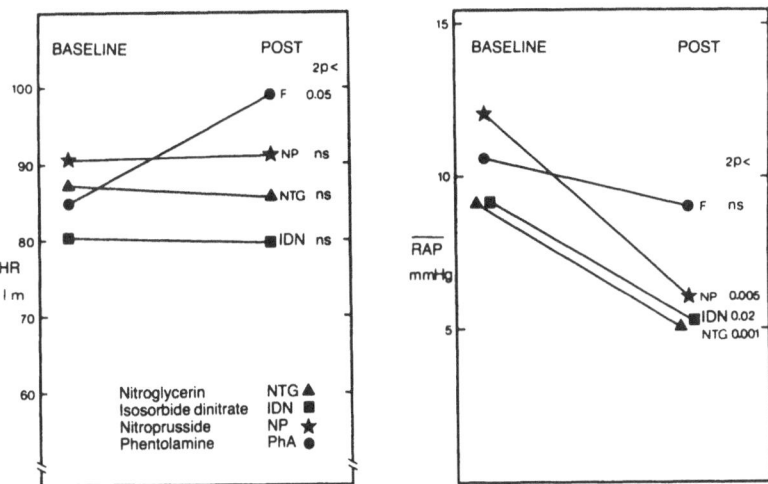

Fig. 4. Variations in heart rate (HR) and mean right atrial pressure (RAP) with arterial, venous and mixed vasodilators. Only phentolamine raises HR and the rest of the vasodilators reduce RAP.

Hemodynamic effects in heart failure

Figs 4 to 6 represent the effects of some arterial, venous and mixed vasodilators on different hemodynamic parameters.

The venous vasodilators mainly reduce biventricular diastolic pressure without modifying the cardiac index or blood pressure [15–18]. Although they do not alter the systemic vascular resistance, blood pressure or cardiac index, pulmonary resistance, mean pulmonary artery pressure, pulmonary capillary and right atrial pressures are reduced. They generally reduce the diastolic work index and do not change heart rate. Although these are the basic features of this group of drugs there are small variations depending on the drug used and the patient's situation. As such, intravenous nitroglycerin used in patients with a normal cardiac index does not significantly vary systemic resistance and the cardiac index. However, if the cardiac index is lowered, resistances decrease and the cardiac index increases with no significant change in blood pressure [19].

Arterial vasodilators mainly reduce systemic and pulmonary vascular resistances. When resistance to ventricular ejection is decreased the cardiac index increases and left ventricular filling pressure declines. Blood pressure is lower because the increase in the cardiac index is proportionally smaller than the reduction in resistances. Venous pressure and the systolic work index have a proportionally smaller decrease, and heart rate does not increase. However,

VASODILATORS IN AMI WITH CHF

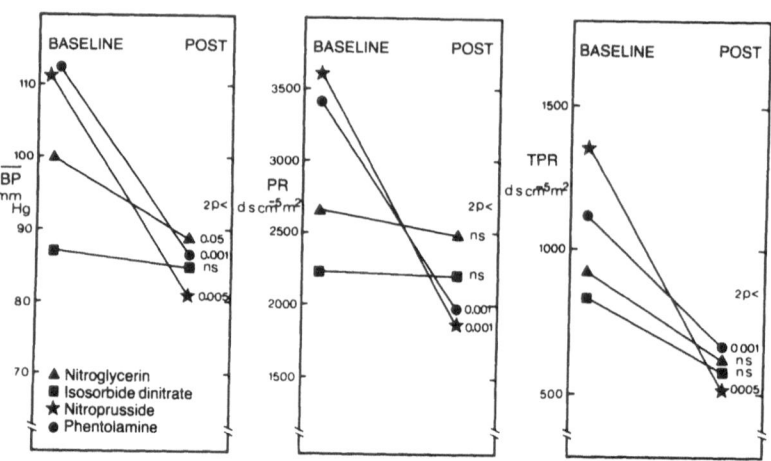

Fig. 5. Variations in mean blood pressure (BP), peripheral resistance (PR) and total pulmonary resistance (TPR). Nitroprusside and phentolamine produce an important reduction in the three parameters, while the venous vasodilators hardly modify them.

heart rate accelerates with hydralazine [20] and phentolamine [21], drugs that also have a positive inotropic effect. In the case of phentolamine it has been demonstrated that the blockade of the α-adrenergic receptors leads to an increase in norepinephrine synthesis and release [22, 23], which in turn explains the tachycardiac and inotropic effects of the drug. The same probably occurs with hydralazine by direct or reflex cardiac stimulation [20].

In contrast, nifedipine exercises a negative inotropic effect that usually does not deteriorate ventricular function because the drug simultaneously reduces systemic vascular resistances [24]. Some authors have even observed a notable hemodynamic improvement [25], while others [26] have described cases of acute pulmonary edema precipitated by nifedipine in aortic stenosis because the negative inotropic effect cannot be counteracted by a reduction in left ventricular afterload. For these reasons, nifedipine is considered to be a second choice vasodilator for treating congestive heart failure and it is contraindicated in some cases.

Mixed vasodilators simultaneously reduce systemic and pulmonary vascular resistances and biventricular filling pressure. The cardiac index increases, blood pressure usually decreases and the pulmonary capillary and right atrial pressures decline, although heart rate remains unchanged [27, 28].

These effects refer to patients with CHF. However, if vasodilators are given to patients with good ventricular function or if pulmonary capillary pressure declines excessively, the cardiac index suffers an important reduction since the ventricle requires a minimum filling pressure to function adequately (Fig. 2).

296

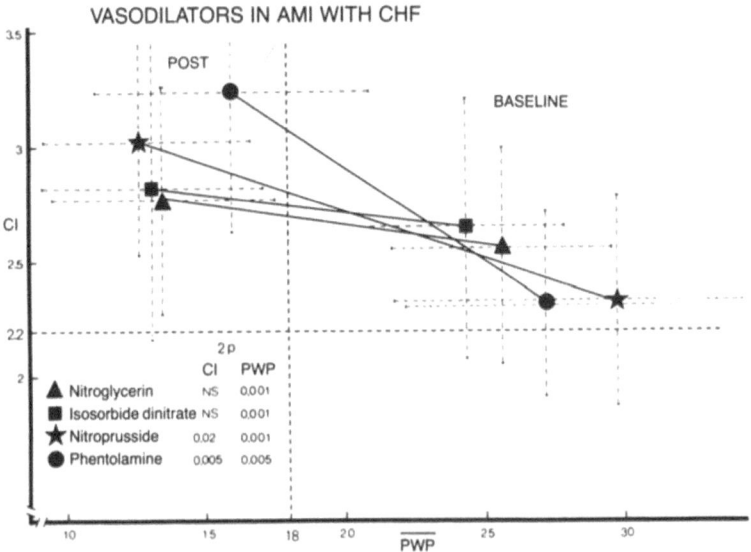

VASODILATORS IN AMI WITH CHF

Fig. 6. Simultaneous variations in cardiac index (CI) and pulmonary capillary pressure (PCP). Most patients were initially in the III of IV stages and passed to I or II, with a notable reduction in PCP.

As a result of the decrease in cardiac index, arterial hypotension and reflex tachycardia appear.

Effect on myocardial oxygen balance

The vasodilators act on the oxygen balance by modifying consumption or supply. They decrease oxygen consumption to a greater or lesser degree by reducing ventricular wall tension: they decrease the radius of the ventricular cavity by reducing the preload and they diminish left ventricular pressure by reducing peripheral resistances. Mixed vasodilators, like nitroprusside, prazosin or captopril, simultaneously reduce preload and afterload, and theoretically produce the greatest decrease in oxygen consumption. Moreover, these drugs do not produce tachycardia and have no direct inotropic effect.

Oxygen supply can be raised or lowered with vasodilators, depending on the patient's disease, the drug used and the dosis given. Most vasodilators have been shown to have a coronary vasodilator effect, but this can be deletereous in some cases. In the presence of obstructive coronary lesion, the ischemic territory is characterized by maximum vasodilation due to hypoxia and can suffer a 'coronary steal' effect [29]. This occurs when the vessels of the healthy territory dilate and part of the blood flow that was directed to the ischemic zone is shifted toward this low pressure zone (Fig. 7). This explains how some

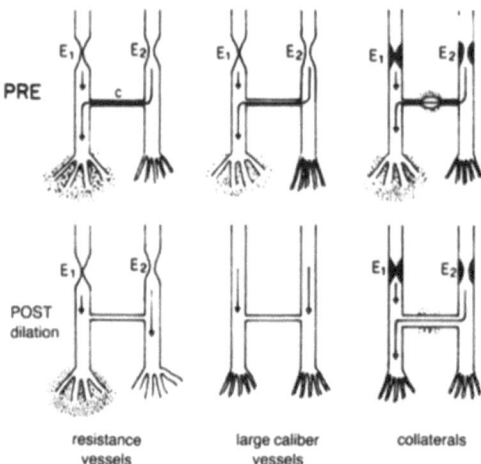

Fig. 7. When there is critical stenosis (E_1) of the coronary blood flow hypoxia produces maximum vasodilation in the arterioles dependent on the vessel. Moreover, collaterals (c) develop and increase the risk in this potentially ischemic zone. If a vasodilator that acts on resistance vessels is administered the arterioles of the nonischemic zone dilate. Coronary steal is produced if there is flow-limiting stenosis (E_2) prior to the branching off of the collateral. If the vasodilator acts on the large caliber vessels suppressing spasm, the blood flow in both territories will increase. If it acts on the collaterals, these dilate in their entire trajectory rather than in the area of contact with the ischemic tissue.

vasodilators can produce angina although they increase the total coronary blood flow and coronary sinus oxygen content [30].

Comparing the respective coronary vasodilator effects of nitroglycerin and nitroprusside, it has been demonstrated that nitroglycerin acts principally on large caliber coronary arteries [31] and collaterals [32], while nitroprusside acts on smaller caliber resistance vessels [31]. It is therefore more probable that nitroprusside will produce a coronary steal. At pharmacologic doses, nitroglycerin does not affect the microvascular self-regulating mechanism [33] and produces increased blood flow to ischemic areas of the myocardium. When comparison is made of the effect of these drugs on ST segment elevation in acute myocardial infarction results are contradictory: in the absence of heart failure ST elevation decreases with nitroglycerin and increases with nitroprusside [34]. In other studies ST elevation decreases with nitroprusside [35], possibly because the coronary steal may be counteracted by a reduction of oxygen consumption in CHF. Isosorbide dinitrate has a similar effect to that of nitroglycerin [36]. Nifedipine also relieves coronary spasm, but its use in angina pectoris is much more extended than in the treatment of heart failure.

Aside from the effect vasodilators have on coronary vascular resistance, they can increase oxygen supply through a reduction in extravascular coronary resistance because they decrease diastolic left ventricular pressure. If diastolic aortic pressure is reduced at the same time, the net effect on oxygen supply will depend on the modification of the myocardial perfusion gradient. Basically, correct adjustment of the drug dosis is required in each case: a well-adjusted dosis improves oxygen supply but an excessive one worsens it, especially if arterial vasodilators are used because they excesively reduce blood pressure. Since the venodilators hardly affect blood pressure and markedly reduce left ventricular filling pressure, these drugs are the ones that most increase the myocardial perfusion gradient. The nitrates are the drugs with the greatest vasodilator effect in large caliber coronary arteries.

On the other hand, the nitrates and nitroprusside produce a certain degree of arterial desaturation [37], probably by altering the alveolar ventilation-perfusion balance. This could be due to a loss of pulmonary capacity for inducing vasoconstriction of the regions with alveolar hypoxia, shifting the perfusion toward better ventilated zones of the lung [38]. Moreover, nitroglycerin overdose can produce methemoglobinemia [39].

Exercise capacity

The hemodynamic effect of the vasodilators has been mainly studied at rest. However, what is really interesting is to improve the exercise capacity of patients with congestive heart failure so normal physical activities can be performed. Improved exercise capacity has been demonstrated in long-term treatment with nitrates [40], prazosin [41], trimazosin [42], captopril [43] and hydralazine [44]. The improvement is evident in the fact that exercise can be prolonged longer and hemodynamic conditions during exercise are better, although systemic oxygen consumption does not increase [45]. The effects are more beneficial when these drugs are used in long-term than in short-term treatments. However, the exercise capacity can be raised by short-term doses: Franciosa and Cohn [46] found that the combination of hydralazine and isosorbide dinitrate improves the hemodynamics of submaximum exercise in patients with congestive heart failure, although the maximum exercise level does not increase, probably because arteriolar vasodilation is complete in these cases. Experimental studies in rats with heart failure support this hypothesis: nitroglycerin infusion in these animals increases blood flow in the renal, splanchnic and cutaneous territories, but not in skeletal muscle [47].

Neuro-endocrine effect

In congestive heart failure, there is usually an exaggerated stimulation of the nervous system and an increase in norepinephrine release and renin-angiotensin-aldosterone system activity. It is generally admitted that the vasodilators that do not possess a direct neuroendocrine effect diminish circulating catecholamine levels. This is a consequence of the alleviation in heart failure, which reduces the compensatory sympathetic discharge [45]. Nonetheless, there are studies that demonstrate elevation in norepinephrine levels after treating heart failure with nitroprusside [48].

Some vasodilators exercise a direct effect on the neuroendocrine system. As a result, the modifications in norepinephrine, angiotensin and aldosterone levels in heart failure differ according to the drug used.

Captopril and teprotide interfere with angiotensin II production and therefore increase plasma renin activity and reduce aldosterone formation [49]. Moreover, it has been confirmed that with these drugs there is a reduction in sympathetic activity and plasma catecholamine concentrations. This effect can be indirectly caused by inhibition of angiotensin II, which stimulates sympathetic activity through a central or peripheral mechanism [50]. Another humoral effect of captopril is the inhibition of bradykinin degradation; increases in plasma levels probably contribute to the vasodilator effect [49].

Prazosin is considered to be a selective inhibitor of the post-synaptic α_1-receptors and theoretically does not block the pre-synaptic α_2-receptors, which inhibit norepinephrine release. However, the selectivity of this substance is not absolute [8] and it produces an increase in plasma norepinephrine, although less intense than that produced by nonspecific α-blockers. In long-term treatment it has been confirmed that prazosin can increase plasma renin, resulting in hyperaldosteronism [51].

Other vasodilators that directly affect smooth muscle fiber, such as hydralazine and isosorbide dinitrate, also elevate renin levels [52]. However, their effect on norepinephrine levels is variable: some authors [52] have observed that patients who are less responsive to vasodilator treatment have higher norepinephrine levels while those who respond adequately tend to have lower levels. The changes in sympathetic activity that occur during treatment may interfere with the effects of these drugs. Other authors [20] have found a chronotropic and inotropic effect in patients with congestive heart failure that is not shared with nitroprusside and improves with hydralazine, raising speculation as to whether it could be due to catecholamine release. Finally, an elevation in norepinephrine, renin and aldosterone levels and a significant increase in epinephrine have been observed with prostacyclin.

Long-term effect; tolerance phenomenon

The vasodilators are highly efficient drugs for the treatment of acute congestive cardiac failure and are also effective when used as initial treatment for chronic heart failure. Most hemodynamic studies compare basal parameters with those obtained after an isolated drug dose, but it has been evidenced that prolongation of this treatment is accompanied by a less satisfactory response, and occasionally, a tolerance phenomenon that requires progressively larger doses to obtain the desired therapeutic effect.

The nitrite tolerance phenomenon has been demonstrated in experiments in animals and in human beings [54]. It is known that tolerance is due to the formation of disulfur links in the vascular smooth muscle at the levels of the nitrate receptors causing the receptors to become temporarily nonresponsive to later administration of the drug [55]. In practice, it has been found that the hemodynamic response to the nitrates continues in prolonged treatments, although it is not as intense as after the first dosis [56]. The same occurs with hydralazine, which is usually used in chronic treatments in association with isosorbide dinitrate: response is still significant after prolonged treatments [57]. When the response to hydralazine is attenuated it is generally due to hydrosaline retention secondary to hyperaldosteronism and can be easily corrected with diuretics [58]. It has also been demonstrated that hydralazine favors the response to diuretics [59].

Probably, the greatest controversy over the tolerance phenomenon has taken place with prazosin. Undoubtedly, attenuation of the effect of prazosin is observed after the first dosis [60, 61], as occurs when it is given to hypertensives, but the drug becomes effective again after 3 or 4 days of treatment [58]. With respect to prolonged use of prazosin, results are contradictory: some authors [62] have detected tolerance and others [63] have obtained good results. It is calculated that the tolerance phenomenon appears in one third of the cases [64]. It is thought to be due to hyperaldosteronism and can be corrected with diuretics, as in the case of hydralazine [58]. In general, it is accepted that reduction in left ventricular filling pressure is maintained somewhat better than the cardiac output [65].

Captopril has been widely tested in prolonged treatments and the results have been excellent [43, 65]. Not only does captopril not induce tolerance, but the drug is more effective in prolonged treatments [43]. Since it exercises an aldosterone inhibiting effect its use does not produce water and salt retention [66] and the diuretic dosage can be reduced. Nonetheless, furosemide is sometimes necessary to avoid hyperpotasemia [67].

Although response to the initial dosis of a vasodilator generally serves to predict long-term response [68], this is not always the case. Packer et al. [69] recently studied the different hemodynamic response patterns to captopril in long-term treatment of advanced heart failure and found the following response variants:

a) no immediate or long-term response;
b) notable improvement maintained for 48 hours and after 2–8 weeks;
c) marked initial improvement, attenuation of the response at 48 hours and spontaneous return to the initial dosis response in long-term treatment; and

d) development of irreversible tolerance 48 hours after onset or in the long-term.

Generally speaking, the type (a) response occurs in patients with decreased renin levels, but not all cases of low renin concentration respond poorly to captopril. This suggests that aside from angiotensin inhibition, there are other vasodilator mechanisms dependent on captopril, such as potentiation of bradykinin, stimulation of prostaglandins or attenuation of the sympathetic nervous system response.

Recently, tests have been made with enalapril [11], another converting enzyme inhibitor that has the same effect as captopril but is longer-lasting. This substance apparently has no adverse collateral effects when used in prolonged treatments.

Indications for the different vasodilators; choice of drug

Selection of a vasodilator should first consider whether heart failure is acute or chronic.

Acute heart failure

In an unstable hemodynamic situation a vasodilator with immediate, short-acting effects should be used because it allows adjustment of the dosis according to patient response. These conditions are met by the vasodilators that can be administered in continuous intravenous perfusion, such as nitroprusside [27] and nitroglycerin [22]. Phentolamine can also be used in continuous perfusion, but when the drug is discontinued its effects last for 60 minutes [22], a disadvantage with respect to nitroglycerin and nitroprusside.

Of all the vasodilators available that can be used intravenously, nitroprusside is generally chosen for hypertensive patients and nitroglycerin for normotensive patients or those with a normal blood pressure because it is much less hypotensive than nitroprusside. Intravenous vasodilators require hemodynamic monitoring and continued monitoring of the patient because these drugs are extraordinarily effective and optimal dosis varies from patient to patient; they may be extremely dangerous if caution is not exercised (Fig. 8).

Chronic heart failure

The choice of a vasodilator in chronic heart failure should be made after considering the compensatory mechanisms in play in each patient [45]. Ideally, plasma renin levels should be measured: If renin is elevated, the response to captopril can be expected to be excellent and the response to nitrates, poor.

302

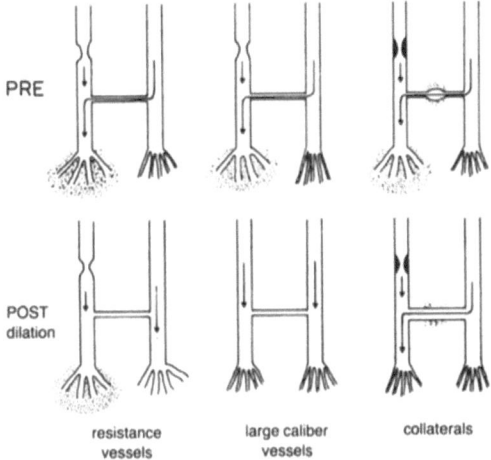

PRE

POST
dilation

resistance   large caliber   collaterals
vessels   vessels

Fig. 8. Hemodynamic effect of intravenous nitroglycerin. If the dosis is excessive because preload is reduced too much, arterial hypotension and a decrease in the cardiac index (CI) appear. PAP: pulmonary artery pressure; PCP: pulmonary capillary pressure; RAP: right atrial pressure; BP: blood pressure.

When plasma renin is low, treatment with arterial (hydralazine), venous (nitrates) or mixed (prazosin) vasodilators can be tried. The choice of one type of vasodilator or another depends on the predominance of venous congestion or tissue hypoperfusion. Usually, both problems exist in advanced heart failure and in practice, mixed vasodilators of the prazosin type or a combination of hydralazine and nitrates are selected. When hydralazine is used as a long-term treatment secondary effects appear in 20% of the cases, often requiring cessation of treatment.

Table 2. Utilization of the most commonly used vasodilators in heart failure.

Drug	Route	Onset effect (min)	Duration effect	Dosis
Nitroglycerin	Sublingual	2–3	15–20 m	0.4–0.8 mg
	Intravenous	2–3	15 m	50–300 μg/m
	Percutaneous	15	6 h	20–25 mg
Isosorbide	Sublingual	5–10	1–2 h	5 mg
dinitrate	Oral	20	4–6 h	20–30 mg
Molsidomine	Oral	30	8 h	4 mg
	Intravenous	10	5 h	4 mg
Nitroprusside	Intravenous	2–3	2–3 m	50–300 μg/m
Prazosin	Oral	30	6–8 h	5 mg
Captopril	Oral	30	6–8 h	25–50 mg
Hydralazine	Oral	30–60	6–8 h	50–100 mg

Table 2 indicates dosage and effect duration of the vasodilators most commonly used in heart failure. Substances that are not extensively employed have been excluded; sometimes because they are not now used for this purpose or because they are still at a trial stage.

Summary

Congestive heart failure (CHF) is characterized by an inadequate cardiac output in relation to venous return and tissue requirements. The organism activates diverse compensatory mechanisms to maintain the blood supply to vital organs. The most immediate mechanism is vasoconstriction, which increases arteriolar resistance and venoconstriction. When afterload increases blood pressure is maintained but the cardiac index declines still more, and when preload increases pulmonary congestion is produced. Moreover, myocardial oxygen consumption (MVO_2) rises and occasionally, supply declines. Treatment of CHF with vasodilators serves to reduce the excessive increase in preload and afterload, limit lung congestion and increase cardiac output. Moreover, the vasodilators lower MVO_2 and sometimes increase supply, thus improving the overall balance. Of the drugs presently available, those most used as venodilators are the nitrates, as mixed dilators, nitroprusside, prazosin and captopril, and as arteriodilators, hydralazine. In acute CHF, the vasodilators are used intravenously, fundamentally nitroglycerin and nitroprusside, and in chronic CHF, orally. If the predominant compensatory mechanism is known, the most appropriate vasodilator can be chosen: In cases with elevated renin levels, captopril is used. In cases with low renin levels, better results are obtained with prazosin or a combination of hydralazine and nitrates. Although long-term effects are usually less satisfactory than for acute CHF, good results are generally obtained with prolonged treatments and exercise capacity improves with the vasodilators.

References

1. López-Sendón J, Coma Canella I: Fisiopatología de la insuficiencia cardiaca. In: Martín Jadraque L, Coma Canella I, González Maqueda I, López-Sendón J (eds) Cardiopatía isquémíca. Norma, Madrid, 1981; 67–379.
2. Starling EG: The Linacre Lecture on the law of the heart. Longmans, Green and Co, London, 1918.
3. Meerson FZ: Development of modern components of the mechanism of cardiac hypertrophy. Circ Res 1974; 35 (Suppl 2): 58.
4. Larag JH: El sistema de la renina en la hipertensión, de la incredulidad a la realidad: bloqueo de la enzima convertidora. Prog Enf Cardiovasc 1979; 19: 223–233.

5. Zelis R, Mason DT, Braunwald E: A comparison of the effects of vasodilator stimuli on peripheral resistance vessels in normal subjects and in patients with congestive heart failure. J Clin Invest 1968; 47: 960–970.

6. Mason DT: Vasodilator and inotropic therapy of heart failure. Am J Med 1978; 65: 101–105.

7. Miller RR, Awan NA, DeMaria AN, Amsterdam EA, Mason DT: Importance of maintaining systemic blood pressure during nitroglycerin administration for reducing ischemic injury. Am J Cardiol 1977; 40: 504–508.

8. U'Prichard DC, Charness ME, Robertson D, Snyder SH: Prazosin: differential affinities for two populations of α- nor adrenergic receptor binding sites. Eur J Pharmacol 1978; 50: 87–89.

9. Gould L, Ramanareddy CV: Phentolamine. Am Heart J 1976; 92: 397–402.

10. Awan NA, Hermanovich J, Whitcomb Ch, Skinner P, Mason DT: Cardiocirculatory effects of afterload with oral trimazosin in severe congestive heart failure. Am J Cardiol 1979; 44: 126–131.

11. Levine TB, Olivari MT, Garberg V, Sharkey SW, Cohn JN: Hemodynamic and clinical response to enalapril, a long-acting converting-enzyme inhibitor, in patients with congestive heart failure. Circulation 1984; 69: 548–553.

12. Gavras H: Congestive heart failure: treatment by angiotensin blockade. Primary Cardiol 1980; Mar: 103–110.

13. Nutter DO, Crumly HJ: Canine coronary vascular and cardiac responses to the prostaglandins. Cardiovasc Res 1972; 6: 217–225.

14. Ebner F, Donath M: Mode of action and efficacy of nifedipine. In: Puech P, Krebs R (eds) Third International Adalat[R] Symposium. Excerpta Medica, Amsterdam 1980; 25–34.

15. Coma Canella I, López-Sendón J: Tratamiento médico de la insuficiencia cardiaca en la cardiopatía isquémica. In: Martín Jadraque L, Coma Canella I, González Maqueda I, López-Sendón J (eds) Cardiopatía Isquémica. Norma, Madrid, 1981; 671–704.

16. López-Sendón J, Coma Canella I, Ruiz Rejon F, Vinuelas J, Garcia Fernandez F, Gonzalez Maqueda I: Efecto hemodinámico de la nitroglicerina sublingual en la fase aguda del infarto de miocardio. Rev Esp Cardiolog 1979; 32: 183–192.

17. Coma Canella I, López-Sendón J, Barahona P, Martin Jadraque L: Efecto hemodinámico de isosorbide sublingual en el infarto agudo de miocardio. Rev Esp Cardiolog 1980; 33: 71–79.

18. Coma Canella I, López-Sendón J: Efecto hemodinámico de la nitroglicerina gel en la insuficiencia cardiaca secundaria a infarto agudo de miocardio. Rev Esp Cardiolog 1983; 36: 43–48.

19. Coma Canella I, López-Sendón J, Benito F, Lacort M: Tratamiento de la insuficiencia cardiaca severa con nitroglicerina intravenosa. Rev Esp Cardiolog 1981; 34: 63–71.

20. Franciosa JA, Pierpont G, Cohn JN: Hemodynamic improvement after oral hydralazine in left ventricular failure. Ann Intern Med 1977; 86: 388–393.

21. Stern MA, Gohlke HK, Loeb HS, Croke RP, Gunnar RM: Hemodynamic effects of intravenous phentolamine in low output cardiac failure. Circulation 1978; 58: 158–163.

22. Dairman W, Gordon R, Spector R, Sjoerdsma A, Udenfriend S: Effect of α-blockers on catecholamine biosynthesis. Federation Proceedings 1968; 27: 240.

23. Bagwell EE, Hilliard CC, Daniell HB, Taylor PL, Walton RP: Studies on the inotropic mechanism of phentolamine (Abstract). Am J Cardiol 1970; 25: 83.

24. Elkayam U, Weber L, Torkan B, Berman D, Rahimtoola SH: Acute hemodynamic effect of oral nifedipine in severe chronic congestive heart failure. Am J Cardiol 1983; 52: 1041–1045.

25. Polese A, Fiorentini C, Olivari MT, Guazzi MD: Clinical use of a calcium antagonist ag t (Nifedipine) in acute pulmonary edema. Am J Med 1979; 66: 825–830.

26. Gillmer DJ, Kark P: Pulmonary edema precipitated by nifedipine. Br Med J 1980; 280: 1420–1421.

27. López-Sendón J, Coma Canella I: Tratamiento de la insuficiencia ventricular izquierda con nitroprusiato sódico. Rev Esp Cardiolog 1979; 32: 435–444.

28. López-Sendón J, Coma Canella I, Lombrera F, Martin Jadraque L: Use of oral prazosin hydrochloride in congestive failure following acute myocardial infarction. Am Heart J 1979; 98: 495–504.

29. Rowe GC: Inequalities of myocardial perfusion in coronary artery disease (coronary steal). Circulation 1970; 42: 193–194.

30. Schanzenbacher P, Deeg P, Liebau G, Kochsiek K: Paradoxical angina after nifedipine: angiographic documentation. Am J Cardiol 1984; 53: 345–346.

31. Macho P, Vatner SF: Effects of nitroglycerin and nitroprusside on large and small coronary vessels in sconscious dogs. Circulation 1981; 64: 1101–1107.

32. Cohen MV, Downey JM, Sonnenblick EH, Kirk ES: The effects of nitroglycerin on coronary collaterals and myocardial contractility. J Clin Invest 1973; 52: 2836–2847.

33. Brown BG, Bolson E, Peterson RB, Pierce CD, Dodge HT: The mechanisms of nitroglycerin action: stenosis vasodilatation as a major component of the drug response. Circulation 1981; 64: 1089–1097.

34. Chariello M, Gold HK, Leinbach RC, Davis MA, Maroko PR: Comparison between the effects of nitroprusside and nitroglycerin in ischemic injury during acute myocardial infarction. Circulation 1976; 54: 766–773.

35. Awan NA, Miller RR, Vera Z, DeMaria AL, Amsterdam EA, Mason DT: Reduction of S-T segment elevation with infusion of nitroprusside in patients with acute myocardial infarction. Am J Cardiol 1976; 38: 435.

36. Cohen MV, Sonnenblick EH, Kirk ES: Comparative effects of nitroglycerin and isosorbide dinitrate on coronary collateral vessels and ischemic myocardium in dogs. Am J Cardiol 1976; 37: 244–249.

37. Pierpont GL, Hale KA, Franciosa JA, Cohn JN: Relationship between pulmonary vascular and hypoxemic effects of vasodilators in left ventricular failure (Abstract). Circulation 1977; 55–56 (Suppl 3): 163.

38. Hales ChA, Westphal D: Hypoxemia following the administration of sublingual nitroglycerin. Am J Med 1978; 65: 911–918.

39. Marshall JB, Ecklund RE: Methemglobinemia from overdose of nitroglycerin. JAMA 1980; 244: 330.

40. Franciosa JA, Nordstrom LA, Cohn JN: Nitrate therapy for congestive heart failure. JAMA 1978; 240: 443.

41. Colucci WS, Wynne J, Holman BL, Braunwald E: Long-term therapy of heart failure with prazosin: a randomized double blind trial. Am J Cardiol 1980; 45: 337–344.

42. Aranow WS, Greendield RS, Alimadadian H, Danahy DT: Effect of vasodilator trimazosin versus placebo on exercise performance in chronic left ventricular failure. Am J Cardiol 1977; 40: 789–793.

43. Topic N, Kramer B, Massie B: Acute and long-term effects of captopril on exercise cardiac performance and exercise capacity in congestive heart failure. Am Heart J 1982; 104: 1172–1179.

44. Chatterjee K, Parmley WW, Massie B, Greenberg B, Werner J, Klausner S, Norman A: Oral hydralazine therapy for chronic refractory heart failure. Circulation 1976; 54: 879–883.

45. Zelis R, Flaim SF, Moskowitz RM, Nellis SH: How much can we expect from vasodilator therapy in congestive heart failure? Circulation 1978; 59: 1092–1097.

46. Franciosa JA, Cohn JN: Immediate effects of hydralazine-isosorbide dinitrate combination on exercise capacity and exercise. Circulation, 1978; 59: 1085–1091.

47. Witzel RL, Flaim SF, Zelis R: Effects of nitroglycerin infusion on the hemodynamic response to exercise in rats in heart failure. Clin Res 1979; 27: 620.

48. Yui Y, Nakajima H, Sakurai T, Wakabayashi A, Kawai C: Adverse increase in plasma norepinephrine during acute vasodilator therapy in congestive heart failure. IX World Cardiology Congress. Moscow, 1982.

306

49. Awan NA, Massie BM: Therapy of severe chronic congestive heart failure. Am Heart J 1982; 104: 1125–1126.
50. Curtis C, Cohn JN, Vrobel T, Franciosa JA: Role of the renin-angiotensin system in the systemic vasoconstriction of chronic congestive heart failure. Circulation 1978; 58: 763–770.
51. Stein L, Henry DP, Weinberger MH: Increase in plasma norepinephrine during prazosin therapy for chronic congestive heart failure. Am J Med 1981; 70: 825–832.
52. Manthey J, Dietz R, Leinberger H, Schmidt-Gayk H, Schomig A, Schwarz F, Kubler W: Vasodilator therapy in heart failure: limited by activation of vasoconstrictor mechanisms? (Abstract). Circulation 1980; 62 (Suppl 3): 259.
53. Yui Y, Nakajima H, Kawai C, Murakami T: Prostacyclin therapy in patients with congestive heart failure. Am J Cardiol 1982; 50: 320–324.
54. Zelis RT, Mason DT: Demonstration of nitrate tolerance: attenuation of the venomotor response to nitroglycerin by the chronic administration of isosorbide dinitrate. Circulation 1969; 39–40 (Suppl 3): 211.
55. Needleman P, Johnson EM Jr: Mechanism of tolerance development to organic nitrates. J Pharmacol Exp Ther 1973; 184: 709.
56. Franciosa JA, Cohn JN: Sustained hemodynamic effects of nitrates without tolerance in heart failure (Abstract). Circulation 1978; 58 (Suppl 2): 28.
57. Fitchett DH, Marin JA, Oakley CM, Goodwin JF: Hydralazine in the management of left ventricular failure. Am J Cardiol 1979; 44: 303–309.
58. Mason DT, Awan NA, Amsterdam EA, Lee G, Joye J, Foerster JM, Laslett LJ, Low RI, DeMaria AN: New therapeutic approaches to the failing heart: recent advances in vasodilators, cardiotonics, and mechanical circulatory assistance. In: Mason DT (ed) Advances in heart disease. Grune and Stratton, New York, 1980; 403–446.
59. Franciosa JA, Cohn JN: Hemodynamic responsiveness to short and long-acting vasodilators in left ventricular failure. Am J Med 1978; 65: 126–133.
60. Packer M, Meller J: Oral vasodilator therapy for chronic heart failure. A plea for caution. Am J Cardiol 1978; 42: 686–690.
61. Chatterjee K: Chronic congestive heart failure and vasodilator therapy. J Contin Educat Cardiology 1978; 13: 17–26.
62. Markham RV, Corbett JR, Gilmore A, Pettinger WA, Firth BG: Efficacy of prazosin in the management of congestive heart failure: a 6 month randomized, double-blind, placebo-controlled study. Am J Cardiol 1983; 51: 1346–1352.
63. Aronow NS, Danahy DT: Efficacy of trimazosin and prazosin therapy on cardiac and exercise performance in outpatients with chronic congestive heart failure. Am J Med 1978; 65: 155–160.
64. Arnold S, Ports T, Chatterjee K, Williams R, Rubin S, Parmley W: Rapid attenuation of prazosin mediated increase in cardiac output in patients with chronic heart failure. Circulation 1978; 58 (Suppl 2): 222.
65. Ader R, Chatterjee K, Ports T, Brundage B, Hiramatsu B, Parmley W: Immediate and sustained hemodynamic and clinical improvement in chronic heart failure by an oral angiotensin-converting enzyme inhibitor. Circulation 1980; 61: 931–937.
66. Sharpe N, Coxon R: Hemodynamic effects of captopril in chronic heart failure: efficacy of low-dose treatment and comparison with captopril. Am Heart J 1982; 104: 1164–1171.
67. Kayanakis JG, Fauvel JM, Giraud P, Bounhoure JP: Long-term treatment of congestive heart failure by captopril: hemodynamic, biological and clinical effects. Eur Heart J 1981; 2: 75–81.
68. Massie B, O'Young J, Ports T, Chatterjee K, Parmley W: Vasodilator therapy of heart failure: results of long-term follow up (Abstract). Circulation 1979; 59–60 (Suppl 2): 231.
69. Packer M, Medina N, Yushak M, Meller J: Hemodynamic patterns of response during long-term captopril therapy for severe chronic heart failure. Circulation 1983; 68: 803–812.

6.4 The New Inotropic Agents

THIERRY H. LEJEMTEL, RICHARD GROSE, JANET STRAIN and
EDMUND H. SONNENBLICK

In the absence of overwhelming valvular or peripheral vascular abnormalities, loss of functioning myocardium and the sequence of events it provokes is the primary pathophysiologic abnormality which leads to myocardial failure, and ultimately to congestive heart failure [1]. Confronted with an increased hemodynamic load, the remaining myocardium hypertrophies and thereby maintains an adequate level of cardiac performance. However, for reasons which are probably not related to the primary process itself, and are still poorly understood, the hypertrophic myocardium eventually fails, leading to depressed cardiac performance. At that point, the peripheral circulation adjusts to the decreased cardiac output by raising arteriolar resistances in order to maintain systemic arterial pressure, and by redistributing blood flow in order to maintain perfusion of essential organs [2].

Severe heart failure cannot be reversed and gradually deteriorates to a point incompatible with life [3–6]. Pharmacologic interventions only improve left ventricular performance and possibly relieve symptoms, but do not replace the loss of functioning myocardium. These interventions are aimed at decreasing the load which the heart has to bear, i.e. afterload reduction with vasodilator agents, and at improving the contractile process, i.e. cardiac stimulation with positive inotropic agents. Inotropic therapy, and especially the use of digitalis glycosides, has been founded on the postulate that further stimulation of the depressed myocardium can substantially improve left ventricular performance and restore blood flow to the different organs to near normal level. To be viable, such a postulate requires that the already depressed myocardium has a contractile reserve which can be mobilized consistently without producing additional myocardial damage. In an experimental model of heart failure, Spann et al. demonstrated that the force developed by the failing heart muscle was reduced but could be somewhat increased by paired pacing or strophanditin [7]. The increments in force produced by inotropic stimulation in the failing heart were, however, markedly lower than those elicited in the normal muscles. To which extent these experimental findings can be applied to patients

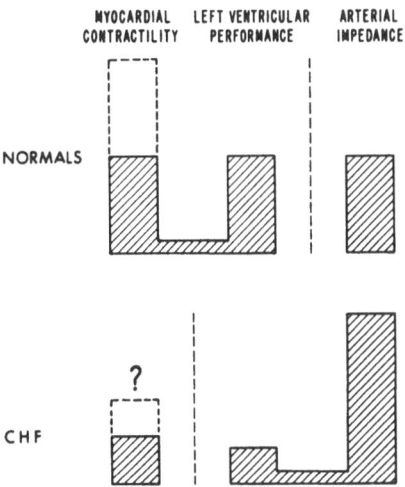

Fig. 1. In normals, a substantial contractile reserve (dashed line) is present, and thus left ventricular performance is not limited by myocardial contractility, nor is it greatly influenced by arterial impedance. In patients with congestive heart failure, contractile reserve, if present, is decreased and left ventricular performance is greatly affected by arterial impedance which is elevated.

with longstanding congestive heart failure is unknown. Indeed, in contrast to patients with coronary artery disease, the presence of contractile reserve has not been systemically appraised in patients with congestive heart failure [8, 9]. Preliminary reports indicate that myocardial contractile reserve appears extremely variable in individuals with heart failure [10].

In normal subjects, left ventricular performance is not limited by myocardial contractility nor is it greatly altered by arterial impedance. However, in patients with congestive heart failure, left ventricular performance is limited by myocardial contractility and greatly affected by arteriolar impedance which, in turn, is elevated (Fig. 1). Consequently, if positive inotropic intervention is to improve left ventricular performance in this clinical setting, it should be preferably used after reduction of the elevated arterial impedance. Vasodilating and inotropic therapy are therefore not exclusive but complementary.

Long-term positive inotropic therapy in patients with congestive heart failure also depends on the premise that the spontaneous deterioration of the disease will not be hastened by overstimulation of an already 'tired' heart. However, there is no data to show that failing myocardium is more sensitive to damage from inotropic stimulation than normal muscle. This does not exclude the possibility that damage and loss of cells may still be proceeding without an as yet known cause or knowledge of what exacerbates it. If the metabolic reserves and resiliency are limited, the concept of intermittent stimulation of the heart by therapy with inotropic agents may be of great interest. Improving left ventricular performance may be most needed when the metabolic requirements of the body are increased, i.e. during physical exercise, and may be superfluous when the metabolic requirements are limited. Moreover, the metabolic cost of positive inotropic therapy may be excessive in hypertrophied and failing hearts which have been shown to have a limited coronary reserve [11]. However, in patients with high left ventricular filling pressures and dilated ventricles, inotropic therapy should lower filling pressures and reduce heart size. This, in turn, should lower myocardial oxygen requirements and possibly offset the increase in oxygen need generated by enhanced myocardial contractility [12].

Lastly, in order to translate inotropic stimulation into symptomatic benefits, the sustained improvement in cardiac performance produced by inotropic therapy should reverse the derangements of the peripheral circulation always present in severe congestive heart failure. Thus, chronic inotropic therapy should enhance renal perfusion and sodium excretion, increase skeletal muscle blood flow during at least submaximal exercise and possibly during maximal exercise, and turn off the neuroendocrine adjustments present in heart failure (i.e. lowering circulating catecholamines and angiotensin II). Failure to generate these beneficial peripheral effects would turn inotropic therapy into a therapeutic intervention of little clinical significance.

Of the new inotropic agents presently under clinical investigation, Milrinone (WIN 47203) appears one of the most promising. In contrast to its precursor, amrinone (WIN 40680) which was associated with multiple side effects during chronic administration, long-term treatment of patients with severe heart failure, i.e. over 2 years in our center, has not been complicated with overt adverse reactions. All these new cardiotonic agents have certain similarities. They all inhibit myocardial phosphodiesterase activity and this inhibition seems more selective than that produced by papavarine or theophylline. For all of them, it is not yet known if phosphodiesterase inhibition alone is responsible for their inotropic action, or whether other mechanisms, such as increased affinity of contractile protein for Ca^{2+}, also play a role. They all exert direct arteriolar vasodilation in the hind limb preparation. The dose response curve of the vasodilating action appears, however, variable from agent to agent: present at low dose in some and at high dose in others.

In patients with severe congestive heart failure, the new inotropic agents consistently improve left ventricular performance, as evidenced by an increase in cardiac output and a decrease in preliminary capillary wedge pressure [13–17]. However, in contrast to the consistent augmentation in cardiac performance, the increase in myocardial contractility as evaluated by the rate of left ventricular pressure rise (dP/dt) is variable (Fig. 2). The effects of ascend-

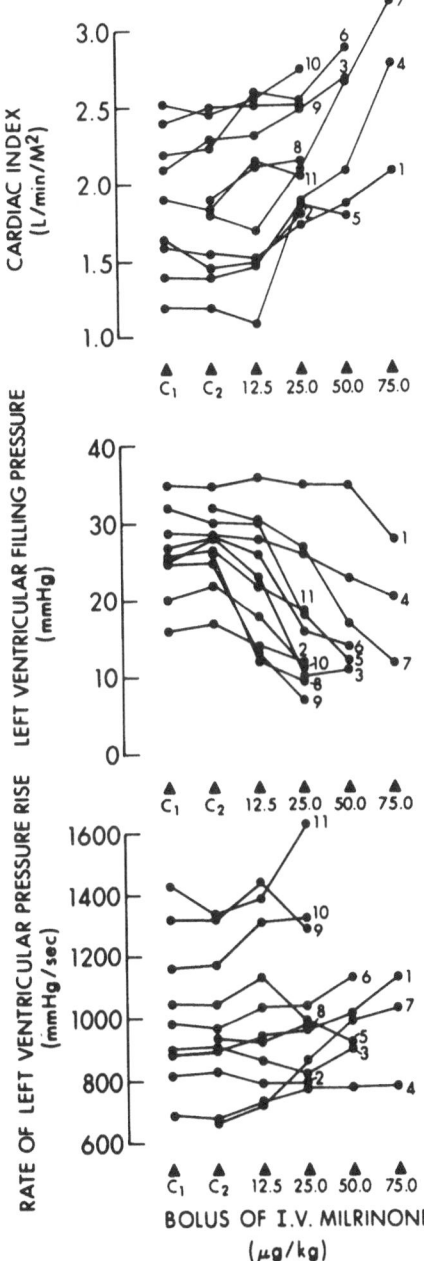

Fig. 2. Changes in cardiac index (top panel), left ventricular filling pressure (middle panel), and rate of left ventricular pressure rise (lower panel) produced by ascending doses of intravenous milrinone in 11 patients. This study was performed during a diagnostic left heart catheterization using a Millar micromanometer-tipped catheter.

ing doses of intravenous milrinone on ventricular performance and myocardial contractility were evaluated in 11 patients with severe congestive heart failure in the catheterization laboratory using a micromanometer-tipped catheter. In 10 of the 11 patients, cardiac index increased and the maximal augmentation averaged 33% and ranged from 4 to 125%. A reduction in left ventricular filling pressure (LVEDP) was noted in every patient. The reduction in LVEDP averaged 47% and ranged from 20 to 72%. Of interest, the only patient who failed (No 9) to demonstrate a significant increase in cardiac index, experienced a major fall in pulmonary wedge pressure to less than 8 mm Hg. This fall in LVEDP may have offset the beneficial effects of milrinone on myocardial contractility and afterload to improve cardiac output. The effects of milrinone on the rate of left ventricular pressure rise varied from patient to patient. It increased significantly in six (Nos 1, 4, 6, 7, 10, 11), did not change significantly in four (Nos 2, 3, 8, 9), and tended to decrease in one (No 5). Of note, in patient 5, the fall in the rate of left ventricular pressure rise occurred despite an increase in cardiac index from 1.4 to 2.9 L/min/M^2 and a decrease in left ventricular pressure from 30 to 12 mm Hg. The fall in the rate of left ventricular pressure rise in this patient does not indicate a real reduction in myocardial contractility, but rather points out the dependence of left ventricular dP/dt on cardiac preload [18]. In patients with moderate increases in myocardial contractility, the improvement in left ventricular performance is likely to predominantly result from a lowering of arterial impedance due to the direct vasodilating property of milrinone. In patients who exhibit substantial increases in myocardial contractility, the beneficial inotropic effect of milrinone to enhance ventricular performance is amplified by the concomitant reduction in cardiac afterload produced by its direct vasodilatory action. In agreement with the dual mechanism of action of milrinone on left ventricular performance is the lack of correlation noted in our 11 patients between the rise on cardiac index and the change in the rate of left ventricular pressure rise (Fig. 3). The hemodynamic evaluation of other new inotropic agents performed in our laboratory has led to results similar to those noted with milrinone. The effects of fenoximone (MDL 17043) in myocardial contractility and ventricular performance were evaluated in seven patients with severe chronic heart failure in the catheterization laboratory. While fenoximone consistently improved left ventricular performance as evidenced by a rise in cardiac output and a fall in pulmonary capillary wedge pressure, the changes in the rate of left ventricular pressure seen were less consistent. Moreover, as illustrated in Fig. 4, the increase in cardiac output produced by successive intravenous boluses of fenoximone seemed to coincide with a fall in systemic arterial pressure suggesting that a direct vasodilator effect of this drug greatly contributed to the improvement in cardiac performance. The dependence of the rate of left ventricular pressure rise on cardiac preload was also documented in this

312

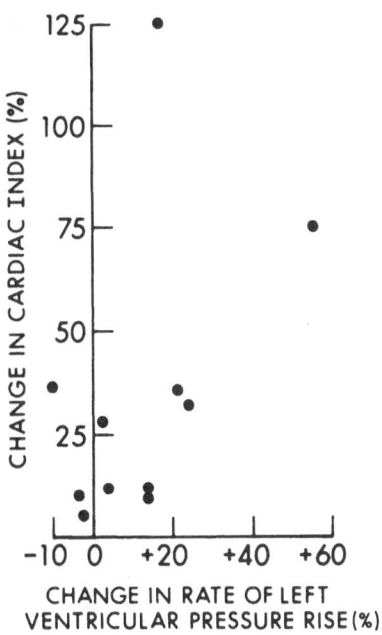

Fig. 3. Lack of correlation between the peak increase in cardiac index (%) and the concomitant change in rate of left ventricular pressure rise (%) in 11 patients who received ascending doses of intravenous milrinone in the catheterization laboratory.

patient as the rate of pressure rise decreased substantially when left ventricular filling pressure fell from 30 to 18 mm Hg. Accordingly, like milrinone, the improvement in ventricular performance produced by fenoximone results from both increased inotropy and direct afterload reduction. While the latter effect seems to be dose dependent and is consistently observed when the dose is increased, the former effect appears variable in magnitude from patient to patient which may reflect the amount of myocardial contractile reserve and the level of myocardial cyclic AMP.

Nevertheless, despite its variability, the positive inotropic action of these new cardiotonic agents appears of great clinical importance for several reasons. First, in contrast to an incidence of 15 to 20% of symptomatic hypotension, which complicates therapy with vasodilators in patients with chronic heart failure, these new cardiotonic agents, from a hemodynamic point of view, are all well tolerated. The rare cases of symptomatic hypotension appear to be related to excessive reduction in cardiac preload in patients who at baseline had borderline elevation of left ventricular filling pressure. Otherwise, hypotension is only observed following administration of high doses of these agents.

Also, in contrast to captopril which does not immediately increase resting

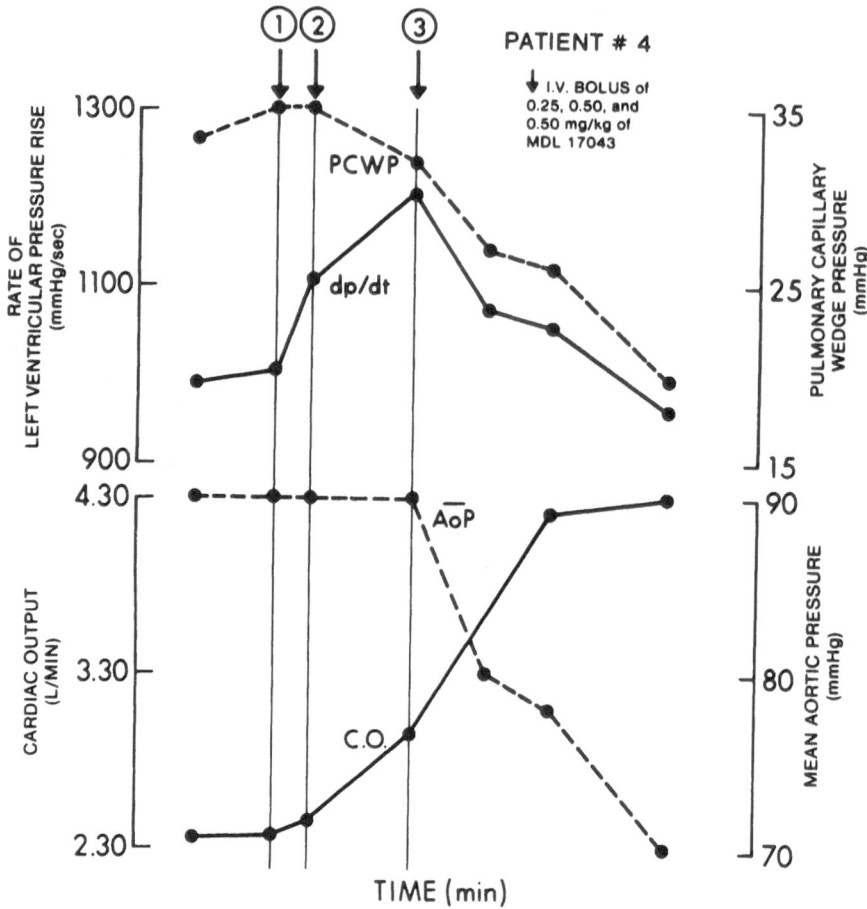

Fig. 4. Time course of changes in rate of left ventricular pressure rise, pulmonary capillary wedge pressure, cardiac output and mean aortic pressure, after three successive intravenous boluses of fenoximone. The increase in cardiac output is concomitant with the reduction in mean aortic pressure, while after an initial increase in the rate of left ventricular pressure rise, it declines in parallel with the fall in pulmonary capillary wedge pressure.

limb blood flow, the new cardiotonic agents, such as amrinone and milrinone, acutely increase resting limb blood flow and tend to delay anaerobic threshold at submaximal load [19]. These acute effects on limb blood flow are most probably responsible for the immediate improvement noted during daily activity by patients who are treated with the new inotropic agents. In addition, improvement in maximal oxygen uptake, i.e. peak aerobic power, is often observed during chronic therapy with these new agents. The lag between the improvement in exercise capacity at *submaximal* and *maximal* workload can be explained by the uncoupling between cardiac performance and peripheral derangements in chronic heart failure. An acute improvement in ventricular function does not immediately reverse the peripheral derangements characteristic of chronic heart failure and vice versa a sudden deterioration in cardiac performance does not acutely give rise in peripheral derangements. To increase maximal oxygen uptake, both an improvement in cardiac performance and an increase in blood flow to the actively metabolizing skeletal muscles are needed.

While at a late stage of chronic heart failure inotropic agents are essentially palliative and do not prevent progression of the disease [20], it is still unknown if, at an earlier stage, they may be more successful and may prevent cardiac dilatation. However, current research in experimental animal models suggests that myocardial preservation may be better accomplished by stabilizing cellular membranes with calcium-channel blockers [21].

References

1. Sonnenblick EH, Factor S, Strobeck JE, Capasso JM, Fein E: The pathophysiology of heart failure: The primary role of microvascular hyperreactivity and spasm in the development of congestive cardiomyopathies. In: Braunwald E, Mock MB, Watson J (eds) Congestive heart failure. Grune and Stratton, 1982.
2. Zelis R, Longhurst J, Capone RJ, Lee G: Peripheral circulatory control mechanisms in congestive heart failure. Am J Cardiol 1973; 32: 481–490.
3. Wilson JR, Schwartz JS, St. John Sutton M, Ferraro N, Horowitz LN, Reicheck N, Josephson ME: Prognosis in severe heart failure: Relation to hemodynamic measurements and ventricular ectopic activity. JACC 1983; 2: 403–410.
4. Convert G, Delaye J, Beaune J, Biron A, Gonin A: Etude prognestique des myocardiopathies primitives non obstructives. Arch Mal Coeur 1980; 73: 227–237.
5. Hamby RI: Primary myocardial disease: A prospective clinical and hemodynamic evaluation in 100 patients. Medicine 1970; 49: 55–78.
6. Franciosa JA, Wilen M, Ziesche S, Cohn JN: Survival in man with severe chronic left ventricular failure to either coronary heart disease or idiopathic dilated cardiomyopathy. Am J Cardiol 1983; 51: 831–836.
7. Spann JF, Buccino RA, Sonnenblick EH, Braunwald EH: Contractile state of cardiac muscle obtained from cats with experimentally produced ventricular hypertrophy and heart failure. Circ Res 1967; 21: 341–354.
8. Dyke SH, Cohn PF, Gorlin R, Sonnenblick EH: Detection of residual myocardial function in coronary artery disease using post-extrasystolic potentiation. Circulation 1974; 50: 691–694.
9. Cohn PF: Evaluation of inotropic contractile reserve in ischemic heart disease using post-extrasystolic potentiation. Circulation 1980; 61: 1071–1075.
10. LeJemtel TH, Sonnenblick EH: Should the failing heart be stimulated? N Engl J Med 1984; 310: 1384–1385.
11. Marehetti GV, Merlo L, Visioli O: Coronary blood flow and oxygen consumption in hypertrophied cardiac muscle in dogs. Adv Cardiol 1976; 18: 93–103.
12. Jentzer JH, LeJemtel TH, Sonnenblick EH, Kirk ES: Beneficial effect of amrinone on myocardial oxygen consumption during acute left ventricular failure in dogs. Am J Cardiol 1981; 48: 75–83.

13. Maskin CS, Sinoway L, Chadwick B, Sonnenblick EH, LeJemtel TH: Sustained hemodynamic and clinical effects of a new cardiotonic agent WIN 47203 in patients with severe congestive heart failure. Circulation 1983; 67: 1065–1070.

14. Uretsky BF, Generalovich T, Reddy PS, Spangenberg RB, Follansbee WP: The acute hemodynamic effects of a new agent MDL 17043 in the treatment of congestive heart failure. Circulation 1983; 67: 823–828.

15. Petein M, Levine BT, Cohn JW: Hemodynamic effects of a new inotropic agent piroximone (MDL 19025) in patients with chronic heart failure. JACC 1984; 4: 364–371.

16. Mancini D, Sonnenblick EH, Latts JR, Olson S, Chadwick B, LeJemtel TH: Hemodynamic and clinical benefits of CI-914 a new cardiotonic agent (Abstract). Circulation 1985; 70 (Suppl II): II 64.

17. Daly P, Viguerat C, Curan D, Dobras F, Parmley W: Improved left ventricular function without increased metabolic cost with RO 13-6438 a non-glycoside, non-catecholamine inotrope vasodilator. Clin Res 1984; 32: 158A.

18. Mahler F, Ross Jr J, O'Rourke RA, Covell JW: Effects of changes in preload, afterload and inotropic state on ejection and isovolumic phase measures of contractility in the conscious dog. Am J Cardiol 1975; 35: 626–634.

19. Siskind SJ, Sonnenblick EH, Forman R, Scheuer J, LeJemtel TH: Acute substantial benefit of inotropic therapy with amrinone on exercise hemodynamics and metabolism in acute congestive heart failure. Circulation 1981; 64: 966–984.

20. Maskin CS, Forman R, Klein NA, Sonnenblick EH, LeJemtel TH: Long-term amrinone therapy in patients with severe heart failure. Am J Med 1982; 72: 113–118.

21. Rouleau JL, Chuck LHS, Hollosi G, Kidd P, Sievers RE, Wikmancoffelt J, Parmley WW: Verapamil preserves myocardial contractility in the hereditary cardiomyopathy of the Syrian hamster. Circ Res 1982; 50: 405–412.

6.5 Right Ventricular Failure in Ischaemic Heart Disease

J. TROUFE, G, HERNANDO, J.M. IRIGOYEN, J. SOLAR and M. PERÉZ

It can no longer be said that little is known about the role of the right ventricle (RV) in ischaemic heart disease, as in recent years many works have been published on the involvement of this ventricle as a consequence of coronary artery lesions.

Progress has been such that clinical, electrocardiographic, echocardiographic or isotopic diagnostic criteria have now been established. The scarce prognostic influence of acute RV infarction (RV-AMI) is described with surprising confidence and the therapy presently used is practically considered as definitive. However, although previously described by pathologists [1, 2], RV-AMI appeared in clinical descriptions only 10 years ago [3], not sufficiently long enough for many aspects to be clarified. In this paper we refer exclusively to RV infarction from a hemodynamic point of view and discuss treatment on this basis. The fact that Cohn's initial work described RV-AMI as ventricular pump failure has perhaps contributed to the fact that this is one of the better studied aspects to date. Nevertheless, there is still much to learn, especially regarding the subacute and chronic phases of the disease.

Acute phase RV infarction

Table 1 lists the diagnostic criteria used in our Coronary Unit to establish RV-AMI diagnosis. The abnormal elevation of right atrial pressure (RAP) in relation to the pulmonary wedge pressure (PWP), is evaluated according to the patterns established by López Sendón et al. [4]. The following criteria correspond to the classical morphologic pattern of loss of ventricular compliance. The mechanical alternance of RV or pulmonary artery, although infrequent (10% in our experience) is a very reliable diagnostic criterion.

To these classical criteria three others can be added, obtained from the right ventricular function curve. By means of rapid venous perfusion of a solution of dextrose 40, left filling pressures are increased to 18–20 mm Hg (of PWP).

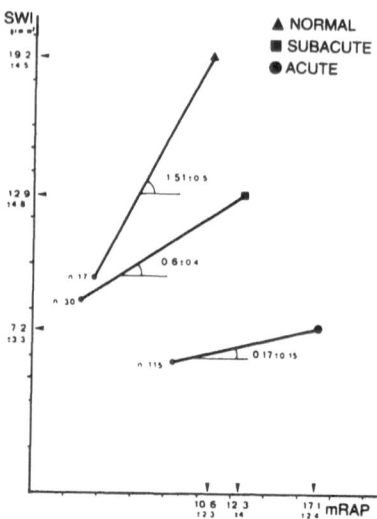

Fig. 1. Comparison of the ascending phase of the function curve, in cases with right ventricular infarction in the acute and subacute phases and cases with normal RV. MRAP = mean right atrium pressure; SWI = systolic work index.

Pressure and cardiac output determinations each time these pressures increase 2–3 mm Hg provide a series of points which give the function curve (FC) of both ventricles.

Fig. 1 shows the ascending phase of the FC in 115 cases of acute RV infarction (lower line), subacute phase in 30 cases and of 17 subjects with normal RV (upper line). The graph correlates the mean RA pressure in abscisa with the systolic work index (SWI) of the RV in ordinate. There is a significant difference (p<0.001) between the RV-AMI and normal subjects, both in the SWI (7 = 2 ± 3 = 3 and 19.2 ± 4.5) and in the ascending slope of the FC (0.17 ± 0.15 and 1.15 ± 0.5). Nevertheless, the pressure necessary to reach the FC peak is significatively higher (p<0.001) in the RV-AMI (17.1 ± 2.4) than in normal subjects (10.6 ± 2.3).

Table 1. RV-AMI: diagnostic criteria.

Similar levels CVP-PWP
Deep $y/_x$ wave of RA
Dip plateau morphology of RV
Mechanical alternance of RV
SWI lower of RV
Smooth function curve
Increased filling pressure at the peak of the ventricular function curve

---

The low level of maximum SWI and the FC slope represents a contractile index of the RV while the abnormal elevation of RA pressure implies a marked impairment of RV compliance. It is interesting to point out that 25 of the 11 cases died, and RV necrosis was demonstrated in all the post-mortem studies. In other words, the specificity of the above criteria, from which at least 4 are required to establish the diagnosis, reached 100%.

RV-AMI in the hyperacute phase

Throughout our studies on right ventricular infarction, our attention was drawn to the fact that one series of patients, in whom signs of RV failure were seen during the first hours of evolution presented the classical data of necrosis of this ventricle 2–4 days later.

The revision of 43 patients with proven RV-AMI admitted within 12 hours of evolution, showed a mean RA pressure in this initial phase of 6.9 ± 3 mm Hg. Without diagnostic or therapeutic manoeuvres to modify the fluid balance, the RA pressure increased between the 2nd and the 4th day to $11,7 \pm 4,1$ mm Hg ($p < 0.001$).

In 11 cases whose evolution confirmed the presence of RV necrosis, function curves were obtained within the first 12 hours. Between 48 and 96 hours and with fluid balance again adjusted, the study was repeated. Results can be seen in Fig. 2. In the early phase of AMI a marked deterioration of the contractile function was detected, shown by the low level of maximal SWI ($6.5 \pm 3 \, g/m^2$) and marked flattening of the ascending phase of the FC (0.16 ± 0.1). In the later study, we found similar SWI (75.3) and ascending slope (0.18 ± 0.2) values. On the other hand, a considerable difference ($p < 0.001$) was detected in the filling pressure of RV at the level of the maximum FC value between the two situations: 13.8 ± 2 in the early phase and 17.5 ± 2 mm Hg between the 2nd and the 4th day.

The role of the pericardium in the diastolic function of RV is a controversial issue and not yet sufficiently clear. However, from our findings we are inclined to think that just as has been proven in LV infarction, in RV-AMI the contractile alteration takes place immediately after coronary occlusion, preceding compliance depression by 48–76 hours. This can be seen graphically in the recordings of RA and RV pressures. In Fig. 3 it is shown how the ventricular diastolic curve, which is normal in the early phase, later gives rise to the typical morphology in 'dip-plateau'.

This finding is of practical as well as of theoretical interest. The most characteristic sign of RV necrosis, that is, the poor compliance pattern, does not appear during the first 12–24 hours. The diagnosis should therefore be based, together with the other clinical data, exclusively on the hemodynamic signs of contractility changes.

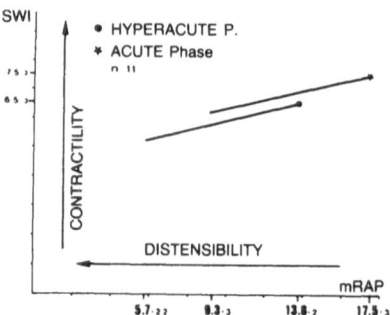

Fig. 2. Ascending phase from the right ventricular function curve of 11 patients suffering RV infarction in hyperacute phase (lower curve) and acute phase (upper curve) (see text).

Experiences of our group not yet published, seem to confirm that the RV-AMI deaths during the first hours present a RV extension of the necrosis larger in size to that of exclusively left infarctions. It seems probable therefore that RV failure is a determining factor of fatal evolution in these cases, thus emphasizing the importance of early diagnosis and aggressive therapy.

RV-AMI in subacute phase

One of the characteristic signs of RV failure following AMI, and which distinguishes this from infarction of the LV, is its rapid recovery in a considerable number of cases. This has been demonstrated by different authors from hemodynamic, echocardiographic or isotopic studies. Thirty of our patients with hemodynamic diagnosis of RV necrosis in the acute phase were re-studied about 2 weeks (13.4 ± 4.2 days) after the infarction. The ascending phase of the FC in these patients is seen in the centre of Fig. 1. The maximum SWI

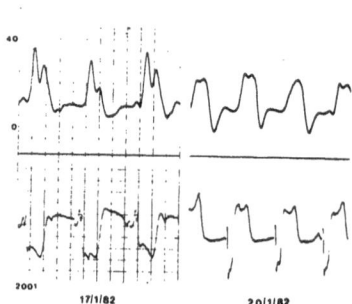

Fig. 3. Right ventricular pressure morphology in one case with RV-AMI during the first hour of infarction evolution (left) and three days later. We can see the deterioration of ventricular distensibility.

values ($12.9 \pm 4.8\,\mathrm{gm^2}$) and the FC slope in this phase (0.6 ± 0.4) were definitively separated ($p<0.001$) from the same parameters in the acute phase. But at the same time they were clearly different from those found in normal cases.

On the other hand, it was proved that the maximum levels of RV output were reached with filling pressures (12 ± 4) statistically similar to those recorded in the cases of normal RV.

It was therefore evident that two weeks after the AMI (although the process began at 7–10 days) a clear recovery of the contractile function of the RV was seen, although this did not reach levels compatible with normality. On the contrary, the ventricular compliance, which was later seen to be affected, showed a practically total recovery, with values clearly equal to normal.

Although the global clinical data suggest a good prognosis, this may not always be the case. In fact, in two weeks, 9 of the 30 cases studied showed contractility and distensibility levels clearly inferior to those we considered as normal. This would indicate that almost one third of patients continue to have RV failure in this phase, although it is maintained in a sub-clinic form due to treatment, control and rest in the Coronary Unit.

'Delayed' pulmonary oedema

There is another interesting point regarding post-infarction RV recovery. It is well-known that very few RV infarctions are limited to this ventricle, but usually involve the LV. However, during the acute phase, signs of left ventricular failure are not usually demonstrated, thus providing one of the diagnostic clues, precisely the radiologic and hemodynamic absence of pulmonary venous hypertension. The reason for this is that the functional deterioration of the RV prevents the appearance of signs of left failure. This situation is known as 'protected lung'.

However, this situation is transitory. At the end of the first week after infarction the RV begins to show signs of recovery, which may be almost total a few days later. If the necrosis of the LV is extensive, especially if fluids have been abundantly administered previously, capillary pressure may be elevated. This situation is sometimes resolved spontaneously with abundant diuresis, but signs and symptoms of increased capillary venous pressure and even clear oedema may be seen. This is the so-called 'delayed pulmonary oedema'.

In 23 of our first patients with RV-AMI, the CP, which had shown basal values of 10.3 ± 5.1 in the acute phase, were later increased to 19.6 ± 2.4. This increase was later avoided by the administration of diuretics guided by the PWP levels. Wedge pressures are systematically monitored during the first week in patients with acute myocardial infarction with high enzymatic levels, or in those who need large amounts of fluid to maintain an adequate hemodynamic condition during the first days.

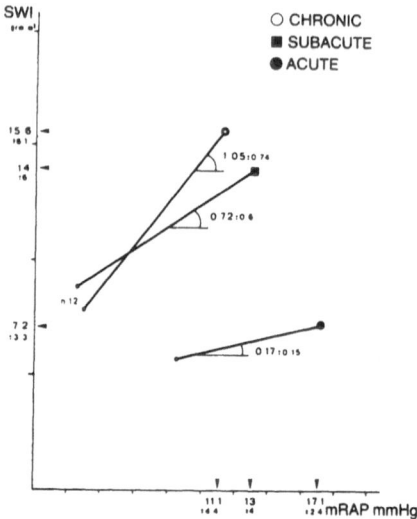

Fig. 4. Function curve of the RV-AMI in acute, subacute and chronic phases. We can see how recovery of RU takes place during the first two weeks after AMI and the hemodynamic situation is exactly the same after several months.

Chronic phase of RV infarction

Study of the RV several months after a RV infarction has received very little attention from clinicians [11]. This is perhaps due to the fact that at this stage, RV is rarely a cause of clinical problems. Only one of our patients was admitted with anasarca eight months after RV-AMI, responding rapidly to treatment. However, another three cases who had not shown right ventricular failure in a basal situation showed evident signs of RV failure in case of RV overload (pneumonia, sustained ventricular tachycardia and anterior LV rein-farction). Fig. 4 shows the FC of 12 patients who were studied in the subacute phase and restudied six months after RV infarction. None of the three param-eters of ventricular function showed significant differences between the two studies, confirming the findings of other authors (11, 12) in the sense that recovery of RV takes place in the first weeks after AMI and that the situation thereafter remains stable. Therefore RV infarction seldom represents a clin-ical problem in the long-term follow-up, and when it does, response to treat-ment with digitalis and diuretics is very satisfactory.

Prognosis of RV-AMI

Although opinion varies, prognosis does not seem to be modified by the occurence of a right infarction [13, 15]. It is possible that when the totality of the cases diagnosed by ECG or isotopic studies is considered, there is no difference between patients with or without signs of RV necrosis. However, when RV-AMI is demonstrated by hemodynamic alterations we believe the prognostic repercussion is clear.

Mortality in our 115 patients with RV-AMI, diagnosed on the basis of the hemodynamic criteria described, was 21.7%, while for the AMI in general within the Coronary Unit it was only 7.8%. Patients who died in the first hours of evolution and in whom it was not possible to make a function curve were excluded from the series (as we believe also occurred in series of other authors).

It would appear that the real rate of mortality due to infarctions with extension to the RV and their significance in the evolution of AMI is yet to be determined. Our experience seems to indicate the clinical repercussion of right ventricular necrosis in AMI is systematically underestimated.

Treatment of RV-AMI

The majority of patients with RV-AMI do not need specific therapy from that used in myocardial infarction. However, the incidence of low cardiac output in this disease is high [16]. Of our cases, 30.4% presented clinical signs of shock or pre-shock and 35% (41 patients) presented a cardiac index less than $2.2 l/min/m^2$.

As we stated in the introduction, the treatment used in this latter group of patients seems to be well established, based on the progressive use of fluid overload, vasodilators and/or inotropic agents. In spite of this, we feel some practical considerations should be made:

1. *Fluid overload:* The pathophysiological basis for the administration of fluids are well-known. The objective is to make maximum use of the Starling law of non-necrotic right ventricular myocardium, and in its absence, increase the right pressure sufficiently to obtain a right-left gradient which facilitates the passive filling of the LV.

   An increase, by means of rapid perfusion of fluids, of the pulmonary wedge pressure to levels of 18–20 mm Hg, produces an increase of CI of 2.45 ± 0.63 to $2.67 \pm 0.75 l/min/m^2$ with a difference of $0.31 \pm 0.32 l/min/m^2$. This difference was equally significant ($p < 0.001$) in the 30 patients with basal CI less than 1.89 ± 0.31 (differences of 0.27 ± 0.23) which confirms our impression that in cases of shock the effect of the fluids is less noticeable. In fact, the CI continued at levels of cardiogenic shock after perfusion.

   The heart's response to the administration of fluids was less in RV-AMI than in isolated left infarction, which is not easy to explain. Perhaps we should investigate whether there is discordance between the pulmonary

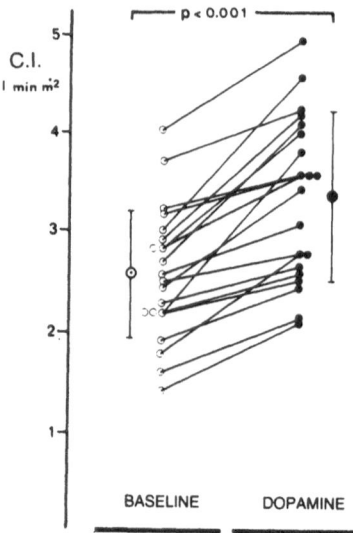

C.I.
l min m²

p < 0.001

BASELINE   DOPAMINE

Fig. 5. The favourable effects of dopamine over the cardiac index (CI) in patients with ventricular right infarction.

wedge pressure and the actual filling pressure of the LV in the presence of RV-AMI, which would alter these results.

2. *Inotropic agents:* it is clinically impossible to compare the effect of inotropic drugs in the two ventricles. However, the effect of dopamine (Fig. 5) in a series of patients with and without cardiogenic shock was surprisingly favourable. The mean CI showed an increase of 0.78 ± 0.30 following a perfusion of 5–8 u/kg/min for 20 minutes. This occured both in basal conditions and following fluid overload. The 4 cases with previous CI inferior to $21/min/m^2$ increased the CI to 2.35 ± 0.33 following administration of the drug.

We would like to emphasize the effect of dopamine. We believe that a more liberal use may be made of this drug in RV-AMI. In over 50% of the patients in whom abundant fluids were needed to maintain an adequate cardiac output, a bilateral pleural effusion occured. This was occasionally severe and required taping. The use of dopamine or another inotropic drugs in controlled dosis greatly helps to avoid this complication by limiting the fluid perfusion.

3. *Pulmonary counterpulsation:* the isolated use of aortic contrapulsation has not been noteworthy in our experience. Recent experimental and clinical works have studied contrapulsation of the pulmonary artery by means of a Dacron tube. The hemodynamic effect of this technique seems to be unquestionable. We believe that in the not very distant future, counter-

pulsation in the pulmonary artery by means of a percutaneously introduced balloon may be of great utility in the treatment of shock due to RV-AMI. This chamber's ability to recover would contribute to the success of this therapeutic method.

References

1. Bennet BW: Infarction of the Heart. III. Clinical and morphological findings. Ann Int Med 1938–1939; 12: 71.
2. Watman W, Hellerstein H: The incidence of heart disease in 2000 consecutive autopsies. Ann Int Med 1948; 28: 41.
3. Cohn JN, Guiha NH, Broder MI, Limas CJ: Right ventricular infarction. Clinical and hemodynamic features. Am J Cardiol 1974; 33: 209.
4. López-Sendón J, Coma-Canella J, Gamallo C: Sensitivity and specificity of hemodynamic criteria in the diagnosis of acute right ventricular infarction. Circulation 1981; 64: 515.
5. Goldstein JA, Vlahakes GJ, Schiller N, Tyberg JV, Chatterjee K: Mechanism of low output in experimental right ventricular infarction (Abstract). Am J Cardiol 1981; 43: 437.
6. Lloyd EA, Gersh BJ, Kennely BM: Hemodynamic spectrum of 'dominant' right ventricular infarction in 19 patients. Am J Cardiol 1981; 48: 1016.
7. Steele P, Kirch D, Ellis J, Huxley R, Vogel R, Battock D: Prompt return to normal of depressed right ventricular ejection fraction in acute inferior infarction. Br Heart J 1977; 39: 1319.
8. Daubert JC, Deplace C, Bourdonnec C, Pony JC, Gouffault J: L'infarctus du ventricle droit. 1. Diagnostic hemodynamic. Correlations anatomiques. Arch Mal Coeur 1977; 70: 243.
9. Croft CH, Nicod P, Huxley R, Lewis S, Willerson JT, Rude RE: Serial analysis of right ventricular function after right ventricular infarction (Abstract). Am J Cardiol 1982; 49: 977.
10. Jugdutt BI, Sussex BA, Sivaram CA, Rossall RE: Right ventricular infarction: Two-dimensional echocardiographic evaluation. Am Heart J 1984; 107: 505.
11. Yasuda T, Okada R, Bingham JB, Golg HK, Leinbach RC, Pohost GM, Srauss HW: Serial evaluation of right ventricular function after right ventricular infarction. Am J Cardiol 1981; 47: 458.
12. Hellman C, Zafrir N, Agmon J: Improvement of ventricular function after acute right ventricular myocardial infarction (Abstract). Circulation 1980; 62 (Suppl 2): 313.
13. Daubert JC, Matteyses M, Fourdilis M, Pony JC, Gouffault J: L'infarctus du ventricle droit. 2. Incidences pronostiques et therapeutiques. Arch Mal Coeur 1977; 70: 257.
14. Legrand V, Smeets JP, Demoulin JC, Rigo P, Kulbertus HE: Right ventricular infarction: clinical course and follow-up (Abstract). Am J Cardiol 1981; 47: 458.
15. Croft CH, Nicod P, Corbertt JR, Lewis SE, Huxley R, Murharji J, Willerson JT, Rude RE: Detection of acute right ventricular infarction by right precordial electrocardiography. Am J Cardiol 1982; 50: 421.
16. Coma-Canella I, López-Sendón J: Ventricular compliance in ischemic right ventricular disfunction. Am J Cardiol 1980; 45: 555.
17. Miller DC, Moreno-Cabral RJ, Stinson EB, Shinn JA, Shumway NE: Pulmonary artery balloon counterpulsation for acute right ventricular failure. J Thorac Cardiovasc Surg 1980; 80: 760.
18. Jett GK, Siwek LG, Picone AL, Applebaum RE, Jones M: Pulmonary artery balloon counterpulsation for right ventricular failure. An experimental evaluation. J Thorac Cardiovasc Surg 1983; 86: 364.

19. Flege JB Jr, Wright CB, Reisinger TJ: Successful balloon counterpulsation for right ventricular failure. Ann Thorac Surg 1984; 37: 167.

6.6 Conclusions

F. MALPARTIDA

Dr R.A. Johnson of Massachusetts General Hospital (Boston, USA) began by indicating that digitalis is still more effective when congestive heart failure is accompanied by atrial fibrillation. The possible causes of digitalis not producing good results in other circumstances can be: poor definition of the diagnosis of congestive heart failure, concealment of the digitalis effect by the efficacy of diuretics and finally, variations in the causes of congestive heart failure, since valvular diseases are surgically treated and arterial hypertension is controlled before they can cause congestive heart failure.

After making a study in 25 patients with congestive heart failure, Dr Johnson reached the conclusion that the variables that predict efficacy with digitalis are the presence of third heart sound, chronic congestive heart failure, left ventricular hypertrophy and reduced ejection fraction. In general, the presence of left ventricular dilation and increased right atrial pressure serve to predict efficacy. However, there are a series of questions that still cannot be answered:

1. Serum digoxin level is important for toxicity, but the relationship it has with the beneficial effects of digitalis are unknown. The effective serum level seems to be 1 ng/ml.
2. The relationship between digitalis toxicity, with its corresponding risk of mortality, and benefits.
3. The role digitalis plays in relation with other associated treatments, such as diuretics or vasodilators.
4. Will the appearance of new inotropic drugs replace digitalis?

The second subject of this chapter was the role of vasodilators in refractory congestive heart failure, with a communication by Dr Isabel Coma of the Ciudad Sanitaria La Paz, Madrid. Dr Coma began by commenting on the classification of vasodilators according to site of action, based on a comparative study of phentolamine, nitroprusside, isosorbide dinitrate and nitroglycerin. She described the principal effects of these substances in accordance with the type of vasodilator. Dr Coma next turned to the cardiac effects of the vasodilators. Subendocardial blood supply is diminished in heart failure, and venous and mixed type vasodilators improve this blood supply. In contrast, arterial vasodilators do not improve subendocardial blood flow and may worsen it. This effect can be important if there is concomitant ischemic heart disease. As to the effect of vasodilators on peripheral coronary resistance, it has been observed that both nitroglycerin and isosorbide dinitrate act on the large caliber coronary vessels, avoiding coronary steal. Captopril seems to have the same effect. In contrast, nitroprusside is more selective for small arteries and can produce coronary steal.

The choice of a vasodilator should be made after considering the pattern of heart failure according to the predominant compensatory mechanism involved. The utility of hemodynamic control is debatable because hemodynamic improvement is not equivalent to functional improvement. Finally, it was observed that there is no relationship between the effect produced by the initial dose and long-term effect.

Dr Coma summarized by saying that the ideal vasodilator should satisfy the following requisites: improvement in functional capacity, prolonged effect, no tolerance or side effects and reduction of mortality. The vasodilator closest to the ideal is captopril, and enalapril, presently under study, may be better. According to Dr Coma, in congestive heart failure, digitalis and the diuretics should be used first, followed by the vasodilators when these fail.

Dr T. LeJemtel of the Albert Einstein Hospital, New York, wrote on the new inotropic drugs. He initiated his communication by asking if there is really a reduction in contractility in chronic congestive heart failure, because if there is, there are important limitations in the possibility of increasing contractility because of the lack of a contractile reserve. This seems to be confirmed by the effects of amrinone, which increases cardiac output and decreases blood pressure similar to captopril, its positive inotropic effect being doubtful. However, the substance apparently acts like a direct vasodilator. The same occurs with another new drug, milrinone (WIN-47203), which increases the cardiac index more than dobutamine and decreases left ventricular end diastolic pressure, but does not raise dP/dt. Dobutamine therefore seems to be more inotropic positive than milrinone. Another agent, MDL-1703, also increases cardiac output and decreases end diastolic pressure, but it only decreases arterial blood pressure and thus appears to affect afterload.

Neither amrinone nor milrinone produces long-term tachyphylaxis, but after a period of time the cardiac index decreases, especially with milrinone. If treatment is interrupted, the resulting hemodynamic situation is worse than at the outset. This also occasionally occurs with the vasodilators.

Finally, a study has been presented in which captopril was used first and milrinone was later added. It was found that the combination is synergistic, both drugs potentiating each other.

To terminate, Dr Jenaro Froufe of Ciudad Sanitaria de Cruces, Bilbao, Spain, presented a report on right heart failure in ischemic heart disease. He initially centered his attention on the diagnosis of right ventricular infarct, principally commenting on the hemodynamic criteria. In his experience, 100% specificity is obtained with 4 of 7 of the usual hemodynamic criteria for right ventricular infarction. In the study of right ventricular function contractility is first impaired and later distensibility. This observation has practical importance because in the first 24 hours there may not be a hemodynamic pattern of right ventricular infarction and the diagnosis can be overlooked. In his large series, it is shown that right ventricular infarction increases mortality, reaching 21.7% in comparison with infarction mortality in general, which is 7.8% in the Coronary Unit. Dr Froufe is of the opinion that aside from conventional treatment with fluids, low doses of inotropics should be used more often since excessive fluid administration can sometimes produce pleural effusions.

Finally, Dr Froufe commented on some of their preliminary experimental and clinical experience of counterpulsation of the pulmonary artery in patients with cardiogenic shock and right ventricular infarction.

7. Heart-Lung Transplantation

7.1 Introduction

L. PLAZA CELEMÍN

After a few years of being somewhat forgotten, interest in heart transplantation has revived thanks to the perseverance of the Stanford University surgical team.

The first heterotopic transplant was performed by Carrel and Guthrie in 1905 [1] in dogs, but it was Shumway's group [2] that systematized the technique of experimental orthotopic heart transplantation and in 1967 Barnard [3] performed the first cardiac transplantation in a human being. Since then, more than 500 transplantations have been done by 60 surgical teams throughout the world. The difficulties in immunologic control of rejection and postoperative infections account for the fact that the results obtained in the early years were not very promising. This was the reason why only four centers were still developing transplant programs in 1980.

The use of cyclosporin A, and the development of other immunosuppressors, like antithymocyte globulin, azathioprine and steroids, have been responsible for a great improvement in the survival rates. Likewise, periodic postoperative endomyocardial biopsy of the right ventricle permits early detection of signs of rejection.

The actuarial survival rate of 51% after 3 years obtained by the Stanford team moves the procedure from the realm of experimental surgery to that of an effective therapeutic method for certain cases of advanced heart disease. The younger the patient submitted to transplantation the better the results; 50 years is considered to be the age limit for heart transplantation.

The aim of cardiac transplantation should not only be to maintain the patient alive, but to improve its quality of life. One hundred six of the Stanford patients who had survived for more than a year had been in functional class IV before surgery and became functional class I after transplantation, most of them returning to their usual activities.

For all these reasons, candidate selection is an essential factor for which the cardiologist is responsible. The main indications [4] for heart transplantation are:

a) Dilated cardiomyopathy with heart failure refractory to medical treatment.
b) Ischemic heart disease with severe myocardial damage and left ventricular akinesia or dyskinesia, severely reduced left ventricular ejection fraction and heart failure resistant to treatment.

Other relative indications are:

a) Hypertrophic cardiomyopathy with heart failure resistant to treatment.
b) Complex congenital heart disease that is not operable by conventional technical procedures without a marked increase in pulmonary vascular resistance.
c) Valvular disease with valvular prosthesis and severe myocardial injury.

In Spain, after the transplant performed by Dr Martínez Bordiu's team more than 10 years ago, the surgical team of the Hospital de la Santa Cruz and San Pablo of Barcelona directed by Dr Caralps and Dr Aris initiated a series of transplants that have had an acceptable survival rate. We thus anticipate further development by other Spanish surgical teams along the lines implemented abroad. In view of the present situation of the cardiologic assistance in Spain, the following suggestions have been proposed to the Administration by the Spanish Cardiology Society:

a) An optimal cost-benefit ratio should be obtained from the material and human resources necessary for heart transplantation surgery, which are costly.
b) A program should be established for sharing experiences accumulated in different centers, with the objective of obtaining valid conclusions for progressively improving the transplant program.

References

1. Carrel A, Guthrie C: The transplantation of veins and organs. Am Med 1905; 11: 1101.
2. Lower R, Shumway NE: Homovital transplantation of the heart. J Thorac Cardiovasc Surg 1961; 196.
3. Barnard CN: Human Cardiac transplantation. Am J Cardiol 1968; 22: 584.
4. Report from the Council of the British Cardiac Society. November, 1983.

7.2 Transplantation of the Heart and Lungs

STUART W. JAMIESON

History of cardiopulmonary transplantation

In 1957 Webb and Howard reported six cardiopulmonary transplants in dogs, with survival ranging from 75 minutes to 22 hours [1]. Subsequent experiments in dogs produced longer survival, with Lower and Shumway achieving 5 days survival [2], and Grinnan et al. reporting survival for up to 10 days in a series of 25 transplants [3]. During this period of early investigation, limited clinical application of the technique was attempted. Prior to the series of patients reported here, the operation was performed in three patients at other centers, with the recipients surviving 14 hours [4], 8 days [5] and 23 days [6].

Successful experimental cardiopulmonary transplantation was carried out in dogs at Stanford in 1959 [2]. In the face of a developing cardiac transplantation program, it then seemed prudent to postpone clinical efforts in this endeavor until immunosuppression had advanced to the point that airway anastomotic healing would be improved.

Cyclosporine was introduced into the ongoing program in clinical cardiac transplantation at Stanford in 1980. The initial results, together with the laboratory experience with heart-lung transplantation in primates treated with cyclosporine, then suggested that a clinical trial of combined heart and lung transplantation would be appropriate [7, 8].

Recipients

All patients had end-stage pulmonary vascular disease, with incapacitating symptoms. All exhibited a rapidly deteriorating clinical course not amenable to additional conventional medical or surgical therapy. Eleven had Eisenmenger's syndrome, and eight suffered from primary pulmonary hypertension. We have transplanted only patients with pulmonary hypertension thus far, feeling that for early clinical trials these patients are most appropriate. The patients are relatively young, and there is almost always significant cardiac involvement even in the primary form of this disease. Other factors that favor these patients are that there is little likelihood of recurrence of disease in the transplanted organs, and the tracheobronchial tree is relatively sterile.

Many patients with Eisenmenger's syndrome have had one or more palliative operations, and most of those with primary pulmonary hypertension have had open lung biopsies. The adhesions caused by previous surgery increase the difficulty of this operation, particularly in Eisenmenger patients who in addition develop very large collateral vessels. In addition, coagulation abnormalities are usual in this group of patients, since they all have hepatic dysfunction. This is more marked in patients with primary pulmonary hypertension, as a result of tricuspid regurgitation.

Donors

The procurement of suitable donors for heart-lung transplantation has proved a considerable difficulty. We estimate that only about 15% of donors suitable for cardiac donation do not have pulmonary damage that precludes pulmonary transplantation. Persons who are brought to the emergency room with critical neurological injury have often aspirated gastric contents, they are generally intubated on an emergency basis, often without optimal sterility, and have a tendency to develop early and severe pulmonary edema. In addition, many have thoracic trauma. A further requirement for heart-lung donors that is not necessary for heart-only donors is a close size-match, since the donor lungs have to fit within the fixed capacity of the recipient's thoracic cage. To compress the donor lungs within the recipient would almost certainly lead to significant atelectasis; the transplantation of smaller donor lungs into a large thoracic cavity is unlikely to be as detrimental provided they were large enough to provide adequate respiration.

Other requirements for donors are that they be certified braindead, and are without a history of cardiopulmonary disease. They must of course be hemodynamically stable, and not have arterial blood gas evidence of significant shunting or have elevated peak inspiratory pressures. A normal chest X-ray and relatively normal electrocardiogram are also required.

The operation

The operative technique has been outlined previously [9]. The patient is cannulated for bypass as for heart transplantation, with high aortic cannulation and two low caval cannulae. The heart is then removed, leaving a posterior cuff of right atrium for subsequent reimplantation. The left lung is then excised, followed by the right lung. The important aspect of this operation is the removal of the recipient cardiopulmonary axis, without injury to the nerves (vagi, phrenic nerves, left recurrent laryngeal), or esophagus, and to attain meticulous hemostasis. The latter is essential particularly in patients with Eisenmenger's syndrome, in whom the bronchial arteries are especially large and tortuous. These vessels must be adequately secured at the time of removal of the recipient organs, since subsequent visualization is difficult.

The donor heart and lungs are then removed. Implantation of the donor organs commences with the tracheal anastomosis, followed by the aortic and atrial anastomoses. All anastomoses are performed with continuous polypropylene sutures.

Postoperative care

There are no doubt many regimens of immunosuppression that would give satisfactory results after heart-lung transplantation; we have been guided by the necessity of using cyclosporine as the primary immunosuppressant, and avoiding regular doses of steroids for the first two weeks, so as to assist tracheal healing. Cyclosporine (15 mg/kg) is given immediately preoperatively, and this dose is resumed immediately postoperatively and modified according to biweekly serum cyclosporine levels determined by radioimmunoassay. All cyclosporine is given orally. Intravenous methylprednisolone (500 mg) is given immediately after cessation of cardiopulmonary bypass; an additional dose of methylprednisolone (125 mg) is given every 8 hours for three doses. No further corticosteroids are then given in the first two weeks. Early immunosuppression is augmented with azathioprine 1.5 mg/kg/day and rabbit antithymocyte globulin given intramuscularly on the day of surgery and for two to three days postoperatively, until the level of circulatory T-lymphocytes falls below 5%. After two weeks, azathioprine is discontinued and replaced with oral prednisone at 0.2 mg/kg/day.

Endomyocardial biopsy is initially performed weekly and later on a less frequent schedule depending on the clinical course. Rejection episodes, as diagnosed by biopsy, are treated with intravenous boluses of methylprednisolone (1 g) daily for three days. Episodes of rejection resistant to this regimen are treated with additional rabbit antithymocyte globulin.

We initially felt that significant pulmonary rejection would not occur in the absence of cardiac rejection [10]. However, our recent experience has shown this not to be the case. The eighteenth patient in the series developed severe respiratory insufficiency in the third week after transplantation, and required reintubation. His pO_2 on an FiO_2 of 1.0 was 20. Cardiac biopsy was normal. A transthoracic pulmonary biopsy showed pulmonary rejection, and he was treated for this. His clinical condition improved, and he was able to be extubated once again three days later. The chest X-ray appearance, which at first showed an almost total diffuse 'white-out' cleared. This patients has now been discharged from hospital.

The frequency of rejection episodes as diagnosed by cardiac biopsy has been less than with cardiac transplantation alone, and it is as yet uncertain whether this is because of the slightly different immunosuppressive protocol used in the latter procedure, or whether transplantation of the lungs in addition to the heart conveys an immunological advantage. The frequency of rejection episodes, as with cardiac rejection, is highest within the first 60 days after transplantation.

Healing of the airway anastomosis has been a major concern in isolated lung transplantation, but thus far there has been no tracheal necrosis, rupture, or late stenosis in our heart-lung recipients. Coronary arteriograms in patients after operation have invariably shown the development of collaterals to the area of the suture-line from the donor coronary circulation. In this regard heart-lung transplantation is likely to be superior to lung transplantation alone, where there is no immediate arterial supply to the airway anastomosis.

Problems in postoperative management specific to these patients relate to the toxicity of cyclosporine and to the so-called 'implantation' response. Cyclosporine is both hepatotoxic and nephrotoxic, and is metabolized almost exclusively by the liver. Hepatic and renal impairment is almost invariable in these patients, and especially so in patients presenting with primary pulmonary hypertension. Reduction in cyclosporine dosage is often required within the first few days, as cyclosporine hepato-toxicity is then superimposed upon existing hepatic impairment aggravated by cardiopulmonary bypass. Several patients have required temporary support with renal dialysis when prior renal impairment has been exacerbated by cyclosporine, often combined with the necessity of giving antibiotics that are also renal toxic.

The 'implantation response' has been defined as a transient and reversible defect in pulmonary gas exchange, compliance, and vascular resistance, coinciding with roentgenographic pulmonary edema early postoperatively. Postulated causes are surgical trauma, ischemia, denervation, lymphatic interruption and other processes. The classical response is seen in animals in the first few days immediately postoperatively, and the above causes exclusive of rejection, may all contribute to this picture. The control of pulmonary vascular resistance in the denervated, transplanted graft certainly remains poorly understood, and it is likely that pulmonary hypertension will be exhibited as part of the response of the lung to ischemia and other forms of injury. In this regard Baranski and associates reported on five cardiopulmonary transplants performed in dogs and found a substantial rise in pulmonary artery pressure after implantation of the graft [11].

In our patients, however, though we have often seen a transient, diffuse and bilateral pulmonary infiltrate, it has generally occurred about ten days post-operatively. It is hard to imagine, if this were due to ischemia, denervation or lymphatic interruption, why the onset would be so late. In light of our more recent experience with isolated pulmonary rejection, it may well be that this late manifestation of pulmonary insufficiency and roentgenographic abnormality may be a reflection of pulmonary rejection though the cardiac biopsy is normal.

Results

Thirteen of the total nineteen patients remain alive at intervals of one to 40 months after operation. Five patients died within one month of surgery, of infection, renal insufficiency or operative complications. The sixth patient died one year after operation from a myocardial infarction, promoted by immune-mediated atherosclerosis of the coronary vasculature.

All surviving patients have undergone serial pulmonary function tests, which showed normal or near normal spirometry, and normal gas exchange shortly after being discharged from hospital. Cardiac catheterization has been carried out in all patients 10–12 months postoperatively. This procedure demonstrated normal pulmonary artery pressures, normal cardiac indices, and normal coronary anatomy at one year. With time, not all these values have remained normal. One patient had a late rejection episode more than a year post-operatively, which manifested as a diffuse infiltrate on the chest X-ray. His pO$_2$ on room air fell to 60, and he was treated with augmented oral steroids. His condition has since normalized. One patient, almost two years postoperatively, has experienced recurrent infections and bronchiectasis, and is colonised with resistant pseudomonas. A third patient presented three years postoperatively with progressive pulmonary failure. Catheterisation demonstrated evidence of pulmonary vascular disease and coronary artery disease, with a normal left ventriculogram but elevated pulmonary artery pressures. He eventually required intubation, and after ventilation for two months had failed to improve his condition he was retransplanted. He remains in hospital, now three weeks after operation, but at the time of writing is doing well.

The long-term outlook for these patients remains uncertain. It is possible that late changes as a result of rejection (manifesting as pulmonary vascular disease and/or bronchiectasis) will limit the usefulness of the procedure. For the present time it would certainly be prudent to continue to regard the operation as palliative rather than curative, though ten patients remain well and asymptomatic at this time.

Discussion

Combined heart and lung transplantation is likely to be superior to the procedure of unilateral lung transplantation, since removal of all diseased pulmonary tissue obviates both the problems of recurrent infection and ventilation-perfusion imbalance. Furthermore, the tracheal anastomosis, with its relatively generous blood supply is more likely to heal than is a bronchial anastomosis, where the only vascular contribution from the donor organ is of pulmonary arterial (deoxygenated) blood.

It is possibly appropriate to consider the application of combined heart and lung transplantation to include other disease processes associated with terminal lung disease, such as cystic fibrosis. The present apparent scarcity of suitable donors, however, makes it difficult to apply this therapy to other than optimal candidates at present.

Summary

Twenty combined heart-lung transplants have now been performed at Stanford University Medical Center. All patients were operated on for end-stage pulmonary failure – eleven had Eisenmenger's syndrome, eight suffered from primary pulmonary hypertension, and one operation was performed in a previously transplanted patient with terminal rejection.

All recipients were treated with cyclosporine postoperatively. Five of the patients died during the first postoperative month, and one died one year after operation. Thirteen patients are now living at intervals of one month to over three years after transplantation.

Cardiopulmonary transplantation has therefore been demonstrated to represent a reasonable therapeutic option for patients with end-stage pulmonary hypertension, with or without associated congenital heart disease. A number of problems remain. Continuing investigation focuses on improved control of the immune response, non-invasive methods of diagnosing pulmonary rejection, the mechanism of changes in pulmonary vascular resistance and pulmonary epithelial permeability after transplantation, and the applicability of the technique to other clinical syndromes associated with advanced pulmonary vascular disease.

References

1. Webb WR, Howard HS: Cardiopulmonary transplantation. Surg Forum 1957; 8: 313.
2. Lower RR, Stofer RC, Hurley EJ, Shumway NE: Complete homograft replacement of the heart and both lungs. Surgery 1961; 50: 842–845.

3. Grinnan GLB, Graham WH, Childs JW, Lower RR: Cardiopulmonary homotransplantation. J Thorac Cardiovasc Surg 1970; 60: 609–615.
4. Colley DA, Bloodwell RD, Hallman GL, Nora JJ, Harrison GM, Leachman RD: Organ transplantation for advanced cardiopulmonary disease. Ann Thor Surg 1969; 8: 30–42.
5. Lillehei CW: Discussion. In: Wildevuur CRH, Benfield JR: A review of 23 human lung transplantations by 20 surgeons. Ann Thor Surg 1970; 9: 515.
6. Barnard CN, Cooper DKC: Clinical transplantation of the heart: A review of 13 years personal experience. J Roy Soc Med 1981; 74: 670–674.
7. Oyer PE, Stinson EB, Jamieson SW, Hunt SA, Billingham M, Scott W, Bieber CP, Keitz BA, Shumway NE: Cyclosporin A in cardiac allografting: a preliminary experience. Transplant Proc 1983; 15: 1247–1252.
8. Reitz BA, Burton NA, Jamieson SW, Pennock JL, Stinson EB, Shumway NE: Heart and lung transplantation: auto and allotransplantation in primates with extended survival. J Thorac Cardiovasc Surg 1980; 80: 360–371.
9. Jamieson SW, Stinson EB, Oyer PE, Baldwin JC, Shumway NE: Operative technique for heart-lung transplantation. J Thorac Cardiovasc Surg 1984; 87: 930–935.
10. Reitz BA, Gaudiani VA, Hunt SA, Wallwork J, Billingham ME, Oyer PE, Baumgartner WA, Jamieson SW, Stinson EB, Shumway NE: Diagnosis and treatment of allograft rejection in heart-lung transplant recipients. J Thorac Cardiovasc Surg 1983; 85: 354–361.
11. Baranski EJ, Scicchitano LP, Camishion RC, Ballinger EG: Pulmonary hypertension following cardiopulmonary transplantation. Surg Forum 1963; 14: 200.

7.3 Heart Transplantation

MANEL BALLESTER RODÉS, MERCÉ CLADELLAS CAPDEVILLA,
LLUISA ABADAL BERINI, DAMIÀ OBRADOR MAYOL, MARÍA
JOSÉ AMENGUAL GUEDÁN, RAMÓN BORDES PRAT, GUILLEM
PONS LLADÓ, MODEST GARCÍA-MOLL, JOSEP M. PADRÓ
FERNÁNDEZ, ALEJANDRO ARÍS and JOSEP M. CARALPS RIERA

Heart transplantation is an established therapy for end-stage heart disease refractory to conventional medical or surgical treatment [1–15]. This method has reached widespread acceptance largely thanks to the pioneering work and ongoing research at the transplantation unit of the Stanford University headed by Dr Norman E. Shumway [16–29].

The recent use of cyclosporin A (CyA) as a selective immunosupressor [30, 31] has improved survival in patients transplanted [32–36], and the number of operations and surgical centers involved in cardiac transplantation are steadily increasing as a consequence [37–39].

Indications and selection of the candidate

Those patients with end-stage heart disease refractory to medical treatment or conventional surgical therapy are eligible as candidates for heart transplantation. The majority suffer from idiopathic dilated cardiomyopathy or heart failure secondary to coronary heart disease [40]. Selection criteria are shown in Table 1. Although the clinical course of unselected patients with dilated cardiomyopathy is variable [41], there is no doubt that certain subgroups of patients with very low ejection fraction and NYHA stage III–IV functional class have an extremely poor prognosis [42, 43]. These patients can benefit most from the operation. Indeed, the probability of survival at 4 years after cardiac transplantation for patients treated with CyA is now 71% [44]. This is a considerable different situation from the survival figures obtained when patients were treated with azathioprine (AZA): 31% at 5 years [44] (Fig. 1).

Not every patient who complies with the above requisites is immediately included in a cardiac transplantation program (Table 2). Some of the contraindications are absolute (e.g.: severe pulmonary hypertension, cancer, psychosis); others are relative (e.g.: age, diabetes without associated cardiovascular complications); finally, there are certain situations that require a delay in the

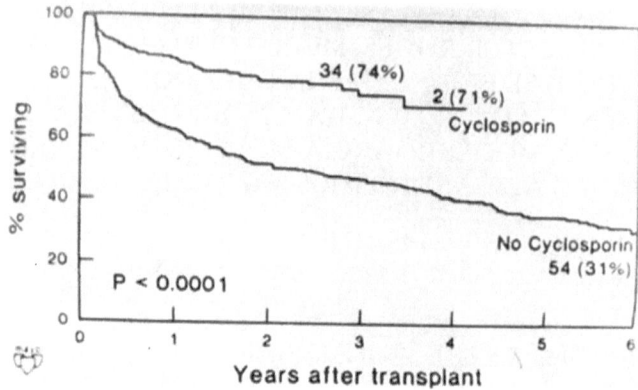

Fig. 1. Six-year survival after heart transplantation recipients. Differences between patients treated with CyA or AZA. (From the International Heart Transplantation Registry [44].)

operative procedure until the underlying condition is solved and no important sequelae are left (e.g.: infection, active peptic ulcer, pulmonary embolism).

The selection process of the candidate is the end result of a series of steps in patient evaluation. Clinical assessment, physical examination, ECG, echocardiogram, lung and kidney function tests, laboratory investigations, immun-

Table 1. Selection criteria of the candidate for cardiac transplantation.

End-stage heart disease refractory to conventional medical or surgical therapy with a low probability of survival at 6 months

Age limit: 15–55 years

Normal hepatic and renal function

Table 2. Contraindications for cardiac transplantation.

Active infection
Recent thromboembolic phenomena or pulmonary infarct
Insulin-dependant diabetes mellitus
Pulmonary vascular units of resistance > 5–6 Wood u.
Diffuse systemic vascular disease
Drug addiction
Active gastrointestinal ulcer
Alcoholic cardiomyopathy
Important obesity
Psychosis
Coexistence of systemic disease that might limit life expectancy

ological studies and psychiatric examination are initially required. Cardiac catheterization to calculate the pulmonary vascular resistance should be undertaken. Wood units of pulmonary resistance above 5–6 may cause the donor's right ventricle to fail during by-pass weaning or a postoperative right sided heart failure with gross tricuspid regurgitation [45–47]. A preoperative endomyocardial biopsy is also required in dilated cardiomyopathy to rule out myocarditis, as these patients can be treated and improved by immunosupressors [48–51].

The patient's determination to undergo a cardiac transplantation, his willingness to accept a very close long-term monitoring, and an enthusiastic family support are important considerations in the selection process [52–54]. The patient must be well informed of what a heart transplantation program entails [55, 56]. In fact, non-compliance has been associated with poor results [57]. On the other hand, a cardiac team must be absolutely commited to these patients [38, 39, 58]. A transplantation program requires 'the extreme dedication of a medical surgical team to closely monitor and meticulously manage patients in the delicate balance between acceptable function of the transplanted organ and the continous threat of rejection or catastrophic infection [59].

Selection of the donor

Selection of the donor heart is made among those patients who have suffered an irreversible head injury and are in a situation of 'brain death'. This represents 1% of all deaths admitted to a general hospital [60].

An adequate assessment of the donor's heart and a good cardiac preservation until implantation are important factors in achieving a successful result [61, 62]. Therefore, a careful evaluation of the potential donor's cardiac status and associated diseases must be made. Table 3 shows the selection criteria of the cardiac donor. Age is regarded as an important factor, as donors above

Table 3. Selection criteria of the donor of heart transplantation.

Age < 35–40 years
Brain death due to:
Cranial trauma (without thoracic trauma)
Spontaneous cerebral hemorrhage
Benign tumor of central nervous system
ABO compatible donor
Body surface are similar to recipient
Negative cross-match

35–40 years appear to limit long-term survival [63, 64]. ABO compatibility is a major selection parameter, as well as the size of the heart. Blood group mismatch and considerable differences in heart size (body surface area) between donor and recipient (small hearts implanted in large recipients can fail when implanted) preclude selection of the donor. A negative crossmatch, where the donor lymphocytes and recipient's serum are tested in search for specific antibodies, is also required [61]. The role of HLA matching in cardiac transplantation is uncertain [65]; due to the time constraint in cardiac transplantation it is not routinely performed.

Main contraindications in the selection of the potential donor are shown in Table 4. Exclusion of cardiac disease in the donor is obviously essential. In our hands, preoperative studies with a portable echocardiograph have been exceedingly useful to rule out cardiac diseases in the donor (Figs 2, 3). Inotropic support can contraindicate the use of a donor heart [61]. However, although fluid administration is preferable, inotropic drugs can be used with care to maintain the donor's blood pressure. Perfusion of dopamine at a rate of 5 ng/kg/min or less for 2–3 days has not been associated with catecholamine-induced myocardial lesions or impaired cardiac function after transplantation [66]. Use of large doses of inotropic drugs is contraindicated, specially in situations where a long ischemic time is anticipated (distant organ procurement).

Surgical procedure

Success of the surgical procedure largely depends on the coordination between the two surgical teams involved in the donor and recipient's operation. The donor's cardiectomy is made through a medial sternotomy. Great vessels are carefully dissected, ascending aorta is occluded and a cardioplegic solution at 4° C is administered. Once the cardiectomy has been performed, the heart is immersed in a bag with such solution and wrapped with a second bath containing 4° C saline and is then transported to theatre where the recipient's operation is being performed. The time limit of cold ischemia is 3–4 hours. Cold

Table 4. Contraindications of the donor for cardiac transplantation.

Clinical, radiological or ECG criteria of heart disease
Abnormal echocardiogram
Long-standing hypotension
Use of high doses of inotropic drugs
Active infection

344

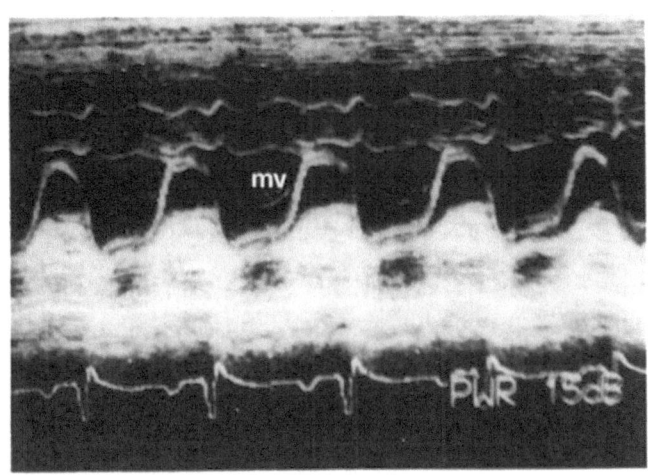

Fig. 2. M-mode echocardiogram of the left ventricular cavity and mitral valve (mv) of a 24-year-old man who suffered severe trauma of the head and was assessed as a potential cardiac donor. The tracing shows a decreased EF slope and a thickened posterior leaflet of the mitral valve indicative of mitral stenosis. Reduction of mitral orifice area by two-dimensional echocardiography was deemed to be moderate. The donor's clinical history, auscultation or ECG did not suggest the presence of such valve lesion.

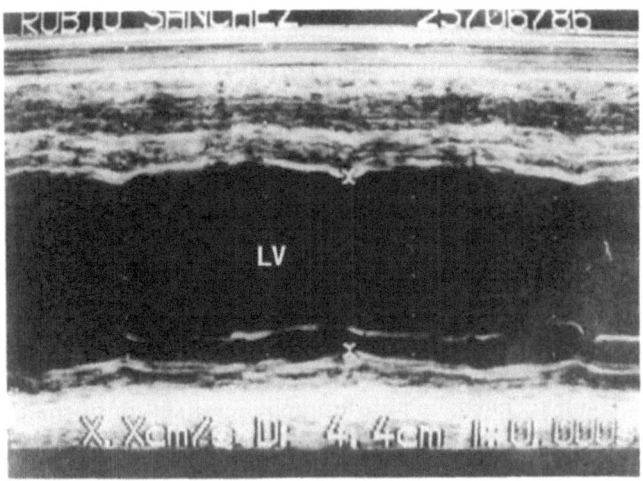

Fig. 3. M-mode echocardiogram of the left ventricular (LV) cavity of a 14-year-old man who suffered a severe head injury and was being assessed as a potential donor for heart transplantation. Note the severe reduction of left ventricular contraction (estimated ejection fraction: 27%). The clinical history, auscultation, chest X-ray, and electrocardiographic tracing were normal. Blood pressure was normal at the time of the clinical assessment and immediately before an M-mode and two-dimensional echocardiogram were performed. The examples shown in Figs 2 and 3 were taken from 28 consecutive assessments of potential cardiac donors, and illustrate the importance of a careful preoperative evaluation of cardiac morphology and function.

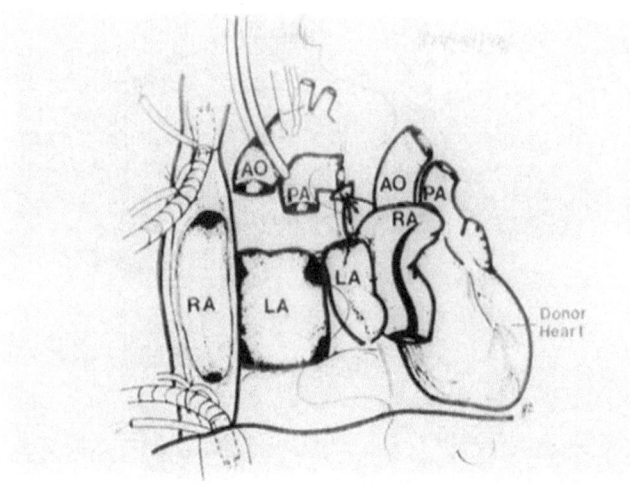

Fig. 4. Orthotopic cardiac transplantation. Donor and recipient hearts. The suture between the two hearts is begun at the atria. (From Cooper DKC and Lanza RP: Heart transplantation [70], with permission of the authors and publishers. AO: aorta; LA: left atrium; PA: pulmonary artery; RA: right atrium.

cardioplegic solution with potassium is used during the operation for preservation [67].

Two types of surgical techniques are currently used: orthotopic and heterotopic, the later pioneered and at present being performed by the South African group at Cape Town [68–70]. In the orthotopic form, the most commonly used, the recipient's atria are left connected to the systemic and pulmonary veins. After the donor's atria have been partially excised, implantation is performed suturing left atrium, right atrium, pulmonary artery and aorta [71–74] (Figs 4, 5). In the heterotopic variety, mainly used in patients with severe pulmonary hypertension or when the donor heart is small [5, 70, 75], the heart is placed in the right side of the chest and then sutured in parallel with the recipient's circulation; a common reservoir is made from left and right atria of the donor and recipient, and a terminolateral suture of the donor great vessels to those of the recipient is performed (Fig. 6).

Immunosuppressive treatment

The heart invariably rejects when implanted if no immunosuppressive treatment is given. There is no doubt, at present, that CyA is the drug of choice in cardiac transplantation [32–36]. The mechanism of action of CyA appears to be basically a selective inhibition of interleukin-2, responsible for T-cell activa-

346

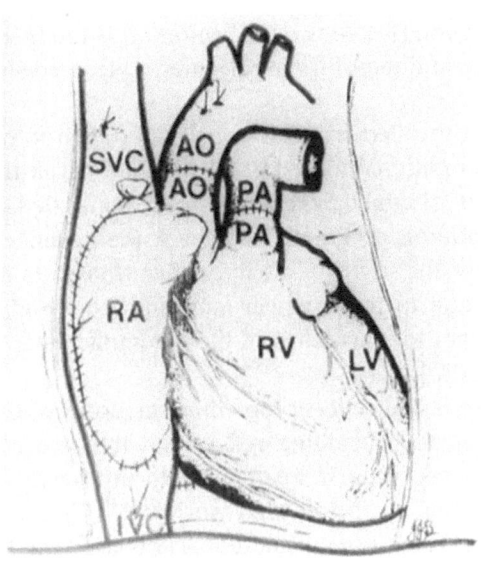

Fig. 5. Orthotopic cardiac transplantation. Complete operation. (From Cooper DKC and Lanza RP: Heart Transplantation [70], with permission of the authors and publishers.) AO: aorta; LV: left ventricle; RA: right atrium; RV: right ventricle; SVC: superior vena cava.

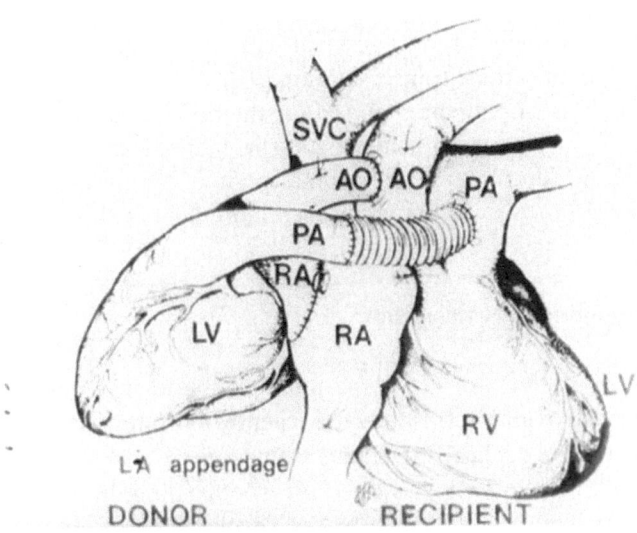

Fig. 6. Heterotopic transplantation. Completed operation. (From Cooper DKC and Lanza RP: Heart Transplantation [70], with permission of the authors and publishers.) Abbreviations as in Fig. 5.

tion and proliferation [31, 76, 77]. Therefore, it is the first *selective* immuno-supressor, sparing antibody-forming B lymphocytes, red blood cells and platelets.

Although no controlled trial has been undertaken to compare CyA with AZA, the drug traditionally used in all forms of organ transplantation, the much better results obtained by several surgical teams that having started their cardiac transplantation programs with AZA then changed to CyA provide sufficient basis for the use of CyA in cardiac transplantation [32–36]. Such improvement is due to reduction in mortality from both rejection and infection, despite that the incidence of these complications has not decreased with the use of CyA [64].

However, there is controversy regarding the doses of CyA that should be used, the convenience of adding AZA, and the role of steroids (CS) or prophylactic initial short course treatment with antithymocyte globulin (ATG) [78]. Several regimes are being used worldwide: CyA + CS, CyA + CS + AZA, CyA + AZA; in some of these, ATG is used the first few days after transplantation. The basic issue being discussed is the degree of immuno-suppression that should be achieved in an individual patient while reducing, at the same time, the risks of exaggerated immunosuppression: infection [79–86], lymphoma [87–90], or other types of neoplasia [91]. Not only is the choice of the immunosuppressive drug, but the doses that should be administered, both immediately after the operation or during long-term follow-up, which is also far from clear [78]. Less controversial is the treatment of moderate and severe rejection episodes, where ATG and high-dose CS bolus seem to be necessary [34, 35, 92]. Enhancement of graft survival with pretransplant blood transfusions is uncertain in cardiac transplantation [93].

The large numbers of patients required for the differences between these immunosupressive protocols to achieve statistical significance is the major stumbling block in determining the optimal regime. Ongoing multicentric analysis of these protocols will hopefully shed more light to this problem.

Side effects of immunosupressor drugs

Of the several side effects of CyA, the most troublesome is renal disease [94–97]. A prospective long-term study has recently indicated that renal function slowly but steadily declines in patients with cardiac transplantation treated with CyA [98]. The question is open on whether long-term survival of transplant patients will be threatened by the development of terminal renal failure [99–102]. The high incidence of acute postoperative renal failure reported in some series [103], seems to be prevented, without additional risk of rejection, if initial very low doses of CyA are used [104, 105]. In some patients with progressive renal failure, conversion from CyA to AZA might be necessary [106]. Lowering CyA doses and adding AZA might also reverse renal disease [107]. Further research is required in the prevention of long-term renal damage; the role of immunosuppressive drug combination, reduction of the 'established' therapeutic blood levels of CyA [107–109], or the introduction of less nephrotoxic cyclosporins [110] are under investigation.

Other side effects of CyA are systemic hypertension [97, 111], the mechanism of which is still obscure [112], hirsutism, gingival hypertrophy, or tremor. Most of them are not severe enough to require drug withdrawal and changing to AZA. Dose-related reversible hepatotoxicity is described [113]. Myocardial fibrosis, initially described to be present in the myocardial biopsies [114, 115], has not been found when CyA levels have been monitored and total CyA doses reduced [116, 117]. Lymphomas have been described with excessive immunosuppression, specially associated with the use of ATG, but its incidence has virtually disappeared with lesser degrees of immunosuppression [36, 88, 89].

Side effects of CS are well known, and can be prevented with low-dose immunosuppressive protocols. In some centers, CS are not used [118].

Control of immunosuppression and detection of rejection

Blood levels of CyA are employed worldwide to adjust doses [28, 119–121]. The therapeutic window of whole blood CyA levels in cardiac transplantation is 500 1000 ng/ml. However, there is no definite proof that blood levels, or the therapeutic window used, are at all useful indicators of the adequacy of immunosuppression.

In monitoring the level of immunosuppression attained by ATG, the role of the rosette formation test, which allows T-cell identification and quantitation [122], seems to be fairly established [123, 124] in that there is a certain relationship between the number of T-cells, or the rate of T-cell rise after ATG withdrawal, and the occurrence of rejection [22, 25, 125].

There is no test that measures the degree of immunosuppression attained by steroids.

Ultimately, control of the immunosuppressive level is achieved by early detection of cardiac rejection, which is done through serial transvenous endomyocardial biopsies [126–132]. Electrocardiographic voltage changes or increased left ventricular wall thickness detected by echocardiography [133–137] were useful when AZA was used as immunosupressor in cardiac transplantation. However, introduction of CyA, which appears to produce less myocardial edema during rejection episodes [32–36] has considerably reduced the diagnostic accuracy of such tests [138, 139].

Therefore, at present, the only reliable method to detect early rejection and to monitor its treatment is the morphologic analysis of the myocardium obtained by serial endomyocardial biopsies. The histological criteria and classification of cardiac rejection on the basis of the endomyocardial biopsy appears to be fairly well established [116, 117, 140–144]. According to varying lymphocyte infiltration rejection is graded as *minimal* or *mild:* detection of myocardial cell damage is considered a *moderate* rejection; necrosis is equated with a *severe* rejection. This classification has become useful in clinical practice, and has shown that:

a) a minimal lymphocytic infiltrate does not require treatment [116];

b) mild infiltrates can spontaneously disappear or evolve to more severe forms of rejection, and their detection calls for a careful surveillance [116, 117, 140];

c) patients with muscle damage have a poor prognosis if not treated with ATG in addition to high-dose bolus of CS [34, 35, 92].

Usually, and specially in patients treated with CyA, acute cardiac rejection occurs before a hemodynamic impairment is obvious [32–36], which underlines the usefulness of the endomyocardial biopsy. However, heart failure can be observed when acute rejection is severe. The incidence of acute rejection is highest at the 3rd or 4th postoperative months, declining thereafter. After the first year, the most common cause of mortality in heart transplantation is so-called chronic (vascular) rejection, which is a diffuse obstruction of the epicardic and intramural coronary arteries [134]. The major determinants in the incidence of chronic vascular rejection are repeat episodes of acute rejection and the doses of CS used [145]. In such situation, clinical symptoms due to myocardial ischemia are lacking because the heart is denervated, and progressive heart failure is the commonest form of clinical presentation. Occasionally, sudden death has been reported [146, 147]. Although this form of coronary artery disease is regarded as fixed, we have documented by coronary angiography and TI-201 isotopic studies the reversibility of such artery obstruction when detected early after transplantation and vigorously treated [148].

Non-invasive diagnosis of rejection

The expense of repeat endomyocardial biopsies, and its being a time-consuming procedure has prompted the search for alternative, non-invasive and less expensive diagnostic tests for early cardiac rejection. In short, analysis of diastolic left ventricular function by ultrasound [138, 139], exercise nuclear studies of global left ventricular contraction [149, 150], TI-201 myocardial imaging [151], search for lymphocytic precursors in peripheral blood [152–155], determination of T-cell subsets in peripheral blood [152–155], blood neopterine [156], nuclear magnetic resonance [157, 158], lymphocyte expression of transferrin receptors [159] expression of class I and II histocompatibility antigens [160], or the use of In-111 labeled antimyosin monoclonal antibodies [157] are being tested for this purpose with varying results [161]. At present, there is no test that provides the near 100% predictive accuracy needed to treat all patients with moderate rejection and to avoid unnecessary and dangerous treatment in those who are not rejecting. The basic problem lies in the fact that the exact moment when the body triggers the rejection process and the mechanisms of rejection itself are largely unknown [162–168].

References

1. Lower RR, Kontos HA, Koser JC, Sewell DH, Graham WH: Experiences in heart transplantation. Technique, physiology and rejection. Am J Cardiol 1968; 22: 766–771.
2. Cooley DA, Bloodwell RD, Hallman GL, Nora JJ, Harrison GM, Leachman RD: Organ transplantation for advanced cardiopulmonary disease. Ann Thorac Surg 1969; 8: 30–46.
3. Editorial. Cardiac transplantation: the second round. Lancet 1980; 687.
4. Hassell LA, Fowles RE, Stinson EB: Patients with congestive cardiomyopathy as cardiac transplant patients. Indications for and results of cardiac transplantation and comparison with patients with coronary artery disease. Am J Cardiol 1981; 47: 1205–1209.
5. Cooper DKC, Novitsky D, Hassoulas J, Barnard CN: Heart Transplantation: The South African experience. Heart Transplantation 1982; 2: 78—84.
6. Hastillo A, Wolfgang TC, Szentpetery S, Lower RR, Hess ML: Cardiac transplantation for intractable heart failure: the Medical College of Virginia experience. Cardiovasc Rev Rep 1982; 3: 1553–1565.
7. Pennock JL, Oyer PE, Reitz BA, Jamieson SW, Bieber CP, Wallwork J, Stinson EB, Shumway NE: Cardiac transplantation in prespective for the future. J Thorac Cardiovasc Surg 1982; 83: 168–177.
8. Cooley DA, Frazier OH, Painvin GA, Boldt L, Kahan BD: Cardiac and cardiopulmonary transplantation using cyclosporine for immunosupression: recent Texas Heart Institute Experience. Transp Proc 1983; 15 (Suppl 1): 2567–2572.
9. Austen WG, Cosimi AB: Heart transplantation after 16 years (Editorial). N Eng L Med 1984; 311: 1436–1438.
10. Copeland JG, Mammana RB, Fuller JK, Campbell DW, McAleer MJ, Sailer JA: Heart Transplantation. JAMA 1984; 251: 1563–1566.
11. Lanza RP, Cooper DKC, Boyd ST, Barnard CN: Comparison of patients with ischemic, myopatic and rheumatic heart disease as cardiac transplant recipients. Am Heart J 1984; 8–12.
12. Wallwork J: Heart and heart-lung transplantation. In: Calne RY (ed) Transplantation immunology. Oxford University Press, Oxford, 1984; 452–482.
13. Salvatierra O Jr: The role of organ transplantation in modern medicine. Heart Transplantation 1985; 4: 285–289.
14. Hardesty RL, Griffith BP, Trento A, Thompson ME, Ferson PF. Mortally ill patients and excellent survival following cardiac transplantation. Ann Thorac Surg 1986; 41: 126–129.
15. Obrador D, Cladellas M, Abadal ML, Ballester M, Pons-Lladó G, García-Moll M, Amengual MJ, Bordes R, Gurguí M, Augé JM, Padró JM, Arís A, Caralps JM. Trasplante cardíaco en el Hospital de Sant Pau, Barcelona. Rev Esp Cardiol 1987; 40 (supl. II): 112–116.

16. Shumway NE, Stinson EB, Dong E Jr: Cardiac homotransplantation in man. Transp Proc 1969; 1: 739–744.

17. Bieber CP, Stinson EB, Shumway NE, Payne R, Kosek J: Cardiac transplantation in man. VII. Cardiac allograft pathology. Circulation 1970; 41: 753–772.

18. Stinson EB, Randall GB, Shroeder JS, Dong E Jr, Shumway NE: Hemodynamic observations one and two years after cardiac transplantation. Circulation 1972; 45: 1183–1193.

19. Stinson EB, Caves PK, Griepp RB, Oyer PE, Rider AK, Shumway NE: Hemodynamic observations in the early period after human heart transplantation. J Thorac Cardiovasc Surg 1975; 69: 264–270.

20. Bieber CP, Hunt SA, Schwinn DA, Jamieson SW, Reitz BA, Oyer PE, Shumway NE, Stinson EB: Complications in long-term survivors of cardiac transplantation. Transpl Proc 1981; 13: 207–211.

21. Griepp RB, Stinson EB, Bieber CP, Reitz BA, Copeland JG, Oyer PE, Shumway NE: Human heart transplantation: current status. Ann Thorac Surg 1976; 22: 171–175.

22. Bieber CP, Griepp RB, Oyer PE, David LA, Stinson EB: Relationship of rabbit ATG serum clearence rate to circulating T-cell level, rejection onset, and survival in cardiac transplantation. Transp Proc 1977; 9: 1031–1036.

23. Oyer PE, Stinson EB, Bieber CP, Reitz BA, Raney AA, Baumgartner WA, Shumway NE: Diagnosis and treatment of acute cardiac allograft rejection. Transp Proc 1979; 11: 296–303.

24. Bieber CP, Stinson EB, Shumway NE: Immunology of cardiac transplantation. In: Zabriskie JB, Engle MA, Villareal H Jr (eds) Clinical immunology of the heart. John Wiley and Sons, New York, 1981; 111–141.

25. Bieber CP: Pharmacokinetics of antithymocyte glubulin (ATG) and cardiac transplant outcome. Heart Transplantation 1981; 1: 22–24.

26. Jamieson SW, Oyer PE, Reitz BA, Baumgartner WA, Bieber CP, Stinson EB, Shumway NE: Cardiac transplantation at Stanford. Heart Transplantation 1981; 1: 86–91.

27. Jamieson SW, Oyer PE, Bieber CP, Stinson EB, Shumway NE: Transplantation for cardiomyopathy: a review of the results. Heart Transplantation 1982; 2: 28–31.

28. Bieber CP, Bleese E, Shorthouse R, Oyer PE, Jamieson SW, Stinson EB. Serum cyclosporine levels in cardiac allograft transplantation. Heart Transplantation 1983; 3: 81–85.

29. Jamieson SW, Stinson EB: Cardiac transplantation for end-stage ischemic heart disease. In: Connor WE, Bristow JP (eds) Coronary heart disease. Lippincott, Philadelphia, 1985; 437–447.

30. Rogers AJ, Kahan BD: Mechanism of action and clinical applications of cyclosporin in organ transplantation. In: Mitchell MS, Fahey JL (eds) Clinics in immunology and allergy. WB Saunders, London, 1984; 217–258.

31. Cohen DJ, Loertscher R, Rubin MF, Tilney NL, Carpenter CB, Strom TB: Cyclosporine: A new immunosupressive agent for organ transplantation. Ann Intern Med 1984; 101: 667–682.

32. Oyer PE, Stinson EB, Jamieson SW, Hunt SA, Billingham M, Scott W, Bieber CP, Reitz BA, Shumway NE: Cyclosporin-A in cardiac allografting: a preliminary experience. Transp Proc 1983; 15: 1247–1252.

33. Oyer PE, Stinson EB, Jamieson SW, Hunt SA, Pelroth M, Billingham M, Shumway NE: Cyclosporine in cardiac transplantation: a $2^1/_2$ years follow-up. Transp Proc 1983; 15 (Suppl 1): 2546–2552.

34. Griffith BP, Hardesty RL, Thompson ME, Dummer JS, Bahnson HT: Cardiac transplantation with cyclosporine: the Pittsburgh experience. Heart Transplantation 1983; 2: 251–256.

35. Hardesty RL, Griffith BP, Denski RF, Bahnson HT: Experience with cyclosporine in cardiac transplantation. Transp Proc 1983; 15 (Suppl 1): 2553–2558.

36. Wallwork J, Cory-Pearce R, English TAH: Cyclosporine for cardiac transplantation: UK trial. Transplant Proc 1983; 15 (Suppl 1): 3135–3141.

37. Evans RW, Anderson A, Perry B: The national heart transplantation study: an overview. Heart Transplantation 1982; 2: 85–87.

38. Oliver ML: Cardiac transplantation in the United Kingdom. Report from the Council of the British Cardiac Society. Heart Bull 1984; 15: 47–50.

39. Kulbertus HE, Limet R: Should we start new programmes of heart transplantation in 1984?. Heart Bull 1984; 15: 44–46.

40. Thompson ME: Selection of candidates for cardiac transplantation. Heart Transplantation 1983; 3: 65–69.

41. Fuster V, Gersh BJ, Giuliani ER, Tajik AJ, Brandenburg RO, Frye RL: The natural history of idiopathic dilated cardiomyopathy. Am J Cardiol 1981; 47: 525–531.

42. O'Connell JB, Gunnar RM: Dilated congestive cardiomyopathy: prognistic features and therapy. Heart Transplantation 1982; 2: 7–17.

43. Franciosa JA, Wilen M, Ziesche S, Cohn JN: Survival in men with severe chronic left ventricular failure due to either coronary heart disease or idiopathic dilated cardiomyopathy. Am J Cardiol 1983; 51: 831–836.

44. The International Heart Transplantation Registry: Heart transplantation 1985; 4: 290–292.

45. Ballester M, Lons-Lladó G, Carreras F, Cladellas M: Reversed Septal motion in right ventricular volume overload: a false negative sign in the presence of increased septal thickness. Clin Cardiol 1986; 9: 623–625.

46. Cladellas M, Abadal ML, Pons-Lladó G, Ballester M, Carreras F, Obrador D, García-Moll M, Padró JM, Arís A, Caralps JM: Early transient multivalvular regurgitation detected by pulsed Doppler in cardiac transplantation. Am J Cardiolog 1986; 1986; 58: 1122–1124.

47. Cladellas M, Abadal ML, Ballester M, Carreras Costa F, Pons G, Obrador D, Faràa-Moll M: Función valvular del corazón donante de trasplante cardíaco. Rev Esp Cardiol 1986; 39 (Supl. II): 32–35.

48. Mason JW, Billingham ME, Ricci DR: Treatment of acute inflammatory myocarditis assisted by endomyocardial biopsy. Am J Cardiol 1980; 45: 1037–1044.

49. Fenoglio JJ, Ursell Ph C, Kellog CF, Drusin RE, Weiss MB: Diagnosis and classification of myocarditis by endomyocardial biopsy. N Eng J Med 1983; 308: 12–18.

50. Zee-Cheng C, Tsai CC, Palmer DC, Codd JE, Pennington DG, Williams GA: High incidence of myocarditis by endomyocardial biopsy in patients with idiopathic congestive cardiomyopathy. J Am Coll Cardiol 1984; 3: 63–70.

51. Obrador D, Bordes R, Cladellas M, Abadal ML, Ballester M, Augé JM: Detección de miocarditis mediante biopsia endomiocárdica en los candidatos a trasplante cardíaco. Rev Esp Cardiol 1987; 40 (supl. II): 14–17.

52. Freeman AM, Watts D, Karp R: Evaluation of cardiac transplant candidates: preliminary observations. Psychosomatics 1984; 25: 197–207.

53. O'Brien VC: Psychological and social aspects of heart transplantation. Heart Transplantation 1985; 4: 229–231.

54. Udina C, Guillamat R, Alvarez E, Casas M: Aspectos psiquiátricos en la valoración de los candidatos a trasplante cardíaco. Rev Esp Cardiol 1987; 40 (supl. II): 22–24.

55. Allender J, Shisslak C, Kasniak A, Copeland J: Stages of psychological adjustment associated with heart transplantation. Heart Transplantation 1983; 2: 228–231.

56. Watts D, Freeman AM, McGiffin DG, Kirklin JK, McVay R, Karp RB: Psychiatric aspects of cardiac transplantation. Heart Transplantation 1984; 3: 243–247.

57. Cooper DKC, Lanza RP, Barnard CN: Noncompliance in heart transplant recipients: The Cape Town experience. Heart Transplantation 1984; 3: 248–253.

58. Copeland JG: Facts to be considered prior to undertaking a heart transplantation program. Heart Transplantation 1984; 3: 275–277.

59. Lower RR, Wolfgang TC, Szenpetery S, Guerraty AJ, Alivizatos PA, Lee HN, Méndez-Picón GJ, Goldman MH, Mohanakumar T, Hastillo A, Hess M: Cardiac transplantation: should its use be expanded? In: McCauley KM, Brest AN, McGoon (eds) McGoon's cardiac surgery: an interprofessional approach to patient care. FA Davis Company, Philadelphia, 1985.

60. Pallis C: ABC of brain stem death. Br Med J 1983.

61. English TAH, Spratt P, Wallwork J, Cory-Pearce R, Wheeldon D: Selection and procurement of hearts for transplantation. Br Med J 1984; 288: 1889–1891.

62. Evans RW, Manninen DL, Gersh BJ, Hart LG, Rodin J: The need for and supply of donor hearts for transplantation. Heart Transplantation 1984; 4: 57–60.

63. Cooper DKC, Boyd ST, Lanza RP, Barnard CN: Factors influencing survival following heart transplantation. Heart Transplantation 1983; 3: 86–91.

64. Hunt SA: Complications of heart transplantation. Heart Transplantation 1983; 3: 70–74.

65. Ting A: The influence of HLA-DR matching on allograft survival in man. Heart Transplantation 1983; 2: 136–142.

66. Ballester M, Cladellas M, Abadal ML, Obrador D, Bordes R, Pons G: Lesión cardíaca en el corazón trasplantado: relevancia clínica de la dopamina administrada al donante. Rev Esp Cardiol 1987; 40 (supl. II): 9–13.

67. Bonnín O, Arís A, Montesinos A, Caralps JM: Trasplante cardíaco experimental: valoración hemodinámica aguda comparando dos métodos distintos de protección miocárdica. Rev Esp Cardiol 1987; 40 (supl. II): 25–30.

68. Barnard CN: Human Heart Transplantation. The diagnosis of rejection. Am J Cardiol 1968; 22: 811–819.

69. Barnard CN, Barnard MS, Cooper DKC, Curchio CN, Hassoulas J, Novitsky D, Wolpowitz A: The present status of heterotopic cardiac transplantation. J Thorac Cardiovasc Surg 1981; 81: 433–439.

70. Cooper DKC, Fraser RC, Rose AG, Azyenberg O, Oldfield GS, Hassoulas J, Novitzky D, Uys CJ, Barnard CN: Technique, complications, and clinical value of endomyocardial biopsy in patients with heterotopic heart transplants. Thorax 1982; 37: 727–731.

71. Lower RR, Shumway NE: Studies on orthotopic homotransplantation of the canine heart. Surg Forum 1960; 11: 18–19.

72. Raney AA, Stinson EB, Oyer PE, Reitz BA, Shumway NE: The technique of cardiac transplantation. In: Hurst JW (ed) The heart, 5th (ed) McGraw-Hill, New York, 1982; 1922–1927.

73. Caralps JM: Técnica quirúrgica del trasplante cardíaco ortotópico. En: Herreros J, Arcas R, Azanza J, Errasti O (eds) Barcelona. Trasplante Cardíaco. Editorial Científico Médica, 1986; 109–1201.

74. Caralps JM, Padró JM, Arís A: El Trasplante cardíaco. Medicine 1986; 52: 60–66.

75. Barnard CN, Barnard MS, Cooper MA et al.: The present status of heterotopic cardiac transplantation. J Thorac Cardiovasc Surg 1981; 81: 433–439.

76. White DJG: Cyclosporin A – Clinical applications and immunology. In: Clinics in immunology and allergy, Vol 3. WB Saunders, London, 1983; 287–304.

77. White DGJ, Calne RY: Chemical immunosupression. In: Calne RY (ed) Transplantation immunology. Oxford University Press, Oxford, 1984; 254–277.

78. Ballester M, Pons-Lladó G, Obrador Mayol F, Carreras F, Cladellas M, Abadal ML, Amengual MJ, Bonnín O, Padró JM, Arís A, Caralps JM: Ciclosporina en el trasplante cardíaco: un tratamiento en evolución. Med Clin 1986; 86: 600–603.

79. Baumgartner WA: Infection in cardiac transplantation. Heart Transplantation 1983; 3: 75–80.

80. Cooper DKC, Lanza RP, Oliver S, Forder AA, Rose AG, Novitzky D, Barnard CN: Infectious complications after heart transplantation. Thorax 1983; 38: 822–828.

81. Mammama RB, Petersen EA, Fuller JK, Siroky K, Copeland JG: Pulmonary infections in cardiac transplant patients: modes of diagnosis, complications and effectiveness of therapy. Ann Thorac Surg 1983; 36: 700–706.

82. Pinching AJ, Cohen J: Infection in the immunocompromised patient: selected topics in prevention and treatment. In: Clinics in immunology and allergy, Vol 3(2). WB Saunders, London, 1983; 305–329.

83. Reece IJ, Painvin GA, Zeluff B et al.: Infection in cyclosporine immunosuppressed cardiac allograft recipients. Heart Transplantation 1983; 3: 239–242.

84. McGregor CGA, Fleck DG, Nagington J, Stovin PGI, Cory-Pearce R, English TAH: Disseminated toxoplasmosis in cardiac transplantation. J Clin Pathol 1984; 37: 74–77.

85. Trento A, Dummer GS, Hardesty RL, Bahson HT, Griffith BP: Mediastinitis following heart transplantation: incidence, treatment and results. Heart Transplantation 1984; 3: 336–340.

86. Andreone PA, Olivari MT, Elick B, Arentzen CE, Bolman RM, Simmons RL, Ring WS: Reduction of infectious complications following cardiac transplantation. Heart Transplantation 1985; 4: 599.

87. Cleary ML, Warnke R, Sklar J: Monoclonality of lymphoprolipherative lesions in cardiac transplant recipients. N Eng J Med 1984; 310: 477–482.

88. Starzl TE, Nalesnik MA, Porter KA, Iwatsuki S et al.: Reversibility of lymphomas and lymphoprolipherative lesions developing under cyclosporine-steroid therapy. Lancet 1984; 1: 583–587.

89. Brumbaugh J, Baldwin JC, Stinson EB, Oyer PE, Jamieson SW, Bieber CP, Henle W, Shumway NE: Quantitative analysis of immunosupression in cyclosporine-treated heart transplant patients with lymphoma. Heart Transplantation 1985; 4: 307–311.

90. Case Records of the Massachusetts General Hospital (Case 4 – 1985). N Engl J Med; 312: 226–237.

91. Penn I: Problems of cancer in organ transplantation. Heart Transplantation 1982; 2: 71–77.

92. Griffith BP, Hardesty RL, Bahnson HT: Powerful but limited immunosupression for cardiac transplantation with cyclosporine and low-dose steroid. J Thorac Cardiovasc Surg 1984; 87: 35–42.

93. Salvatierra O, Vicenti F, Amend WJC Jr, Garovoy MR, Feduska NJ: The enhancement of graft survival with pretransplant blood transfusions. Heart Transplantation 1983; 2: 181–187.

94. Devineni R, McKenzie N, Duplan J, Keown P, Stiller C, Wallace AC: Renal effects of cyclosporine: clinical and experimental observations. Transpl Proc 1983; 15: 2695–2698.

95. Engel J, Greenberg A, Thompson ME et al.: Renal failure in heart transplant receiving cyclosporine. Transpl Proc 1983; 15: 2706–2707.

96. McKenzie N, Keown P, Stiller C, Kostuk W, Campbell C, Keith F: Early and late effects of cyclosporine on renal function following orthotopic cardiac transplantation. Heart Transplantation 1985; 4 (Suppl): 146.

97. Rottenbourgh J, Mattei MF, Cabrol A, Leger P, Aupetit B, Beaufils H, Gluckman JC, Pavie A, Gandbakhch I, Cabrol C: Renal function and blood pressure in heart transplant recipients treated with cyclosporine. Heart Transplantation 1985; 4 (Suppl): 147.

98. Myers BD, Ross J, Newton L, Luetscher J, Pelroth M: Cyclosporine-associated chronic nephropathy. N Eng J Med 1984; 311: 699–705.

99. Hesse UJ, Sutherland DER, Mauer SM, Najarian JS (Letter). N Eng J Med 1984; 312: 49.

100. Merion RM, White DJG (Letter). N Eng J Med 1984; 312: 49.

101. Strom TB, Loertscher R: Cyclosporine-induced nephrotoxicity. N Eng J Med 1984; 311: 728–729.

102. Chomette G, Auriol M, Beaufils H, Rottenbourg J, Cabrol C: Morphology of cyclosporin nephrotoxicity in human heart transplant recipients. Heart Transplantation 1985; 4: 617.

103. McGiffin DC, Kirklin JK, Naftel DC: Acute renal failure following cardiac transplantation with cyclosporine. Heart Transplantation 1985; 4 (Suppl): 145.

104. Spratt P, Esmore DS, Baron DW, Harrison K, Shanahan MX, Farnsworth AE, Chang VP: Effectiveness of minimal dosage cyclosporine in limiting toxicity and rejection. Heart Transplantation 1985; 4: 588.

105. Cladellas M, Sánchez JM, Abadal ML, Ballester M, Obrador D, Amengual JM, Quintana E, Net A, Cámara ML, Padró JM, Arís A, Caralps JM: Estudio de la función renal en el postoperatorio inmediato del trasplante cardíaco utilizando dosis iniciales muy bajas de ciclosporina A. Rev Esp Cardiol 1987; 40 (Supl. II): 70–73.

106. McGiffin DC, Kirklin JK, Logic JR, Edwards ME, McVay RF, Diethelm AG: Conversion of patients from cyclosporine to azathioprine immunosupression following cardiac transplantation. Heart Transplantation 1985; 4: 596.

107. Miller LW, McBride LR, Pennington DG: Reversibility of cyclosporine A nephrotoxicity. Heart Transplantation 1985; 4: 615.

108. Cavarocchi N, Hakim M, Cory-Pearce R, English TAH, Wallwork J: A prospective randomised trial of cyclosporine and low dose prednisolone versus cyclosporine and azathioprine. Heart Transplantation 1985; 4: 591.

109. Bolman RM, Elick B, Olivari MT, Ring WS, Arentzen CE: Improved immunosuppression for heart transplantation. Heart Transplantation 1985; 4: 315–318.

110. Hoyt EG, Billingham ME, Masek MA, Morris RE, Baldwin JC, Jamieson SW: Assessment of cyclosporin G, a new immunosupressant agent. Heart Transplantation 1985; 4: 616.

111. Greenberg ML, Uretsky BF, Reddy S, Bernstein RL, Griffith BP, Hardesty RL, Thompson ME, Bahnson HT: Long-term hemodynamic follow-up of cardiac transplant patients treated with cyclosporine and prednisone. Circulation 1985; 71: 487–494.

112. Thompson ME, Shapiro AP, Johnsen AM, Reeves R, Itzkoff J, Ginchereau E, Hardesty RL, Griffith BL HT, McDonald Jr R: New onset of hypertension following cardiac transplantation: a preliminary report and analysis. Transp Proc 1983; 15 4 (Suppl 1): 2573–2577.

113. Klintmalm GBG, Iwatsuki S, Starzl TE: Cyclosporin A hepatotoxicity in 66 renal allograft recipients. Transplantation 1981; 32: 488–489.

114. Cohen RG, Hoyt EG, Billingham ME, Bieber CP, Jamieson SW, Shumway NE: Myocardial fibrosis due to cyclosporine in rat heterotopic heart transplantation. Heart Transplantation 1984; 3: 355–358.

115. Humen DP, McKenzie FN, Kostuk WJ: Restricted myocardial compliance one year following cardiac transplantation. Heart Transplantation 1984; 3: 341–345.

116. Stovin PGI: The morphology of myocardial rejection and transplantation pathology. In: Calne RY (ed) Transplantation immunology. Oxford University Press, Oxford, 1984; 78–100.

117. Pomerance A, Stovin PGI: Heart transplant pathology: the British experience. J Clin Pathol 1985; 38: 146–159.

118. Yacoub M, Alivizatos P, Radley-Smith R, Khanagi K, Mitchell A: Early and medium term results of cardiac transplantation with minimum or no oral steroids. Proc British Card Soc, London, 1984; 19.

119. Bowers LD, Canafax DM: Cyclosporine: experience with therapeutic monitoring. Drug Monit 1984; 6: 142–147.

120. Faynor SM, Moyer TP, Sterioff S, McDonald MW: Therapeutic drug monitoring of cyclosporine. Mayo Clin Proc 1984; 59: 571–572.

121. Loisance D, Hamberger C, Barre J, Tavolaro O, Tillement JP, Cachera JP: Preoperative evaluation of optimal cyclosporine therapy in heart transplantation. Heart Transplantation 1984; 3: 295–299.

122. English TAH, McGregor C, Wallwork J, Cory-Pearce R: Aspects of immunosupression for cardiac transplantation. Heart Transplantation 1982; 4: 280–284.

356

123. Thomas FT, Szenpetery SS, Wolfgang TC, Quinn JE, Thomas J, Lower RR: Improved immunosupression for cardiac transplantation: Immune monitoring and individual modulation of recipient immunity by in vitro testing. Ann Thorac Surg 1979; 28: 212–221.

124. Wallwork J: The use of anti-lymphocytic sera in transplantation. In: Calne RY (ed) Transplantation immunology. Oxford University Press, Oxford, 1984; 304–318.

125. Goldman MH, Mohanukumar T, Hess ML, Méndez-Picón G, Lee HM, Wolfgang TC, Szentpetery SS, Hastillo A, Lower RR: Antithymocyte globulin and immunologic monitoring in cardiac transplantation. Heart Transplantation 1981; 1: 18–21.

126. Caves PK, Stinson EB, Billingham ME et al.: Diagnosis of human allograft rejection by serial cardiac biopsy. J Thorac Cardiovasc Surg 1973; 66: 461–466.

127. Caves PK, Stinson ED, Billingham ME, Shumway NE: Serial transvenous biopsy of the transplanted human heart improves management of acute rejection episodes. Lancet 1974; 821–826.

128. Cooper DKC, Fraser RC, Rose AG, Azyenberg O, Oldfield GS, Hassoulas J, Novitzky D, Uys CJ, Barnard CN: Technique, complications, and clinical value of endomyocardial biopsy in patients with heterotopic heart transplants. Thorax 1982; 37: 727–731.

129. Spiegelhalter DJ, Stovin PGI: An analysis of repeat biopsies following cardiac transplantation. Statistics in Medicine 1983; 2: 33–40.

130. Laser JA, Fowles RE, Mason JW: Endomyocardial biopsy. In: Schroeder JS (ed) Invasive cardiology. Cardiovascular Clinics. FA Davis, Philadelphia, 1985; 141–163.

131. Cladellas M, Augé JM, Crexells C, Oriol A: Biopsia endomiocárdica. Medicine 1986; 52: 69–75.

132. Imakita M, Tazelaar HD, Billingham ME: Heart allograft rejection under varying immunosuppressive protocols as evaluated by endomyocardial biopsy. Heart Transplantation 1986; 5: 279–285.

133. Lower RR, Dong E, Glazener FS: Electrocardiograms of dogs with heart homografts. Circulation 1966; 33: 455–460.

134. Lower RR, Kosek JC, Kemp VE, Graham WH, Sewell DH, Lim F: Rejection of the cardiac transplant. Am J Cardiol 1969; 24: 492–499.

135. Popp RL, Schroeder JS, Stinson EB, Shumway NE, Harrison DC: Ultrasonic studies for the early detection of acute cardiac rejection. Transplantation 1971; 11: 543–550.

136. Hess ML, Hastillo A, Wolfgang TC, Lower RR: The noninvasive diagnosis of acute and chronic allograft rejection. Heart Transplantation 1981; 1: 31–38.

137. Sagar KB, Hastillo A, Wolfgang TC, Lower RR, Hess ML: Left ventricular mass by M-mode echocardiography in cardiac transplant patients with rejection. Circulation 1981; 64 (Suppl 2): 216–220.

138. Dawkins KD, Oldershaw PJ, Billingham ME, Hunt SA, Oyer PE, Jamieson SW, Stinson EB, Shumway NE: Changes in diastolic function as a noninvasive marker of cardiac allograft rejection. Heart Transplantation 1984; 3: 286–294.

139. Abadal ML, Cladellas M, Ballester M, Obrador D, Ballester R, Pons-Lladó G: Estudio ecocardiográfico del corazón trasplantado tratado en ciclosporina A. Rev Esp Cardiol 1987; 40: (Supl. II): 45–51.

140. Billingham ME: Some recent advances in cardiac pathology. Prog Hum Pathol 1979; 10: 367–386.

141. Billingham ME: Diagnosis of cardiac rejection by endomyocardial biopsy. Heart Transplantation 1981; 1: 25–30.

142. Rose AG, Uys CJ: Pathology of acute rejection. In: Cooper DKC, Lanza RP (eds) Heart transplantation. MTP Press, Lancaster, 1984; 157–176.

143. Ueda K, Baumgartner WA, Beschorner WE, Borkon MA, Soule LM, Reitz BR, Herskowitz A: Histologic pattern of early heart allograft rejection under cyclosporine treatment. Heart Transplantation 1985; 4: 296–301.

144. Bordes R, Cladellas ML, Abadal ML, Obrador D, Ballester M: Biopsia endomiocárdica en los pacientes trasplantados cardíacos tratados con ciclosporina A. Rev Esp Cardiol 1987; 40 (Supl. II): 36–40.

145. Zusman DR, Stinson EB, Oyer PE, Baldwin JC, Jamieson SW, McGregor CG, Hunt SA, Schroeder JS, Shumway NE: Determinants of accelerated graft atherosclerosis in conventional and cyclosporine treated heart transplant recipients. Heart Transplantation 1985; 4: 587.

146. Mackintosh AF, Carmichael DJ, Wren C, Cory-Pearce R, English TAH: Sinus node dysfunction in first three weeks after cardiac transplantation. Br Heart J 1982; 48: 584–588.

147. Abadal ML, Ballester M, Cladellas M, Obrador D, Badía F, Rodriguez C, Bordes R, García-Moll M, Padró JM, Arís A, Caralps JM: Muerte súbita como manifestación inicial del rechazo cardíaco en un paciente tratado con ciclosporina A. Rev Esp Cardiol 1987; 40 (Supl. II): 52–54.

148. Abadal ML, Ballester M, Cladellas M, Obrador D, Carrió I, Bordes R, Serra R, Augé JM, Padró JM, Arís A, Caralps JM: Vasculitis coronaria aparecida precozmente después del trasplante cardíaco: diagnóstico y tratamiento. Rev Esp Cardiol 1987; 40 (Supl. II): 74–78.

149. McGiffin DC, Karp RB, Logic JR, Tauxe WE, Ceballos R: Results of radionucleide assessment of cardiac function following transplantation of the heart. Ann Thorac Surg 1984; 37: 382–386.

150. Reilmann L, Schüller S, Ötting G, Warnecke H, Kotzerke J, Gratz KF, Schober O, Creutzig H, Hertzer R, Hundeshagen H: Serial MUGA studies in the follow-up of the heart transplanted patients. Proc Eur Nucl Med Congr. London, 1985; 174.

151. Richter J, Herreros J, Serena A, Pardo J, Azanza JR, Charvet MA, Honorato J, Arcas R: 201-TI Myocardial imaging in a cardiac rejection episode. Eur J Nucl Med 1986; 11: 368–370.

152. Ertel W, Reichenspurner H, Hammer C, Welz, Uberfuhr P, Hemmer W, Reichart B, Gokel M: Immunologic monitoring in dogs after allogenic heterotopic heart transplantation. Heart Transplantation 1984; 3: 268–273.

153. Ertel W, Reichenspurner H, Lersch C, Hammer C, Plahl M, Lehman M, Kemkes BM, Osterholzer G, Reble B, Reichart B, Brendel W: Cytoimmunological monitoring in acute rejection and viral, bacterial or fungal infection following transplantation. Heart Transplantation 1985; 4: 390–394.

154. Hammer C, Reichenspurner H, Ertel W, Lersch C, Plahl M, Brendel W, Reichart B, Uberfuhr P, Welz A, Kemkes BM, Reble B, Funccius W, Gokel M: Cytological and immunologic monitoring of cyclosporine-treated human heart recipients. Heart Transplantation 1984; 3: 228–232.

155. Amengual MJ, Abadal ML, Cladellas M, Ballester M, Obrador D, Agustí M, Rodríguez JL: Subpoblaciones linfocitarias en sangre periférica en el diagnóstico de rechazo cardíaco en pacientes tratados con ciclosporina A. Rev Esp Cardiol 1987; 40 (Supl. II): 41–44.

156. Havel MP, Laczkovics AMD, Preiss PS, Müller MM, Wolner E: Neopterin as a new marker to detect acute rejection after heart transplantation. Heart Transplantation 1985; 4: 594.

157. Hall TS, Baumgartner WA, Borkon AM, La France ND, Traill TA, Jacobus WE, Norris S, Hutchins GM, Braun J, Reitz BA: Diagnosis of acute cardiac rejection utilizing phosporus nuclear magnetic resonance, antimyosin monoclonal antibody, 2-D echocardiography and endomyocardial biopsy. Heart Transplantation 1985; 4: 595.

158. Lechat P, Eugène M, Hadjiisky P, Tcillac A, Grosgogeat Y, Cabrol C: Nuclear magnetic resonance and detection of rejection in experimental heart transplantation. Heart Transplantation 1985; 4: 593.

159. Hoshinaga K, Pascoe EA, Wood NL, Szentpetery S, Mohanakumar T, Lower RR: Expression of transferrin receptors on lymphocytres and its correlation with rejection in cardiac transplant recipients. Heart Transplantation 1985; 4: 589.

358

160. Steinhoff G, Wonigeit K, Haverich A, Schäfers J, Kemnitz J, Borst HG: Class I MCH-antigen induction on myocytes in acute rejection after orthotopic heart transplantation: reversibility by steroid treatment. Proc Int Symp Inflam Heart Dis. Würzburg, 1986; 78.

161. Ballester M, Obrador D: Diagnóstico incruento del rechazo cardíaco: perspectivas y futuro. Med Clin 1988 (in press).

162. Brenner MK, Munro AJ: The major histocompatibility system, antigen presentation and graft rejection. Heart Transplantation 1982; 1: 268–274.

163. Rabin BS: Immunological aspects of human cardiac transplantation. Heart Transplantation 1983; 2: 188–191.

164. Hall BM: The cellular immune basis of cardiac allograft rejection. Heart Transplantation 1984; 3: 260–264.

165. Forbes RDG, Lowry RP, Gomersall M, Blackburn J: Cellular mechanisms of cardiac allograft rejection. Heart Transplantation 1984; 3: 300–311.

166. Roser BJ: Mechanisms of graft rejection. In: Calne RY (ed) Transplantation immunology. Oxford University Press, Oxford, 1984; 186–194.

167. Roser BJ: Approaches towards donor-specific immunosupression (DSI). In: Calne RY (ed) Transplantation immunology. Oxford University Press, Oxford, 1984; 201–207.

168. Rabin BS, Griffith BP, Hardesty RL: Vascular endothelial cell HLD-DR antigen and myocyte necrosis in human allograft rejection. Heart Transplantation 1985; 4: 293–295.

8. Valvulopathies

8.1. Introduction

P. ZARCO GUTIERREZ

The problem of valvular disease is determined by three basic variables:
a) its natural history;
b) the operative mortality of valve substitution and
c) the duration of the prosthesis.
In this introduction, we will only refer to two aspects of the natural history of valvular diseases. The first is cardiac hypertrophy, a fundamental occurrence concerning which our knowledge is incomplete. The universal response to mechanical overload is cardiac hypertrophy. Assuming that the hypothesis diagrammed in Fig. 1 is accurate and that hypertrophy is the response to increased systolic stress and dilation is the response to diastolic stress, there are elementary facts that still remain unknown. We do not know what the humoral stimulus for hypertrophy is, nor what difference there is between physiologic and pathologic hypertrophy, or whether atrial hypertrophy is of

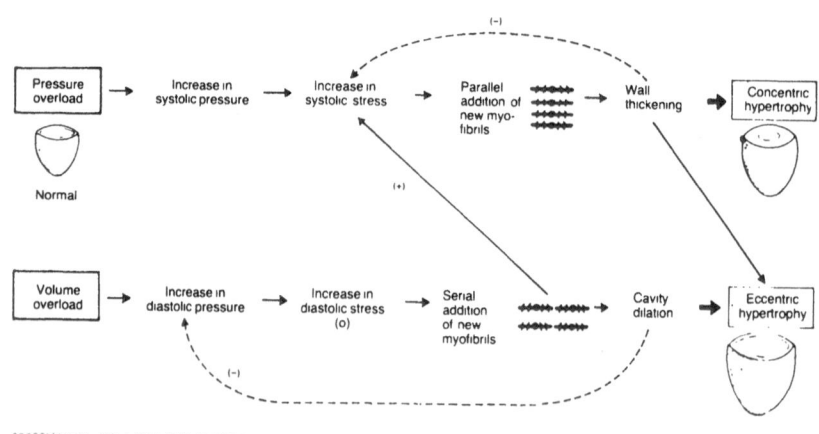

GROSSMAN. W AM J MED 1980 69 576-84

Fig. 1. Hypothesis of the development of left ventricular (LV) hypertrophy. (From: Grossman W: Am J Med 1980; 69: 576–584.)

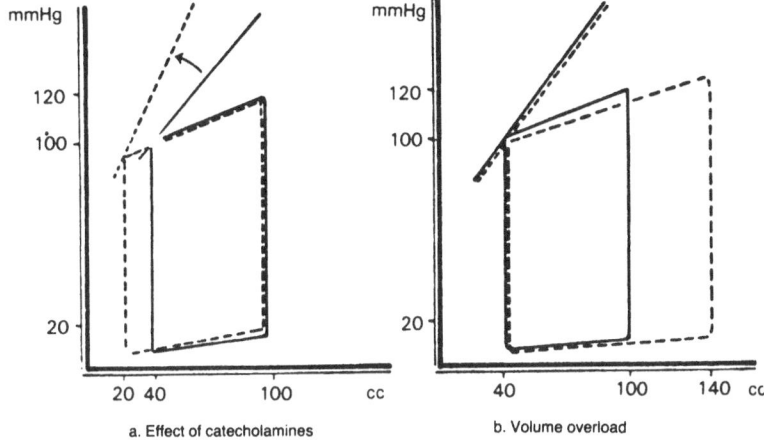

a. Effect of catecholamines

b. Volume overload

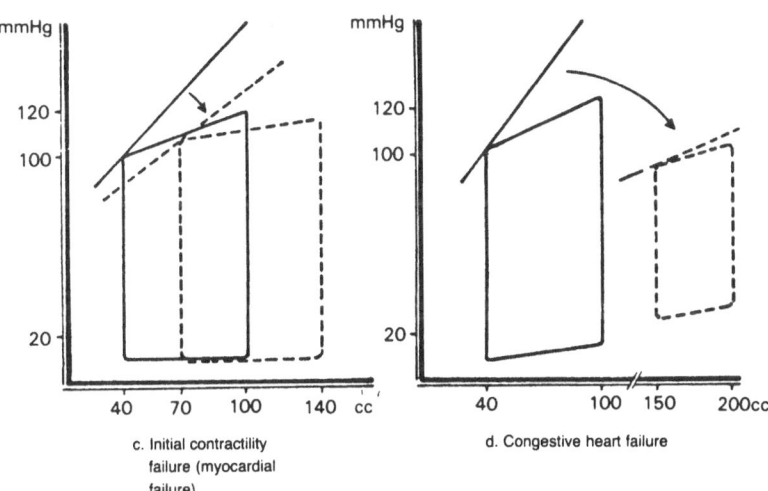

c. Initial contractility
failure (myocardial
failure)

d. Congestive heart failure

Fig. 2. Graphs of the natural history of left ventricular function as reflected by the Starling curve. a. Effect of catecholamines. b. Volume overload. c. Initial contractility failure (myocardial failure). d. Congestive heart failure.

the same type as ventricular hypertrophy. Moreover, we do not even know if hypertrophy is useful, nor when it regresses, or under what circumstances.

In connection with this problem, Fig. 2 illustrates the natural history of left ventricular function as reflected by the Starling curve as the ratio of maximum pressure/end-systolic volume.

Fig. 2a and d represent the adaptation of the normal heart to stress and the final stage of congestive heart failure. Fig. 2b shows excentric hypertrophy produced by volume overload; the end-diastolic volume, end-systolic volume and ejection fraction remain normal and the maximum systolic pressure/end-systolic volume ratio is also normal.

Fig. 2c shows the onset of contractility failure. The final systole marks the radical difference between these two situations and that indicated by the alteration in cardiac systolic function, and the descent in maximum pressure/end-systolic volume ratio and ejection fraction. Diastolic volume does not differentiate graphs 2b and 2c.

8.2 Bioprosthesis Versus Mechanical Devices

BERNARD R. CHAITMAN

Introduction

Choice of a valve device in patients requiring cardiac valve replacement is a major consideration addressed by cardiovascular surgeons and cardiologists in the management of patients with valvular heart disease. The large choice of valve substitutes can be classified into 2 major categories (Table 1). Several valve designs have been modified since their introduction. An example is the Starr-Edwards caged ball prosthesis initially introduced in 1960 and modified several times to reduce thrombogenicity and improve hemodynamic function. The central disk design is not a satisfactory valve substitute. Central disk valves tend to be semiocclusive, resulting in increased hemolysis, suboptimal hemodynamic function, and increased thrombogenicity. Among tilting disk valve design, the Omniscience, St. Jude, and Medtronic prostheses are relative newcomers and long term experience does not exceed five years at the time of this report. The Delrin disc of the Bjork Shiley valve, introduced in 1969 was replaced by a pryrolytic carbon disc in 1971 to improve disc durability and in 1978, the shape of the disc was changed to convexo-concave to reduce thrombogenicity. Preliminary results with the convex-concave Bjork-Shiley valve indicate reduced thrombogenicity. The sewing ring and opening angle of the mitral valve disc was also modified in the mid 1970s. However, the change in valve design is associated with an increased risk of strut fracture at the minor strut, particularly in the larger stent sizes. This unusual complication has been observed as early as 2 weeks postoperatively and is frequently fatal. This complication has led to the monostrut valve in which an integral post has replaced the minor strut to abolish the problem of minor strut fracture and disc embolization. F.D.A. approval for this change has not yet been received in the United States.

Among bioprostheses, the use of homograft valves are limited by availability and limited widespread surgical experience. Porcine xenografts are widely used in Europe and North America, with the Hancock valve first introduced in the United States in 1970, and the Carpentier-Edwards valve in 1976. Both Hancock and Carpentier-Edwards valve have been modified since their introduction to improve hemodynamic function, primarily in the smallest stent sizes. The Angell-Shiley valve was withdrawn from the North American market because of suboptimal hemodynamic function.

Pericardial xenografts differ from porcine xenografts in that the stent mounted tissue is bovine pericardium rather than a porcine aortic valve. The Ionescu-Shiley pericardial valve in use since 1970, is bulky, and has recently been modified to a lower profile design. The pericardial xenograft valve introduced by Vascor, and Edwards Laboratories respectively, is not yet available in the United States.

Comparison of different valve devices is difficult, since duration of follow-up, statistical reporting techniques, definitions of an event, patient population, and number of valve design modifications during follow-up, differ among the many reported series. Randomized trials which compare one valve to another are not currently available, although several studies are currently in progress which compare mechanical prostheses to bioprostheses [1]. Retrospective analyses can be of help in assessing the results of the different reports, however, and can be used to formulate appropriate guidelines for choice of valve device in individual patients. This review will compare long term results with mechanical prostheses to bioprostheses with special emphasis on thromboembolic rates, hemodynamic function, and valve durability.

Table 1. Selected cardiac valve devices.

MECHANICAL DEVICES		
Caged ball	*Central disc*	*Tilting disc*
Starr-Edwards	Starr-Edwards	Bjork-Shiley
Smeloff-Cutter	Kay-Shiley	Lillehei-Kaster
Braunwald-Cutter	Beall-Surgitool	Omniscience
Magovern-Cromie	Cooley-Cutter	St Jude
DeBakey-Surgitool		Medtronic Hall-Kaster
BIOPROSTHESES		
Homografts	*Porcine xenografts*[a]	*Pericardial xenografts*[b]
Aortic valve	Hancock-Vascor	Vascor
Dura mater	Carpentier-Edwards	Carpentier-Edwards
	Ionescu-Shiley	
	Angell-Shiley	
	Liotta Low Profile	Ionescu-Shiley

[a] Glutaraldehyde-treated porcine aortic valve.
[b] Glutaraldehyde-treated bovine pericardium.

Thromboembolism

Variables which influence the thromboembolic rate include type and position of cardiac valve device, the time frame of implementation, adequacy of anticoagulant control, cardiac rhythm, left atrial size, and definition of an embolic event. In general, thromboemboli are more common in valves in mitral position, particularly in patients who are in atrial fibrillation. The incidence of thromboemboli is increased in patients with large left atrium and in those patients who have had previous thromboembolic phenomenon. All mechanical valve devices require lifetime anticoagulant therapy. Failure to anticoagulate patients with a mechanical valve device can increase the risk of thromboembolism 3–6 times more than patients who are adequately anti-coagulated [2]. An example of the risk of poor anticoagulant control in patients with a Bjork-Shiley mitral valve is illustrated in Table 2. Thrombotic valve obstruction and death occurred in a significant number of patients over a relatively short follow-up period [3–9]. The majority of patients stopped their anticoagulant therapy or were poorly controlled. The actuarial incidence of valve thrombosis is 0.8% per year in the aortic position and 1–3% per year in the mitral position.

The actuarial determined thromboembolic rates for the Bjork-Shiley, Starr-Edwards Models no 6120 and no 2320, and bioprostheses in the mitral and aortic valve positions are compared in Table 3. When mechanical valves are compared, the thromboembolic rate is greater for the Starr-Edwards than the Bjork-Shiley prosthesis [3, 9–16]. Horstkotte et al., in a 6 year randomized follow-up study of Bjork-Shiley versus Starr-Edwards mitral prostheses reported a cumulative thromboembolic rate of 8.2% for the Bjork-Shiley valve versus 13.9% for the Starr-Edwards (p<0.05) [17]. The Starr-Edwards model 2400 and 6400 is reported to be less thrombogenic than model 6120 and 2320; however, the length of follow-up is substantially less.

Table 2. Bjork-Shiley mitral prosthesis; incidence of thrombotic obstruction.

	N	Number of occluded valves	Deaths	Months of follow-up
Murphy [3]	105	8	3	63
Copans [4]	224	12	1	17
Lepley [5]	230	13	11	43
Bjork [6]	302	17	15	51
Mattingly [7]	54	6	3	51
Moreno-Cabral [8]	85	6	5	28
Karp [9]	167	3	2	38

The thromboembolic rate for bioprostheses is substantially less than with mechanical valve devices, and ranges from 1–2% per year for bioprostheses in the mitral position and less than 1% per year in the aortic position [18–30]. In our experience approximately 5% of patients with an aortic bioprosthesis and 20–30% of patients with a mitral bioprosthesis require lifetime oral anti-coagulant therapy [19]. Our indications for continuing anticoagulants in patients with a bioprosthesis are atrial fibrillation, moderate to severely large left atrium, or a previous bioprosthetic thromboembolic event. The difference in thrombogenic potential between mechanical valves and bioprostheses is further accentuated by the fact that lifetime oral anticoagulant therapy is standard in patients with mechanical prostheses.

Table 3. Actuarially determined thromboembolic rates for mechanical and biological valves.

	N	Actuarial method		
		5	10	15 yrs
MITRAL VALVE DEVICE				
Bjork Shiley				
Karp [9]	167	18		
Starr-Edwards (no 6120)				
Miller [10]	509	38	45	
Starr [11]	259	30	47	53
Bioprostheses				
Gallucci [18]	257	13	17	
Pelletier [19]	205	7		
Ionescu [20]	246	1	4	
AORTIC VALVE DEVICE				
Bjork-Shiley				
Karp [9]	379	15		
Starr-Edwards (no 2320)				
Murphy [3]	440	10		
Starr [11]	507	23	34	44
Bioprostheses				
Gallucci [18][a]	69	2	5	
Pelletier [19][b]	182	3		
Ionescu [20][c]	279	1	2	

[a] Hancock.
[b] Carpentier-Edwards.
[c] Ionescu-Shiley.

Hemodynamic performance

The hemodynamic performance of cardiac valve devices can be assessed in vitro using steady or pulsatile flow techniques, by intraoperative gradient measurements, and by postoperative hemodynamic catheterization studies; the latter is preferable since this experimental approach most closely approximates valve performance under normal physiologic conditions and endothelialization of the valve has occurred. Stress hemodynamic studies (exercise, isuprel, pacing) are preferable to only rest studies to allow assessment of valve performance at different flow levels.

The best hemodynamic method to assess valvular performance is to use catheter techniques which do not cross the valve; i.e. transseptal catheter in the left ventricle and aortic catheter in the ascending aorta for the aortic valve; transeptal catheter in the left atrium and a left ventricular catheter retrograde across the aortic valve for the mitral valve. These techniques are not constant among the many different valve series and should be considered when comparisons are made.

In a randomized trial of mechanical versus bioprosthetic valve devices, Hammermeister et al. evaluated 6 month postoperative hemodynamics in 55

Table 4. Hemodynamic performance of mechanical and biological valves.

Aortic valve device	Stent size			
	21–23 mm		25–27 mm	
	Grad (mm Hg)	Area (cm^2)	Grad (mm Hg)	Area (cm^2)
Bjork-Shiley	19	1.5	16	2.4
Starr-Edwards	18	1.5	21	1.5
St. Jude	10	2.0	8	2.9
Hancock	20	1.0	19	1.5
Carpentier-Edwards	13	1.1	11	1.6
Ionescu-Shiley	13	1.4	9	2.0
Mitral valve device	27–29 mm		31 mm	
	Grad (mm Hg)	Area (cm^2)	Grad (mm Hg)	Area (cm^2)
Bjork-Shiley	4	2.5	4	2.9
Starr-Edwards	4	2.4	5	2.7
St. Jude	3	3.0	2	3.2
Hancock	6	2.3	5	2.4
Carpentier-Edwards	7	2.3	5	2.7
Ionescu-Shiley	6	2.0	–	–

patients with a Hancock valve to 42 patients with a Bjork-Shiley valve [1]. The effective orifice area of the Bjork-Shiley valve was significantly greater than the Hancock valve in aortic stent sizes from 23–27 mm. The orifice area for the 23 mm stent size was 1.3 cm^2 for the Hancock versus 2.3 cm^2 for the Bjork-Shiley valve. In the mitral position, no significant differences were observed between the 2 valves in stent sizes of 29–33 mm.

In general, the hemodynamic performance of mechanical or bioprosthetic valve devices are acceptable when stent sizes exceeds 25 mm in the aortic (21 mm or less) position and 29 mm in the mitral position (Table 4). In smaller stent sizes which account for a smaller percentage of valve devices inserted in adults, higher gradients are observed and calculated effective orifice areas are reduced [6, 19, 31–39]. Since the effective orifice area is determined from flow divided by the square root of the transvalvular pressure gradient (Torricelli equation) small differences in effective orifice area in the smaller stent sizes can result in large differences in gradient. We have reported larger effective orifice areas for bioprostheses and others have reported larger orifice areas for tilting disc valves during exercise when transvalvular flow rates are higher [6, 34]. Tissue leaflet or disc inertia results in a slightly smaller calculated valve area at rest.

Mechanical valve devices usually have better hemodynamic characteristics than bioprostheses in 21–23 mm stent sizes in the aortic position. In these small valve sizes, the St Jude valve has the largest effective orifice area among the machanical valves and the Ionescu-Shiley pericardial xenograft among the currently available bioprostheses.

In the mitral position, the St Jude valve offers the largest effective orifice area in the smaller stent sizes. The effective orifice area of 3.0 cm^2 is larger than the 2.0–2.3 cm^2 reported for bioprostheses. The effective orifice area of the new generation of bioprostheses is improved in the smaller stent sizes. A recent in vitro comparison by Gabbay and colleagues, reported the new 21 mm and 25 mm pericardial xenograft produced by Edwards Laboratories, and Vascor respectively, have substantially better hemodynamic performance than each of the companies' standard valve design [39].

Minor degrees of regurgitation are common with the Bjork-Shiley and St Jude valves inherent to valve design. Minor degrees of regurgitation are also common in bioprostheses as a result of slight imperfections in leaflet coaptation. The incidence of parvalvular leaks is mainly related to sweing ring design, sewing techniques, and aortic root and mitral valve apparatus anatomy and appears to be similar among mechanical valves and bioprostheses.

Valve durability

The major concern for the use of bioprostheses are related to valve longevity. Early experience with formaldehyde-treated bioprostheses was disappointing and resulted in an inordinately high degree of valve failure between 5–10 years. Changes in tanning techniques and substitution of glutaraldehyde to replace formaldehyde improved tissue durability. Other techniques such as the development of a flexible stent, variable position of the aortic valve leaflets during the fixation procedure, and better selection of tissue valves for mounting may also have improved tissue valve durability.

Comparison of the failure rates of mechanical valve devices to bioprostheses is difficult because of the lack of a uniform definition for valve failure. Perhaps the best definition of valve failure is that put forth by the Stanford Group in which a valve failure is classified as an event which causes reoperation or death. Thus, prosthetic valve occlusion, multi-thromboembolism requiring reoperation, prosthetic valve endocarditis, severe hemodynamic dysfunction, hemolysis or periprosthetic leaks, and anticoagulant-related hemorrhage are all classified as a valve failure if the event caused reopeartion or death.

In children, mechanical prostheses appear to offer an advantage over bioprostheses. Table 5 illustrates the result of six series in children aged 20 or less. The incidence of valve failure is unacceptably high regardless of whether porcine or pericardial xenografts are used [40–45]. The five year actuarial incidence of valve replacement ranges from 41–90%. New techniques to reduce tissue calcification are currently under investigation and preliminary observations are encouraging for porcine xenografts [46]. However, the new decalcification techniques have not been tested in humans. Until the problem of early calcification of bioprosthetic valves in children is resolved, mechanical devices such as the St Jude valve, which offers good hemodynamic function, a relatively low profile, and perhaps a lower thromboembolic rate than other tilting disc valves, may be the valve of choice in the younger age group. The

Table 5. Bioprostheses in children; valve failure rate.

	Age cut-off	Valve	N	No valves replaced	Duration of follow-up (mo)
Williams [40]	18	Hancock	46	8	34
Sanders [41]	20	Hancock	44	8	22
Rocchini [42]	17	Hancock	17	6	42
Geha [43]	20	Mixed	31	7	36
Antunes [44]	20	Mixed	135	71	60
Walker [45]	16	Ionescu-Shiley	30	7	31

Five year actuarial incidence of valve replacement: 41–90%.

precise age cutoff whereby early bioprosthetic calcification occurs has not been clearly identified. However the 5 year survival rate for bioprostheses in patients under 20 is dismal.

In adults, the 10 year survival rate of bioprostheses is not unlike that of mechanical devices (Table 6). Mechanism of valve failure is an important consideration when comparing the two types of valves. Bioprostheses usually require replacement for either stenoses because of progressive calcification [47] or severe regurgitation as a result of leaflet tear [48]. The onset of symptoms is often gradual when stenoses is the failure mode but can be abrupt when a leaflet tear occurs. In contrast, the failure mode for caged ball and tilting disc prostheses, particularly in the mitral position, is multiple thromboemboli with secondary target organ damage or acute thrombosis. Paravalvular leaks and anticoagulant-related hemorrhage are other major modes of valve failure for mechanical devices. The incidence of anticoagulant-related hemorrhagic events approximates 3–5% per year, and the incidence of fatal

Table 6. Actuarially determined valve failure rate for mechanical and biological valves.

	N	Actuarial method		
		5	10	15 yrs
MITRAL VALVE DEVICE				
Bjork-Shiley				
Murphy	90	12		
Starr-Edwards (no 6120)				
Miller	509	22	29	
Starr	259	8	18	28
Bioprostheses				
Schoen[a]	373	2	21	
Pelletier[b]	205	1		
Ionescu[c]	246	2	8	
AORTIC VALVE DEVICE				
Bjork-Shiley				
Murphy	97	6		
Starr-Edwards (no 2320)				
Murphy	440	5		
Starr	507	5	11	19
Bioprostheses				
Schoen[a]	519	2	9	
Pelletier[b]	182	1		
Ionescu[c]	279	2	11	

[a] Hancock
[b] Carpentier-Edwards
[c] Ionescu-Shiley

anticoagulant-related events can be as high as 0.3% per year [9]. The Starr-Edwards and original Bjork-Shiley valve are extremely durable and are rarely replaced because of a mechanical fault. However, both valves usually fail because of coexisting morbidity.

The incidence of bioprosthetic valve failure is confounded by inclusion of children with adults in reporting results. The 10 year rate of valve failure ranges between 20–30% for the aortic position and 10–20% for the mitral position [18–22, 24, 25, 28–30]. The failure rate is substantially less for adults over 35 years. Magilligan et al. report a 9 year valve failure rate of 14% for patients over 35 years versus 46% for patients less than 35 years (p<0.01) [25]. At 10 years, between 10–20% of aortic and 5–10% of mitral bioprostheses have clinical evidence of dysfunction not requiring immediate valve replacement (new or changing murmur, decreased exercise tolerance, etc.).

Considerations in choice of valve device

Clearly, the choice of a valve device is a complicated issue which can be approached by consideration of both patient and valve related factors. Mechanical valves are the device of choice in childhood or in patients with abnormalities of calcium metabolism (chronic hemodialysis). In older, child-bearing women over 30 years a bioprosthetic valve might be an acceptable choice in order to avoid anticoagulant usage during pregnancy. Occupation is generally not a major consideration in choice of valve device, although socio-economic conditions may play a major role in deciding which valve to insert. When anticoagulant control is difficult or the patient unreliable, a bioprostheses may be preferable. Long-standing cardiac arrhythmias such as atrial fibrillation would normally require anticoagulant therapy following surgery regardless of the valve device inserted. Under these conditions, a mechanical device would be preferable although a bioprosthesis might still be preferable in certain patients if a contraindication to long-term oral anticoagulants is present. Operative mortality rate increases with the number of previous cardiac operations. Thus, a mechanical valve device would be preferable in a patient who has had two or more cardiac operations unless the patient was elderly and bioprosthetic valve survival would exceed the lifespan of the patient.

Quality of life with a well functioning bioprosthetic valve is better than with a mechanical prosthesis, which can be noisy and requires lifetime anticoagulant therapy. In smaller stent sizes, mechanical devices offer a hemodynamic advantage which may be important for younger individuals with an active and vigorous lifestyle.

Valve durability is a major consideration which cannot be completely answered at the present time. Randomized trials comparing bioprosthetic to mechanical valve devices have not yet been reported. Clearly, the 10–20 year period following bioprosthetic valve replacement will be critical and should answer most of the important questions regarding durability [49]. The life span of some of the newer valve devices, both biological and mechanical, may exceed older valves. Improved hemodynamic function and chemical preservation of biological tissue may reduce leaflet stress and improve tissue durability. Improved mechanical valve design may reduce blood stasis and thromboembolism.

Surgical preference and experience are perhaps the greatest determinant of which valve is inserted in an individual patient. Selection of the appropriate valve substitute should be based on all of the above considerations with an open mind towards new developments in valve design and results of recent randomized trials of bioprostheses versus mechanical devices soon to be reported.

References

1. Khuri S, Folland E, Hammermeister F, Sethi G, Souchek J: Late postoperative hemodynamics of the Hancock heterograft and the Bjork-Shiley prosthesis: results of a national prospective randomized trial (Abstract). Circulation 1983; 68 (Suppl 3): 320.
2. Edwards LH Jr: Thromboembolic complications of current cardiac valvular prostheses. Ann Thorac Surg 1981; 34: 96.
3. Murphy DA, Levine FH, Buckley MJ. Swinski L, Daggett WM, Akins CW, Austen GW: Mechanical valves: a comparative analysis of the Starr-Edwards and Bjork-Shiley prostheses. J Thorac Cardiovasc Surg 1983; 86: 746–752.
4. Copans J, Lakier JB, Kinsley RH, Colsen PR, Fritz VU, Barlow JB: Thrombosed Bjork-Shiley mitral prostheses. Circulation 1980; 61: 169–174.
5. Lepley D, Flemma RJ, Mullen DC, Singh H, Chakravarty S: Late evaluation of patients undergoing valve replacement with the Bjork-Shiley Prosthesis. Annals Thorac Surg 1977; 24: 131–139.
6. Bjork VO, Henze A: Ten year's experience with the Bjork-Shiley tilting disc valve. J Thorac Cardiovasc Surg 1979; 78: 331–342.
7. Mattingly WT, O'Connor W, Ziok JV, Todd EP: Thrombotic catastrophe in the patient with multiple Bjork-Shiley prostheses. Annals Thorac Surg 1983; 35: 253–256.
8. Moreno-Cabral RJ, McNamara JJ, Mamiya RT, Brainard SC, Chung GKT: Acute thrombotic obstruction with Bjork-Shiley valves. J Thorac Cardiovasc Surg 1978; 75: 321–330.
9. Karp RB, Cyrus RJ, Blackstone EH, Kirklin JW, Kouchoukos NT, Pacifico AD: The Bjork-Shiley valve. J Thorac Cardiovasc Surg 1981; 81: 602–614.
10. Nicoloff DM, Emery RW, Arom KV, Northrup WF, Jorgensen CR, Wang Y, Lindsay WG: Clinical and hemodynamic results with the St. Jude medical cardiac valve prosthesis. J Thorac Cardiovasc Surg 1981; 82: 674–683.
11. Teply JF, Grunkemeier GL, Sutherland HD, Lambert LE, Johnson VA, Starr A: The ultimate prognosis after valve replacement: an assessment at twenty years. Annals Thorac Surg 1981; 32: 111–119.
12. Daenen W, Nevelsteen A, Van Cauwelaert P, De Maesschalk E, Willems J, Stalpaert G:

374

Nine years' experience with the Bjork-Shiley prosthetic valve: early and late results of 932 valve replacements. Annals Thorac Surg 1983; 35: 651–663.

13. Macmanus Q, Grunkemeier GL, Lambert LE, Starr A: Non-cloth-covered caged-ball prostheses. J Thorac Cardiovasc Surg 1978; 76: 788–794.

14. Sala A, Schoevaerdts JC, Jaumin P, Ponlot R, Chalant CH: Review of 387 isolated mitral valve replacements by the Model 6120 Starr-Edwards prosthesis. J Thorac Cardiovasc Surg 1982; 84: 774–750.

15. McGoon MD, Fuster V, McGoon D, Pumphrey CW, Pluth JR, Elveback LR: Aortic and mitral valve incompetence: long-term follow-up (10 to 19 years) of patients treated with the Starr-Edwards prosthesis. JACC 1984; 3: 930–938.

16. MacManus Q, Grunkemeier G, Housman L, Maloney C, Harlan B, Lambert L, Starr A: Early results with composite strut caged ball prostheses. Am J Cardiol 1980; 46: 566–569.

17. Horstkotte D, Loogen F, Haerten K, Schulte HD, Birck W: Six to eight years follow-up after prospective, randomized mitral valve replacement (Abstract). Circulation 1983; 68 (Suppl 3): 320.

18. Gallucci V, Valfre C, Mazzucco A, Bortolotti U, Milano A, Chioin R, Dalla Volta S, Cevese PG: Heart valve replacement with the Hancock bioprosthesis: a 5–11 year follow-up. In: Cohn LH, Gallucci V (eds) Cardiac bioprostheses. Yorke Medical Books, New York, 1982; 9–24.

19. Pelletier C, Chaitman BR, Baillot R, Val PG, Bonan R, Byrda I: Clinical and hemodynamic results with the Carpentier-Edwards porcine bioprosthesis. Annals Thorac Surg 1982; 34: 612–624.

20. Ionescu MI, Tandon AP, Saunders NR, Chidambaram M, Smith DR: Clinical durability of the pericardial xenograft valve: 11 years, experience. In: Cohn LH, Gallucci V (eds) Cardiac bioprostheses. Yorke Medical Books, New York, 1982; 42–60.

21. Duran CMG, Gallo I, Ruiz B, Revuelta JM, Ochoteco A: A thousand porcine bioprostheses revisted. Do they conform with the expected pattern? In: Cohn LH, Gallucci V (eds) Cardiac bioprostheses. Yorke Medical Books, New York, 1982; 35–41.

22. Deloche A, Perior P, Bourezak H, Chavaud S, Donzeau-Gouge PG, Dreyfus G, Fabiani JN, Massoud H, Carpentier A, Dubost C: A 14-year experience with valvular bioprostheses: valve survival and patient survival. In: Cohn LH, Gallucci V (eds) Cardiac bioprostheses. Yorke Medical Books, New York, 1982; 25–34.

23. Betriu A, Chaitman BR, Almazan A, Val GP, Pelletier C: Preoperative determinants of return to sinus rhythm after valve replacement. In: Cohn LH, Gallucci V (eds) Cardiac bioprostheses. Yorke Medical Books, New York, 1982; 184–191.

24. Oyer PE, Stinson EB, Miller DC, Jamieson SW, Reitz BA, Baumgartner W, Shumay NE: Clinical analysis of the Hancock porcine bioprosthesis. In: Cohn LH, Gallucci V (eds) Cardiac bioprostheses. Yorke Medical Books, New York,, 1982; 539–551.

25. Magilligan DJ, Lewis JW, Stein PD, Lakier J, Smith DR: Decreasing incidence of porcine bioprosthetic degeneration. In: Cohn LH, Gallucci V (eds) Cardiac bioprostheses. Yorke Medical Books, New York, 1982: 559–571.

26. Gonzalez-Lavin L, Tandon AP, Chi S, Blair TC, McFadden PM, Lewis B, Daughters G, Ionescu M: The risk of thromboembolism and hemorrhage following mitral valve replacement. J Thorac Cardiovasc Surg 1984; 87: 340–351.

27. Geha AS, Hammond GL, Laks H, Stansel HC, Glenn WWL: Factors affecting performance and thromboembolism after porcine xenograft cardiac valve replacement. J Thorac Cardiovasc Surg 1982; 83: 377–384.

28. Cohn LH, Mudge GH, Pratter F, Collins JJ: Five to eight-year follow-up of patients undergoing porcine heart-valve replacement. New Eng J Med 1981; 304: 258–262.

29. Gallo I, Ruiz B, Duran G: Isolated mitral valve replacement with the Hancock porcine

bioprosthesis in rheumatic heart disease: analysis of 213 operative survivors followed up 4.5 to 8.5 years. Am J Cardiol 1984; 53: 178–181.

30. Schoen FJ, Collins JJ, Cohn LH: Long-term failure rate and morphologic correlations in porcine bioprosthetic heart valves. Am J Cardiol 1983; 51: 957–964.

31. Kloster FE, Herr RH, Starr A, Griswold HE: Hemodynamic evaluation of a cloth-covered Starr-Edwards valve prosthesis. Circulation 1969; 39/40 (Suppl 1): 119–125.

32. Brown JW, Myerowitz PD, Cann MS, Colvin SB, McIntosh CL, Morrow AG: Clinical and hemodynamic comparisons of Kay-Shiley, Starr-Edwards No 6520, and Reis-Hancock porcine xenograft mitral valves. Surgery 1974; 76: 983–991.

33. Rothkopf M, Davidson T, Lipscomb K, Narahara K, Hillis LD, Willerson JT, Estrera A, Platt M, Mills L: Hemodynamic evaluation of the Carpentier-Edwards bioprosthesis in the aortic position. Am J Cardiol 1979; 44: 209–214.

34. Chaitman BR, Bonan R, Lepage G, Tubau JF, David PR, Dyrda I, Grondin CM: Hemodynamic evaluation of the Carpentier-Edwards porcine xenograft. Circulation 1979; 60: 1170–1182.

35. Lee G, Grehl TM, Joye JA, Kaku RF, Harter W, DeMaria AN, Mason DT: Hemodynamic assessment of the new aortic Carpentier-Edwards bioprosthesis. Cath Cardiovasc Diag 1978; 4: 373–381.

36. Gray RJ: Hemodynamic function of St. Jude aortic valves: comparison with a porcine and Bjork-Shiley prostheses. In: Cohn LH, Gallucci V (eds) Cardiac bioprostheses. Yorke Medical Books, New York, 1982; 247–256.

37. Bjork VO, Book K, Holmgren A: The Bjork-Shiley mitral valve prosthesis. Annals Thorac Surg 1974; 18: 379–390.

38. Morris DC, King SB, Douglas JS, Wickliffe CW, Jones EL: Hemodynamic results of aortic valvular replacement with the porcine xenograft valve. Circulation 1977; 56: 841–844.

39. Gabbay S, Wasserman F, Bortolotti U, Frater RWM: In vitro hydrodynamic corparison of the new generation of heart valve bioprostheses (Abstract). Eur Heart J 1983; 4: 21.

40. Williams DB, Danielson GK, McGoon DC, Puga FJ, Mair DD, Edwards WD: Porcine heterograft valve replacement in children. J Thorac Cardiovasc Surg 1982; 84: 446–450.

41. Sanders SP, Levy RJ, Freed MD, Norwood WI, Castaneda AR: Use of Hancock porcine xenografts in children and adolescents. Am J Cardiol 1980; 46: 429–438.

42. Rocchini AP, Weesner KM, Heidelberger K, Keren D, Behrendt D, Rosenthal A: Porcine xenograft valve failure in children: an immunologic response. Circulation 1981; 64 (Suppl 2): 162–171.

43. Geha AS, Laks H, Stansel HC, Cornhill JF, Kilman JW, Buckley MJ, Roberts WC: Late failure of porcine valve heterografts in children. J Thorac Cardiovasc Surg 1979; 78: 351–364.

44. Antunes MJ, Med M, Santos LP: Performance of glutaraldehyde-preserved porcine bioprosthesis as a mitral valve substitute in a young population group. Annals Thorac Surg 1984; 37: 387–392.

45. Walker WE, Duncan JM, Frazier OH, Livesay JJ, Ott DA, Reul GJ, Cooley DA: Early experience with the Ioenscu-Shiley pericardial xenograft valve. J Thorac Cardiovasc Surg 1983; 86: 570–575.

46. Arbustini E, Jones M, Moses RD, Eibdo EE, Carrol RJ, Ferrans VJ: Modification by the Hancock T6 process of calcification of bioprosthetic cardiac valves implanted in sheep. Am J Cardiol 1984; 53: 1388–1396.

47. Milano A, Bortolotti U, Talenti E, Valfre C, Arbustini E, Valente M, Mazzucco A, Gallucci V, Thiene G: Calcific degeneration as the main cause of procine bioprosthetic valve failure. Am J Cardiol 1984; 53: 1066–1070.

48. Pomar JL, Bosch X, Chaitman BR, Pelletier C, Grondin CM: Late tears in leaflets of porcine bioprostheses in adults. Annals Thorac Surg 1984; 37: 78–83.

49. Miller DC, Oyer PE, Stinson EB et al.: Ten to fifteen year reassessment of the performance characteristics of the Starr-Edwards model 6120 mitral valve prosthesis. J Thorac Cardiovasc Surg 1983; 85: 1–20.

8.3 Conservative Mitral Valve Surgery

C.M.G. DURAN, I. GALLO, J.F. NISTAL, A. FIGUEROA and
J.L. UBAGO

Once extracorporeal circulation became safe to use, surgical treatment of
mitral stenosis under direct vision was recommended and progressively implemented. Initially, only open heart commissurotomy was performed, rapidly
followed by papillary myotomy of the subvalvular apparatus. When there was
significant mitral incompetence, the patient was considered to be a candidate
for valve replacement. The description of new valvular reconstruction techniques [1, 2] aimed mainly at treating mitral incompetence has progressively
modified the concept of open heart mitral surgery. At the present, a new
attitude toward all mitral surgery is taking place; it is considered as such from
the simple mitral commisurotomy to valve substitution that includes more or
less complex valvular reconstruction procedures. It is the anatomic status of
the valve that determines the selection of a certain technique and its re-
strictions rather than the preoperatory functional diagnosis of the valve as
stenotic or incompetent.

Surgical techniques

Some technical points are essential when contemplating this type of surgery.
Satisfactory exposure of the mitral valve is indispensable to clearly identify the
pathological process involved in each valve. We always make an atriotomy
behind the atrial septum and well extended posterior to both venae cava. We
use two separators that adapt to the configuration of each left atrium and
angled cannulas that simplify the exposure and improve visibility of the tricuspid valve, which we have found to be implicated in approximately 30% of
the mitral patients operated. In second place, cardioplegia is a prerequisite,
not only to attain cardiac relaxation and a better view of the mitral apparatus,
but to give enough time to study and apply the different reconstructive techniques without haste. In third place, a method for intraoperative quality
control of the repair is needed. Although a number of methods are described

in the literature [3, 4], all have limitations. Experience with a method is required to safely assess the results obtained. This is necessary because poor results are therefore secondary to poor surgical technique either in forming the indication or in its realization. We use a method based on pressurized injection of blood through the left ventricular apex connected to the arterial line [4]. The entire mitral apparatus must be carefully explored and each element individually evaluated. The state of the leaflets, location and extension of calcified deposits and leaflet retraction and mobility have to be assessed. The commissural fusion line should be identified from both the atrium and ventricle and the points of implantation of the tendinous chords studied. The subvalvular structure is probably the most critical area for producing shortening and fusion of chords, especially in stenotic mitral lesions. The existence of papillary muscle hypertrophy, the degree of annular dilation and whether the dilation is symmetric or asymmetric must also be considered. A clear comprehension of the pathology of the valve to be repaired is the condition *sine qua non* for applying any reconstructive procedure.

Specific surgical techniques have been extensively described in the literature [5, 6]. They consist mainly in commissurotomy, papillary myotomy, separation of chords and excision of calcified nodules in predominantly stenotic lesions. In predominantly incompetent lesions, selective annuloplasty, shortening of tendinous chords and leaflet resection are performed. We perform annuloplasty with a totally flexible ring (Durán Flexible Ring, Hancock Lab, California) that adapts to the continuous changes in the mitral ring during the cardiac cycle [2].

Results

With this attitude toward open heart mitral surgery, from June 1974 to June 1984 we substituted 1175 mitral valves and preserved 817 (41%). Basically, conservative surgery can be divided into 426 isolated commissurotomies, including all types of conservative procedures without annuloplasty, and 391 procedures with annuloplasty.

To analyze the surgical results, we decided to study patients with isolated mitral pathology, to avoid interference by other valvular disorders, at 6 to 10 years of follow-up. All the patients operated on between June 1974 and June 1984 were included. They were divided into three groups:

1. Commissurotomy group (C): 116 cases of commissurotomy accompanied by any other type of conservative surgery, except for annular interventions.
2. Flexible ring group (Flx): 90 cases of isolated annuloplasty or annuloplasty with any other reconstructive procedure.
3. Valve substitution group (VSub): 236 isolated mitral valve substitutions with Hancock prostheses.

Hospital mortality

Hospital mortality (in the first 30 days of postoperatory or the initial hospitalization) was 2.6% in the C group, 1.1% for the Flx group and 10% for the VSub group. It has always been assumed that the patients in whom the valve is replaced are in a more deteriorated condition than those submitted to conservative surgery, mainly because of the presence of long-term mitral incompetence. Nonetheless, it is interesting to note that in 267 annuloplasties performed from 1975 to 1982, the hospital mortality was similar for the cases with mitral stenosis and those with pure mitral incompetence (2.6% versus 2.9%) (Table 1). In an earlier study [8], we found that even among patients in functional class III–IV, hospital mortality was much higher when the valve was replaced by a prosthesis than when annuloplasty was performed. The fact that in the annuloplasty group the union between papillary muscle and mitral ring is preserved, which is not the case with mitral replacement, may explain this difference in hospital mortality.

Thromboembolism

The incidence of thromboembolism was 0.51% patient/years for the C group, 2.67% for the Flx group and 1.87% for the VSub group. The high incidence of thromboembolic accidents in the annuloplasty group is surprising, especially in view of the fact that our anticoagulation regimen is the same for all mitral surgery, with the exception of mechanical valve replacement. According to our policy all patients in sinus rhythm receive only antiaggregant drugs for 3 months and all those in atrial fibrillation receive anticoagulants for only 3 months. Only patients with a giant left atrium or intraatrial thrombi are given permanent anticoagulant therapy. This policy is really only hypothetic, considering that each cardiologist is naturally free to decide on anticoagulant therapy. Table 2 reflects the true situation, with the percentages of patients receiving different anticoagulant regimens according to whether they have

Table 1. Flexible ring mitral annuloplasty. Hospital mortality.

Type of lesion	Patients	Mortality
Predominantly stenosis	171	(5) 2.9%
Pure	76	(2) 2.6%
Double	95	(3) 3.1%
Predominantly incompetence	96	(4) 4.1%
Pure	34	(1) 2.9%
Double	62	(3) 4.8%

undergone prosthetic or conservative surgery. Nine per cent of the patients with bioprosthesis were not receiving atiembolic therapy, in comparison with 85.7% of the patients with flexible rings who did not.

Late mortality

The incidence of late mortality was 0.5% patient/year in group C, 1.1% for group FLx and 1.3% for group VSub. In contrast with hospital mortality, there did not seem to be any significant difference in late mortality between the three groups.

Reoperation

As we just saw, late mortality apparently did not differ for the three types of mitral surgery studied. It is also clear that there was no functional difference between the three groups. However, it is interesting to study the differences in reoperation incidence. Comparison of these three groups shows that in 113 cases with open heart commissurotomy, 3 required reoperation in the 6 to 10 years of follow-up. Six of 89 (6.8%) annuloplasties and 17 of 213 (7.9%) valve substitutions required reoperation during this follow-up period. If we examine more closely the incidence of reoperation in the group that had conservative surgery with annuloplasty between 1975 and 1982 and a minimum follow-up of 2 years, 15 of the 267 (5.6%) patients had to be operated. All the patients reoperated had rheumatic disease. Two required reoperation, one for bacte-

Table 2. Permanent antiembolic treatment.

	Flx (no 267)	Hck (no 221)
Antiaggregant drugs	2.6%	24%
Anticoagulants	11.6%	67%
Untreated	85.7%	9%

Table 3. Flexible ring mitral annuloplasty. Reoperations.

Reoperations	
Predominantly stenosis	4.8% (9/166)
Pure	0% (0/74)
Mixed	9.7% (9/92)
Predominantly incompetence	4.3% (4/92)
Pure	9% (3/33)
Mixed	1.7% (1/59)

rial endocarditis and an aortic bioprosthesis and one for massive tricuspid incompetence. In the other 13, reoperation was necessary for dysfunction of the mitroplasty. In 6 incompetence reappeared as a result of ring dehiscence and in 7 mitral dysfunction was present from the moment of the initial surgery. In 3 patients there was significant mitral stenosis and in 4 regurgitation persisted. During reoperation it was found that this regurgitation was due to elongation of the tendinous chords that had been overlooked; annuloplasty therefore did not satisfactorily correct mitral incompetence. Analysis of the underlying disorder of the 13 patients who required reoperation for mitral dysfunction (Table 3) showed that none pertained to the group with pure mitral stenosis and 9% (3/33) had pure mitral incompetence (one due to ring dehiscence and two to unsuspected elongation of the tendinous chords). The other 10 patients had mixed mitral lesions, either predominantly stenotic (9/92) or incompetent (1/59).

Condition of the mitral valvular apparatus

It is important to emphasize the effect the condition of the mitral apparatus has on results. We have analyzed the whole group of patients with flexible ring mitral annuloplasty operated on from 1975 to 1982 with a minimum follow-up of two years. The patients were divided into two groups on the basis of presence or absence of calcified nodules (Table 4). There was no clear difference in hospital or late mortality between both groups, and the incidence of reoperation was higher in cases without calcified nodules. All the patients were divided into two groups according to the type of surgery (Table 5): those

Table 4. Flexible ring mitral annuloplasty. Calcified nodules.

Calcified nodules	+(30)	−(237)
Hospital mortality	(1) 3.3%	(8) 3.3%
Late mortality	(2) 6.9%	(10) 4.3%
Reoperations	(1) 3.7%	(12) 5.2%

Table 5. Flexible ring mitral annuloplasty. Surgical procedures.

Surgical procedures	Simple (207)	Complex (60)
Hospital mortalilty	(5) 2.4%	(4) 6.6%
Late mortality	(10) 4.9%	(2) 3.5%
Reoperations	(10) 4.9%	(3) 5.3%)

with a 'simple' surgery, annuloplasty alone or with commissurotomy and papillary musculotomy, and those with more 'complex' surgery, that included procedures such as chordal shortening, leaflet resection, secondary chord resection, etc. The incidence of reoperation was higher in the 'complex' surgery group, as could be expected, although the late mortality was lower. These results can be interpreted as an indication that the condition of the valvular apparatus has little effect on the results. The quality of the surgery performed has more influence on the short- and long-term results. This becomes more evident when we consider that 7 of 13 patients required reoperation for dysfunction of the annuloplasty, that is, they were reoperated for an unsatisfactory surgical correction. However, it is obvious that a poor valvular condition requires a more complex surgical procedure, implying a longer period of ischemia and suboptimal functional results.

Hemodynamic evaluation

Hemodynamic results of the reconstruction techniques are intimately related to the condition of the mitral valve apparatus. If candidates with valves in good condition are selected, excellent results can be expected, and if the valve is in poor condition mediocre hemodynamic results can be anticipated.

This is especially meaningful in cases of predominantly stenotic lesions with rigid cusps and a deformed subvalvular apparatus. We attempted to correlate hemodynamic results with the condition of the mitral valve apparatus in 110 patients who were recatheterized after annuloplasty. Forty patients who had a flexible ring of 84 mm circumference were chosen. The preoperatory angiograms were reviewed to study two anatomic parameters:

1. Mitral valve condition. We studied cusp thickening during recirculation, valvular mobility and the subvalvular apparatus.
2. Angiographic dimensions of the mitral ring. We measured the distance

Table 6. Mitral annuloplasty (28 mm Flx ring). Hemodynamic results.

Preoperative		Postoperative	
Ring size	Valve condition	MVA (cm^2/m^2)	RMI (%)
Increased	Good (n = 7)	2.33 ± 1.1	0
	Poor (n = 5)	1.3 ± 0.2	65
Normal	Good (n = 6)	1.5 ± 0.3	0
	Poor (n = 5)	0.95 ± 0.4	0

Predominantly incompetent (n = 23); MVA: mitral valve area (index); RMI: residual mitral incompetence.

between the posterior commissure and the anterior part of the mitral ring adjacent to the aortic valve. This measurement probably does not correspond to the anatomic diameter of the mitral valve but it is easy to measure angiographically. The normal size is approximately $2.5\,cm/m^2$. Patients with larger rings were considered to have mitral ring dilation.

Twenty-three patients had predominant mitral incompetence and 17 predominant stenosis. Preoperatively, those with predominant incompetence (Table 6) were divided on the basis of ring size into enlarged, normal or reduced groups. Postoperative hemodynamic data were analyzed for each of these groups. Patients with an enlarged ring and a good mitral valve condition had a mitral area of $2.3\,cm/m^2$ and no mitral regurgitation. Those with dilated ring and poor valvular condition had an area of $1.3\,cm/m^2$, which is satisfactory, but accompanied by a very high incidence of postoperative mitral regurgitation (65%). Patients with mitral incompetence, normal size ring and good valvular condition had a mitral area of $1.5\,cm/m^2$ and no residual mitral regurgitation; if the mitral valvular apparatus was in poor condition, the postoperative area was $0.95\,cm/m^2$ and the valve was stenotic but there was no residual regurgitation.

Undoubtedly, excellent results can be obtained when the cause of mitral incompetence is a dilated ring with a mitral valvular apparatus of good quality. When it is in poor condition, the ring has to be significantly reduced to obtain a competent valve, which results in stenosis, or a residual incompetence has to be allowed.

The group of patients with stenotic or predominantly stenotic lesions corrected with an 84 mm circumference ring was also divided according to valvular ring size and valvular apparatus condition (Table 7). The patients with enlarged ring and good mitral valve condition obtained a postoperative area of $1.5\,cm/m^2$ without risidual incompetence and the patients with a valve in poor condition achieved an area of $1.1\,cm/m^2$ and 25% residual incompetence.

Table 7. Mitral annuloplasty (28 mm ring). Hemodynamic results.

Preoperative		Postoperative	
Ring size	Valve condition	MVA (cm^2/m^2)	RMI (%)
Increased	Good (n = 4)	1.56 ± 1.2	0
	Poor (n = 3)	1.16 ± 0.6	25
Normal	Good (n = 5)	1.0 ± 0.3	0
	Poor (n = 5)	1.1 ± 0.5	40

Predominantly stenotic (n = 17); MVA: mitral valve area (index); RMI: residual mitral incompetence.

Patients with predominantly stenotic valve, normal ring size and valve in good condition had a postoperative area of $1\,cm/m^2$, but 40% residual incompetence. The clear conclusion is that patients with predominantly stenotic mitral lesions and a valve in good condition can attain valvular competence at the expense of a reduction in area, which will be satisfactory if there is annular dilation but will produce stenosis if it is normal. If valve condition is poor, independent of ring size, there will be an elevated percentage of stenosis or residual incompetence. The condition of the valvular apparatus therefore plays a primordial role in late hemodynamic results.

Conclusions

1. Open heart mitral surgery should be considered as a whole that extends from simple commissurotomy to valve replacement and includes more or less complex surgical procedures.
2. When surgery is reconstructive, rarely does a simple technique suffice to correct the lesion. It is essential that the alterations in each valve be individually identified.
3. To satisfactorily perform this type of surgery certain technical details are essential, such as perfect visibility of the mitral valve, good cardioplegia and a method for intraoperatory quality control of the reconstruction.
4. The comparative results of commissurotomy, annuloplasty and valvular substitution by bioprosthesis shows that there is a lower hospital mortality and a low incidence of reoperation for conservative surgery as compared to substitution. The increased incidence of thromboembolism in patients with annuloplasty is due to the difference in anticoagulant regimens used in each case; only 9% of the patients with bioprosthesis did not receive any type of permanent antithrombotic treatment; 85% of those with annuloplasty did not receive this treatment.
5. Study of the incidence of reoperations required by patients with annuloplasty showed that reconstruction techniques are very stable as long as a satisfactory surgical correlation is achieved.
6. Postoperative hemodynamic studies show that global analysis of results is not very reliable in this type of surgery. The dispersion of the results is secondary to variations in valve condition and surgery. A thorough evaluation of individual lesions, correct indication for each surgical procedure and intraoperative evaluation of the results obtained are imperative.

References

1. Carpentier A, Deloche A, Dauptain J, Soyer R, Blondeau P, Piwnica A, Dubost C: A new reconstructive operation for correction of mitral and tricuspid insuffiency. J Thorac Cardiovasc Surg 1971; 61: 1–13.
2. Duran CMG, Ubago JL: Clinical and hemodynamic performance of a totally flexible prosthetic ring for atrioventricular valve reconstruction. Ann Thorac Surg 1976; 22: 458.
3. Hetzer R, Warnecke H: Intraoperative assessment of the reconstructed mitral valve using a low pressure crystalloid infusion. Thorac Cardiovasc Surgeon 1981; 29: 100–104.
4. Pomar JL, Cuchiara G, Gallo JI, Duran CMG: Intraoperative assessment of mitral valve function. Ann Thorac Surg 1978; 25: 354–355.
5. Carpentier A, Chauvaud S, Fabiani JN et al.: Reconstructive surgery of mitral valve incompetence. Ten-year appraisal. J Thorac Cardiovasc Surg 1980; 79: 338–348.
6. Duran CMG: Reconstructive procedures of the mitral valve including annuloplasty. In: Cohn LH (ed) Modern techniques in surgery, 2nd ed. Futura Publishing, Mt Kisco, NY, 1979; 20.1–20.10.
7. Duran CMG, Ubago JL: Conservative mitral valve surgery. Problems and development in the techniques of prosthetic ring annuloplasty. In: Kalmanson D (ed) The mitral valve. A multidisciplinary approach. Publishing Science Group, Acton, MA, 1975; 549–557.
8. Duran CMG, Pomar JL, Revuelta JM, Gallo I, Poveda J, Ochoteco A, Ubago JL, Cohn LH: Conservative operation for mitral insufficiency. Critical analysis supported by postoperative hemodynamic studies of 72 patients. J Thorac Cardiovasc Surg 1980; 79: 326–337.

8.4 Chronic Valvular Heart Disease: Timing of Surgery

VALENTIN FUSTER

Up until the last decade, one of the main challenges to the clinical cardiologist was to be capable of making the exact clinical diagnosis in the office or at the bedside, just based on a clinical history, physical examination, chest x-ray and electrocardiogram. With the recent wide availability of sensitive non invasive diagnostic procedures, that diagnostic challenge has greatly dissipated.

Today, probably the main challenge to the clinical cardiologist is to choose the exact timing for therapeutic cardiac intervention, with surgery or other invasive therapeutic procedures. In this context cardiologists should:

a) be aware of the new emerging knowledge on the natural history of disease with intervention as compared without intervention (medical therapy); and

b) they should also be aware of the important emerging role of the noninvasive procedures for the detection of certain parameters of myocardial dysfunction that lead to an earlier and more appropriate timing for intervention when compared with the past.

We will add, however, that such noninvasive procedures should not be over-utilized, but rather used with specific reasons and at appropriate times within the clinical course of the patient.

In this paper we will briefly outline the above issues as they apply today to the timing of surgery for isolated chronic valvular heart disease.

Aortic valvular stenosis

Natural history and pathophysiology

The severity of aortic valvular stenosis tends to be progressive. When the valvular orifice area is less than a third of normal, symptoms usually appear in the form of angina pectoris, exertional dyspnea or exertional syncope [1]; in the younger age groups particularly with congenital aortic stenosis, symptoms tend to appear only with a more severe degree of stenosis [2]. Most important-

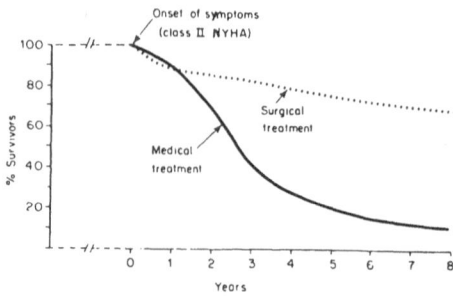

Fig. 1. Aortic valvular stenosis. Graph obtained from Mayo Clinic experience on the long-term survival of medical vs surgical treatment. Observe, from the moment of onset of symptoms, the rapid decline in survival of those patients treated medically as compared with those treated surgically.

ly, in aortic valvular stenosis, once symptoms appear, there is a rapid downhill course (Fig. 1).

From a pathophysiological point of view, the obstruction produces left ventricular pressure overload which eventually leads to left ventricular hypertrophy. The left ventricular pressure overload and left ventricular hypertrophy both increase cardiac work and oxygen consumption which can lead to left ventricular failure with the exertional dyspnea or exertional syncope. The increase in cardiac work and oxygen consumption also explain the frequent development of angina pectoris, reflecting an unmet oxygen demand in the absence of coronary artery disease (only one-third of these patients with angina have associated coronary artery disease). Increased electrical instability of the hypertrophied and pressure overloaded left ventricle may lead to ventricular fibrillation which is the main cause of sudden death in patients with severe aortic stenosis; in the adult sudden death tends to occur in the previously symptomatic patient [3], while in children may be the first and only symptom of severe aortic stenosis [4].

Timing and indications of surgery (Fig. 1, Table 1)

According to the above information it is now established that in aortic valvular stenosis, the appearance of symptoms is definitive indication for surgical intervention [5]. Symptoms are usually the manifestation of significant valvular obstruction, with a peak systolic pressure gradient across the aortic valve of greater than 50 mm Hg; the gradient is lower if the cardiac output is reduced in which case the calculated aortic valve area is about less than 0.7 cm². It is at this late stage of the disease that the prognosis for nonoperative management is very poor, whereas the prognosis with surgical intervention is generally good [6, 7]. Patients with significant associated coronary disease should be considered for coronary bypass surgery at the same time as valve surgery.

In valvular aortic stenosis, there is a lack of specific indications for valve replacement in the absence of clinical symptoms; this is because the patient with severe stenosis and, therefore, at risk of sudden death rarely remains symptomatically silent. Nevertheless, in future years, as the long-term results of valve replacement are better established and improved, and as the noninvasive techniques for evaluating left ventricular function are also improved and serially evaluated, it is anticipated that valve replacement will be recommended on the basis of a certain severity of stenosis and ventricular dysfunction, perhaps prior to the patient becoming symptomatic. In fact there are two uncommon clinical situations of aortic stenosis in which surgical intervention is probably indicated prior to clinical symptoms. The first is in the patient whom despite of severe aortic stenosis may remain asymptomatic; this tends to occur in the younger age group and the possibility of sudden death before ventricular dysfunction deserves surgical consideration; thus, in our practice, we intervene to such young asymptomatic patients when the aortic systolic gradient is over 75 mm Hg.

The second uncommon clinical situation is in older patients in whom the first manifestation of significant aortic stenosis is not the clinical symptomatology, but either cardiomegaly with a cardiothoracic ratio of over 0.6, frequent ventricular extrasystoles at rest which increase with exercise, or a limited exercise capacity detected on a cautiously performed treadmill test; in such asymptomatic patients, if indeed severe aortic stenosis is documented, with an aortic systolic gradient over 75 mm Hg and a valve area of less than $0.6\,cm^2$, surgical intervention is probably indicated for the prevention of sudden death and irreversible left ventricular dysfunction.

What we can expect from the surgical intervention with aortic valve
replacement [8]

This can be performed at an operative mortality of about 5% or less [9–12]. Left ventricular hypertrophy regresses towards, but not to, normal. Surviving patients are functionally improved. The ten-year survival after aortic valve replacement is 60% or better and the 15-year survival is 50% or better. Nevertheless, in the future the results might be improved by offering operation at an earlier stage of the disease prior to the development of symptoms. As discussed previously in this section, subgroups of such asymptomatic patients potential for earlier operation are now beginning to be identified.

Regarding higher risk patients, valve replacement in patients with aortic stenosis and heart failure can be performed at an operative mortality of 10% or less. Although this rate is increased when compared with patients who are not in heart failure, the operative mortality is reasonable because late survival in those who live through the operation is far superior to that which can be expected with medical therapy. The impaired left ventricular function improves in all such patients – provided there has been no perioperative myocardial damage – and becomes normal at rest in two thirds of the patients [13]. In addition, the operative survivors are functionally much improved. Left ventricular dilatation (if present preoperatively) regress towards normal.

In patients age 60 years and older, the operative mortality is increased (possibly 5–10%). The late survival is far superior to that which can be expected with medical therpay [14]; one third of the late deaths are from noncardiac causes. The majority of the survivors are functionally improved.

Mitral stenosis

Natural history and pathophysiology

The natural history of mitral stenosis is that it takes about 10 years from the time of the attack of rheumatic fever before abnormal auscultatory signs, 10 years before symptoms occur, and another 10 years before total disability ensues [15, 16]. Marked variations from this history occur in two settings. First, in some areas like Alaska, India, and Malaysia, severe mitral stenosis may develop at a young age, while mitral stenosis may be quite mild in older patients in the United States. The course of the patient with mitral stenosis is quite different from that of aortic valve stenosis where there is often a long period without symptoms followed by a very short, serious course of progressive symptoms. In mitral stenosis, there is usually gradual progression, frequently interrupted by episodes of acute symptomatic difficulty, precipitated by the onset of atrial fibrillation, unusual physical stress, pregnancy, respiratory infections, or pulmonary emboli.

From a pathophysiological point of view [7, 17], the increased left atrial pressure associated with mitral stenosis is transmitted back to the pulmonary veins and capillaries and may be associated with transudation of fluid into the interstitial space. This accounts for the dyspnea, orthopnea, nocturnal dyspnea, and dyspnea associated with pulmonary edema. It also accounts for the hemoptysis which results from rupture of small bronchial veins or in association with pulmonary edema. In the later stages, pulmonary arteriolar constriction associated with intimal and medial hyperplasia protects the pulmonary capillaries and interstitial tissue and consequently prevents recurrent pulmonary edema. It leads, however, to pulmonary arterial hypertension with right ventricular hypertrophy and finally right ventricular failure with symptoms of fatigue (low cardial output), hepatic congestion, ascites, and peripheral edema. The most common late complication is pulmonary embolism and infarction with hemoptysis. Two additional common complications of mitral stenosis are atrial fibrillation which occurs in more than 50% of patients and systemic emboli which occur in 10–20% of patients.

Timing and indications of surgery (Table 2)

In mitral stenosis, we first should briefly comment about when the operation is not indicated. Thus, with the onset of mild symptoms no special treatment is indicated, except that there is a need for the physician to carefully evaluate the life-style and occupation of the patient and to periodically review his clinical status. If the shortness of breath slowly progresses, we advise salt restriction or a mild diuretic regimen. An initial episode of pulmonary edema related or unrelated to atrial fibrillation may direct the physician to consider surgical treatment if other clinical data indicate the presence of a severe mitral stenosis. In a significant number of such patients, however, it is apparent that they can continue with a reasonable good life style for a number of years before surgical treatment may be necessary. Finally, in patients with systemic emboli, when considering surgical treatment for the prevention of new emboli, it is important to realize that the operation will not lessen the likelihood of thromboembolic complications when prosthetic replacement of the mitral valve is necessary; in fact, the tendency for thromboembolism is probably increased [18]. Also, in the patient with relatively mild stenosis that has been essentially asymptomatic there has been no evidence that mitral valvoltomy will reduce the tendency to thromboembolism if this occurred preoperatively. It has been considered probable, however, that in the patient with severe mitral stenosis who has had a thromboembolic complication, a well-performed and successful mitral valvotomy may lessen the likelihood of thromboembolic events; on theoretical grounds this seems a reasonable proposition, but remains to be proven. Our approach in these patients with previous emboli is the use of oral anticoagulants since their benefit is well established [18].

The indication for mitral operation is often clear, as for the patient with mitral stenosis having progressive, severely limiting dyspnea and fatigue on exertion. Thus, most patients who are not approaching senility and have no other serious limitations to their anticipated longevity are definite candidates for operation if they begin to exhibit Class III status (New York Heart Association classification). Since clinical symptoms of mitral stenosis can also occur as a result of other associated conditions, like chronic obstructive pulmonary disease or hyperventilation, clinical or hemodynamic confirmation of significant mitral stenosis should be ascertain before operation is offered; thus, if a confirmatory hemodynamic study becomes necessary, a significant transmitral diastolic pressure gradient at rest and/or exercise and a valve area of less than $1.5–2 \, cm^2$ should be established. There are important technical

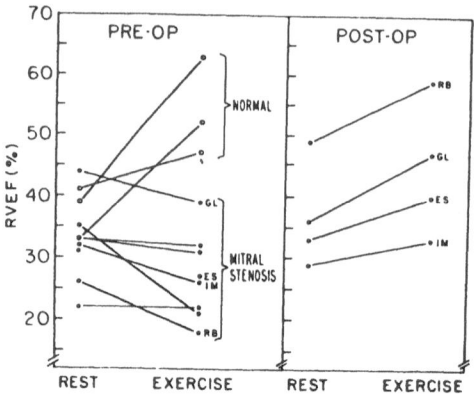

Fig. 2. The preoperative (PRE-OP) right ventricular ejection fraction (RVEF %) at rest and at exercise is depicted for three control patients (open circles) and eight mitral stenosis patients (closed circles) with significant pulmonary hypertension. The panel on the right depicts the postoperative (POST-OP) exercise response of the four patients who underwent corrective mitral surgery. (they are identified by their initials); observe that two of these postoperative patients have a low right ventricular ejection fraction at rest or on exercise. (with permission from J Am Coll Cardiol [20]).

factors in deciding about commissurotomy versus valve replacement, but they are out of the scope of this chapter.

There is a second group of patients with mitral stenosis in whom operation is probably indicated. These are asymptomatic or minimaly symptomatic patients with severe pulmonary hypertension who show clinical or radionuclide evidence of significant right ventricular dysfunction. Despite of operation releaving the right ventricular pressure overload, if the right ventricular dysfunction becomes irreversible, some of these patient may suffer postoperative low cardiac output with fatigue as well as reduced long term survival. At present, we are investigating and defining this problem of significant and irreversible right ventricular dysfunction (Fig. 2) [19, 20].

What we can expect from the surgical intervention [8, 17]

It is recognized that when surgically indicated, palliation from 'open' commissurotomy will probably be limited to a 10 or 20 year period, because of re-stenosis or residual incompetence [21]. However, with our present state of knowledge and with presently available prosthetic valves, which have been tested in humans for less than 20 years, a good result from commissurotomy of only 10 to 20 years would still appear to be preferable to a prosthetic valve [22]. The low risk of repair of such mitral valves is another positive factor because there is no more than 2% mortality for the properly selected patients and may be near 5% for valve replacement. It is essential not to allow induced mitral incompetence to go unrecognized, since postoperative results can be poor [23]. Our recent approach, which appears to be most sensitive and specific, is the use of contrast 2-D echocardiography [23]. At the end of operation, the echocardiogram is performed by applying a $5MH_2$ transducer directly on the heart during agitated saline injections via an apical ventricular sump or transseptal needle, generating contrast microbubbles which can be imaged in the left atrium if the mitral valve is not competent; thus, if there is significant mitral incompetence, further valve reconstruction or valve replacement can be undertaken within the same operative session.

There is an overall clinical impression that the small number of patients with poor surgical results following mitral valve replacement for mitral stenosis are mainly those with significant residual right ventricular dysfunction (with or without associated tricuspid incompetence) preoperatively and postoperatively. It is for this reason that in mitral valve disease with pulmonary hypertension, noninvasive assessment of right ventricular dysfunction is becoming an important area of interest and investigation.

Aortic valvular incompetence

Natural history and pathophysiology

The specifics of patients with aortic incompetence secondary to disease of the ascending aorta, in the form of chronic aneurysm or acute dissection, and of patients with aortic incompetence secondary to intrinsic acute valvular infective endocarditis are not discussed in this section. Therefore, we will focus primary attention to those patients with intrinsic chronic valvular incompetence, the main cause being rheumatic.

In rheumatic aortic incompetence, a diastolic murmur may occur with the onset of rheumatic fever. The degree of regurgitation may be minimal, and longevity may not be affected, barring complicating events such as infectious endocarditis. More often, after a period of about one decade, in which the only sign is a diastolic murmur, the aortic regurgitation becomes hemodynamically significant, but with the exception of the patient's awareness of the overactivity of the heart and neck vessels this condition is usually well tolerated for periods ranging from one to three decades [24–27]. Ultimately, significant symptoms of left ventricular failure appear, consisting of exertional shortness of breath with episodic nocturnal dyspnea, followed by progressive deterioration over one to ten years; angina pectoris is an infrequent and late event, occurring in about 20% of patients. Thus, our study in patients with significant symptoms, in class III or IV indicated that after 10 years, 90% of patients had

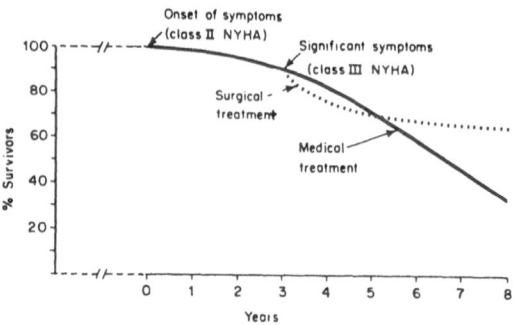

Fig. 3. Chronic aortic incompetence. Graph obtained from Mayo Clinic experience on the long-term survival of medical vs. surgical treatment. Observe that, from the moment patients develop significant symptoms, the long-term survival is better for patient who undergo surgical treatment.

died (Fig. 3) [7, 28]. Other investigators found that over 80% of high risk patients (those with a systolic blood pressure over 140 and diastolic blood pressure under 40 mm Hg, left ventricular strain on the electrocardiogram, and moderate or marked cardiomegaly) experienced either severe heart failure, angina or death within 6 years, while only 8% of those without any risk factors had similar outcomes [29].

From the pathophysiological point of view [30], the fundamental hemodynamic abnormality in aortic incompetence is the diastolic regurgitation of blood from the aorta into the left ventricle. In patients with significant chronic aortic incompetence, the diastolic runoff of blood into the left ventricle results in a large total systolic stroke volume. These two events explain the aortic diastolic and systolic murmurs, the characteristically dynamic carotid pulses, the wide pulse pressure and the detection by palpation of a hyperdynamic left ventricle displaced to the left. At rest, effective stroke volume is maintained by the Starling's law; that is, there is ejection of the increased left ventricular enddiastolic volume (which results from the diastolic regurgitation), with concomitant increase in total stroke volume and ejection fraction. The increased left ventricular volume and dilatation leads to myocardial fiber stretching and elongation and so to an increased wall stress. However, sarcomere replication and hypertrophic thickening tend to normalize left ventricular wall stress as described by the law of Laplace ($\sigma = Pa/2h$, where σ = circumferential wall stress, P = intraventricular pressure, a = intraventricular radius, and h = wall thickness).

Left ventricular decompensation at rest and/or exercise may be manifested:
a) by a decreased ejection fraction leading to an increase in endsystolic volume; this adds in diastole to the increased diastolic volume related to the

394

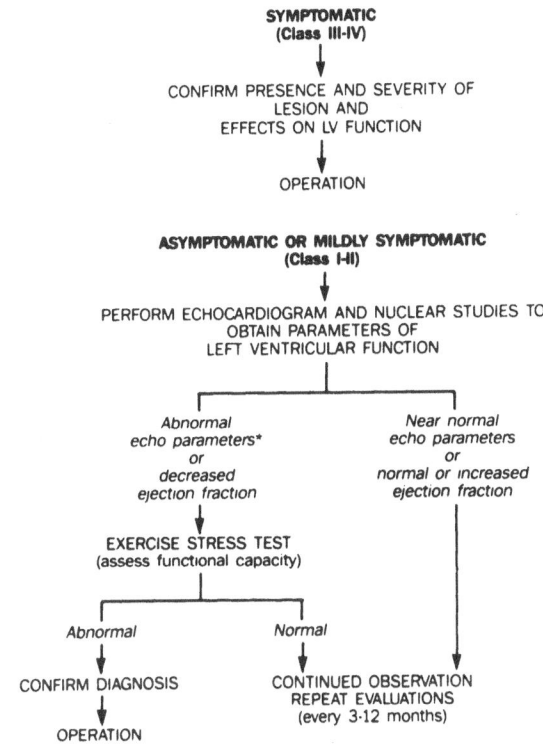

CHRONIC AORTIC VALVULAR INCOMPETENCE

SYMPTOMATIC
(Class III-IV)

CONFIRM PRESENCE AND SEVERITY OF
LESION AND
EFFECTS ON LV FUNCTION

OPERATION

ASYMPTOMATIC OR MILDLY SYMPTOMATIC
(Class I-II)

PERFORM ECHOCARDIOGRAM AND NUCLEAR STUDIES TO
OBTAIN PARAMETERS OF
LEFT VENTRICULAR FUNCTION

*Abnormal
echo parameters**
or
decreased
ejection fraction*

*Near normal
echo parameters
or
normal or increased
ejection fraction*

EXERCISE STRESS TEST
(assess functional capacity)

Abnormal

Normal

CONFIRM DIAGNOSIS

CONTINUED OBSERVATION
REPEAT EVALUATIONS
(every 3-12 months)

OPERATION

* FS <25%, ESD >55mm, Abnormal wall stress

diastolic regurgitation, all resulting in increased left ventricular end diastolic pressure and shortness of breath [31–35]; and

b) decompensation may also be manifested by an abnormal wall stress [36, 37], which may contribute to the angina. That is, increased left ventricular myocardial mass and, in advanced cases, increased wall stress augment total myocardial oxygen consumption; in addition, elevated wall stress decreases the subendocardial perfusion gradient by exerting extravascular compression on intramyocardial coronary arterioles; coronary blood flow, which occurs predominantly during diastole, is also reduced by the lower diastolic aortic pressure caused by the regurgitant valvular lesion. Likely, all or either of these factors explain the anginal symptoms in some of these patients.

Timing and indications of surgery (Fig. 3)

Optimal timing of aortic valve replacement in patients with significant aortic

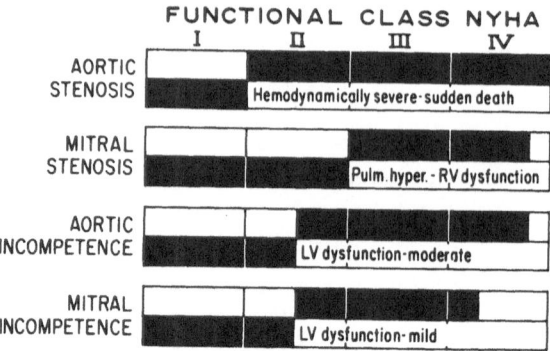

Fig. 5. Schematic surgical approach to the four conditions described in this chapter. Within each condition, the solid bar on the top represents the classical indication for operation according to the functional class of the patient. The solid bar on the bottom is representative of additional recent indication for surgery, the reasons being stated on the right.

incompetence remains elusive. Truly optimal timing of surgical intervention implies maximizing total overall life span and minimizing left ventricular dysfunction and symptoms. Our approach to the timing of aortic valve replacement has been summarized in Fig. 3. It is accepted that patients with moderate to severe symptoms (Class III and IV) deserve aortic valve replacement both for symptomatic relief and prolongation of life (Fig. 5) [28, 38–40]. It is widely felt, however, that results would be enhanced if operation were performed before significant symptoms develop, and that timing of operation should be based on the severity of aortic incompetence and degree of left ventricular dysfunction.

A number of recent studies suggest that intervention is reasonable in asymptomatic or minimally symptomatic patients with left ventricular systolic dysfunction [32, 39, 42–43]. Specifically, asymptomatic or minimally symptomatic patients (Class I–II) with evidence of left ventricular dysfunction (i.e. endsystolic diameter greater than 55 mm or fractional shortening less than 25–29%) and abnormal wall stress (enddiastolic radius/myocardial wall thickness ratio greater than 4.0) have a high likelihood of developing postoperative symptoms and shortened long term survival [44–46], suggesting that operation should be performed soon in these patients. In addition, a decreased radionuclear ejection fraction (lower than 45%) may also be considered in the operative range [47, 48]. Recent radionuclear studies indicate that left ventricular exercise dysfunction may be present in up to two-thirds of asymptomatic patients with a normal resting ejection fraction [49]. However, this indicator may be too sensitive to warrant operation since long-term prognosis may still be excellent [39]; nevertheless, may be a first warning to the physician for a closer follow up of the patient.

Based on all the above information, our approach in the asymptomatic or minimally symptomatic patient is to advise operation when two conditions are present:
a) the above specific degree of left ventricular dysfunction at rest, and
b) an impaired exercise capacity.
That is, in these asymptomatic or minimally symptomatic patients with some left ventricular dysfunction at rest, if preoperative exercise capacity is preserved, prognosis is better and operation might be temporarily deferred [39].

What can be expected from the surgical intervention with
aortic valve replacement?

There is growing information on the beneficial effects of aortic valve replacement in patients with significant aortic incompetence; this refers to survivorship, symptomatology and left ventricular function.

A reasonable estimate of perioperative mortality for patients with symptomatic predominant aortic incompetence at present would be 6–8%, and for minimally disabled patients, 2% [50]. We examined the long-term status of very symptomatic patients (Class III–IV) undergoing aortic valve replacement with Starr-Edwards prosthesis. Among the surgical survivors, probability of surviving to one year was 84%, to 10 years 52%, and to 15 years 40% [52]. In this group of very symptomatic patients with aortic incompetence, the surgical survivorship was significantly better than in similar patients treated medically [28]. However, such long term surgical survivorship in patients with aortic incompetence tends to be somewhat worse than in patients with aortic stenosis [53]. Regarding symptomatology, in our long term study the majority (80%) of patients with aortic valve replacement for aortic incompetence who were alive at the time of follow-up had improved symptomatically by at least one functional class. Regarding left ventricular function, about 60% of the patients with chronic aortic incompetence demonstrate normal left ventricular diastolic diameter eight months after operation; this outcome appears to be related to the degree of preoperative left-ventricular dysfunction as defined previously. Approximately half of operated patients demonstrate electro- and echocardiographically documented complete regression of left ventricular hypertrophy, especially those with relatively less ventricular dilatation preoperatively [54].

In summary, although early operation, in terms of postoperative clinical status and left ventricular function, appears to be of benefit, it is not yet exactly established when in the clinical course of the disease operation should be recommended. Nevertheless, important prognostic parameters of left ventricular function are emerging. In addition, emerging pathological and ultrastructural findings of irreversible myocardial changes, in the form of fibrosis and/or cellular degeneration [55–57] offer promise for the future understanding and better approach of these patients.

Mitral valve incompetence

Natural history and pathophysiology

Mitral incompetence may occur as a result of three general anatomic abnormalities:
a) primary alteration of the mitral valve leaflets or commisures;
b) anatomic or functional defects of the tensor apparatus; or
c) alteration of left ventricular and left atrial function.
Not uncommonly mitral incompetence may be produced by two or more of these anatomic abnormalities acting simultaneously. From a clinical point of view the three anatomical varieties can present:
a) as a chronic variety, or
b) as an acute or subacute variety [17].
In this section we will focus primary attention to chronic mitral incompetence as a result of primary alteration of the mitral valve or of the tensor apparatus.

Those patients with the insidious onset and gradual progression of mitral regurgitation, as occurs in chronic rheumatic mitral incompetence, have a prolonged asymptomatic interval of up to 20 years or more after the initiating event [58, 59] , and symptoms first appear in middle age or beyond [60]. In most cases, left atrial compliance and size increases to accommodate the regurgitant volume and effectively protects against marked elevation of pulmonary vascular pressure. Consequently, symptoms of pulmonary congestion are less prominent and occur late in the course of the disease [61]. Lassitude, fatigue, and generalized weakness reflecting low cardiac output as a result of the large regurgitant volume of blood ejected into an enlarged left atrium, tend to predominate as early symptoms, rather than frank dyspnea or pulmonary edema which are more likely to occur with mitral stenosis. Similarly, the intercurrent and frequent development of atrial fibrillation in about three-fourths of the patients [60] and the non infrequent occurrence of systemic emboli tend to be associated with an enlarged left atrium ($\geqslant 5$ cm) at echocardiography [62]. As left ventricular function deteriorates, exertional dyspnea, orthopnea, and paroxysmal nocturnal dyspnea become more prominent. Longevity of patients with chronic mitral incompetence depends, in part, on the point in the disease process from which follow-up is initiated. Patients in functional class III-IV had a 5-year survival of about 40% and 10-year survival of about 15%) [63, 64].

From the pathophysiological point of view, in mitral incompetence the systolic escape of blood into the left atrium with its subsequent diastolic return results in a large total left ventricular systolic stroke volume. Both events explain the detection by palpation of a hyperdynamic left ventricle displaced to the left (left ventricular enlargement), a quick upstroke of the pulse in the carotid artery, the ausculatory features of a diastolic filling sound (S_3, which does not necessarily imply left ventricular failure), and an apical holosystolic and short middiastolic murmur. In significant mitral incompetence the large total left ventricular systolic stroke volume is accomplished, like in aortic incompetence, by the Starling's law-compensatory ejection in the increased ventricular volume and by the development of left ventricular hypertrophy.

In contradistinction to aortic incompetence, in mitral incompetence of comparable severity the increase in left ventricular volume is less pronounced [65, 66], but most importantly, the diastolic acceptance of large volumes is without proportionate elevation of filling pressure. Thus, in addition to the left ventricular enddiastolic pressure which in relation with increased in volume may be relatively normal, in significant chronic mitral incompetence left ventricular hypertrophy develops concomitantly with dilatation of the chamber, so that the chamber volume to wall mass-ratio remains normal, thereby minimizing wall tension by the Laplace relationship [67]. The result of these factors is that myocardial oxygen consumption in mitral incompetence is less perturbed than in aortic incompetence. Thus, compensated state may be preserved for an extended period during which parameters of myocardial function, such as ejection fraction or velocity of fiber shortening remain normal or supranormal, and ventricular emptying is augmented. With time, left ventricular function deteriorates slowly, concomitant with the late development of symptoms. However, because of the persistent low resistance pathway for ejection, (opened mitral valve and low impedance left atrial chamber), the actual extent of left ventricular myocardial depression may not be apparent until elimination of the pathway by operation [68]. Indeed, conventional ejection phase parameters of myocardial function may be near normal in markedly decompensated patients, reflecting the fact that despite 'normal' left ventricular function, an inadequate proportion of stroke volume contributes to effective forward flow. Thus, only mildly reduced or even normal ejection fractions in patients with chronic mitral incompetence should be regarded as poor prognostic indicators [69, 70].

Our histologic studies of myocardial tissue from patients with chronic mitral incompetence and severe left ventricular failure have shown an increased proportion of interstitial fibrotic tissue [55]. This may explain, in part, the mechanism by which irreversible decompensation occurs. However, our most recent study suggest that in less severe but irreversible left ventricular failure interstitial fibrotic tissue is not necessarilly increased and, therefore, irreversible myocardial cell metabolic or ultrastructural changes have occurred [57].

Regarding significant pulmonary arterial hypertension leading to right ven-tricular hypertrophy and right ventricular failure, these are much less frequent in chronic isolated mitral incompetence than in mitral stenosis. This is because of the increased compliance of the large left atrium which, as discussed earlier, tends to accommodate the systolic regurgitant flow; and, by doing so, prevents a significant elevation of the pulmonary venous pressure, pulmonary vascular resistance and, therefore, of the pulmonary arterial pressure.

Timing and indication of surgery (Fig. 6)

The above observations imply that operation, either mitral valve repair or replacement, should be undertaken before the disease has progressed to an irreversible state. Nevertheless, precise hemodynamic and volumetric criteria to determine truly optimal timing have not been established and substantial controversy still exists. Also, the technical considerations favoring mitral valve repair versus mitral valve replacement are not fully established and out of the scope of this chapter; nevertheless, with the help of intraoperative contrast echocardiography for the assessment of competence of the mitral valve [23], valve repair will be more frequently attempted before considering mitral valve replacement.

Our approach (Fig. 6), which is in general agreement with other groups, is to offer operative intervention for patients who are clearly symptomatically limited [71], particularly those in functional Class III or IV [60]. However, because of the increased operative mortality and poor postoperative results, and until further data are available, we are reluctant to recommend surgery routinely for patients with ejection fraction below 25–30%. Pending new data, these patients should be treated vigorously with digitalis, diuretics, and vasodi-lators. If they make a good improvement with this therapy, they should be reevaluated for surgery and, in such case, if at all possible, preservation of the chordae tendinaeae and papillary muscles, should be attempted since it ap-pears to provide better hemodynamic results than with conventional valve replacement [73, 74].

Asymptomatic patients or patients with mild symptoms, but with normal or low ejection fraction, might be considered surgical candidates, particularly if associated with certain echocardiographic parameters. Thus, in chronic mitral incompetence, probably, an accurate echocardiographic assessment of global left ventricular function is based on estimates of ventricular systolic wall stress (e.g. radius-thickness ratio) and ventricular systolic volume as assessed echo-cardiographically [70, 75]; that is, the so called endsystolic wall stress-end-systolic volume index ratio (ESWS/ESVI), takes into account ventricular function under possible preload and afterload changing conditions. Therefore, a left ventricular ESWS/ESVI of less than 2.5 [70, 75] and fractional shortening

400

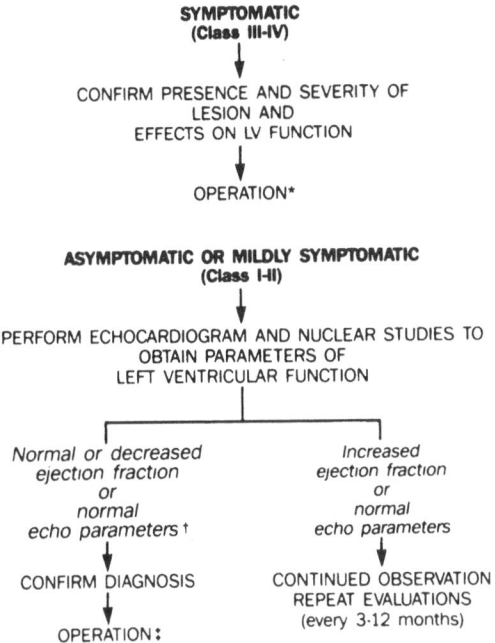

CHRONIC MITRAL VALVE INCOMPETENCE

SYMPTOMATIC
(Class III-IV)
↓
CONFIRM PRESENCE AND SEVERITY OF
LESION AND
EFFECTS ON LV FUNCTION
↓
OPERATION*

ASYMPTOMATIC OR MILDLY SYMPTOMATIC
(Class I-II)
↓
PERFORM ECHOCARDIOGRAM AND NUCLEAR STUDIES TO
OBTAIN PARAMETERS OF
LEFT VENTRICULAR FUNCTION

Normal or decreased | Increased
ejection fraction | ejection fraction
or | or
normal | normal
echo parameters † | echo parameters
↓ | ↓
CONFIRM DIAGNOSIS | CONTINUED OBSERVATION
↓ | REPEAT EVALUATIONS
OPERATION: | (every 3-12 months)

* Questionable if ejection fraction <25-30%
† FS <30%. Wall stress/Volume
‡ Also consider in atrial fibrillation or pulmonary hypertension with
  RV dysfunction

of less than 30% [76], when associated with normal or low ejection should lead to surgical consideration; on the other hand, patients with increased ejection fraction may be observed serially every 6 to 12 months. Finally, the development of atrial fibrillation [76, 77] or significant pulmonary hypertension with right ventricular dysfunction should be considered late manifestations also leading to surgical consideration.

What can be expected from the surgical intervention?

Details of the postoperative course and follow-up after mitral valve reconstruction are presently evolving [78]. More body of information is available regarding valve replacement. Thus, there is now good information on the beneficial effects of mitral valve replacement in patients with significant mitral incompetence; this refers to survivorship, symptomatology and left ventricular function.

Reports of postoperative survival of isolated mitral incompetence employ various operative techniques (repair or replacement) and variable patient selection. In general, patients with mitral incompetence have lower survival than those with mitral stenosis [79, 80]. Operative mortality has been reported in the 5–12% range [71, 79, 81, 82]. Our study patients undergoing valve replacement between 1963 and 1971 for very symptomatic isolated mitral incompetence had a postoperative survivorship of about 70% at 5 years, 50% at 10 years and 40% at 15 years [52]. Such surgical survivorship was much better than in similar disabled patients treated medically [63]. Regarding symptomatology, in our study a large majority (72%) of patients with mitral valve replacement for mitral incompetence who were alive at the time of follow-up had improved symptomatically by at least one functional class. Regarding left ventricular function the postoperative hemodynamic response may depend on the degree to which ventricular function is depressed by chronic irreversible myocardial damage [83]. As previously discussed, the majority of patients demonstrate a decline in ejection fraction following successful valve replacement [68, 71, 84], probably due to the net effect of two factors: cumulative permanent myocardial damage, and the increase of the afterload by the valve replacement which eliminates the low resistance pathway as mentioned, preservation of the chordae and papillary muscles ameliorates this problem. In general, estimation of the postoperative ejection fraction should allow for a likely decrease of 10–20% early after valve replacement; also, in mitral incompetence, unlike aortic incompetence, the ejection fraction is more likely to remain depressed late postoperatively as well [85].

In summary, as in chronic aortic incompetence, in chronic mitral incompetence early operation appears to be of benefit, but is not yet exactly established when in the clinical course of the disease operation should be recommended. Again, emerging pathological and ultrastructural findings of irreversible myocardial changes, in the form of fibrosis and/or cellular dysfunction, offer promise for the future understanding and better approach of these patients.

Tricuspid valve incompetence

Natural history and pathophysiology

In acquired valvular heart disease, tricuspid disease usually takes the form of incompetence; and if stenosis is present, it is commonly associated with some degree of incompetence. In addition, acquired tricuspid disease is commonly associated with disease in one or two of the other cardiac valves. In this section we will specifically discuss acquired chronic tricuspid incompetence [17, 86, 87].

Usually, acquired tricuspid incompetence is a functional derangement secondary to dilatation of the right ventricle, which occurs in response to pulmonary hypertension from rheumatic mitral valve disease or, less often, chronic cor pulmonale. In a minority of patients, chronic tricuspid incompetence is organic in nature and tends to be of rheumatic origin, which is almost always associated with mitral valve disease and, often, with aortic valve disease also. Chronic tricuspid incompetence of congenital origin, in the form of Ebstein's anomaly or atrioventricular canal defect, subacute tricuspid incompetence secondary to carcinoid syndrome, and acute or subacute tricuspid incompetence secondary to bacterial endocarditis in narcotic addicts are out of the scope of this chapter.

The natural history and clinical course of acquired chronic tricuspid incompetence is not well established since generally is dictated by the left heart lesions. From a pathophysiological point of view, in chronic tricuspid incompetence some of the hemodynamics of the right ventricle and right atrium are probably similar to the hemodynamics of the left ventricle and left atrium as discussed in the section of mitral incompetence; however, as mentioned before, the assessment and understanding of right ventricular function are still at a very early stage of our knowledge. The symptoms of significant tricuspid disease include fatigue related to reduced cardiac output and dyspnea that probably is primarily related to the associated mitral and aortic valvular disease. The presence of edema, ascites, and hepatic congestion with right upper quadrant or epigastric discomfort are all late manifestations of significant tricuspid incompetence or severe right ventricular failure. The most important physical sign of tricuspid incompetence is prominent systolic venous pulsation of the neck veins, and if the incompetence is severe, a pulsatile enlarged liver can be detected by manual palpation.

Timing and indications of surgery

Usually, the management of patients with acquired tricuspid incompetence is determined by the more severe left-sided valvular lesions. If the tricuspid disease results in significant hepatic congestion and ankle edema, treatment with diuretics will be started. However, with the diuretic treatment, the improvement in the signs and symptoms of systemic venous hypertension is frequently associated with an increasing feeling of tiredness because of further reduction of the low cardiac output.

Tricuspid valvular surgery should be definitely considered at the time of operation for the left-sided valvular lesions (which produce pulmonary hypertension leading to the incompetent valve), if there is evidence of symptomatic (Class III–IV) systemic venous congestion, and the clinical diagnosis of significant tricuspid incompetence is confirmed by the surgical examination and intraoperative contrast echocardiography [88]. Operation should also probably be performed even in the patient without significant systemic venous congestion but, when at the time of operation for the left sided valvular lesions (again causing pulmonary hypertension and the incompetent valve), the diagnosis of significant tricuspid incompetence is made by the surgical examination and intraoperative echocardiography [88]. Finally, operation should be considered when the tricuspid incompetence is the only significant valvular lesion and the patient continues to be very symptomatic despite a good diuretic regimen; these are patients with organic tricuspid incompetence or with residual tricuspid incompetence following previous left sided valvular surgery or tricuspid repair. The problem with such patients is that operation by increasing the right ventricular afterload can lead to further decompensation, particularly if there is significant preoperative right ventricular dysfunction. Unfortunately, as discussed previously in the chapter, in the context of indications for surgical interventions, preoperative assessment and definition of right ventricular dysfunction are still in the very early stage of development.

The operation of choice for functional tricuspid incompetence is the De Vega annuloplasty, and the operation of choice for organic tricuspid incompetence and stenosis is a wide commissurotomy followed by the annuloplasty [89]. Such reconstructive procedures are usually successful because of the lack of calcification of the tricuspid valve [90]; in addition, if possible, valve replacement should be avoided because of the incidence of prosthetic dysfunction and thrombosis, even of the porcine valve, which is one of the prosthesis of choice if valvular reconstruction cannot be accomplished.

What we can expect from the surgical intervention

There is a clinical impression that when significant tricuspid incompetence is associated to mitral or aortic valve disease and pulmonary hypertension, amelioration of the pulmonary hypertension by the operation on the left-sided valve plus additional repair of the tricuspid valve tend to lead to a good surgical result. On the other hand, without amelioration of the pulmonary hypertension and with significant preoperative right ventricular dysfunction, repair of the tricuspid valve may lead to a poor surgical result. When tricuspid incompetence is the only significant valvular lesion, the repair of the tricuspid valve may provide a poor surgical result if there is significant right ventricular dysfunction.

As mentioned, when, instead of tricuspid valve repair, valve replacement is performed the results appear to be less good. Nevertheless, part of the morbidity and mortality in these patients is also dependant from the left sided valvular surgery. Our recent study of 86 patients with triple valve replacement indicates that perioperative mortality whilst high is declining; actuarially determined 10-year survival in perioperative survivors was 54% with excellent symptomatic improvement in these patients. Arrhythmia or sudden unexpected death was the major cause of late death, with thromboembolism and prosthetic valve dysfunction (particularly involving the tricuspid valve) the major cause of late morbidity [91].

References

1. Wood P: Aortic stenosis. Am J Cardiol 1: 553, 1958.
2. Wagner HR, Weidman WH, Ellison RC, Miettinen OS: Indirect assessment of severity in aortic stenosis. Circulation 56: 1–20, 1977.
3. Ross J Jr, Braunwald E: Aortic stenosis. Circulation 37–38: V–61, 1968.
4. Wagner HR, Ellison RC, Keane JF, Humphries JON, Nadas AS: Circulation (Suppl 1) 56: 47.
5. Frank S, Johnson A, Ross J: Natural history of valvular aortic stenosis. Br Heart J 1973; 35: 41.
6. Barnhorst DA, Oxman HA, Conolly DC et al.: Isolated replacement of the aortic valve with the Starr-Edwards prosthesis. J Thorac Cardiovasc Surg 1975; 70: 113.
7. Brandenburg RO, Fuster V, Giuliani ER: Valvular heart: When should the patient be referred? Pract Cardiol 1979; 5: 8: 50.
8. Rahimtoola SH, Chandraratna PAN: Valvular Heart Disease. In: John A. Spittell Jr (ed) Clinical medicine, Harper and Row 1983; pp 1–51.
9. Barnhorst DA, Oxman HA, Connolly DC, Pluth JR et al.: Long-term follow-up of isolated replacement of the aortic or mitral valve with the Starr-Edwards prosthesis. Am J Cardiol 1975; 35: 228.
10. Starr A, Grunkemeier G, Lambert LE, Thomas DR et al.: Aortic valve replacement: A ten-year follow-up of non-cloth-covered vs. cloth-covered caged ball prosthesis. Circulation 1977; 56 (Suppl 2): 11–133.
11. Oyer PE, Miller DC, Stinson EB, Reitz BA et al.: Clinical durability of the Hancock porcine bioprosthetic valve. J Thorac Cardiovasc Surg 1980; 80: 824.
12. Bjork VO, Henze A: Ten years experience with the Bjork-Shilley tilting disc valve. J Thorac Cardiovasc Surg 1979; 78: 331.
13. Smith N, McAnulty JH, Rahimtoola SH: Severe aortic stenosis with impaired left ventricular function and clinical heart failure: Results of a valve replacement. Circulation 1978; 58: 255.
14. Murphy E, Lawson RM, Starr A, Rahimtoola SH: Severe aortic stenosis in patients 60 years and older: State of left ventricular function and result of valve replacement on 10 year survival. Circulation 1981; 64 (Suppl 2): 184.
15. Wood P: An appreciation of mitral stenosis. Br Med J 1954; I: 105.
16. Rowe JC, Bland F, Sprague HB et al.: Course of mitral stenosis without surgery: ten and twenty year perspectives. Ann Intern Med 1960; 52: 741.
17. Fuster V, Brandenburg RO, Giuliani ER, McGoon DC: Clinical approach and management of acquired valvular heart disease. In the Adult Cardiovasc Clinics 1980; 10: 3, 125.
18. Pumphrey CW, Fuster V, Chesebro JH: Systemic thromboembolism in valvular heart disease and prosthetic heart valves. Mod Con Cardiovasc Dis 1982; 51: 131.
19. Cohen M, Fuster V: What do we gain from the analysis of right ventricular function? J Am Coll Cardiol 1984; 3: 1082.
20. Cohen M, Horowitz SF, Machac J, Mindich BP, Fuster V: The response of right ventricle to exercise in isolated mitral stenosis: observation before and after surgical correction. J Amer Coll Cardiol (in press).

21. Logan A, Lowther CP, Turner RWD: Reoperation for mitral stenosis. Lancet I: 433, 1962.
22. Heger JJ, Wann LS, Weyman AE et al.: Long-term changes in mitral valve area after successful mitral commissurotomy. Circulation 1979; 59: 433.
23. Goldman ME, Mindich BP, Teichholz LE, Burgess N, Staville K, Fuster V: Intraoperative contrast echocardiography for the evaluation of mitral valve operations. J Am Coll Cardiol 1985; 6: 370–376.
24. Rotman M, Morris JJ, Behar VS et al.: Aortic valvular disease: Comparison of types and their medical and surgical management. Am J Med 1971; 51: 241.
25. Magida MG, Streitfeld FH: The natural history of rheumatic heart disease in the third, fourth, and fifth decades of life. II. Prognosis and special reference to morbidity. Circulation 1957; 16: 713.
26. McDonald: Circulation 1980; 61: 1291.
27. Hegglin R, Scheu H, Rothlin M: Aortic insufficiency. Circulation 1968; 38 (Suppl 5):77.
28. McGoon MD, Fuster V, Pluth JR, McGoon DC: Medical and surgical long term follow-up (10–21 years) of chronic aortic incompetence. Circulation 1981; 64: IV–76.
29. Spagnuolo M, Kloth H, Taranta A, Doyle E, Pasternack B: Natural history of rheumatic aortic regurgitation: Criteria predictive of death, congestive heart failure, and angina in young patients. Circulation 1971; 44: 368.
30. Laniado S, Yellin EL, Yoran C et al.: Physiologic mechanisms in aortic insufficiency. I. The effect of changing heart rate on flow dynamics. II. Determinants of Austin-Flint murmur. Circulation 1982; 66: 226.
31. Dehmer GJ, Firth BG, Hillis LD, Corbett JR, Lewis SE, Parkey RW, Willerson JT: Alterations in left ventricular volumes and ejection fraction at rest and during exercise in patients with aortic regurgitation. Am J Cardiol 1981; 48: 17.
32. Ricci DR: Afterload mismatch and preload reserve in chronic aortic regurgitation. Circulation 1982; 66: 826.
33. Osbakken M, Bove AA, Spann JF: Left ventricular function in chronic aortic regurgitation with reference to end-systolic pressure, volume and stress relations. Am J Cardiol 1981; 47: 193.
34. Thompson R, Ross I, McHaffie D, Leslie P, Easthope R, Elmes R: Left ventricular function in asymptomatic patients with severe aortic regurgitation: Relation to clinical parameters and exercise performance. Clin Cardiol 1982; 5: 523.
35. Schuler G, Von Olshausen K, Schwarz F et al.: Noninvasive assessment of myocardial contractility in asymptomatic patients with severe aortic regurgitation and normal left ventricular ejection fraction at rest. Am J Cardiol 1982; 50: 45.
36. Goldman ME, Packer M, Horowitz SF, Meller J, Patterson RE, Kukin M, Teichholz LE, Gorlin R: Relation between exercise-indiced changes in ejection franction and systolic loading conditions at rest in aortic regurgitation. J Am Coll Cardiol 1984; 3: 924.
37. Kumpuris AG, Quinones MA, Waggoner AD, Kanon DJ, Nelson JG, Miller RR: Importance of preoperative hypertrophy, wall stress and end-systolic dimension as echocardiographic predictors of normalization of left ventricular dilatation after valve replacement in chronic aortic insufficiency. Am J Cardiol 1982; 41: 1091.
38. Samuels DA, Curfman GD, Friedlick AL, Buckley MJ, Austeu WG: Valve replacement for aortic regurgitation: long-term follow-up with factors influencing the results. Circulation 1979; 60: 647.
39. Bonow RO, Rosing DR, Kent KM, Epstein SE: Timing of operation for chronic aortic regurgitation. Am J Cardiol 1982; 50: 325.
40. Smith, Neutz, Roche, Agnew, Barrott-Boyer BG: The natural history of rheumatic aortic regurgitation and the indications for surgery. Br Heart J 1976; 38: 147.
41. Forman R, Firsth BG, Bernard MS: Prognostic significance of preoperative left ventricular

eyection franction and valve lesion in patients with aortic valve replacement. Am J Cardiol 1980; 45: 1120.

42. Herreman F, Amewz A, deVernejoul F et al.: Pre- and postoperative hemodynamic and cineangiographic assessment of left ventricular function in patients with aortic regurgitation. Am Heart J 1979; 98: 63.

43. Rahimtoola SH: Valve replacement should not be performed in all asymptomatic patients with aortic incompetence. J Thorac Cardiovasc Surg 1980; 79: 163.

44. Gaasch WH, Carroll JD, Levine HJ, Criscitiello MG: Chronic aortic regurgitation: prognostic value of left ventricular end-systolic dimension and end-diastolic radius/thickness ratio. J Am Coll Cardiol 1983; 1: 775.

45. Cunha CLP, Giuliani ER, Fuster V, Seward JB, Brandenburd RO, McGoon DC: Preoperative M-mode echocardiography as a predictor of surgical results in chronic aortic insufficiency. J Thorac Cardiovas Surg 1980; 79: 2: 256.

46. Henry WL, Bonow RO, Rosing DR, Epstein SE: Observation on the optimum time for operative intervention for aortic regurgitation: II. Serial echocardiographic evaluation of asymptomatic patients. Circulation 1980; 61: 484.

47. Fioretti P, Roelandt J, Bos RJ, Meltzer RS, Hoogenhuuze DV, Serruys PW, Nauta J, Hugenoltz PG: Echocardiography in chronic aortic insufficiency: Is valve replacement too late when left ventricular end-systolic dimension reaches 55 mm? Circulation 1983; 67: 216.

48. Greves J, Rahimtoola SH, McAnulty JH et al.: Preoperative criteria predictive of late survival following valve replacement for severe aortic regurgitation. Am Heart J 1981; 101: 300.

49. Borer JS, Bacharach SL, Green MV et al.: Exercise-induced left ventricular dysfunction in symptomatic and asymptomatic patients with aortic regurgitation: Assessment with radionuclide cineangiography. Am J Cardiol 1978; 42: 351.

50. McGoon DC: Editorial: Valve replacement for aortic incompetence. J Thorac Cardiovasc Surg 1980; 79: 169.

51. Huxley RL, Gaffney FA, Corbett JR, Firth BG, Peshock R, Nicod P, Rellas JS, Curry G, Lewis SE, Willerson JT: Early detection of left ventricular dysfunction in chronic aortic regurgitation as assessed by contrast angiography, echocardiography, and rest and exercise scintigraphy. Am J Cardiol 1983; 51: 1542.

52. McGoon MD, Fuster V, McGoon DC, Pumphrey CW, Pluth JR, Elveback LR: Aortic and mitral valve incompetence: Long-term follow-up (10 to 19 years) of patients treated with the Starr-Edwards prosthesis. J Am Coll Card 1984; 3: 4, 930.

53. Murphy E, Lawson RM, Starr A, Rahimtoola SH: Severe aortic stenosis in patients 60 years and older: State of left ventricular function and result of valve-replacement on 10 year survival. Circulation 1981; 64 (Suppl 2): 184.

54. Carroll JD, Gaasch WH, Naimi S, Levine HF: Regression of myocardial hypertrophy: electrocardiographic-echocardiographic correlations after aortic valve replacement in patients with chronic aortic regurgitation. Circulation 1982; 65: 980.

55. Fuster V, Danielson MA, Robb RA, Broadbent JC, Brown AL: Quantitation of left ventricular myocardial fiber hypertrophy and of interstitial tissue in human hearts with pressure and volume overload. Circulation 1977; 55: 504.

56. Donaldson RM: Left ventricular hypertrophy in aortic valve disease: regression of ventricular mass and volume following surgery for chronic volume overload. Eur Heart J 1983; 3: A: 179.

57. Pumphrey CW, Fuster V, Pluth JR: Myocardial histology in patients with pressure and volume overload of the left ventricle: Relationships to preoperative parameters and postoperative results (in preparation).

58. Magida MG, Streitfeld FH: The natural history of rheumatic heart disease in the third fourth and fifth decades of life. II. Prognosis and special reference to morbidity. Circulation 1962; 16: 713.

59. Wilson MG: The life history of systolic murmurs in rheumatic heart disease. Prog Cardiovasc Dis 1962; 5: 145.

60. Selzer A, Katayama F: Mitral regurgitation: Clinical patterns, pathophysiology and natural history. Medicine 1972; 51: 337.

61. Braunwald E, Awe WC: The syndrome of severe mitral regurgitation with normal left atrial pressure. Circulation 1962; 27: 29.

62. Sherrid MR, Clark RD, Cohn K: Echocardiographic analysis of left atrial size before and after operation in mitral valve disease. Am J Cardiol 1979; 43: 2, 171.

63. Fuster V, Pluth JR, Giuliani ER, Brandenburg RO, McGoon DC: Medical and surgical long term follow-up (10–19 years) of chronic mitral incompetence. Circulation 1980; 62: 111.

64. Muñoz S, Gallardo J, Diaz-Gorrin JR, Medina O: Influence of surgery on the natural history of rheumatic mitral and aortic valve disease. Am J Cardiol 1975; 35: 234.

65. Urschel CW, Covell JW, Sonnenblick ED et al.: Myocardial mechanics in aortic and mitral valvular regurgitation: the concept of instantaneous impedance as a determinant of the performance of the intact heart. J Clin Invest 1968; 47: 867.

66. Braunwald E: Mitral regurgitation: physiologic, clinical and surgical considerations. N Engl J Med 1969; 281: 425.

67. Sasayama S, Kubo S, Kusukawa R: Hemodynamic and angiocardiographic studies on cardiodynamics. Experimental mitral insufficiency. Jpn Circ J 1970; 34: 513–530.

68. Wong CYH, Spotnitz HM: Systolic and diastolic properties of the human left ventricle during valve replacement for chronic mitral regurgitation. Am J Cardiol 1981; 47: 40.

69. Schuler G, Peterson KL, Johnson A et al.: Temporal response of left ventricular performance to mitral valve surgery. Circulation 1979; 59: 1218.

70. Carabello BA, Nolan ST, McGuire LB: Assessment of preoperative left ventricular function in patients with mitral regurgitation: Value of the end-systolic wall stress-end-systolic volume ratio. Circulation 1981; 64: 6, 1212.

71. Kay JH, Zubiate P, Méndez MA et al.: Mitral valve repair for significant mitral insufficiency. Am Heart J 1978; 96: 253.

72. Fowler NO, Van der Bel-Kahn JM: Indications for surgical replacement of the mitral valve with particular reference to common and uncommon causes of mitral regurgitation. Am J Cardiol 1979; 44: 148.

73. David TE, Uden DE, Strauss HD: The importance of the mitral apparatus in left ventricular function after correction of mitral regurgitation. Circulation 1983; 68 (Suppl 2): 76.

74. David TE, Druck MM, Burns RJ: Mitral valve replacement for mitral regurgitation with and without preservation of chordae tendinae. Proceedings of the Sixty-fourth Annual Meetings of the American Association of Thoracic Surgeons, May 1984; 52.

75. Carabello BA, Spann JF: The uses and limitations of end-systolic indexes of left ventricular function. Circulation 1984; 69: 5, 1058.

76. Cunha CLP, Giuliani ER, Fuster V, Brandenburg RO, McGoon DC: Preoperative M-mode echocardiography as a predictor of surgical results in chronic mitral insufficiency (Abstract). Am J Cardiol 1980; 45: 442.

77. Bonchek LI: Indications for surgery of the mitral valve. Am J Cardiol 1980; 46: 155.

78. Carpentier A, Chavraud S, Fabiani JN et al.: Reconstructive surgery of mitral valve incompetence: Ten year appraisal. J Thorac Cardiovasc Surg 1980; 79: 338.

79. Salomon NW, Stinson EB, Greipp RB et al.: Patient-related risk factors as predictors of results following isolated mitral valve replacement. Ann Thorac Surg 1977; 24: 519.

80. Rahimtoola SH: Valvular heart disease: A perspective. J Am Coll Cardiol 1983; 1: 199.

81. Dalby AJ, Firth BG, Forman R: Preoperative factors affecting the outcome of isolated mitral valve replacement: At 10 year review. Am J Cardiol 1981; 47: 826.

82. Starr A, Grunkemeier G, Lambert L et al.: Mitral valve replacement: A ten-year follow-up of

non-cloth-covered vs. cloth-covered caged-ball prostheses. Circulation 1976; 54 (Suppl 3): 47.

83. Phillips HR, Levine FH, Carter JE et al.: Mitral valve replacement for isolated mitral regurgitation: Analysis of clinical course and late postoperative left ventricular ejection fraction. Am J Cardiol 1981; 48: 647.

84. Kennedy JW, Doces JG, Steward DK: Left ventricular function before and following surgical treatment of mitral valve disease. Am Heart J 1979; 97: 592.

85. Boucher CA, Bingham JB, Osbakken MD et al.: Early changes in left ventricular size and function after correction of left ventricular volume overload. Am J Cardiol 1981; 47: 991.

86. Glancy DL, Marcus FI, Cuadra M et al.: Isolated organic tricuspid regurgitation. Am J Med 1969; 46: 989.

87. Sbar S, Dariceff G, Nightgale D et al.: Chronic tricuspid insufficiency. South Med J 1973; 66: 917.

88. Goldman G, Mindich B, Guarino T, Fuster V: Intraoperative contrast echo: A new method to evaluate tricuspid regurgitation (In preparation).

89. De Vega NF: La anuloplastia selectiva, regulable y permanente. Rev Esp Cardiolog 1972; 25: 6.

90. Reed GE, Bod AD, Spencer FC et al.: Operative management of tricuspid regurgitation. Circulation 1976; 54 (Suppl 3): 96.

91. Vatterott PJ, Gersh BJ, Fuster V, Schaff HV, Danielson GK, Pluth JR, McGoon DC: Long-term follow-up (2–20 years) of patients with triple valve replacement (Abstract). J Am Coll Cardiol 1983; 1: 586.

8.5 Diagnosis of Prosthetic Dysfunction by means of Echocardiography and Doppler Ultrasound

P. YUSTE PESCADOR

For more than 10 years, since M-mode echocardiography began to be used, attempts have been made to visualize the mobility and characteristics of valvular prostheses. Since then, numerous valve models have appeared on the market and the changes echocardiographic technique have undergone are profound; today, echocardiography is based on M-mode recording, bidimensional examination and Doppler scanning.

Mitral prostheses

M-mode echocardiography is used to visualize the echoes that correspond to the fixed (implantation ring and cage) and mobile portions (disk or disks) of any metallic prosthesis model. The peculiarities of each system are well known and deviations from normality are easily discovered. In addition, there are *secondary anomalies* due to changes in rhythm, alterations in intracavitary pressures, reduced flow due to cardiomyopathy, etc. On the other hand, there are *primary anomalies* due to intrinsic prosthetic malfunction. An increase in echo density in the zone corresponding to the prosthesis and the absence of occlusor element movement indicate prosthetic thrombosis. In other cases, observation of a delay in valve opening or closure, or a reduction in valve mobility reflects the existence of an impediment to normal mobility caused by a thrombus or wear and deformation of the prosthetic material. A sign we described more than 10 years ago is a protodiastolic bobbing of the prosthesis which suggests the existence of suture dehiscence, although the sign also may appear in other circumstances.

In biological prostheses the echoes corresponding to the implantation ring and the movement of the sigmoid cusps of the prosthesis can be studied. These images recall the echo of the aortic (tricuspid) valve implanted in mitral position. Ring mobility does not seem to be a useful criteria for discriminating between the different functional anomalies – prosthetic stenosis or incompe-

BIOLOGICAL MITRAL PROTHESIS

Vmax = 1,8 m/s   Initial grad. 13 mmHg   Diastolic area 1,1 cm²

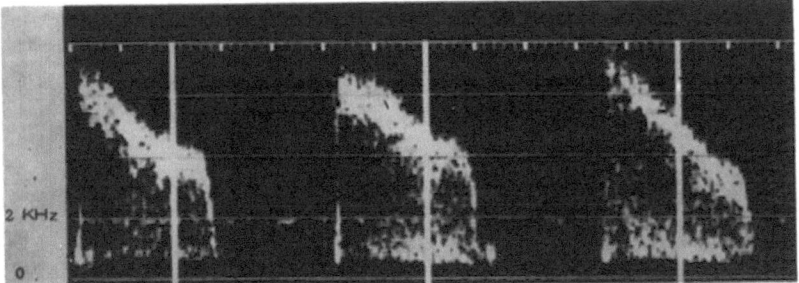

Fig. 1. Doppler recording of atrioventricular flow through a biological mitral prosthesis. From the maximum initial diastolic velocity, the initial gradient is calculated with the Bernouilli formula. The Hatle method serves to deduce functional diastolic area, which is decreased in this case.

tence. Examination of the echo density of the sigmoids, which is related to degeneration and fibrosis of the valvular cusps, is more interesting. As for the peculiarities of cusp movement, diastolic fluttering of the cusps does not indicate dysfunction, but reflects only the anatomic integrity of the cusps and absence of fibrosis, which would be related to sigmoid eversion

Bidimensional echocardiography obtains a cross-section of the heart. Different views should be used, the most useful being the apical parasternal or the four-chamber view. Metal prostheses are very reflective and produce abnormal and cyclic echoes that should be identified as artifacts. This does not occur with biological prostheses, in which the sigmoid cusps can be visualized. The bidimensional technique is also useful to study the left ventricle. The technique is of great importance to diagnose valvular eversion of a biological valve.

The Doppler technique is today important in evaluating the different models of prosthesis in mitral position. The acustic focus window is apical to obtain a good image of all four chambers. As such, the Doppler beam is emitted at the same angle over left atrioventricular flow, thus facilitating a reliable calculation of the Doppler velocities. A postoperative study is necessary for each patient and there should be successive follow-up studies, that can be compared with the control study. Using the pulsed Doppler technique, flow direction can be localized, which depends on the prosthesis model or the placement of the prosthetic occlusor element in each case. Once this is found, a good recording of the different diastolic transprosthetic flow speeds must be obtained, which requires utilization of pulsed Doppler with sample multiplication or continuous Doppler. The next step consists in extrapolating transprosthetic pressures from the speeds obtained using Bernouilli's reduced formula. As a

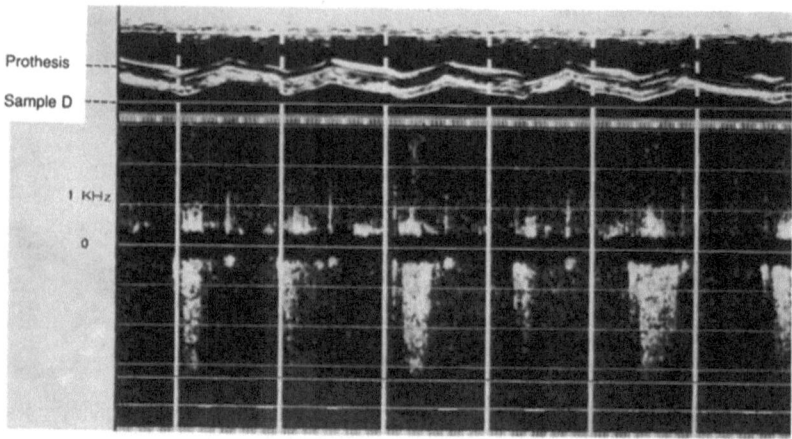

Fig. 2. Left atrial scanning with a Doppler sample volume (Sample D) in a patient with an Angell-Shilley mitral prosthesis and eversion of a prosthetic sigmoid. A turbulent regurgitation, variable in intensity and duration is detected during systole. This finding concurred with cardiac auscultation that found a variable systolic 'cackle'.

complement to this information, functional diastolic area can be calculated with the Hatle technique. These two types of calculation, pressure and area, should be obtained with every model or type of prosthesis (Fig. 1).

Another application of interest for pulsed Doppler is to detect regurgitation flow. To do so, the left atrium with the sample volume has to be scanned. A serious drawback observed is the reverberation phenomenon of metallic prostheses, which produce sound artifacts in the left atrium and impedes correct Doppler scanning. In some cases, this phenomenon can be palliated by studying the patients from the parasternal focus. In the biological prostheses, which do not produce reverberation, the apical plane continues to be the most indicated focus (Fig. 2).

Aortic prostheses

Examination with *M mode echocardiography* of the prosthesis in aortic position is more difficult. From the parasternal area, the movement of the occlusor element of metallic prostheses is not always correctly recorded, requiring use of the suprasternal, supraclavicular and even apical views. The normofunctional prosthesis exhibits systolic occlusor aperture and diastolic closure movements. Biological prostheses offer images similar to those of the normal aortic valve, with a reinforced echo density proceding from the implantation ring. Anomalies in the movement of mobile elements should be carefully evaluated, because images of abnormality determined by the position of the transducer

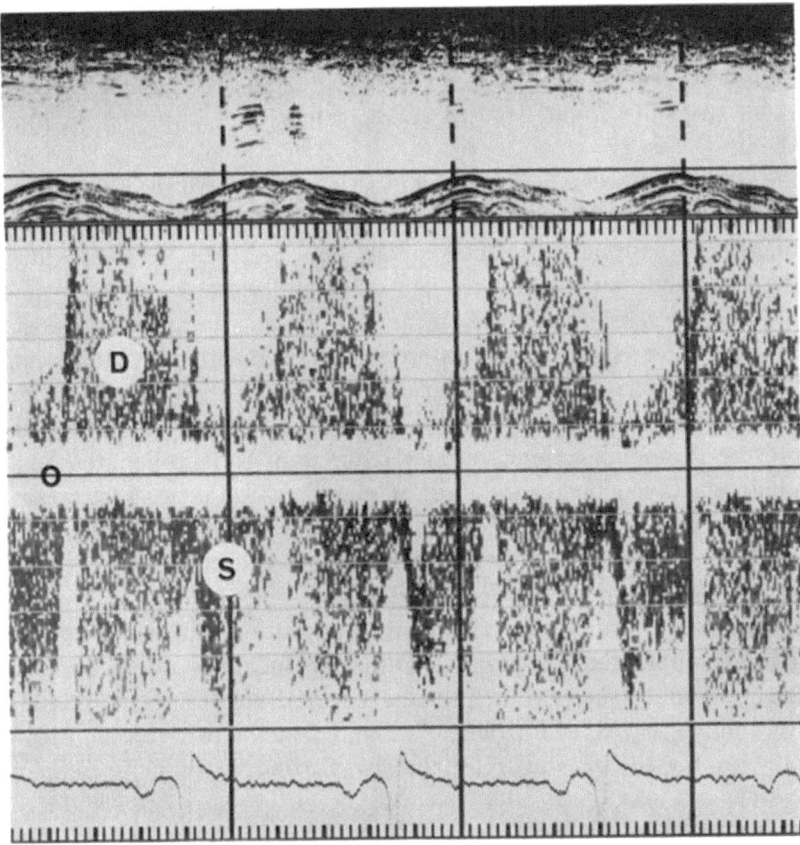

Fig. 3. Examination from the apex of the left ventricular outflow tract in a case with incompetent metallic prosthesis. In systole (S), the left ventricular outflow is recorded. In diastole (D), diastolic turbulence occupying the entire diastole is demonstrated and prosthetic regurgitation is evidenced.

and its incidence on the prosthesis are frequent. In biological prostheses, the malfunction criteria are similar to those described for bioprostheses in the mitral position. *Bidimensional echocardiography* affords few new data. In general, the M-mode technique helps to better direct the sound wave beam and to individually examine sigmoid cusp movement in biological models.

The Doppler technique is used to study aortic outflow from the suprasternal view. The study angle is appropriate for obtaining a systolic velocity curve. It is indispensable to scan the aortic supravalvular zone to determine maximum outflow near the prosthetic valve and to calculate the 'peak' gradient from the maximum volocity. However, it must be kept in mind that the finding of elevated systolic aortic flow velocities may not necessarily imply obstruction, as in cases of an increased cardiac output. The presence of prosthetic regurgitation also increments flow. For this reason, it is important to determine the delay in the maximum flow peak with respect to the onset of ventricular ejection. In view of this, it seems more advisable to calculate the mean gradient from the complete flow curve, rather than from the endsystolic gradient.

It is simple to ascertain if regurgitation is present with the Doppler technique. From the parasternal area, the left ventricular outflow tract can be scanned and diastolic turbulence can be detected. This view provides an inadequate study angle, but the aim of its utilization is qualitative. The four-chamber section which also includes the aorta is useful to correct the study angle. The regurgitation flow produces a turbulence that can be quantified by various criteria. One criterion is time, specified by the period in diastole where turbulence appears (remembering that many models of metallic prosthesis produce a slight 'normal' regurgitation). Another method is by mapping, classifying the regurgitation as mild when turbulence is located in the subvalvular area, moderate when it is detected in a more extensive section of the outflow tract near the free edge of the mitral septal cusp, and severe when it is detected in the rest of the ventricular cavity (Fig. 3).

In conclusion, sequential and combined utilization of M-mode, bidimensional and Doppler techniques in their different modalities provide substantial information on the status of the prosthesis in different positions. The state of the techniques allows hemodynamic estimations to be made by approximate calculation of gradients and areas, and also provides real-time images.

8.6 Conclusions

E. ASIN CARDIEL

In this chapter we have had reports on four aspects of great clinical interest concerning valvular disease.

Choice of a prosthesis for patients with valvular disease should be individualized, giving consideration to different aspects of the valve and the patient. Various factors must be weighed, such as patient age, activity, possibility of pregnancy, size of left atrium, persistence of atrial fibrillation, need for anticoagulant treatment and facility of control, valvular ring size, etc. The most recent biological valve models have improved their hemodynamic function and chemical stability, making them more durable. Perfection of mechanical valve design is oriented toward reducing thromboembolic phenomena. These factors offer promising perspectives for this field.

Conservative surgery has extended the possibility of surgical treatment of mitral valve disease. The reduction in mortality rates and elimination of certain prosthesis-related problems mean that this treatment should be attempted whenever possible. A more precise study of the mitral valve using techniques such as echocardiography helps in the selection of the surgical treatment to be realized.

Choosing the moment for establishing the surgical indication of valvular patients is still difficult in many cases. Careful evaluation of the patient can now be based on nuclear ergometric echocardiographic parameters and hemodynamics, allowing us to make the surgical correction before hemodynamic deterioration leads to failure of surgery. This fact and improvements in prosthesis quality mean that surgery is probably indicated in an earlier functional situation than has been traditionally admitted.

Echocardiography provides interesting findings for the diagnosis of prosthetic dysfunction, but the procedure has various limitations that reduce its utility. There are dysfunction criteria for mechanical prostheses in mitral position. In prosthetic obstruction, signs related to disk movement are less reliable. For biological prostheses in mitral and aortic position, assessment of the evolution of sigmoid cusp thickness is probably the most useful sign. For dysfunction of mechanical prosthesis in aortic position, echocardiographic findings are not very sensitive. Other indirect signs, such as evolution in cavity size, can help in the diagnosis. The Doppler method permits detection of regurgitation. Measurement of ejection speed may be useful for aortic prostheses, continuous Doppler being more useful for this purpose.

9. Surgical Correction of Tetralogy of Fallot: Mid-term Results

9.1 Introduction

J.I. HERRAIZ SARACHAGA

In 1954, Dr Lillehei performed the first total correction of tetralogy of Fallot [1]. Nine years later, this author published a report of the experience obtained in postoperatory cardiac catheterization studies [2]. In the sixties, Dr Rábago performed the first total correction in Spain [3]. In the 30 years since then, operative mortality has declined to 5–10% [4–7] and experience has accumulated in the long-term followup of these patients [8, 9] thanks to technological advances and surgeons' ability.

We will enumerate the points of controversy that will emerge in the course of our discussion. Surgically (Table 1), the debate over single-stage correction as compared with correction after establishing a preliminary fistula is conditioned mainly by the following factors: age, cardiac anatomy (size of the pulmonary arteries and left cavities), presence of important associated cardiac anomalies [10]. As to surgical technique (Table 2), there has been debate on myocardial protection, circulatory support, hypothermia, etc., different techniques for relieving outflow tract obstruction or the problems occasioned by the large ventriculotomy scar. AV block and coronary artery damage are less common [11].

The other subject for discussion is follow-up of the postoperated patient. The postoperated patient is a new type of patient, the consequence of the high survival rates achieved by surgery. These patients pose new situations that can be examined under the section of residual lesions, sequelae and late complications [12]. Among them, we must emphasize (Table 3) the electrocardiographic alterations evidenced by dynamic electrocardiography, on which Dr Paul

Table 1. Total correction of tetralogy of Fallot. Surgical problems.

Single stage correction vs. two-stage correction:
Age
Anatomy
Associated anomalies

420

Table 2. Total correction of tetralogy of Fallot. Surgical problems.

Technique:
Myocardial protection – Circulatory support
Resolution RV outflow tract obstruction
Ventricular scar in repair site
AV block
Impaired coronary blood supply due to arterial injury

Table 3. Total correction of tetralogy of Fallot, residual lesions, sequelae and late complications.

I.	ECG alterations:
	Conduction disorders
	Rhythm disorders
II.	Alterations in response to exercise
III.	Anatomic alterations:
	Pulmonary stenosis and incompetence
	Ventricular septal defect
	Tricuspid incompetence
	Pulmonary hypertension
	Ventricular function

Gillette will speak, and objective assessment by ergometric tests of response to exercise [13]. Anatomic lesions, sequelae or residual lesions (Table 3) should be evaluated noninvasively (echocardiography, Doppler and cardiac isotopes) [8, 9], if possible. The most significant alterations are pulmonary stenosis and incompetence, ventricular septal defect, tricuspid incompetence, pulmonary hypertension and late complications derived from ventricular malfunction [14]. The need for cardiac catheterization to study the postoperated patient must be considered in view of the availability of noninvasive technology, and the balance of this panel's efforts would be positive if it established indications for catheterization in these patients.

References

1. Lillehei CW, Cohen M, Warden HE, Read RC, Aust JB, Dewall RA, Warco RL: Direct vision of the tetralogy of Fallot, pentalogy of Fallot and pulmonary atresia defects. Report of first cases. Ann Surg 1955; 142: 418.
2. Lillehei CW, Lery M, Adams P, Anderson RL: Corrective surgery for tetralogy of Fallot. Long-term follow-up by postoperative recatheterization in 69 cases and certain surgical considerations. J Thorac Cardiovasc Surg 1964; 48: 556.
3. Urquia M, Castillon L, Perez Leon J, Rabago G: Actitud quirúrgica ante la tetralogía de Fallot. Rev Esp Cardiolog 1968; 21: 528.

4. Daily PO, Stinson EB, Griepp RB, Shunway NE: Tetralogy of Fallot: Choice of surgical procedure. J Thorac Cardiovasc Surg 1978; 75: 358.
5. Pacifico AD, Kirklin JW, Blackstone EH: Surgical management of pulmonary stenosis in tetralogy of Fallot. J Thorac Cardiovasc Surg 1977; 74: 382.
6. Arciniegas E, Farooki AQ, Hakim M, Perry L, Green EN: Early and late results of total correction of Fallot. J Thorac Cardiovasc Surg 1980, 80: 770.
7. Castaneda AR, Freed MD, Williams RG, Norwood WI: Repair of tetralogy of Fallot in infancy. J Thorac Cardiovasc Surg 1977; 74: 372.
8. Fuster V, McGoon DC, Kennedy MA, Kitter DG, Kirklin JW: Long-term evaluation (12–22 years) of open heart surgery of tetralogy of Fallot. Am J Cardiol 1980; 46: 635.
9. Rosenthal A, Behrendt D, Sloan H, Ferguson P, Snedecor SM, Schorck MA: Long-term prognosis (15 to 26 years) after repair of tetralogy of Fallot: I. Survival and symptomatic status. Ann Thorac Surg 1984; 38: 151.
10. Kirklin JW, Blackstone EH, Pacifico AD, Brown RN, Bargeron LM Jr: Routine primary repair vs. two stage repair of tetralogy of Fallot. Circulation 1979; 60: 373.
11. Kirklin JW, Karp RB: The tetralogy of Fallot from a surgical viewpoint. Saunders, Philadelphia, 1970.
12. Graham TP: Assessing the results of surgery for congenital heart disease: A continuing process. Circulation 1979; 60: 1049.
13. Gillette PC, Yeoman MA, Mullins CE, McNamara DG: Sudden death after repair of tetralogy of Fallot. Electrocardiographic and electrophysiologic abnormalities. Circulation 1977; 56: 566.
14. Lorgevil M, Friedli B, Assimacopoulos A: Factors affecting left ventricular function after correction of tetralogy of Fallot. Br Heart J 1984; 52: 536.

9.2 Mid-term Postoperative Cardiac Catheterization Study after Corrective Surgery for Tetralogy of Fallot

J.I. HERRAIZ SARACHAGA, J.C. FLORES,
R. BERMUDEZ-CANETE and M. QUERO JIMENEZ

A study was made of the results of cardiac catheterization in 25 children who underwent total corrective surgery for tetralogy of Fallot between January 1978 and November 1981. Age at the time of corrective surgery ranged from 19 months to 10 years (a mean of 4 years and one month). In the 3 patients under 2 years the following procedures were performed: one infundibulectomy, one valvulotomy and one transannular patch. In all the children from 2 to 5 years, the largest patient group, a patch was inserted: 12 transannular and 4 infundibular. Finally, in the 6 patients from 5 to 10 years, a patch was made in 5: 3 transannular and 2 infundibular. Sixty four percent of the patients required a transannular patch.

The indication for postoperative catheterization was presence of residual lesions in 3, assessment of correction of major associated anomalies in 2 and quality control in 20.

The time lapse between operation and postoperative catheterization was less than a year in 5 patients and more than a year in 20. In the latter group, elective catheterization was performed as a quality control. The mean time lapse was 3 years 10 months.

In all patients, right and left catheterization was done according to our laboratory's routine, and left ventricular, right ventricular and pulmonary artery angiographies were made. Dodge's biplanar method was used to assess ventricular function.

The hemodynamic results (Table 1) were classified as excellent, good or poor [1–3]. Results were considered excellent when right ventricular systolic pressure was less than 40 mm Hg, transpulmonary systolic gradient was under 20 mm Hg and there was no ventricular shunt; 10 (40%) of our patients satisfied all these requisites. Results were considered good when right ventricular pressure was 40–60 mm Hg, transpulmonary systolic gradient was 20–40 mm Hg, ventricular shunt was inferior to 1.5 or when pulmonary systolic pressure was less than 40 mm Hg.

Thirteen (52%) patients met some of these requisites. Finally, results were considered poor when any of the following appeared: right ventricular systolic pressure over 60 mm Hg, transpulmonary systolic gradient of more than 40 mm Hg, Qp/Qs greater than 1.5 or systolic pulmonary artery pressure over 40 mm Hg. Two of our patients (8%) presented some of these data.

The relationship between surgical procedure, hemodynamic classification and Qp/Qs is shown in Table 2; the first line indicates data from patients in whom only infundibulectomy was done. The second line shows the patients with infundibular patch and the third patients with transannular valved tube patch. The proportion of excellent and good results obtained with infundibulectomy and transannular patch were similar; however, in the patients with a patch extending to the ring there were two cases with poor results. Table 3 compares the hemodynamic results of one or two-stage (with prior shunt) surgery. The first line shows the results of single-stage surgery and the second line, that of two-stage surgery with preliminary shunt. Sixty-eight per cent of the patients were corrected in one stage, with poor results in one case; the remaining 32% was corrected in two stages, with poor results in one case. It can be deduced that the proportional failure rate of two-stage surgery was

Table 1. Postoperative hemodynamic classification.

	Hemodynamic result	No of patients	Percentage
Excellent	PSRV ≤ 40 mm Hg		
	$\triangle$ RV-PA < 20 mm Hg		
	No ventricular short circuit	10	40
Good	PSRV 40–60 mm Hg		
	$\triangle$ S PV-PA < 20–40 mm Hg		
	PS PlmA ≤ 40 mm Hg	13	52
Poor	PSRV > 60 mm Hg		
	$\triangle$ S RV-PA > 40 mm Hg		
	Qp/Ps > 1.5		
	PS PlmA > 40 mm Hg	2	8
Total		25	100

Table 2. Intracardiac surgical procedures and postoperative hemodynamic classification.

Surgery	Total	Excellent	Good	Poor	Qp/Qs < 1.5	Qp/Qs > 1.5
Infundibulectomy	2	1	1	–	2	0
Patch to ring	7	2	3	2	5	2
Transannular patch or valved conduct	16	7	9	–	16	–
Total	25	10	13	2	23	2

twice as high as for one-stage surgery. Respiratory failure was evaluated (Table 4) attending these parameters: differential pulmonary artery pressure ratio divided by systolic pulmonary artery pressure more than or less than 0.75; diastolic pulmonary artery pressure more than or less than right ventricular

Table 3. Relationship between one- or two-stage surgery and postoperative hemodynamic classification.

Surgery	Total	Excellent	Good	Poor	Qp/Qs < 1.5	Qp/Qs > 1.5
1 Stage with corrective surgery	17 (68%)	6	10	1	16	1
2 Stages with prior shunt	8 (32%)	3	4	1	7	1
Total	25	9	14	2	23	2

Table 4. Evaluation of respiratory failure.

		Patients	Percentage
Mild/moderate			
$\dfrac{\text{Differ. Pulm. Art. Pr.}}{\text{Syst. Pulm. Art. Pr.}}$	< 0.75		
Diast. Pulm. Art. Pr.	> RVEDP		
Regurgitation fraction	< 20%	11	44
Severe			
$\dfrac{\text{Differ. Pulm. Art. Pr.}}{\text{Syst. Pulm. Art. Pr.}}$	< 0.75		
Diast. Pulm. Art. Pr.	≤ RVEDP		
Regurgitation fraction	> 20%	14	56
Total	25		100

$$\text{Regurgitation fraction} = \frac{\text{RV Ejection Vol.} - \text{LV Ejection Vol.}}{\text{RV Ejection Vol.}}$$

Table 5. Relationship between respiratory failure (RF) and hemodynamic results.

	Severe RF	Mild-moderate RF	Total
Excellent	6	4	10
Good	5	8	13
Poor	–	2	2
Total	11	14	25

enddiastolic pressure; and right ventricular regurgitation fraction, determined by angiography, less or more than 0.20 [2–3]. Respiratory failure was mild or moderate in 44% and severe in 56%.

We compared (Table 5) the degree of respiratory failure with excellent, good or poor hemodynamic results, and found that the proportion of severe and mild respiratory failure was similar in excellent and good cases. It is notable that the two cases with poor hemodynamic results had mild respiratory failure.

As could be anticipated, none of the cases with infundibulectomy presented severe respiratory failure. Five of the seven (71%) patients with a patch from infundibulum to ring had severe respiratory failure, and 8 of 16 (50%) with a transannular patch presented severe respiratory failure. Left ventricular end-diastolic volume was increased in 12 patients (48%), less than half of whom had had a preliminary shunt operation. There was no clear relationship between elevated left ventricular enddiastolic pressure and postoperative hemodynamic results [5, 6]. Left ventricular ejection fraction declined to less than 90% of the normal expected value in 10% of cases, but there was no relationship with the hemodynamic classification or the time between correction and postoperative hemodynamic study [7]. As regards to left ventricular mass, no relationship between variations in mass (increase, decrease or normal) and previous shunt was demonstrated [5]; one case had decreased left ventricular mass and prior shunt.

Our conclusions were the following:

a) Only the group with infundibular patch to the ring had poor hemodynamic results.
b) The degree of respiratory failure was unrelated to hemodynamic results or type of surgery.
c) When resolving right ventricular outflow tract obstruction, care should be taken in designing the patch because respiratory failure does not necessarily have to worsen, but even if it does, the hemodynamic results are good, at least at mid-term [1, 3, 8, 9].

References

1. Ruzyllo W, Nihill MR, Mullins ChE, McNamara DG: Hemodynamic evaluation of 221 patients after intracardiac repair of tetralogy of Fallot. Am J Cardiol 1974; 34: 565–576.
2. Garson JR, McNamara DG: Postoperative tetralogy of Fallot. In: Angle MA (ed) Pediatric cardiovascular disease. FA Davies, Philadelphia, 1981; 407–449.
3. Garson JR, McNamara MD, Cooley BA: Tetralogy of Fallot in adults. In: Roberts WC (ed) Congenital heart disease in adults. FA Davies, Philadelphia 1979; 341–364.
4. Albertal G, Swan HJC, Kirklin JW: Hemodynamic studies two weeks to six years after repair of tetralogy of Fallot. Circulation 1964; 29: 583.

5. Bermudez-Canete R, Merino G, Herraiz I, Quero M, Brito JM, Campillo A: Left ventricular volumes and function in children with tetralogy of Fallot before and after surgery. Prospective protocol and analysis of 22 cases (Abstract 245). World Congress of Paediatric Cardiology. London, 1980.
6. Nomoto SH, Murakoa R, Yokota M, Aoshimia M, Kyokn I, Nakano H: Left ventricular volume as a predictor of postoperative hemodynamics as a criterion for total correction of tetralogy of Fallot. J Thorac Cardiovasc Surg 1984; 88: 389.
7. Lorgevil M, Friedli B, Assimacopoulus A: Factors affecting left ventricular function after correction of tetralogy of Fallot. Br Heart J 1984; 52: 536.
8. Fuster V, McGoon DC, Kennedy MA, Ritter DG, Kirklin JW: Long-term evaluation (12 to 22 years) of open heart surgery for tetralogy of Fallot. Am J Cardiol 1980; 46: 635.
9. Rosenthal A, Behrendt D, Sloan H, Ferguson P, Snedecor SM, Schork MA: Long-term prognosis (15 to 26 years) after repair of tetralogy of Fallot: I. Survival and symptomatic status. Ann Thorac Surg 1984; 38: 151.

9.3 Mid- and Long-term Postoperative Results of Tetralogy of Fallot Cases Operated on in the Hospital Infantil, Ciudad Sanitaria 'Vall d'Hebron' (1971–1983)

J. CASALDALIGA

Introduction

Since 1954, when the first surgical correction of tetralogy of Fallot (TF) was performed [1], diverse studies and publications have attempted to assess long-term results [2–11].

Cardiac rhythm or conduction disorders secondary to surgery and residual anatomic anomalies resulting from the operative technique can condition the future of these patients [12–19].

Different variables, such as age at intervention, surgical technique or the need for previous palliative surgery can modify a priori the later evolution of these patients [2, 5, 12, 13].

To evaluate the results of the surgical correction of tetralogy of Fallot, the postoperative, mid- and long-term evolution of the patients treated in our center since pediatric cardiac surgery commenced (1971–1983) was reviewed.

Material and methods

From 1971 to 1983, 205 children with tetralogy of Fallot were operated on in our center: 184 of them survived and were discharged from hospital.

We reviewed the cardiologic follow-up reports of these patients, which had been made with a mean yearly frequency. Of the 184 patients, 137 were seen in the year before our study. In 10 cases we did not follow up, an updated record of the patient's condition prepared by the responsible cardiologist was used. In 34 cases, there was no follow-up in the year before study and they were excluded from this review. The remaining three patients died after hospital discharge. One hundred forty-seven patients with known clinical status (137 controlled by us and 10 evaluated according to our indications) were included in this study.

Mean age of these 147 patients at the time of study was 9 ± 4 years (2.5–22).

The patients were operated on at 3.5 ± 2 years (0.5–11.4). The mean time since operation was 6.2 ± 3.6 years (0.5–13.2). In only 2 cases had the operation been performed less than a year earlier.

The surgical correction techniques used in these patients consisted of ventricular septal defect (VSD) closure in every case and different modalities of repair of the right ventricular (RV) outflow obstruction, as determined by the anatomy of the malformation: infundibulectomy with enlargement of the right ventricular outflow tract (RVOT) to the pulmonary artery trunk (PAT) in 85 cases (57.8%); infundibulectomy and pulmonary valvulotomy in 15 (10.2%); infundibulectomy and limited RVOT enlargement in 13 (8.8%); infundibulectomy, pulmonary valvulotomy and RVOT enlargement in 6 (4.1%); variants of the previous procedure in 14 (9.5%) and suture of a valved tube between RV and PAT in one (0.7%) (Table 1). Pericardium was used for the enlargment in 35.7% of cases and synthetic material in 64.3%.

Preliminary palliative surgery was performed in 50 cases (34% of the total): Blalock-Taussig technique in 27 cases (18.3% of the total), Waterston procedure in 22 (14.9% of the total) and Cooley procedure in one (0.6% of the total).

Intraoperative pressures after correction of the cardiac malformation were: $53.6 \pm 12.3 \, mm \, Hg$ (25–100) in RV; RV: aortic (Ao) pressure ratio 0.50 ± 0.1 (0.2–0.9). Conventional extracorporeal circulation and moderate hypothermia were used in all patients.

In every case, clinical evaluation consisted of assessment of daily quality of life, clinical examination, plain chest films and conventional ECG.

In 97 selected cases, bidimensional and pulsed Doppler echocardiography were performed. Enddiastolic diameter of the RV, left ventricle (LV), pulmo-

Table 1. Tetralogy of Fallot (1971–1983). Surgical technique.

Closure of ventricular septal defect and	Cases	Percentage
Infundibulectomy + RVOT enlargement. Ring and PAT	85	57.8
Infundibulectomy + P valvulotomy	15	10.2
Infundibulectomy	13	8.8
Infundibulectomy + RVOT enlargement	13	8.8
Infundibulectomy + P valvulotomy + RVOT enlargement	6	4.1
Valved tube from RV to PAT	1	0.7
Variants of the above	14	9.5
Total	147	
Enlargement with pericardium		35.7
Enlargement with synthetic material		64.3

RVOT: right ventricular outflow tract. P: pulmonary. PAT: pulmonary artery trunk. RV: right ventricle.

nary artery ring and aortic ring were measured: Residual anomalies were sought, for example, pulmonary stenosis (PS), pulmonary branch stenosis (PBS), pulmonary incompetence (PI), ASD and tricuspid incompetence (TI). Residual PS or PBS were considered to be present when there was more than 50% reduction in the caliber of the pulmonary trunk, ring and branches [20] and Doppler flow analysis of the zone distal to the obstruction revealed a turbulent and more rapid flow. PI was accepted when Doppler echocardiography of the RVOT detected retrograde diastolic flow from the PAT [21]. TI was present when Doppler flow analysis of the right atrium demonstrated retrograde holosystolic flow from the RV. There was residual ASD when a clear loss of ventricular septal continuity was observed and/or Doppler scanning of the area disclosed turbulent systolic flow.

In 26 cases postoperative hemodynamic studies were available. These studies were performed under the suspicion of residual anomalies. The time between surgery and catheterization was 2.9 ± 2.2 years (1 month to 7 years).

On the basis of present clinical status and presence of associated anomalies with possible risk, the patients were functionally staged as follows:

Stage A1: this category included the patients who led normal lives with no limitations, did not require treatment, had a normal plain chest film and no ECG anomalies other than right bundle branch block (RBBB).

Stage A2: these patients satisfied all the requisites of group A1, except that the chest film could not be considered normal because of prominence of the pulmonary artery sector, although there is no cardiomegaly.

Stage B1: all the patients with any of the following:
a) functional limitation that does not preclude social integration,
b) plain chest film showing cardiomegaly, or
c) need for cardiac medication.

Stage B2: patients who satisfy the same premises as B1, but exhibit some cardiac conduction or rhythm disorder in the ECG (with the exception of RBBB) that was not present in preoperatory studies.

Stage C: all patients with evident functional limitation or poorly compensated heart failure (Table 2).

To determine if there is a significant relationship between postoperatory results and several variables, such as age at intervention, previous palliative surgery, surgical technique, intraoperative pressures and reoperation, we carried out statistical studies (Pearson's correlation coefficient, variance analysis and contingency table) to correlate them with the clinical parameters presently considered most significant, such as radiologic findings, echocardiographic RV/LV diameter ratio, existence of cardiac rhythm or conduction disorders and classification by functional stage.

430

Table 2. Tetralogy of Fallot (1971–1983). Postcorrectional functional stages.

Stage A1. Presence of all the following:	
Normal activities without limitations	
Normal chest film	
Normal ECG or only RBBB	
Medical treatment not required	
Number of cases	25 (17%)
Stage A2. The same features as A1 except for:	
Prominent pulmonary sector but no cardiomegaly in the chest film	
Number of cases	27 (18.4%)
Stage B1. Presence of any of the following:	
Some limitation in activity	
Cardiomegaly in the chest film	
Medical treatment required	
Number of cases	57 (38.8%)
Stage B2. The same features as B-1, except:	
ECG with rhythm or conduction alterations (not including RBBB)	
Number of cases	34 (23.1%)
Stage C. Uncompensated heart failure	
Number of cases	2 (1.4%)

RBBB: Right bundle branch block.

Results
Of the three patients who died after hospital release, this occurred 1.5 months, 13 months and 2.2 years after surgery. Cause of death was heart failure in two and bronchopneumonia in the third, who had Pierre Robin syndrome and hemidiaphragmatic paralysis secondary to the operation. The surgical technique used in the patients who died of heart failure was ASD closure and infundibulectomy, with valvulotomy in one and RVOT enlargement to the PAT with pericardium in the other. Both had residual VSD and PI. In the patient who died of bronchopneumonia 1.5 months after surgery, the technique was VSD closure and suture of a valved tube from the RV to the PA because there was a coronary artery crossing the RVOT and it had to be enlarged. In all three cases, there had been preliminary palliative surgery, consisting of Blalock-Taussig, Cooley and Waterston systemic-pulmonary shunts, respectively.

The present clinical situation of our 147 cases is the following: 87% (128 cases) lead normal lives with no limitations; 11% (17 cases) have some limitation (dyspnea with great effort, hemiplegia secondary to thromboembolic surgical problems in two, etc.), but this does not impede them from being well-integrated into their social context; and 1.3% (2 cases) are invalids because of heart failure.

Auscultation detected a soft pulmonary ejection murmur in every case. In

114 patients (77%), there was an early diastolic murmur suggestive of PI. In 12 (8%), there was a holosystolic murmur of residual VSD. In 6 (4%), a harsy systolic murmur was heard in the pulmonary focus, in 2 cases irradiated to both hemithoraces, suggesting residual PS and/or stenosis of the pulmonary artery branches.

The plain chest film was normal in 29 cases (19%). There were different degrees of cardiomegaly in 88 (59%) and dilation of the pulmonary artery arch in 77 (51%). Cardiomegaly and pulmonary arch dilation were associated in 47 cases (32%).

Conventional ECG showed right bundle branch block (RBBB) in 141 cases (96%). The frontal plane QRS axis was deviated to the left in 20 cases (13%), suggesting left anterior hemiblock (LAH). Different degrees of atrioventricular block (A-V B) were recorded in 16 (11%), one of whom had a pacemaker implanted for this reason. In 5 (3.4%), ventricular extrasystoles (VE) were detected. Only 3 patients (2.1%) presented a normal ECG or incomplete block of the right bundle branch. ECG alterations were sometimes associated in the same patient, the most frequent associations being those listed in Table 3.

In 26 cases (17%), the postoperative hemodynamic study was indicated by a clinical suspicion of residual anomalies. The results obtained were: 66.4 ± 21.6 mm Hg (31–100 mm Hg) in RV; RV/Ao pressure ratio 0.7 ± 0.3 (0.07–1.02). The residual anomalies found are specified in Table 4.

After cardiac catheterization, reoperation was considered to be indicated in 8 patients (5.4% of the total series). Residual pulmonary stenosis in 4 cases (50% of reoperations) was the most frequent cause. Residual VSD led to reoperation in 2 cases (25%) and the persistence of palliative systemic-pulmonary shunt patency after surgery in the last 2 cases (25%). The mean time between the corrective operation and reoperation was 2.6 years (9 days to 7.4 years).

Bidimensional echocardiography with pulsed Doppler technique was performed in 96 patients, demonstrating residual PS in one case (1% of the group

Table 3. Tetralogy of Fallot (1971–1983) – postcorrectional ECG anomalies and the most common associations.

RBBB + LAH	19 cases	(13.0%)
RBBB + LAH + VE	1 case	(0.7%)
RBBB + A-VB	16 cases	(10.8%)
RBBB + LAH + A-VB	4 cases	(2.7%)
RBBB + VE	4 cases	(2.7%)

RBBB: right bundle branch block. LAH: left anterior hemiblock. A-VB: atrioventricular block. VE: ventricular extrasystoles.

432

studied with echocardiography), PBS in 7 (7.2% of this group), PI in 87 (90.6% of this group) and residual VSD in 7 (7.2%). These anomalies had been clinically syspected or hemodynamically confirmed. Bidimensional and Doppler echocardiography proved to be very useful in discovering TI (23 cases) (24% of those studied by echocardiography) undetected by clinical manifestations. Enddiastolic RV diameter was increased in all patients with a RV diameter/LV diameter ratio of 0.7 ± 0.2 (0.1–1.5) and the parameter was demonstrated to have a good correlation (p = 0.005) with the clinical classification by functional studies.

Patient classification by functional stages (Table 2) showed the following results:

Stage A: 52 patients (35.4%) subdivided into stage A1, 25 cases (17%), and stage A2, 27 cases (18.4%). Stage B: 91 cases (61.9%) divided into 2 subgroups: stage B1 with 57 cases (38.8%) and stage B2 with 34 cases (23.1%). Stage C: 2 cases (1.4%). Two patients could not be classified because there were inconsistencies in the report of present status and previous reports.

Study of the statistical correlation between postoperative findings and the variables indicated produced the following results: there was a statistically significant (p = 0.01) correlation between functional staging and need for preliminary palliative surgical shunt before definitive correction; there was a higher percentage of patients with shunt in the groups with the most deteriorated functional state (20% in group A, 40% in group B and 100% in group C). It was also significant (p = 0.02) that the patients who required reoperation were preferentially classified in the group with the worst functional status (0% reoperation in group A, 8% in group B and 50% in group C). Of the patients

Table 4. Tetralogy of Fallot (1971–1983). Postcorrectional hemodynamic study of 26 cases (17.6% of total).

Residual anomalies	Cases	Cases studied (%)
PS	12	46.1
VSD	7	26.9
TI	7	26.9
PBS	5	19.2
'Aneurysmal' RVOT dilation	4	15.3
'Aneurysmal' PA dilation	2	7.6
RV dysfunction	2	7.6
LV dysfunction	2	7.6
Persistent S-P fistula	2	7.6

PS: pulmonary stenosis. VSD: ventricular septal defect. TI: tricuspid incompetence. PBS: pulmonary branch stenosis. RVOT: right ventricular outflow tract. PA: pulmonary artery. RV: right ventricle. LV: left ventricle. S-P: systemic-pulmonary.

who presently have cardiomegaly, most (73%) needed enlargement of the pulmonary ring (p = 0.02). No significant statistical correlation (p>0.05) was found between present clinical status and age of the patient at operation. Existence of cardiac rhythm or conduction disorders did not correlate significantly. The intraoperative pressures (RV pressure, RV pressure/Ao pressure ratio) had no significant correlation with postoperative catheterization pressures (p = 0.13), reoperation (p = 0.87) or present patient status (p = 0.11).

Discussion and conclusions

From this study of 147 patients, and 3 patients who died after hospital discharge treated in the course of a 12-year interval in surgical correction of tetralogy of Fallot, we have reached the following conclusions:

1. The postoperative mortality after hospital release was 2%. The absence of sudden deaths in our series in comparison with other series [10, 14] is noteworthy, but we should recall that 34 cases (18% of those who survived surgery) were excluded from the study because their situation in the year before our review was unknown.
2. Mid-term results of corrective surgery for tetralogy of Fallot were good: 98% of the patients who survived surgery could carry out their normal activities and were well-integrated in their social context.
3. The most frequent functional situation was that classified as stage B (61%), in which the present patient status is good, but there are abnormal objective findings (cardiomegaly and/or electrocardiographic alterations) that may represent a future risk. To understand this problem better, we think it is necessary to conduct longer studies using more functional assessment techniques (Holter ECG, exercise tests, etc.) that would help predict the future situation of these patients.
4. The presence of different degrees of cardiomegaly and/or dilation of the pulmonary artery arch was the most common radiologic finding in these patients.
5. RBBB was the most common electrocardiographic alteration (96%). RBBB with left axis deviation in the frontal plane, suggestive of bifascicular block, was present in 13% of our cases. VE in the conventional ECG, probably the most important risk factor in these patients [14, 15], was present in 3.4% of our cases.
6. The most frequent residual anomaly, PI (82%), was well-tolerated at mid-term follow-up, although a longer appraisal is needed to determine the true tolerance. The fact that TI was frequently detected (18% of the total) should caution us to not be overly optimistic that these favorable results indicate future tolerance.

434

7. The most frequent cause for reoperation at short- and mid-term was residual PS (3% of all patients and 50% of reoperations). The prognosis for the patient's future functional status was worse for those who were reoperated.
8. Intraoperative pressures considered acceptable are not useful to predict postoperative catheterization pressures, need for reoperation, or future functional status of the patient.
9. Patient age at operation does not condition postoperative functional status.
10. The patients with the best postoperative functional status were those who did not require palliative surgical techniques, pulmonary ring enlargement during corrective surgery, or reoperation. However, preoperative anatomy, which conditions the selection of a surgical technique, is probably what really determines the patients' future evolution.

References

1. Lillehei CW, Cohen M, Warden HE. Read RC, Aust JB: Direct vision intracardiac surgical correction of tetralogy of Fallot, pentalogy of Fallot and pulmonary atresia defects. Ann Surg 1955; 142: 418–445.
2. Alderson PO, Boonvisut S, McKnight RC, Hartman AF: Pulmonary perfusion abnormalities and ventilation-perfusion imbalance in children after total repair of tetralogy of Fallot. Circulation, 1976; 53: 332–337.
3. Buhlmeyer K, Lorenz HP, Sebening F: Early repair of tetralogy of Fallot: clinical results. XVIIIth Annual General Meeting of the Association of European Paediatric Cardiologists. Milan, 1981 (Abstract). Ped Cardiol 1982; 3: 80–81.
4. Fancini P, Vignati G, Figini A, et al.: Fallot tetralogy: a postoperative study. XVIIIth Annual General Meeting of the Association of European Paediatric Cardiologists. Milan, 1981 (Abstract). Ped Cardiol 1982; 3: 81.
5. Graham TP, Cordell D, Atwood GE et al.: Right ventricular volume characteristics before and after palliative and reparative operation in tetralogy of Fallot. Circulation 1976; 54: 417–423.
6. Hamilton DI, Eusanio G, Piccoli GP, Dickinson DF: Eight years' experience with intracardiac repair of tetralogy of Fallot. Early and late results in 175 consecutive patients. Br Heart J 1981; 46: 144–151.
7. James FW, Kaplan S, Schwartz DC, Techuan Chou, Sandker MJ, Naylor V: Response to exercise in patients after total surgical correction of tetralogy of Fallot. Circulation 1976; 54: 671–679.
8. Katz NM, Blackstone EH, Kirklin JW, Pacifico AD, Bargeron LM: Late survival and symptoms after repair of tetralogy of Fallot. Circulation 1982; 65: 403–410.
9. Perez Martinez VM, Garcia Aguado A, Benito F, Fernandez Ruiz A, Burgueros M, Cabo J: Evaluación hemodinámica tras la corrección completa de la tetralogía de Fallot. Indicaciones y resultados en 83 pacientes. Communication for the II Reunión Nacional de la Sociedad Española de Cardiología. Barcelona, 1984. Rev Esp Cardiolog 1984; 37 (Suppl 2): 2–53.
10. Quattlebaum TG, Varghese PJ, Neill CA, Donahoo JS: Sudden death among postoperative

patients with tetralogy of Fallot. A follow-up study of 243 patients for an average of twelve years. Circulation 1976; 54: 289–293.

11. Uretzky, Puga FJ, Danielson GK, Hagler DJ, McGoon DC: Reoperation after correction of tetralogy of Fallot. Circulation 1982; 66 (Suppl 1): 202–208.
12. Benito F, Aguado A, Fernandez A et al.: Arritmias tras la corrección quirúrgica de la tetralogía de Fallot por método de Holter. Communication at the II Reunión Nacional de la Sociedad Española de Cardiología. Barcelona, 1984. Rev Esp Cardiolog 1984; 37 (Suppl 2): 2–34.
13. Benito F, Aguado A, Fernandez A et al.: Arritmias inducidas por el esfuerzo tras la corrección quirúrgica de la tetralogía de Fallot. Communication at the II Reunión Nacional de la Sociedad Española de Cardiología. Barcelona, 1984. Rev Esp Cardiolog 1984; 37 (Suppl 2): 33–34.
14. Gillette PC, Yeoman MA, Mullins ChE, McNamara DG: Sudden death after repair of tetralogy of Fallot. Electrocardiographic and electrophysiologic abnormalities. Circulation 1977; 56: 566–571.
15. James FW, Kaplan S, Te-Chuan Chou: Unexpected cardiac arrest in patients after surgical correction of tetralogy of Fallot. Circulation 1975; 52: 691–695.
16. Neches WH, Park SC, Mathews RA, Lenox CC, Marin-Garcia J, Zuberbuhler JR: Tetralogy of Fallot. Postoperative electrophysiologic studies. Circulation 1977; 56: 713–719.
17. Niederhauser H, Simonin Ph, Friedli B: Sinus node function and conduction system after complete repair of tetralogy of Fallot. Circulation 1975; 52: 214–220.
18. Yabek SM, Jarmakani JM, Roberts NK: Diagnosis of trifascicular damage following tetralogy of Fallot and ventricular septal defect repair. Circulation 1977; 55: 23–27.
19. Friedli B, Bolens M: Significance of PR prolongation and right bundle branch block after surgical correction of tetralogy of Fallot. XVIIIth Annual General Meeting of the Association of European Paediatric Cardiologists. Milan, 1981 (Abstract). Ped Cardiol 1982; 3: 82.
20. Tinker DD, Nanda NC, Harris JP, Manning JA: Two-dimensional echocardiographic identification of pulmonary artery branch stenosis. Am J Cardiol 1982; 50: 814–820.
21. Patel AK, Rowe GG, Dhanani SP, Kosolcharden P, Lyle LEW, Thomsen JH: Pulsed Doppler echocardiography in diagnosis of pulmonary regurgitation: its value and limitations. Am J Cardiol 1982; 49: 1801–1805.

9.4 Cardiac Dysrhythmias after Surgical Treatment of Tetralogy of Fallot

PAUL C. GILLETTE

Introduction

Tetralogy of Fallot is the most common cyanotic congenital heart defect [1]. It is estimated that in the United States 2,700 patients are born each year with tetralogy of Fallot. The surgical treatment of tetralogy of Fallot now consists of an anatomical repair of the defects. It is estimated that 2,400 patients per year with tetralogy of Fallot will survive into their teenage years in the United States alone.

Patients who have had surgical repair of tetralogy of Fallot have been found to be prone to sudden death and to various cardiac dysrhythmias. The two dysrhythmias which have been noted with the greatest frequency clinically are premature ventricular contractions and right bundle branch block, left axis deviation pattern. It has been speculated that one or both of these abnormalities was responsible for the sudden deaths which occur after correction of tetralogy of Fallot [2–5]. The frequency of late deaths in several series of patients with tetralogy of Fallot is 5–6% [1, 6, 7].

Clinical correlates of sudden death after tetralogy of Fallot

Several investigators have attempted to correlate clinical findings with sudden death in tetralogy of Fallot. Wolff et al. [4] noted that surgically induced right bundle branch block and left anterior hemiblock were particularly common in their group of patients with tetralogy of Fallot repair who died. Although not stressed by the authors, these patients also had a high incidence of premature ventricular contractions. Krongrad et al. [8] found that transient complete AV block, right bundle branch block, and left anterior hemiblock carried a higher incidence of either sudden death or late onset complete heart block than any other combination of conduction defects. However, very few patients in this review actually had sudden death. In patients with right bundle branch block

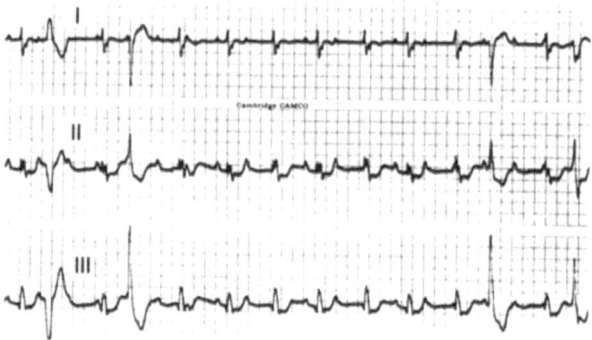

Fig. 1. Simultaneous ECG leads I, II and III showing multiform PVC's in a patient with atrioventricular dissociation post operative tetralogy of Fallot. There is no evidence of atrioventricular conduction. The 'normal beats' have a right bundle branch block pattern.

and left anterior hemiblock without transient complete AV block, only 1.5% went on to late complete heart block or sudden death. This study did not address the problem of PVC's. Garsons [1] review correlated a high right ventricular pressure and the presence of premature ventricular contractions with later onset of sudden death (Fig. 1). Kavey et al. [9] found a correlation with PVC's and dilatation of the right ventricle.

Etiology and incidence of conduction defects after repair of tetralogy of Fallot

The incidence of right bundle branch block, after repair of tetralogy of Fallot, ranges from 60–91% [10, 11]. The incidence of left axis deviation ranges from 9–23%. Right bundle branch block can be caused either by incision of the free wall of the right ventricle or by direct trauma to the right bundle branch [11–13]. A 44% incidence of right bundle branch block occurs if the ventricular septal defect (VSD) is closed through the tricuspid valve without a ventriculotomy.

Electrophysiological studies after repair of tetralogy of Fallot

Several investigations have been performed to determine if electrophysiological studies can be predictive of later dysrhythmic events after tetralogy of Fallot repair. Gillette et al. [12] studied 51 patients who had had previous repair of tetralogy of Fallot. Ninety-four per cent had right bundle branch block, 16% had right bundle branch block and left anterior hemiblock. Nine had premature ventricular contractions. Diffuse abnormalities of the conduc-

438

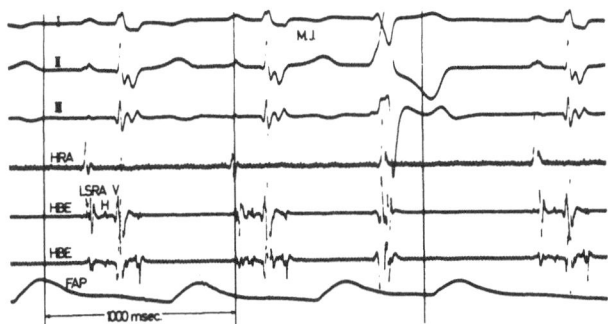

Fig. 2. Simultaneously recorded surface ECG I, II, and III together with the high right atrium and His bundle electrograms in a patient after repair of tetralogy of Fallot. The conduction intervals from HRA to low septal LSRA and from LSRA to H and H to V are normal. The third beat is premature ventricular contraction as shown by the fact that there is no H bundle depolarization preceding it. FAP: femoral artery pressure; H: His; HBE: His bundle electrograms; HRA: high right atrium; LSRA: low septal right atrium; V: ventricle.

tion system were found. Six of 30 had intra-atrial conduction delay, 5 of 51 had slowing of atrioventricular nodal conduction, 4 of 51 had prolonged His-Purkinje conduction. No differences were found in the groups of patients with and without left anterior hemiblock. Eight patients had abnormally prolonged sinus node recovery times. Thus, there was evidence for diffuse damage to the electrical system of the heart. In follow-up, 3 of these patients died suddenly. One was documented to have ventricular fibrillation and the others were undocumented. Each had premature ventricular contractions on resting electrocardiogram. One of the 3 had prolonged H:V interval, but this was the one that was documented to have ventricular fibrillation secondary to multiform PVC's. In a study on a different group of patients, Garson and Gillette et al. [13] found 41% to have abnormal sinus node recovery time, 15% to have abnormal AV node conduction, 41% had a lower than normal rate at which second degree AV block occurred during pacing, 22% had a prolonged HV interval, and 48% had a prolonged V to RV apex interval indicating that their right bundle branch block was central (Fig. 2). The second group of patients also had attempted induction of ventricular tachycardia (VT) by single and double PVC's into the right ventricular apex. Fourteen patients, 52% had one or more re-entrant beats induced. Seven or 26% had bundle branch reentrant beats which are considered a normal variant. Of these 27 patients, 13 were undergoing testing as part of routine follow-up, whereas 14 were being studied because of suspected electrophysiological abnormalities or symptoms. There were no differences in these groups of patients in the proportion that had conduction system abnormalities. Twice as many patients, however, in the symptomatic group had induced ventricular dysrhythmias. Sustained VT occurred only in the symptomatic group. Two of the 14 symptomatic patients had induction of sustained VT. When comparing clinical and noninvasive testing to electrophysiologic data it was found that 44% of patients with induced VT had syncope, whereas none of the patients without induced arrhythmia had syncope. Of the patients with induced VT, 67% had either very frequent uniform PVC's, multiform PVC's, couplets, or VT on 24-hour electrocardiogram vs. none having these criteria in the noninducible group. Fifty-six per cent of the patients with induced VT had a right ventricular systolic pressure greater than 70 mm Hg, whereas none had this right ventricular pressure in the group who did not have VT induced. There was also significantly higher proportion of the patients with induced VT who had a low right ventricular ejection fraction or a prolonged H:V interval when compared to the ones who did not have an arrhythmia induced. Other studies have found the bradycardia-tachycardia syndrome to occur in a symptomatic fashion after correction of tetralogy of Fallot. Fox et al. [14] documented this in a 13-year-old boy, 8 years after correction of tetralogy of Fallot who had atrial flutter and depression of sinus node function, eventually requiring pacemaker implantation. These authors point out, that sinus bradycardia or bradycardia-tachycardia syndrome might be responsible for a proportion of the deaths after tetralogy of Fallot. Findings of abnormalities of sinus node function on routine electrophysiologic testing indicate that this is a real possibility.

Effects of age at correction

The great majority of the studies mentioned have been done in patients who were relatively old at the time of repair, that is between 4 and 9 years of age. The current practice in many centers is to operate patients with tetralogy of Fallot very early in life at the age of 1 or 2 years. It may be that by performing surgery earlier, many of the post operative dysrhythmic problems may be avoided. It is also possible, that operating on smaller hearts will result in more conduction disturbances. The effects of cardioplegia also remain largely unstudied. Thus, studies are needed in patients who have undergone early repair of tetralogy of Fallot to compare to the original studies.

Recommendations

In order to try and prevent sudden deaths and symptomatic dysrhythmias in patients after repair of tetralogy of Fallot, an aggressive diagnostic approach is necessary. Hemodynamic abnormalities after repair of tetralogy of Fallot such as high right ventricular pressure, decreased right ventricular contractility and

440

right ventricular dilatation seemed to be related to dysrhythmias and to severity of dysrhythmias. A hemodynamic catheterization should be carried out in each patient after repair of tetralogy of Fallot. Patients with elevated right ventricular systolic or diastolic pressure, decreased contractility or dilitation are at higher risk for symptomatic dysrhythmias. Patients with elevated right ventricular systolic pressure also seemed to be at higher risk for sudden death.

Twenty-four hour ambulatory electrocardiographic monitoring correlated with symptomatic dysrhythmias in one study. Therefore, 24-hour electrocardiograms should be done one year after repair of tetralogy of Fallot and approximately every 3 to 5 years thereafter, to observe for onset of dysrhythmias.

It is not yet certain whether electrophysiological testing is predictive of later dysrhythmias. Early results indicate that it is. Therefore, electrophysiological evaluation with programmed ventricular stimulation and recording intracardiac intervals is probably indicated as part of the hemodynamic catheterization.

Exercise testing has not been found to be completely predictive. Patients who did not have PVC's during exercise or who have their PVC's suppressed during exercise may still go on to have significant ventricular dysrhythmias. On the other hand, patients who have ventricular tachycardia induced at exercise are at significant risk. Therefore, exercise testing is recommended as part of the postoperative evaluation of patients after tetralogy of Fallot.

Treatment

It is not yet certain which patients after repair of tetralogy of Fallot require antidysrhythmic treatment. Patients who have both an elevated right ventricular systolic pressure and PVC's on resting electrocardiogram have been shown to be at an increased risk of sudden death and we, therefore, recommend treating them with Phenytoin. Phenytoin has been shown to suppress PVC's and to prevent sudden death [15]. Patients with high grade ventricular ectopy, such as multiform PVC's, couplets or triplets, should also be treated. Patients with exercise induced ventricular dysrhythmias should be treated. In some of these patients propranolol would be effective. Patients with ventricular tachycardia should all undergo treatment. Phenytoin and propranolol are the drug choices in this group. Patients with syncope should undergo complete evaluation including electrophysiologic testing and treatment should be based on the findings of electrophysiological testing. Patients with right bundle branch block and left anterior hemiblock do not require pacemaker treatment, even if the HV interval is mildly prolonged. Markedly prolonged H:V intervals over 90 msec probably require pacemaker treatment. Patients with second or third degree block after tetralogy of Fallot should each have implantation of a pacemaker. Physiological pacemakers which sense the atrium and pace the ventricle are recommended.

Summary

Surgical repair of tetralogy of Fallot results in diffuse electrophysiological abnormalities which may in some cases result in death. A careful history combined with noninvasive and invasive testing can predict which patients are at the greatest risk. Poor hemodynamic result and PVC's are the two most significant risk factors. Treatment with phenytoin supresses PVC's and reduces the incidence of sudden death. The influence of recent refinements in surgical technique such as infant surgery and cardioplegia are yet to be defined.

References

1. Garson A Jr, Nihil MR, McNamara DG, Cooley DA: Status of the adult and adolescent after repair tetralogy of Fallot. Circulation 1979; 59: 1232–1240.
2. Quattlebaum TG, Varghese PG, Neill CA, Donahoo JS: Sudden death among post operative patients with tetralogy of Fallot. Circulation 1976; 54: 289.
3. James FW, Kaplan S, Chou TC: Unexpected cardiac arrest in patients after surgical correction of tetralogy of Fallot. Circulation 1975; 52: 691.
4. Wolff GS, Rowland TW, Ellison RC: Surgically induced right bundle branch block with left anterior hemiblock. Circulation 1972; 45: 587.
5. James EW, Kaplan S, Schwartz DC, Chou TC, Sandler MJ, Naylor V: Response to exercise in patients following total surgical correction of tetralogy of Fallot. Circulation 1976; 54: 671.
6. Fuster V, McGoon DC, Kennedy MA: Long-term evaluation (12 to 22 years) of open heart surgery for tetralogy of Fallot. Am J Cardiol 1980; 46: 635–641.
7. Deanfield J, McKenna W, Yen S, Hallidie-Smith K, Anderson R, Allwork S: Sudden death after correction of tetralogy of Fallot: a clinical pathological study (Abstract). Am J Cardiol 1982; 49: 998.
8. Krongrad E: Prognosis of patients with congenital heart disease and post operative intraventricular conduction defects. Circulation 1978; 57: 867.
9. Kavey REW, Blackman MS, Sondheimer HM: Ventricular dysrhythmias after repair of tetralogy of Fallot: incidence and severity. Circulation 1980; 62 (Suppl 3): 72.
10. Okoroma EO, Guller B, Maloney JD, Weidman WH: Etiology of right bundle branch block pattern after surgical closure of ventricular septal defects. Am Heart J 1975; 90: 14–18.
11. Sung RJ, Tamer DM, García OL, Castellanos A, Myerburg RJ, Gelband H: Analysis of surgically induced right bundle branch block pattern using intracardiac recording techniques. Circulation 1976; 54: 442–446.
12. Gelband H, Waldo AL, Kaiser GA, Bowman FO Jr, Malm JR, Hoffman BF: Etiology of right bundle branch block in patients undergoing total correction of tetralogy of Fallot. Circulation 1971; 44: 1022.

13. Krongrad E, Hefler SE, Bowman FO Jr, Malm JR, Hoffman BF: Further observations on the etiology of right bundle branch block pattern following right ventriculotomy. Circulation 1974; 50: 1105.
14. Fox K, Evans T, Rowland E, Krikler D: Bradycardia-tachycardia syndrome 8 year after correction of Fallot's tetralogy. Eur J Cardiol 1979; 10: 109–115.
15. Garson A, Kugler JD, Gillette PC, Simonelli A, McNamara DG: Control of late post operative ventricular arrhythmias with phenytoin in young patients. Am J Cardiol 1980; 46: 290–294.

9.5 Tetralogy of Fallot: Present Status of Corrective Surgery and Mid-term Follow-up

J.M. BRITO

The results of surgery for tetralogy of Fallot vary and generally depend on the center where it is performed. We review our experience with special attention to risk factors, morbidity and late results. From March 1978 to December 1984, a total of 278 children with tetralogy of Fallot were operated on. In 163 cases, corrective surgery was performed, and in 115 cases palliative procedures were used. Results are shown in Table 1.

The results of corrective surgery are listed in Table 2.

Among the most statistically significant ($p < 0.05$) risk factors were:

1. Presence of associated anomalies (summarized in Table 3).
2. Degree of anatomic severity and its technical implications, summarized in Table 4.
3. Year in which surgery was performed, child's age at the time of operation and need for previous palliative surgery.
4. Surgical management before, during and after operation (Table 5).

These findings become evident in comparison of the results of our first 50 cases (operated on 1978–1979), which had a hospital mortality of 14%, with those obtained in our last 67 cases (1982–1984), in which mortality decreased mark-

Table 1. Palliative surgery in 115 children with tetralogy of Fallot (1978–1984).

	1978–1984	1978–1981	1982–1984
Hospital mortality	4/115 (3.4%)	2/49 (4%)	2/66 (3%)
Number of survivers	111	47	64
Follow-up period	8	5	3
Number of children followed-up	103	42	61
Follow-up (mean)	3–71 (21.8) mo	3–71 (26) mo	3–35 (19) mo
New shunt required	13/103 (12.6%)	10/42 (23%)	3/61 (3.2%)
Total late mortality	6/103 (5.8%)	4/42 (9.5%)	2/61 (3.2%)
Severe heart failure	1/103 (0.9%)	1/42 (2.3%)	0/61

Sixty-six per cent were infants and 23% newborns.

444

edly, to 2.9%. The 5-year results of the 50 cases operated on before 1980 are summarized in Table 6. We consider it important that 90% of the survivers are presently asymptomatic and do not require any type of treatment.

We summarize our present guidelines for establishing the surgical indication for tetralogy of Fallot in Table 7, although we emphasize the need for individual evaluation of each case, mainly on the basis of age and anatomy.

Table 2. Corrective surgery in 163 cases, March 1978 to December 1984.

Present hospital mortality (last 30 mos)	2/67	2.9%
Hospital follow-up (entire series)	139	
Lost for follow-up	9/139	
Followed-up 3–72 mos (mean 25 mos)	130/139	
Reoperated for residual lesions	10/130	7.6%
Asymptomatic w/o medical treatment	114/130	87.6%
Asymptomatic with medical treatment	10/130	7.6%
Symptomatic	6/130	4.6%
Hemodynamic situation (routine catheterization):		
Good-excellent 5 years after correction	20/20	100%

Table 3. Tetralogy of Fallot. Corrective surgery for associated anomalies.

	Number	Mortality
Pulmonary valve agenesia	5	2
Pulmonary artery anomalies	5	1
Complete AV canal	3	
Mitral stenosis	1	1
Mitral incompetence	1	
Tricuspid incompetence	1	1
Aortic stenosis	1	
Anomalous pulmonary vein drainage	1	
Total	18	5 (27.7%)

Table 4. Unfavorable anatomic factors for corrective surgery of tetralogy of Fallot.

Severe pulmonary artery anomalies: hypoplasia and/or nonconfluence
Hypoplastic pulmonary ring and trunk
Great aortic dextroposition
Severe hypoplasia or absence of the infundibular septum
Anomalous coronary crossing the right ventricular infundibulum
Very small left ventricle
Severe associated anomalies

Table 5. Tetralogy of Fallot. Variations in corrective surgery with time.

	1978–1981	1982–1984
Myocardial protection	Intermittent Ao unclamping	Cardioplegia
VSD closure	Interrupted sutures	Continuous suture
	+	+
	Continuous suture	Reinforcement sutures
Type of patch used to enlarge infundibulum	PTFE	Equine pericardium
	Goretex-Impra	Goretex
Anatomic evaluation (coronary anomalies)	General	Meticulous
Immediate postoperative	Classic treatment	Routine: dopamine nitroglycerin

Table 6. Tetralogy of Fallot. Evolution at 5 years.

50 cases corrected in 1978–1979		
Initial mortality	7	14%
	2	Residual shunt
Morbility	3	
	1	Respiratory failure
		Reoperation
Symptomatic	1	Arrhythmia
Asymptomatic	Without treatment	39/43 90%
	With treatment	3/43 6%

Table 7. Corrective surgery for tetralogy of Fallot. Surgical guidelines presently followed in our service.

Age	Indication	
0–12 months	1st	Palliative surgery
	2nd	Surgery to correct unfavorable anatomy or associated pulmonary agenesia
12–36 months	1st	Corrective surgery
	2nd	Palliative surgery for very unfavorable anatomy
> 36 months	*Elective* corrective surgery	
Any age	In severe pulmonary artery abnormalities: right ventricle-pulmonary artery connection	

10. Angina Pectoris (I)

10.1 Introduction

M. GARCIA MOLL

The advances made in medical and surgical treatment of angina pectoris in the last decade have enabled us not only to eliminate or ameliorate symptoms, principally pain in most patients, but to prolong survival. Advances in therapy were one of the most influential factors contributing to the important reduction in mortality due to ischemic heart disease observed in the United States in recent years. We are gradually approaching our ideal objective: prolonging the patient's life and improving the quality of his life.

In the seventies, therapeutic progress was centered mainly on diffusion of myocardial revascularization surgery by aortocoronary bypass. In the first half of the eighties, the principal break-throughs have been in medical treatment. These advances have been largely possible because new physiopathologic findings have allowed development of novel areas of pharmacologic study or more effective use of those previously known. The contributions of Maseri and colleagues have been fundamental in confirming the existence of a dynamic obstructive factor. Specchia and Waters have recently demonstrated that this factor participates in some forms of effort angina. Correct identification of these forms is a prerequisite for their treatment.

Pharmacologically, progress has concentrated on extending use of the different calcium antagonists (introduced by Fleckenstein in 1971) and on improving the efficacy of the nitrites by intravenous or transdermal administration of nitroglycerin.

The increase in the effectiveness of pharmacologic treatment, a tendency initiated in 1968 with the introduction of β-blocking agents, has not only enhanced control of anginal pain, but has produced a notable increment in the survival rate of these patients, who have an global yearly mortality of 1.6% in the CASS study. This improvement has also been observed in high risk subgroups; as such, patients with severe three-vessel disease had an annual mortality of 11.4% at the end of the sixties, 4.8% in the mid-seventies, 3.5% at the end of that decade, and 2.1% at the beginning of the eighties. One of the first consequences of the prolongation of patient life expectancy by medical treatment has been a critical review of certain surgical indications designed to improve the prognosis of patients who are asymptomatic or have controlled angina.

It is a reasonable assumption that the near future will bring further progress in nonsurgical treatment of angina patients. Likewise, this progress will continue to derive from elucidation of the pathophysiological mechanisms involved. However, it cannot be ignored that greater use and perfection of techniques for treating coronary obstruction (conventional or laser percutaneous transluminal coronary angioplasty) will lend increasing importance to these procedures.

10.2 Coronary Reserve and Angina Therapy

M. IRIARTE EZKURDIA, J.M. AGUIRRE SALCEDO,
J. BOVEDA ROMEO, E. MOLINERO DE MIGUEL and
J. URRENGOETXEA MARTINEZ

Introduction

Several studies have confirmed that patients with vasospastic angina have a variable ischemia threshold for exercise [1–3]. In our group, Molinero has demonstrated [4, 5] that variable ischemia threshold, identified by different serial electrocardiographic effort tests, is frequent (12/20 cases) in patients with angina at rest and with exertion (mixed angina). Servi [1] identified a significant increment in exercise tolerance and regional coronary flow after administration of nifedipine in patients with effort angina and variable electrocardiographic threshold. Parting from these findings, our study had a double objective:

a) identification of the vasospastic component of effort angina by evaluating coronary reserve, and

b) appraisal of the therapeutic value of identifying this component.

Maseri [6–9] classified transitory ischemia as *primary* and *secondary* according to its relation with metabolic demand. Using this criterion, effort angina is secondary when it appears at fixed metabolic demand levels and primary when it is produced at different levels, these levels being indicated by the 'double product' (DP). Angina at rest is secondary when it appears after an increase in DP and primary if it presents without modifications in this index.

The beneficial effects of antianginal medication are the result of two general mechanisms: reduction in metabolic oxygen demand and/or increased supply by improvement in coronary blood flow. β-blocking agents act through the first mechanism and calcium antagonists and nitrites by both. Considering that variations in coronary vasomotor tone are the main known determinant of primary angina, identification of these variations has great therapeutic significance.

452

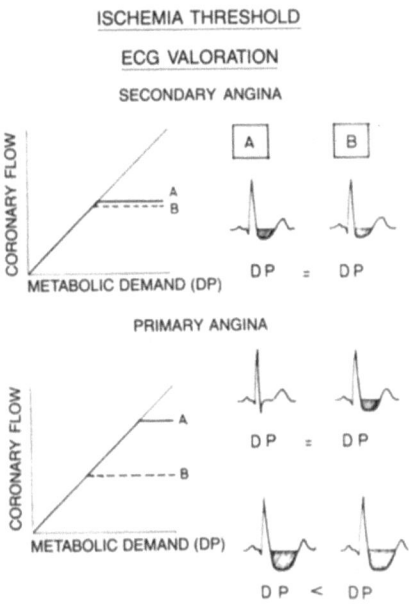

ISCHEMIA THRESHOLD

ECG VALORATION

SECONDARY ANGINA

PRIMARY ANGINA

Fig. 1. Determination of the ischemia threshold by two consecutive electrocardiographic exercise tests (A and B). DP: double product. (See text.)

Ischemia threshold (Fig. 1)

The ischemia threshold and its variability can be determined by serial electro-cardiographic effort tests. If we graph coronary flow (ordinate) and metabolic demand or DP (abscissa) on a Cartesian coordinate system, the ischemia threshold can be defined as the DP increment required to produce stabilization of coronary flow. In secondary angina the threshold is stable in two or more consecutive tests, while it varies in primary angina.

If ischemia is quantified in terms of the magnitude of S-T segment depression during exercise, in secondary angina it is identical for the same DP in several effort tests. In contrast, in primary angina one test may be positive and another negative for the same level of metabolic demand or there may be the same degree of positivity for different DP magnitudes.

Identification of variations in the myocardial ischemia threshold with thallium-201 perfusion studies

The electrocardiographic exercise test has limited sensitivity and specificity for identifying myocardial ischemia and consequently, little utility for quantifying

METHOD

1 – Coronary angiogram

2 – Ergonovin test (up to 0.4 mg i.v.)

3 – Serial gammagraphic perfusion with Tl-201

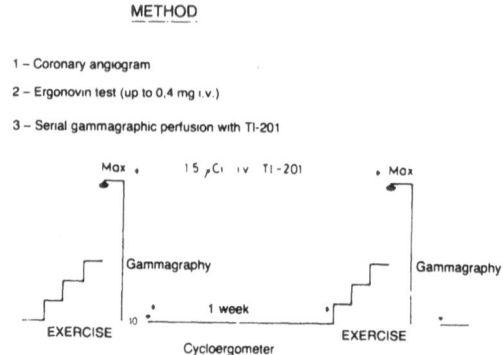

Fig. 2. Methodology of the electrocardiographic effort tests. Max: maximum. (See text.)

it. Identification and quantification of myocardial ischemia by gammagraphic perfusion (Tl-201) is more precise because myocardial capture of the radio-active cation is directly related to the fractional distribution of coronary blood flow.

In view of this, we proposed to assess modifications in myocardial ischemia in serial effort tests in stable and probable vasospastic angina by computer-quantified thallium-201 perfusion studies.

Material and methods

We studied 26 male patients (mean age 54 ± 56 years) with and without previous angina. These patients were divided into two groups:

Group A: 10 patients with stable effort angina, significant coronary lesions (at least one proximal stenosis >70%) and negative ergonovine test.

Group B: 16 patients with clinical evidence of vasospastic angina (3 variant angina, 4 angina at rest and with mixed angina (in SF II)) in whom there was S-T depression during spontaneous angina. Fourteen had significant coronary disease and 2 had normal coronary arteries. In 7 the ergonovine test was positive.

Two maximum effort tests on an ergometric bicycle were performed within a one-week interval. At peak of exercise, 1.5 mCi of Tl-201 were intravenously injected. Ten minutes after terminating the exercise images were obtained in anteroposterior, left oblique and left lateral position (Fig. 2).

Perfusion was quantified with Silber's [10] computerized method, which records segmental Tl-201 distribution as a histogram representing the respective percentage of maximum activity (Fig. 3).

Heart rate, blood pressure and DP were recorded in each test. In each

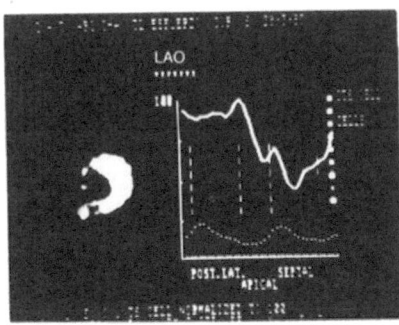

Fig. 3. Silber's computerized method for quantifying segmental activity as a percentage of the segment with the highest activity. On the left, the left anterior oblique view shows marked reduction in septal activity. On the right, the histogram shows a 40% reduction of the activity of the septum compared with that of posterolateral segment.

ischemic segment, maximum ischemia, mean ischemia and mean ischemia normalized for DP (NI) were determined. NI *variability* was calculated as the difference between the values obtained in two tests expressed as percentage of the maximum value (Fig. 4).

The *fixed threshold* was defined as a function of findings in 10 patients with stable angina (group A), in whom NI variation attained a mean value of $12.2 \pm 8.8\%$.

By increasing this mean value by two standard deviations, we obtained a variability of 30%; above this level was the *variable threshold* with a margin of raliability of 95% (p<0.0005) (Fig. 5).

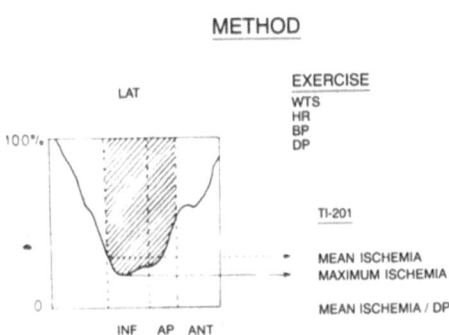

Fig. 4. Method for determining maximum ischemia, mean and mean normalized for double product. LAT: lateral. INF: inferior. AP: anteroposterior. WTS: watts. HR: heart rate. BP: blood pressure. DP: double product. (See text.)

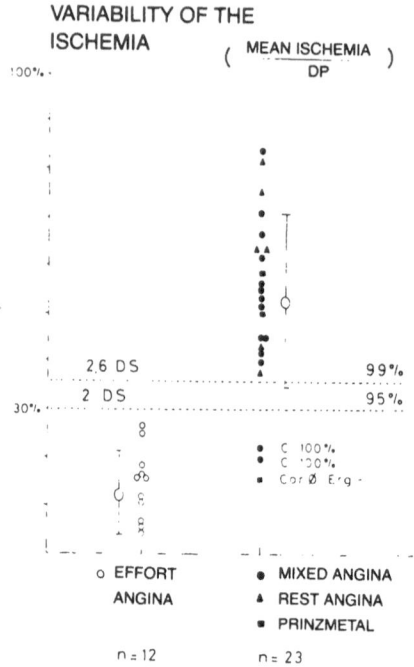

VARIABILITY OF THE ISCHEMIA

$\left(\dfrac{\text{MEAN ISCHEMIA}}{\text{DP}} \right)$

o EFFORT ANGINA

• MIXED ANGINA
▲ REST ANGINA
■ PRINZMETAL

n = 12

n = 23

Fig. 5. Study of the variability of the ischemia index in patients with secondary angina (effort angina) and primary angina (mixed, rest and Prinzmetal angina). The response of the 10 patients with effort angina allows determination of the limit of threshold variability. (See text.)

Results (Fig. 5)

NI variability in group B was $50.2 \pm 18\%$, as compared with $12.2 \pm 8\%$ for group A ($p < 0.001$). In all the patients in group B except for three, NI was superior to 30%. In the 3 patients in whom vasospastic angina was suspected, but no *variable ischemia threshold* was found, one had variant angina and normal coronary arteries and the disease was not in the active phase. The other two presented angina at rest with subocclusive stenosis and scant coronary reserve.

In stable effort angina, the reproducibility of the method was very good, as illustrated by the example in Fig. 6 of a patient with severe right coronary artery stenosis. In this patient, the DP histograms were similar and variability was 6% (Fig. 6). In the group B patients, the *variable threshold* may appear with the same or different DPs, as can be observed in a patient with angina in a test – the smaller the DP, the greater the ischemia (Figs 7 and 8).

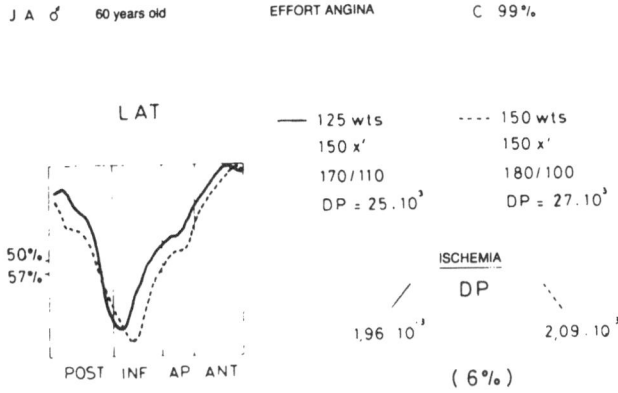

Fig. 6. Gammagraphic expression of a fixed ischemia threshold in a patient with effort angina. Observe the similarity of the diagrams in two consecutive effort tests in which there were no evident variations in the double products.

Discussion

Reflex stimulation of the sympathetic system and catocholamine release during physical effort are a potential origin of coronary vasoconstriction. However, exercise-mediated vasospasm is not easily comprehended because local vasodilator factors [11] normally counteract the neurogenic and humoral vasoconstrictor effects. A possible explanation would be that epicardial arteries are less affected by local vasodilator metabolites [12].

It has been experimentally demonstrated that coronary vasoconstriction

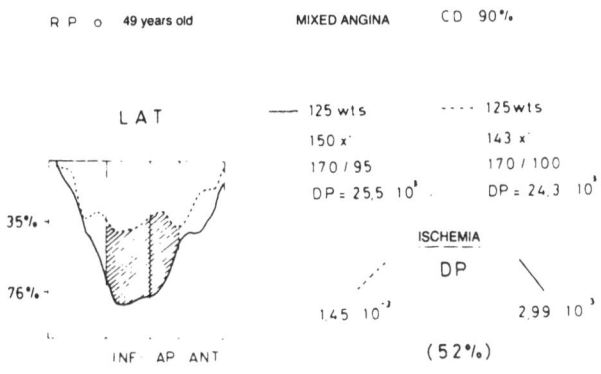

Fig. 7. Isotopic study of a patient with mixed angina and variable ischemia threshold (52%). It can be seen that for a similar double product there is an evident difference in ischemia (shaded area) from one test to another.

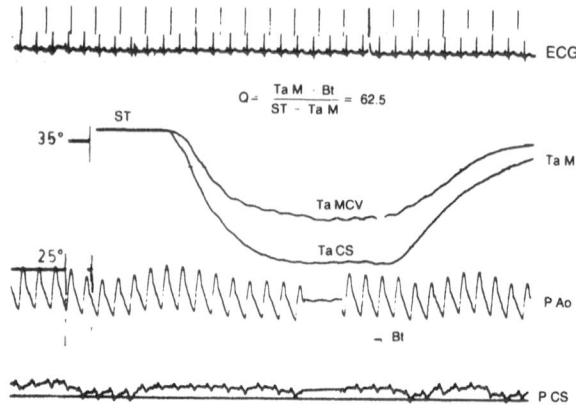

Fig. 8. Bain method for determining blood flow in the coronary sinus (CS) and major coronary vein (MCV) by introducing 2 termistor in these structures. Q: blood flow. TM: temperature of the mixture. BT: blood temperature. ST: serum temperature. AoP: aortic pressure. CSP: coronary sinus pressure.

occurs during effort because α-adrenergic block during effort produces a greater decrease in resistance with respect to the basal situation.

It has been clinically confirmed that isotonic exercise can produce vaso-spasm in patients with variant angina. Theroux [13] encountered an incidence of 30% positive effort tests with S-T segment elevation in these patients during the active disease phase. The real incidence is probably higher since vasospasm can occur without producing electrogram modifications or ST depression.

Several authors [13, 14] have angiographically confirmed coronary spasm during effort. Yasue [15] encountered a circadian rhythm for effort capacity in coronariographies made during serial effort tests in a group of patients with variant angina. Coronary vessel diameter was smaller during morning exercise than for afternoon exercise.

A relationship has also been observed between the phase of activity of vasospastic disease and positive effort test results [15]: effort tests that were positive during active disease phases became negative in latent phases.

Following Conti [16], the pathophysiological scheme of angina has two clearly defined ends of the spectrum: one with patients with slight or absent coronary lesions, angina at rest and spasm-induced coronary ischemia; and the other are patients with fixed severe coronary lesions and stable effort angina, the ischemic mechanism being restriction of supply due to the structural lesions. In the latter patients, the ischemia threshold would be fixed and highly reproducible; as the disease progresses and exercise tolerance changes, the threshold would still be fixed, but lower. Between these two extremes is wide continuum of intermediate situations in which organic lesions and associated vasospasm participate in a variable degree.

Several authors [3, 4, 6] have observed a lack of reproducibility in the ischemia threshold of patients with effort angina. In the anamnesis it is not rare to encounter patients with angina at rest and with great effort. In these patients, a mixed pathophysiological mechanism evidently has to be invoked. Yasue [17] has demonstrated that this tolerance, different from effort tolerance, is due to coronary vasospasm. Analyzing tolerance to effort with electrocardiographic ergometric tests, various authors [6, 18] find that in an elevated percentage of cases of vasospastic angina, the DP level at which ischemia is produced changes from one test to another. This different effort tolerance can be manifested two ways, by alternation of positive and negative test results or with positive test results at different double products. What these authors did not analyze were the differences in DP level from which the ischemia threshold can be considered to be variable.

Molinero et al. [4], aside from taking a different approach (they analyzed the predictive value of variable ischemia threshold instead of sensitivity), normalized ischemia for DP and established the limits of normal variability for normalized ischemia in a group of patients with stable effort angina. Although electrocardiographic methods are useful to detect ischemia, it is questionable that they are useful to quantify it; the magnitude of ST segment depression in a lead is not a good parameter for evaluating the severity and extension of ischemia. The study by Molinero et al. parted from this limitation.

In our study we used a more accurate method to evaluate myocardial ischemia: T1-201 perfusion imaging and computerized (Silber) quantification of the degree of segmental ischemia. Although these images cannot directly quantify flow, there is a linear relation with the intensity of isotope distribution. Since what we analyze are the variations in isotope distribution in different effort tests, it is presumible that modifications in the distribution can only be attributed to variations in coronary flow. We described the precision and reproducibility of this method earlier [19]. Moreover, by normalizing segmental ischemia for DP, we establish a precise limit for establishing variable ischemia threshold.

The hypothesis that best explains variable ischemia threshold in patients with primary component angina is that of Epstein and Talbot [3]. These authors attribute it to alterations in coronary vasomotor tone prior to beginning exercise because it is difficult to imagine that the sympathetic stimulus produced by effort would vary from one test to another.

We selected our 16 patients by clinical criteria, on the basis of suspicion of a primary component in angina that appeared at rest and showed electrocardiographic signs of ischemia during pain. The main disadvantage of this selection process is that we may label a patient with severe atherosclerotic lesions and scant coronary reserve as primary resting angina, when angina is induced by small DP increments at rest, making it secondary. This possibility may explain our findings in two patients in whom we could not demonstrate variable ischemia threshold although they presented angina at rest and had a positive T1-201 image for ischemia. Both patients presented subtotal coronariographic obstruction of the circumflex artery without infarction.

The third patient who did not have variable ischemia threshold had variant angina with minimal coronary lesions and the disease was inactive at the time of study.

With variable ischemia threshold determination using the method described, we detected vasoactivity in 81% of the patients in our study group. In these same patients, the incidence of positive ergonovine test was 41%. In the light of these results, variable ischemia threshold determination is more sensitive than the ergonovine test to detect vasoactivity, at least in patients with mixed angina. This finding entails a review of the concept of active vasospastic disease. Primary angina was considered to be active when evidenced as Prinzmetal angina or when vasospasm could be induced by the ergonovine test. Nonetheless, vasospastic disease may clinically manifest itself by lower vasoconstriction levels or increased coronary tone, which might not be sufficiently intense for the ergonovine vasoconstrictor stimulus to induce spasm. This hypothesis is based on the observation that in some patients, physiological stimuli like effort are potentially more vasoconstrictive than ergonovine. Of our patients, all those with positive induction tests presented variable ischemia threshold, but several patients with negative test results had a variable ischemia threshold.

Of the two patients with normal coronary arteries, one had variant angina and the other had angina at rest. Variable ischemia threshold was detected in one, although T1-201 activity was lower than in patients with organic coronary stenosis.

Fig. 7 shows the isotopic results of a patient with mixed angina and 90% stenosis of the RC. In two consecutive effort tests of similar magnitude and similar DP there was a net difference in the ischemia of lower segments and 52% NI variability.

T1-201 allows segmental identification of the ischemic process, thus allowing us to identify both temporal and spatial variations in the vasomotor tone. In a patient who had mixed angina and two-vessel disease, ischemia of the territory irrigated by the anterior descending coronary artery was seen in an ET and ischemia of the inferior myocardium supplied by the right coronary artery was seen in another, despite equal DP.

We can therefore conclude that variable ischemia threshold is a more sensitive indicator than the ergonovine test for modifications in coronary vasomotor tone. This is independent of the state of the coronary network, since we demonstrated variable ischemia threshold in patients with normal coronaries and a negative ergonovine test.

Although the Tl-201 images quantified by computer provided sufficient evidence to attribute variable ischemia threshold to changes in coronary circulation, unequivocal demonstration of this fact requires precise quantification by thermodilution techniques that enable appraisal of global and segmental coronary flow. At the present, our group is orienting their research along these lines.

Variations in coronary blood flow in relation with ischemia threshold and nifedipine administration (Figs 9, 10 and 11)

To demonstrate that *variable ischemia threshold* is related to modifications in coronary blood flow independent of metabolic demand, we correlated DP with *coronary flow* in serial effort tests (morning/afternoon) in 2 patients with severe anterior descending coronary artery stenosis, one with a fixed ischemia threshold and the other with a variable one.

We calculated blood flow in the coronary sinus and major coronary vein with the BAIN thermodilution technique [12]. In the patient with a fixed threshold, the 'flow/DP' curves in different tests were practically the same, while the variable threshold patient had appreciably higher flow levels for each DP in the second test than in the first.

After concluding exercise and reestablishing basal hemodynamic conditions, both patients were given 20 mg nifedipine sublingually. In both cases, the medication produced a 20% decrease in systolic blood pressure, increasing major coronary vein blood flow from 63 to 109 ml/min in 40 minutes (73%) in the variable threshold patient. The fixed threshold patient did not experience any change. These findings suggest that the calcium antagonist modified coronary vasomotor tone at rest in the patient with variable threshold, increasing the blood flow in the ischemic territory, while it had no effect on the other patient.

Specchia recently studied [19] the effect of nifedipine on coronary circulation in 14 patients with predominant effort angina and severe stenosis of the anterior descending coronary artery. Two modalities of response were observed:

In 7 patients nifedipine did not modify main coronary vein blood flow at rest or during exercise; all presented a fixed ischemia threshold in the electrocardiographic effort test. The drug did not improve exercise tolerance or decrease the degree of ST segment displacement in any. In the rest of the patients nifedipine induced an increase in main coronary vein flow at rest and during exercise, enhanced exercise tolerance and reduced the magnitude of the ST displacement. Although threshold variability was not verified in this group because the second exercise test was performed under the influence of nifedi-

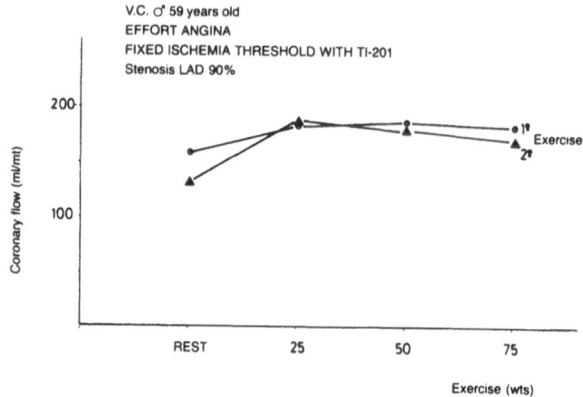

Fig. 9. Correlation between coronary blood flow (ml/min) and the work developed during exercise (watts) in two consecutive tests. The patient with effort angina and fixed threshold has two diagrams with the same trajectory.

pine, we invoke this substance's effect on vasomotor tone to explain the increase in coronary flow and clinical and electrocardiographic improvement. In any case, this improvement could not be attributed to a descent in the hemodynamic determinants of O_2 consumption (DP and contractility). Similarly, nifedipine was reported to improve the angina threshold in two patients with effort angina with a vasospastic component; the drug produced a notable increase in coronary blood flow [1]. In any case, earlier investigations have not clarified why this calcium antagonist has a beneficial effect in some patients

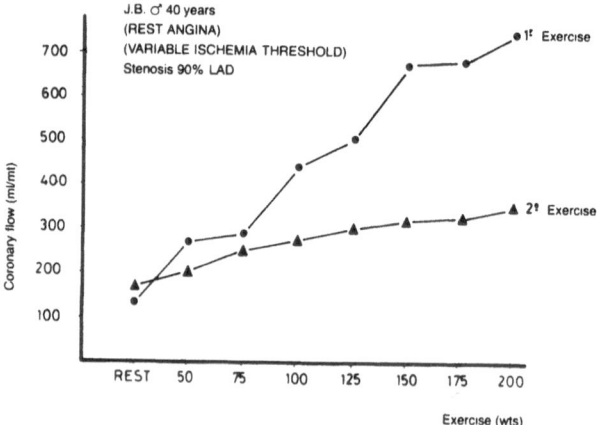

Fig. 10. Correlation between coronary flow and work expressed in watts in a patient with angina at rest and variable threshold. Note how during the first exercise the coronary flow is notably greater for each work level achieved.

462

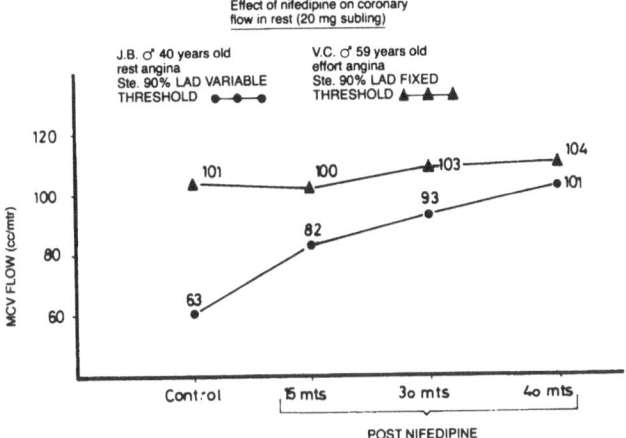

Fig. 11. Effect of nifedipine on coronary flow at rest in the patients in figs 9 and 10. It can be seen that nifedipine increases blood flow in the major coronary vein in the patient with variable threshold but not in the carrier of fixed threshold.

and not in others [19]. Our findings, quantified by T1-201 studies, suggest that clinical manifestations have a high predictive value for identifying the existence of variable ischemia threshold, since 81% of our patients with mixed angina or angina at rest presented it. On the other hand, fact that main coronary vein blood flow only increased after nifedipine administration in patients with variable ischemia threshold provides a possible explanation for Specchia's findings of no clinical or hemodynamic improvement in 7 of 14 patients with predominant effort angina and fixed threshold [19] and improvement in 7 in whom the threshold was not assessed. Like Specchia, we detected a favorable effect on blood flow at rest, corroborating the hypothesis of Epstein et al. [3], who attribute the primary nature of certain effort anginas that occur before initiating exercise to changes in vasomotor tone.

Conclusions

1. The ischemia/DP ratio is highly reproducible in secondary angina.
2. The presence of variable ischemia threshold serves to differentiate primary from secondary ischemia ($p<0.001$).
3. Identification of a vasospastic component, which may also be found in effort angina, suggests that the calcium antagonists could be useful for many of these patients.
4. Our results suggest that nifedipine will benefit patients with variable threshold (rest and mixed angina) more than patients with fixed threshold (stable effort angina).

References

1. DeServi S, Specchia G, Falcone C, Gavazzi A, Mussini A, Angali C, Bramucci F, Ardissino B, Vaccari L, Salerno J, Bobba P: Variable threshold exertional angina in patients with transient vasospastic myocardial ischemia. Am J Cardiol 1983; 51: 397.
2. Lentenegger F, Rafflenbeul W, Gahl K: Quantitative koronaroespasmen nach nifedippine. Schw Med Wschr 1980; 110: 1703.
3. Epstein SF, Talbot TL: Dynamic coronary tone in precipitation, exacerbation and relief of angina pectoris. Am J Cardiol 1981; 48: 797.
4. Molinero E, Terradillos P, Faus JM, Fernandez L, Aguirre JM: Aproximación al diagnóstico fisiopatológico de la angina a través de las pruebas de esfuerzo seriadas. Rev Esp Cardiolog 1983; 36 (Suppl 2): 4.
5. Molinero E: Tesis doctoral. Universidad del País Vasco, Bilbao, 1983.
6. Maseri A, Chierchia S: Coronary artery spasm: demonstration, definition, diagnosis and consequences. Prog Cardiovasc Dis 1982; 25: 169–189.
7. Maseri A, L'Abbate A, Chierchia S, et al.: Significance of spasm in the pathogenesis of ischemic heart disease. Am J Cardiol 1979; 42: 1019–1035.
8. Maseri A, L'Abbate S, Denes M, et al.: Variant angina: one aspect of a continuous spectrum of vasospastic myocardial ischemia. Am J Cardiol 1975; 42: 1019–1035.
9. Maseri A, L'Abbate A, Pesola A, et al.: Coronary vasospasm in angina pectoris. Lancet 1977; 1: 1034.
10. Iriarte MM, Boveda FJ, Aguirre JM, Faus JM, Martinez G, Molinero E, Negueruela J: Utilidad diagnóstica en la cardiopatía isquémica de la gammagrafía con T1-201 a través de un programa de cuantificación con ordenador. Rev Esp Cardiol 1985; 38: 92–99.
11. Heyndrickx GR, Myulaert P, Mabilde C, Pannier JL: Role of coronary α-receptors in the regulation of the coronary flow during exercise in dogs (Abstract). VIII European Congress of Cardiology. Paris, 1980: 135.
12. Murray PA, Vatner SE: α-receptor atentuation of coronary vascular response to severe, spontaneous exercise (Abstract). Fed Proc 1978; 37: 235.
13. Waters DD, Szlachcic J, Bourassa MG, Scholl JM, Theroux P: Exercise testing in patients with variant angina: results, correlation with clinical and angiographic features and prognostic significance. Circulation 1982; 65: 265–274.
14. Fuller CM, Raizner AE, Chachine RA, et al.: Exercise-induced coronary arterial spasm: Angiographic demonstration, documentation of ischemia by myocardial scintigraphy and results of pharmacologic intervention. Am J Cardiol 1980; 46: 500–506.
15. DeServi S, Specchia G, Curti MT, Falcone C, Gavazzi A, Bramucci E, Mussini A, Angoli L, Salerno J, Bobba P: Variable threshold of angina during exercise: a clinical manifestation of some patients with vasospastic angina. Am J Cardiol 1981; 48: 188–192.
16. Conti RC, Pepine CJ, Felman RL: Coronary artery spasm by heart. Cardiol Ser 1981; 4: 7.
17. Yasue H, Omote S, Takizawa A, Nagao M, Miwa K, Tanaka S: Circadian variation of exercise capacity in patients with Prinzmetal variant angina: role of exercise-induced coronary arterial spasm. Circulation 1979; 59: 938–948.
18. Aguirre JM, Boveda FJ, Molinero E, Cid M, Arrillaga M, Urcengoetxea J, Iriarte M: Serial thallium 201 imaging: quantitative variable ischaemia threshold at rest and effort angina (Abstract). Eur Heart J 1984; 5 (Suppl 1).
19. Specchia G, DeServi S, Colomba F, Angeli L, Gavazzi A, Bramucci E, Mussini A, Ferrario M, Salerno J, Montemartini C: Effects of tidipine in coronary hemodynamic dinings during exercise in patients with stable exertional angina. Circulation 1983; 68: 5. 1035–1043.

10.3 Nitrates in the Treatment of Angina Pectoris

A. CABADÉS O'CALLAGHAN, J. COSÍN AGUILAR,
A. SALVADOR SANZ and V. PALACIOS MOTILLA

More than a century has passed since nitrates began to be used in the treatment of angina pectoris, but in the last two decades, the therapeutic arsenal for this disease has been spectacularly enlarged by the introduction of new drugs, coronary surgery and pecutaneous transluminal angioplasty. Moreover, a more precise knowledge of the pathophysiology of angina guides the selection of the most appropriate procedure, therapy or drug for each modality of the disease. In view of these facts, what role do the nitrates now play in angina therapy? What can we say about the mechanism of action of the nitrates and what advantages do innovative forms of administration offer?

Mechanisms of action of the nitrates

The main pharmacologic effect of the nitrates is relaxation of the smooth muscle of vein and artery walls [1]. Two possible antianginal mechanisms derive from this effect: restoration of O_2 supply to areas of O_2 depletion (direct local coronary dilator effect) and reduction of myocardial O_2 consumption to levels within the limits of the possibilities of supply (indirect global hemodynamic effect) (Tables 1 and 2). This serves to prevent and interrupt anginal attacks, enhance exercise tolerance and ameliorate electrocardiographic signs of myocardial ischemia [2].

This effect on the vascular wall is also the source of the proanginal mechanisms of the nitrates:
a) reduction in O_2 supply to ischemic zones as a consequence of hypotension or the 'steal' mechanism; and
b) increased O_2 consumption by reflex increments in heart rate and myocardial contractility (Table 3).

The biochemical mechanism of this effect is not exactly known, although various possibilities have been considered:
a) modification of calcium currents [3] (thus acting like a specific calcium

465

antagonist on smooth, not striated, fiber);
b) activation of guanosincyclase, analogous to the effect of hydralazine [4], which increases cyclic *guanosin*-monophosphate concentration; and
c) stimulation of the specific vascular smooth muscle nitrate receptors [5].

With this array of possibilities (direct, indirect and proanginal effects), two fundamental questions should be asked: what is responsible for the antianginal effect of the nitrates? Under what circumstances can the combination of effects invert the beneficial pharmacologic effects?

At the beginning of the 70s, Ganz and Marcus [6] demonstrated that intracoronary nitroglycerin (NTG) does *not* suppress anginal pain induced by electrical stimulation. This study is cited by most researchers in this field [2, 7, 8] and constitutes the theoretical basis for assigning preponderance to systemic mechanisms rather than to direct coronary vasodilator effects. Aronow [2]

Table 1. Antianginal effects on coronary circulation (O_2 supply).

1. Reduction of resistance in arteries with organic stenosis
2. Antispasm effects
3. Incremented small artery resistance
4. Improvement in distribution of the subendocardial blood supply (by decreased LVEDP, filling pressure and extravascular resistance)

Table 2. Antianginal effects on systemic circulation (O_2 savings).

1. Venodilation with decreased enddiastolic and filling pressures
2. Reduction of ventricular volume
3. Fall in peripheral resistances due to arterial dilation
4. Decline in mean aortic pressure and the peak systolic pressure

Table 3. Proanginal effects.

1. Reduction in O_2 supply
   a. Hypotension
   b. 'Coronary steal' phenomenon
   – by collaterals
   – by epicardial vessels
   – by dilation of the arterial capillary bed
   c. Decrease in O_2 content in blood
2. Increase in O_2 consumption
   a. Tachycardia
   b. Increased contractility

considered the local coronary wall effects of the nitrates to be counterproductive; since it had not been demonstrated that arteriosclerotic vessels dilate under the effect of these substances, the increased coronary blood flow had occur in the healthy arteries, thus stealing the blood supply and increasing the ischemia in the zones already affected.

The improved quality of coronariography and use of highly sensitive and reproducible computerized methods for measuring the coronary lumen and its modifications contributed to the demonstration at the onset of the 80s that nitroglycerin *does* increase coronary vessel section in stenotic zones.

Brown et al. [7] favor that the effects of nitroglycerin mainly depend on coronary vessel size and drug concentration in blood. In normal vessels of 1.6–2.3 mm in diameter the lumen can dilate 35%, while vessels of more than 4–5 mm in diameter only increase their lumen by 9%. In diseased vessels the arteriosclerotic lesions do not occupy the entire vessel wall nor are they homogeneous; lumen modifications are therefore excentric and intermittent. The magnitude of the dilation is small in absolute terms: vessel diameter increases by an average of 0.15 mm and 0.2 mm in moderately and severely stenotic vessels, respectively. However, this represents a reduction in coronary flow resistance in the diseased area of 25% and 38%, respectively, an important increase.

In view of this reevaluation of local nitroglycerin antianginal effects, Brown et al. [7] ask: why did NTG fail in the Ganz and Marcus series? After repeating the analysis, they arrived at the following conclusions:

a) Pharmacological doses of NTG dilate large coronary arteries and stenotic segments but do not affect the distal vascular bed, resulting in an increase in poststenotic perfusion pressure.

b) At elevated dosages (Marcus and Ganz [6] reached doses that were 200 times pharmacological levels), microvascular autoregulation mechanisms are affected and the large arteries do not dilate, but intramyocardial vascular bed resistance fall.

Consequently, poststenotic pressure does not improve and may decline, worsening subendocardial perfusion and maintaining or aggravating anginal manifestations.

The importance of these direct antianginal effects was confirmed definitively [7, 9] by the finding that the subendocardial perfusion and contractile function of affected zones remain within physiologic limits as long as pressure distal to the coronary stenosis does not fall below 60 mm Hg at rest.

Direct coronary effects

In pathophysiological terms, the coronary vascular tree is constituted by two types of vessels (Fig. 1):

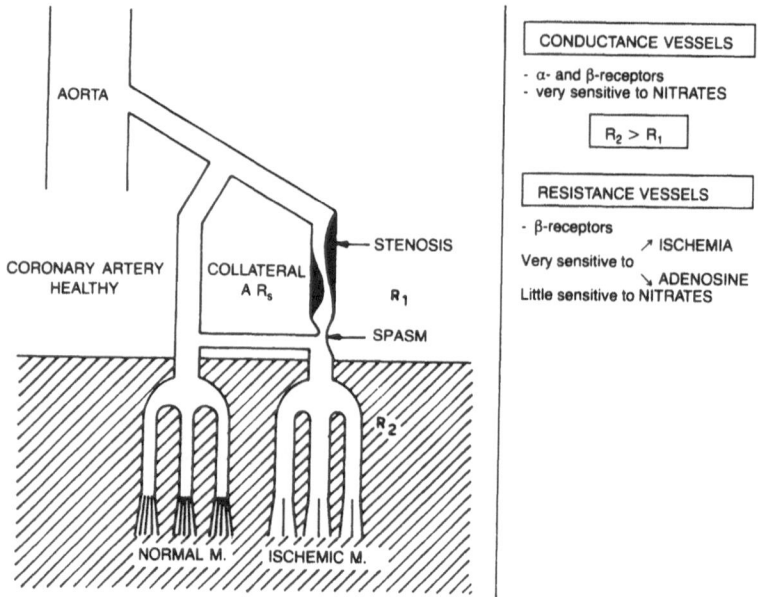

Fig. 1. Diagram of the two types of coronary vessels. Organic lesions and spasms usually occur in conductance vessels. To maintain adequate subendocardial perfusion pressure, the resistance in the conductance vessels would be less than that of the resistance vessels ($R_2 > R_1$).

a) *Epicardial conductance vessels:* large caliber, low resistance (R_1) vessels that supply blood to the myocardium. The walls of these vessels respond very well to nitrates, even at low concentrations, but they are relatively insensitive to metabolic stimuli [8, 10, 11] and their tone is regulated by α- and β-receptors.

b) *Resistance vessels:* small caliber intramyocardial and subendocardial arteries and arterioles with high resistance to flow (R_2). These vessels depend fundamentally on myocardial metabolic state, probably mediated by local adenosine concentration, and they are very sensitive to local ischemia and dipyridamol. It has not been demonstrated that they respond to α-stimulants [8, 10, 11]. Only elevated doses of nitrates dilate them, as was found in the study by Marcus and Ganz [6].

Changes in conductance artery flow resistance (R_1) can produce reciprocal changes in resistance vessels (R_2) to keep constant the circuit resistance ($R_1 + R_2$) and adequate subendocardial perfusion pressure. This explains (Fig. 2) [8, 10, 11]:

a) completely normal coronary flow in the presence of significant stenosis of the conduction vessels (fall in R_2);

b) nitrate antianginal effects unaccompanied by a significant increment in coronary flow (fall of R_1); and

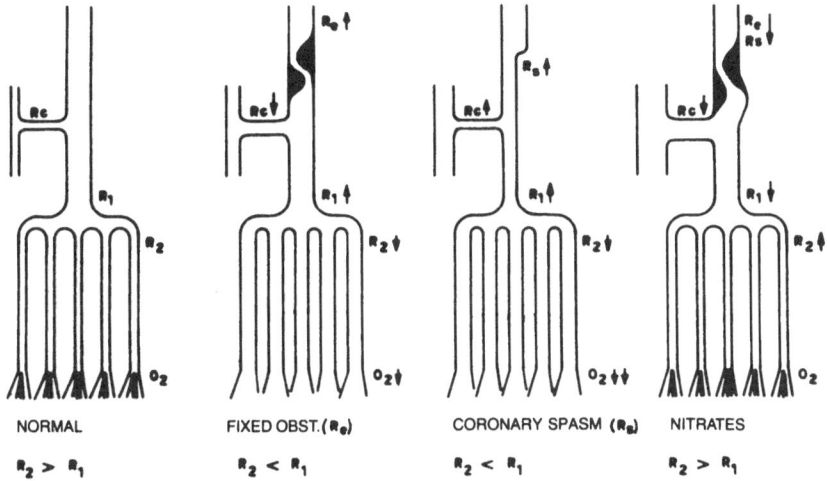

NORMAL   FIXED OBST.(R_e)   CORONARY SPASM (R_s)   NITRATES

$R_2 > R_1$ $R_2 < R_1$ $R_2 < R_1$ $R_2 > R_1$

Fig. 2. Diagram of direct nitrate effect on coronary vessels. From left to right: Normal situation with no stenosis or spasm and $R_2 > R_1$. Fixed stenosis (fixed obstruction) in which conductance vessels resistance ($R_1 \uparrow$) increases at the expense of stenosis ($R_e \uparrow$); to compensate, there is a fall in collateral resistance ($R_c \downarrow$) and dilation of the resistance vessels ($R_2 \downarrow$); in this case, these mechanisms are not capable of maintaining an adequate subendocardial perfusion pressure ($R_2 < R_1$) and the underlying muscle is ischemic ($O_2 \downarrow$). A similar situation is produced with coronary spasm ($R_5 \uparrow$), in the diagram also affecting collateral circulation ($R_c \uparrow$), thus increasing conductance vessel resistance ($R_1 \uparrow$); in spite of intramyocardial vessel dilation ($R_2 \downarrow$), the muscle is still ischemic ($O_2 \downarrow$). Finally, the nitrates can produce excentric dilation at the level of organic lesions ($R_1 \downarrow$), making the spasm disappear or preventing it ($R_p \downarrow$) and dilating other epicardial and collateral vessels ($R_c \downarrow$), thus restoring adequate subendocardial perfusion pressure, since no dilation is produced in the coronary bed by nitrates (at pharmacologic doses) or ischemic stimuli, with which $R_2 > R_1$ is maintained.

c) failure of high nitrate doses to produce an antianginal effect, although they increase coronary flow (fall of R_1 and R_2) (rupture of autoregulation).

Nitrate effects involve the conduction vessels, specifically in the sites most often affected by atherosclerotic lesions of the vascular wall, where coronary spasm is usually produced. The nitrate-induced fall in R_1 increases poststenotic pressure and maintains the subendocardial flow of the ischemic area.

Nitroglycerin can depress the coronary vessel constrictive reflexes normally induced by internal organ stimulation; this means that it can inhibit the vascular component of nociceptive reactions [12]. The efficacy of nitroglycerin in patients with variant angina is due to its direct effect on the coronary vessels, where it prevents vasospasm, not only by antagonism to coronary artery α-receptors, but by an intracellular effect that detains smooth muscle cell contraction in response to different types of stimuli [13].

The nitrates also dilate the rest of the coronary vessels and their collaterals [14], thus incrementing blood flow toward the ischemic myocardium (Fig. 2).

Systemic or indirect effects

The vasodilator effects on the walls of extracardiac veins and arteries can reduce myocardial oxygen consumption, which benefits zones with coronary ischemia. Various authors are of the opinion that the effect of nitrates may be greater on the venous wall than on the arterial wall [13, 15, 16].

Venodilation decreases end-diastolic pressure [7, 8], thus reducing subendocardial compression and improving the coronary flow gradient to the endocardium [8]. The fall in filling pressure can decrease ventricular volume, which according to the Laplace law reduces oxygen needs. Naturally, these effects are most intense in angina with high left ventricular diastolic pressure, that is, in situations with a certain degree of hemodynamic failure [8]. Likewise, this effect is less marked lying down than standing or sitting up, because of the greater venous return in this position [16]. Reduced stroke volume (as a result of the fall in ventricular volume) shortens the ejection time and diminishes O_2 consumption [16].

The arterial effects produce a fall in peripheral resistance and decrease peak systolic pressure, mean aortic pressure and general afterload, resulting in lower O_2 consumption [7, 8, 16]. In Table 4, we summarize the hemodynamic effects of nitroprusside in an experimental series. Fig. 3 illustrates diverse experimental systemic effects of isosorbide dinitrate.

The improvement in subendocardial flow produced by the direct effects of nitrates on coronary circulation, combined with the reduction in extravascular resistance as a result of effects on preload and afterload, helps to improve [17]

Table 4. Hemodynamic effects of nitroprusside.

	Control	Nitroprusside (μg/min)		
		5	10	15
peak LVP (mm Hg)	145 ± 6	128 ± 7[a]	115 ± 5[a]	109 ± 5[a]
LVEDP (mm Hg)	6.6 ± 0.5	4.6 ± 0.6[a]	3.6 ± 0.4[a]	3.0 ± 0.3[a]
APm (mm Hg)	122 ± 5	104 ± 7[a]	91 ± 4[a]	84 ± 5[a]
$(dP/dt)_{max}$ (mm Hg/sec)	2520 ± 351	2820 ± 330[b]	2879 ± 320[b]	3039 ± 358[b]
$(dP/dt)_{min}$ (mm Hg/sec)	− 3366 ± 575	− 3019 ± 367[b]	− 2747 ± 317[a]	− 2601 ± 280[a]
T (msec)	25.3 ± 2.3	20.9 ± 1.8[a]	20.5 ± 2.0[a]	19.1 ± 4.4[a]

Experimental effects in 5 dogs with closed chest and anesthetized. *Abbreviations:* LVP = left ventricular pressure; LVEDP = left ventricular end-diastolic pressure; APm = mean aortic pressure; T = T relaxation index (semilogarithmic method) [21].
[a] $p<0.01$ vs. control. [b] $p<0.05$ vs. control.

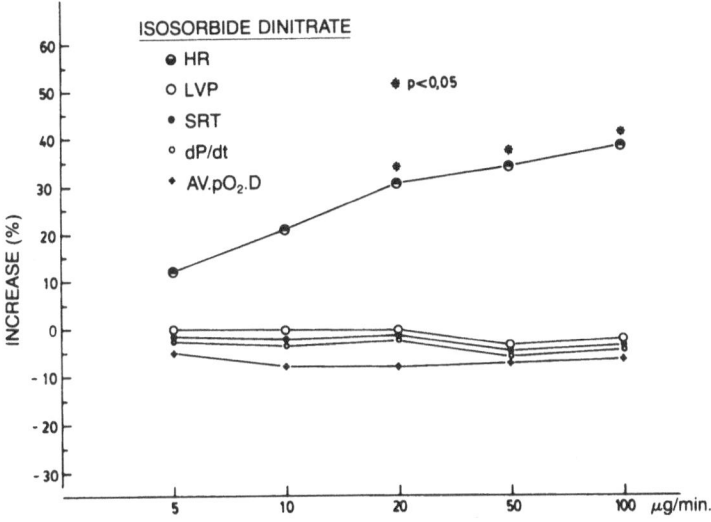

Fig. 3. Effects of different doses of isosorbide dinitrate on isolated guinea pig heart preparations. In the absence of systemic circulation, reflex effects disappear. Successive doses of the nitrate do not modify sinus frequency (studied by SRT – sinus recuperation time), maximum positive dP/dt, or left ventricular pressure peak (LVPP). No variations are produced in myocardial O_2 consumption (estimated by A-V PO_2 D – arteriovenous PO_2 difference). However, local effects on coronary circulation persist and coronary flow (CF) increases parallel to drug dose up to and average of more than 30%.

left ventricular function in patients with coronary stenosis and segmental contraction abnormalities. This phenomenon enhances coronary blood flow distribution and reduces ventricular volume.

As for improving left ventricular function, some studies suggest that reversible asynergy may coexist with reversible myocardial ischemia, which demonstrates that severe coronary stenoses can produce reversible asynergy at rest in zones of histopathologically normal myocardium [18, 19]. Nitroglycerin causes the asynergy to disappear as a consequence of a favorable alteration in the supply-demand relationship in the ischemic myocardium. Although it has not been clearly demonstrated, nitroglycerin seems to act on these asynergies by reducing afterload and preload, improving distribution of coronary blood flow [20].

Proanginal effects

The proanginal effects are usually amply counteracted by the therapeutic effects. As mentioned earlier, a reduction in O_2 supply can appear with use of large intracoronary doses of NTG or oral dipyridamol. This produces resist-

471

Table 5. Hemodynamic effects of nitroprusside after autonomic block.

	Control	Autonomic block	Nitroprusside (μg/min) 5	10	15
LVP peak (mm Hg)	143 ± 8	141 ± 9	114 ± 7[d]	102 ± 13[d]	94 ± 15[d]
LVEDP (mm Hg)	7.5 ± 3.4	12.8 ± 3.5[b]	10.3 ± 4.6[c]	8.8 ± 3.4[d]	3.8 ± 2.3[d]
APm (mm Hg)	110 ± 8	116 ± 9	91 ± 6[d]	81 ± 10[d]	73 ± 13[d]
(dP/dt)$_{max}$ (mm Hg/sec)	3696 ± 405	2361 ± 483[b]	1858 ± 346[d]	1623 ± 332[d]	1623 ± 281[d]
(dP/dt)$_{min}$ (mm Hg/sec)	−3074 ± 454	−2974 ± 460[a]	−2338 ± 432[d]	−2091 ± 570[d]	−1961 ± 452[d]
T (msec)	22.8 ± 1.4	28.6 ± 6.7[b]	27.1 ± 5.3	25.6 ± 5.3[c]	21.8 ± 5.1[c]

Experimental effects in 4 dogs with closed chest and under anesthesia. Autonomic block was realized with propanolol (0.4 mg.kg) and atropine (0.2 mg/kg). *Abbreviations:* As in Table 4.
[a] p<0.005 vs. control. [b] p<0.001 vs. control. [c] p<0.005 vs. autonomic block. [d] p<0.001 vs. autonomic block.

ance vessel dilation and steal phenomenon, increasing coronary flow and diminishing perfusion to the ischemic areas [8].

The increment in flow through patent epicardial vessels and collaterals, together with other sublingual NGT effects, can in some way 'steal' blood flow from ischemic areas [7]. In a critical situation, the fall in aortic pressure could lead to a decline in subendocardial perfusion pressure [2], which reduces O_2 supply.

The use of nitrates can also reduce O_2 supply, although not significantly, by displacing O_2 in blood through metahemoglobin production [7].

The nitrates can enhance oxygen consumption, not only by improving supply to zones poor in oxygen (direct therapeutic effect), but by increasing heart rate and contractility as a reflex response to hypotension [2, 7, 14]. These effects disappear if a β-blocking agent is given first (Table 5).

Nitrates in effort angina

The role of the 'long-acting' oral nitrates in preventing effort angina attacks has received attention in recent years, after an initial period of doubt as to the capacity of these drugs to reach systemic circulation in active form [22]. Lately, a series of effects that are dose-related in magnitude and duration has been demonstrated [23]. These effects would be responsible for the evident increase in effort capacity produced in coronary disease patients by these drugs.

The efficacy of the nitrates in effort angina is related to their mechanism of action. They improve oxygen supply to ischemic areas by dilating stenotic conduction arteries [7, 24, 25] and collaterals. Likewise, they reduce the tone of normal and stenotic coronary arteries, thus reducing the incidence of effort-induced coronary spasm [26, 27]. Nonetheless, the systemic effects seem to contribute more than local effects to the antianginal efficacy of the nitrates. Their venodilator effect is accompanied by a reduction in left ventricular filling pressure [28] and wall tension, lowering myocardial oxygen consumption and subendocardial coronary capillary flow resistance [11]. All these effects, which improve the exertional capacity of angina patients, are only partially neutralized by the reflex tachycardic effect of nitrates.

Long-acting nitrates

The use of long-acting nitrates was initially criticized because it was thought that their rapid metabolization would prevent reaching sufficient drug concentrations in blood to produce significant hemodynamic changes [29]. Nonetheless, numerous studies in the last decade have demonstrated the utility of these drugs in the treatment of effort angina [30–32].

The drugs used, their respective administration route, recommended dosage and duration of effect are shown in Table 6 [32–34]. There is a clear relationship between dosage and response, as reflected in: duration of the antianginal effect, exercise tolerance assessed by bicycle or treadmill ergometry and reduction of post-exercise ST depression [15, 33–36]. As such, the dosage of 5 to 10 mg isosorbide dinitrate (ISDN) *per os* originally suggested has been found to be insufficient to sustain increased effort capacity for more than 45 minutes. In contrast, 20 mg [35] produced beneficial effects for 3 hours and 40 mg of a slow release ISDN preparation was effective for 8 hours [33].

The antianginal efficacy of the oral nitrates usually parallels their hypotensive and tachycardiac effects. It has been recommended that a large enough dosage be given to reduce blood pressure by 10 mm Hg and increase heart rate by 10 beats/min [37], as long as patients are not simultaneously taking β-blocking agents [34]. In practice, this recommendation should only be taken into account to establish initial dosage, but not dose intervals, which should be determined by the duration of the angina-free period after each drug dosis [34].

Tolerance

One of the major problems of long-term nitrate therapy is development of tolerance. The phenomenon was initially detected in in vitro experiments with vascular strips [22] and was found to be related to chemical reactions between the nitrates and sulfhydryl groups in the cell membrane, forming disulfur bonds that act on the vascular smooth muscle nitrate receptors to decrease their nitrate affinity.

In the human being, the phenomenon of nitrate tolerance was described in 1888 for nitroglycerin [38]. In 1967, cross tolerance between nitroglycerin and other nitroderivates was documented [4]. In 1975, this phenomenon was observed in ISDN treatment [40]. It was later found that in spite of devel-

Table 6. Long-acting nitrates. Recommended dosages.

Drug	Dosage	Duration of effect (hrs)
Oral nitroglycerin	6–20 mg/4–6 hr	4–6
2% nitroglycerin gel	1.5–5 cm/4–6 hr	3–6
Isosorbide dinitrate		
Sublingual	2.5–10 mg/2–4 hr	1.5–3
Oral	10–60 mg/4–6 hr	4–6
Retarded	20–40 mg/6–8 hr	6–8
Oral tetranitrate		
Pentaeritritol	40–80 mg/4–6 hr	3–5

opment of ISDN hemodynamic tolerance, no reduction in its antianginal effectiveness was observed during prolonged treatment [37, 41]. It has been observed that the effects on blood pressure and duration are dose-dependent only after acute administration of ISDN; in contrast, long-term administration of the drug every 6 hours reduces the antianginal effect in the first four hours after oral administration, then supresses it but is restored in subsequent hours. There is little dose-dependence in this phenomenon [36], the same circulatory and antianginal effects being obtained with 15–30 mg as with larger doses.

The nitrate tolerance phenomenon seems to appear fairly rapidly, at least for hypotensive effects. Partial tolerance has been demonstrated to occur within 48 hours of administration. Reversion of tolerance when the drug is interrupted is also rapid, beginning 24 hours after cessation and being complete in 48 hours [42].

ISDN tolerance is unrelated to plasma concentrations, since these are similar or somewhat higher in long-term treatments than with the first dosis [36, 42].

The pharmacologic mechanism of tolerance may be related to the fact that the metabolites produced by ISDN denitration (2-mononitrate and 5-mononitrate) are less active vasodilators than dinitrate and may alter the vascular dinitrate-receptor union, consequently reducing vasodilator response during long-term treatment [43]. It has been demonstrated that vasodilator therapy activates the sympathetic nervous system and renin-angiotensin system, partially activating the vasoconstrictor forces opposed to its therapeutic effects [44] in long-term treatment [43]. In any case, the mechanisms involved in the nitrate tolerance phenomenon are still hypothetical and it is only clear that they are unrelated to a decrease in absorption rhythm or acceleration of drug elimination [43]. The existence of cross-tolerance to ISDN for the antianginal and hemodynamic effects of sublingual nitroglycerin has been demonstrated [45]: two hours after giving ISDN, effort capacity is unaffected by administration of nitroglycerin. However, when ISDN effects have subsided (6 hours after administration), sublingual nitroglycerin again produces a significant antianginal effect.

In view of the rapid onset and decline in tolerance with administration and suppression of oral nitrates, specifically ISDN, some patients with effort angina could benefit from treatment limited to the work day (6 to 10 hours) with an interval of 14 to 18 hours between the last dose of the day and the first of the next. This would minimize tolerance and permit daily reversion of the phenomenon [43].

Nitrate dependence has also been described, especially in workers in nitro-derivatives industries (explosives) who leave work after at least a year of exposure to nitroglycerin [46, 47]. There is an abnormally high incidence (4–5%) of angina without atherosclerotic heart disease in these workers. For this reason, it is advisable that when treatment must be discontinued nitrate dosage be gradually reduced [2].

Nitroglycerin patches

These are preparations in the form of multilayered adhesive patches containing nitroglycerin designed to release it into the skin in predetermined quantities [16, 48, 49].

The patches are generally elaborated from polymers impregnated with nitroglycerin and joined to an adhesive film for skin application; the external surface is impermeable and the internal surface releases nitroglycerin. The control of nitroglycerin release varies with different preparations, including by interposition of a semipermeable membrane between the drug reservoir and skin [49, 50]. Dose depends on patch size, but generally speaking a patch provides from 0.5 to 1 mg/cm² and day and the recommended dosage is 5–10 mg/day [49, 50]. Therapeutic levels are attained 30–60 minutes after application and are maintained at least 30 minutes after removal. After an initial stage of optimism in which the first studies indicated therapeutic levels and antianginal effects lasting 24 hours [48, 51], recent publications seriously question the possibility that the antianginal effect of these patches lasts more than 7 hours [49, 52, 53]. Moreover, elevated doses of nitroglycerin (more than 20 mg/24 hr) are needed to obtain antianginal effects that are often less intense than those obtained with oral nitrates [53]. Further studies are required to clarify the utility of nitroglycerin patches in the treatment of angina.

Present role of the nitrates in effort angina

Nitroglycerin has been used as an antianginal agent for more than 100 years and is still the drug of choice (0.3 mg sublingual) for treating angina attacks. It is also a useful prophylaxis prior to undertaking an activity that might precipitate angina. Since it does not produce tolerance when given sporadically, it can be prescribed as the only drug in patients with few attacks of effort angina (at intervals of 1 to 2 weeks). When attacks are more frequent, they can be controlled with high doses of oral nitrates, nitroglycerin gel, slow release oral preparations or very slow release transdermal preparations, which increase exercise capacity to more or less prolonged time periods.

In patients whose functional situation requires use of other drugs, such as β-blockers, there is evidence that nitrates produce an additive antianginal effect [34]. The existence of tolerance, and perhaps dependence, the possibility of inducing a 'steal' phenomenon in the arterioles supplying ischemic areas, and the fact that side effects (usually headache) are fairly frequent mean that chronic prescription and abrupt suppression of oral nitrates should be done cautiously. In these situations, addition or alternation with β-blockers or calcium antagonists helps to control anginal episodes in an elevated percentage of cases.

Nitrates in angina at rest

Intravenous nitrates

Intravenous nitrate perfusion is a valuable tool for controlling painful attacks of angina at rest, some authors considering intravenous nitroglycerin (IVNTG) to be the drug of choice for controlling angina before coronary surgery [16, 54]. Although isolated publications have shown interest in this form of administration, recent studies have appeared that examine larger series with a more strict methodology [56–62] (Table 7).

IVNTG administration. IVNTG should be administered in a glass bottle using a polyethylene catheter. Polyvinyl systems can absorb the drug [60].

Perfusion begins at 5–10 μg/minute and is gradually increased. Blood pressure and heart rate are checked until the angina attack is under control [60], or until there is a 20% decrease in basal systolic blood pressure [61], a 20 mm Hg reduction of previous systolic blood pressure [57] or appearance of adverse effects [61].

Hemodynamic effects of IVNTG. In most series IVNTG administration does not produce important changes in heart rate or blood pressure within the dosage range used to obtain therapeutic effects and when perfusion is done gradually with 5–10 μg/min (Table 7).

Since coronary blood flow occurs mainly during diastole, maintenance of adequate diastolic pressure and duration is important in these patients. The apparent adaptation of the circulatory apparatus to progressively larger IVNTG doses contrasts with the abrupt changes produced in heart rate by sublingual NTG [60]. The absence of tachycardia after IVNTG does not seem to be related to the β-blocking agents which many of the patients in these series were simultaneously receiving [60], or to the number of cases of heart failure in the series, a circumstance that would allow left ventricular filling pressure to decline without reaching levels that would provoke tachycardia and hypotension.

Results of IVNTG in resting angina. An analysis was made of the results of intravenous nitrate administration in 187 patients (175 IVNTG, 12 ISDN) with unstable angina at rest distributed in 6 series (Table 7). There were favorable

Table 7. IVNTG and resting angina.

	Dauwe [55]	Distante [56]a	Mikolich [57]	Page [59]	Kaplan [60]	Curfman [61]
No. of cases	14	12	45	67	35	14
Improvement b angina episodes	12	9	40	64	33	9
	2.7–0.69	8.33–1.08	?	9.83–1.2	3.5–0.3	3.3–1
Mean dosage c	47	?	54.4	31.4	140	82
(Max.-min.)	(20.8–83.31)	(20.8–83.31)	(5–267)	(128–51.4)	(50–130)	(10–200)
HR	57–>60	72–>75	69.8–>69.5	70–>72	84–>86	?
SBP (mm Hg)	?	135–>129	129–>124	140–>126	?	138–>108
DBP (mm Hg)		85–>81	78–>78	84–>82	?	78–>62
MBP (mm Hg)	85.8–>79.3	101–>97	95–>93	102–>96	79–>77	98–>77
Adverse effects	1 headache	2 headache	2 hypotens. 11 headache	2 hypotens. 14 headache	15 headache	3 hypotens. 3 headache

a Intravenous ISDN. b Abolition angina attacks or >50% reduction. c Expressed in μg/minute.

478

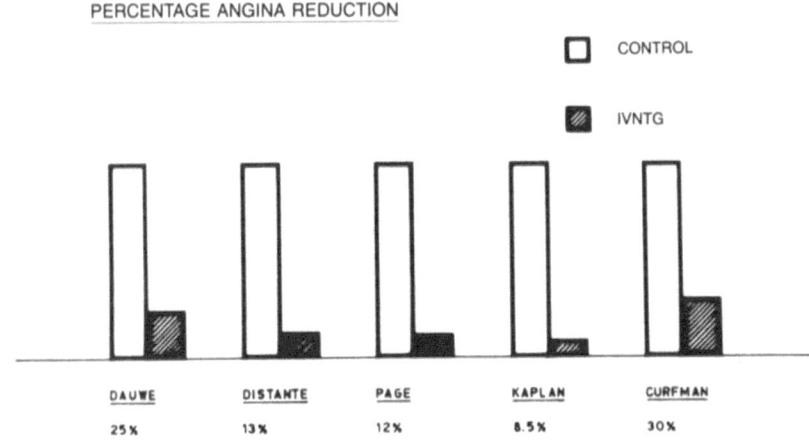

PERCENTAGE ANGINA REDUCTION

☐ CONTROL

▨ IVNTG

| DAUWE | DISTANTE | PAGE | KAPLAN | CURFMAN |
| 25% | 13% | 12% | 8.5% | 30% |

Fig. 4. Effectiveness of IVNTG administration in the series in Table 7. The shaded area represents the percentage of patients whose anginal symptomatology did not improve with IVNTG (abolition of attacks or a decrease of more than 50% in their frequency).

effects in 89% of cases, consisting in abolition of angina or a reduction by more than 50% in the frequency of its ocurrance (maximum 92%, minimum 65%) (Fig. 4). The decrease in the number of episodes of angina was statistically significant in every series (Table 7). These results are more striking considering that many of these patients were taking other antianginal medications (oral nitrates, β-blocking agents, calcium antagonists) that had proved to be ineffective in treating anginal attacks. The dosis required to obtain these beneficial effects varies widely, from 5 to 350 μg/min, probably because the series are not necessarily homogeneous and comparable. Our initial experience (unpublished data) with 19 cases of unstable angina treated with 25–200 μg IVNTG according to Kaplan's system [60] produced results similar to those described: complete abolition of attacks in 63% of cases and improvement in 21% (reduction of more than 50% of the pain attacks) (Fig. 5).

The time required to attain the dosis that abolishes angina at rest varies from 6 hours to 27 days in the series in Table 7. In one study [60], the maximum dosis of IVNTG needed to control the episodes of angina was unrelated to the patient's age, sex, body weight, extension of coronary disease, the existence of previous myocardial infarct or previous administration of β-blocking agents.

Why IVNTG was effective in some cases in which adequate doses of oral isosorbide dinitrate or nitroglycerin in gel or orally did not produce favorable results is not well known. The fact that IVNTG gave better results could be related to more stable blood concentrations, which avoid the fluctuations that occur in other forms of administration. The possibility of attaining new therapeutic levels and sustaining the therapeutic effect indefinitely [57] may be

EFFECTIVENESS OF IVNTG

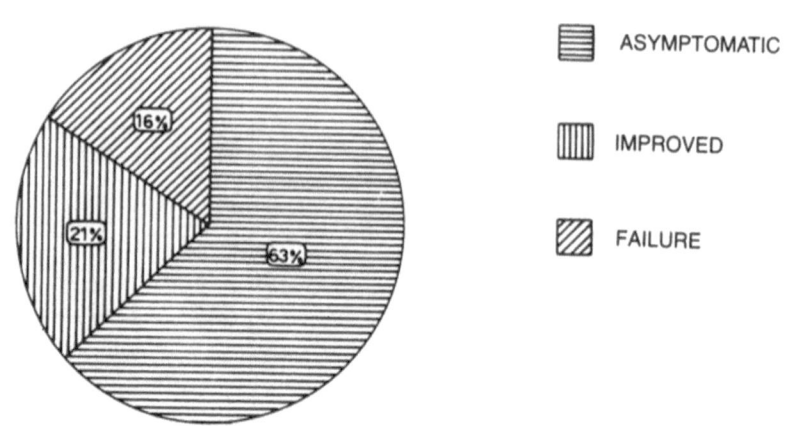

Fig. 5. Effectiveness of IVNTG administration in one of the author's series [63].

reasons for the greater effectiveness of IVNTG. However, in a study by Curfman [61] comparing the effectiveness of IVNTG and ISDN, when ISDN was given in sufficient quantity to produce the same effects on blood pressure as IVNTG, the effects of these drugs were almost identical.

IVNTG results have only been assessed for reduction or abolition of pain attacks, which is more frequently achieved in the first 48 hours [16, 61]. In some series [61] the effect sometimes relapses after this time. Whether IVNTG contributes to the prevention of myocardial infaction in these patients has not been sufficiently clarified. On the other hand, many of these studies were not crossed and their methodology can be criticized. Only Distante's study [56] with intravenous ISDN was double blind and crossed, and it clearly demonstrated the efficacy of this drug in vasospastic angina.

IVNTG side effects. Among the potential complications of IVNTG are hypotension and bradycardia, hypoxemia due to ventilation-perfusion imbalance, metahemoglobinemia, nausea, vomiting and headache [58, 62]. Of the 187 cases in Table 7, headache was present in 46 and hypotension in 10. The incidence of headache seems to be fairly high, but in only 3 of 46 cases of headache did the dosis have to be reduced, as compared with 7 of 10 cases of hypotension. Thus, in contrast with the early idea that administration of IVNTG in unstable angina would require hemodynamic monitoring and perhaps a Swan-Ganz catheter, there are now sufficient data to affirm that with the regimen described (Table 7) IVNTG can be safely given without invasive hemodynamic monitoring [58]. Only when hypovolemia is suspected, in which case the vasodilator effect of IVNTG could precipitate abrupt and severe hypotension, should invasive hemodynamic monitoring be done before initiating therapy. Likewise, IVNTG is contraindicated in endocranial hypertension [62]. It has not been clearly demonstrated that there is a rebound effect after abruptly terminating nitrate perfusion. In some cases in which perfusion rhythm was accidentally decreased, anginal attacks reappeared [60] (unpublished data). In any case, it is recommended that IVNTG be gradually withdrawn [60].

Oral nitrates in resting angina

The nitrates were the first drugs available for treatment of angina at rest and still constitute the mainstay of medical therapy of unstable angina at rest [16, 54]. Medical treatment of unstable angina was at first based on bed rest and nitrates, resulting in control of 61% of cases [59], and later complemented with β-blocking agents. This combination of drugs increased effectiveness to 70–85% of cases [59]. The calcium antagonists were later shown to be useful for treating vasospastic forms of angina at rest [16].

What is the role now of oral nitrates in the treatment of angina at rest? The information presently available can be summarized as follows:
1. Oral nitrates are generally accepted to be beneficial if they are given in adequate doses, sufficient to reduce systolic blood pressure by 15 mm Hg or to 100–110 mm Hg, as long as these levels do not represent a large reduction in previous values [16, 63]. If they produce excessive tachycardia it is helpful to add β-blocking agents.
2. Nitrates have been shown to be very effective in angina at rest with a confirmed vasospastic component. In two studies [64, 65] in which nitrates were compared with nifedipine for this type of angina, both drugs were effective and there were no significant differences between them. Some patients with angina attacks refractory to nifedipine responded favorably to treatment with oral nitrates. In contrast, some cases of refractory angina were controlled with nifedipine. Nonetheless, the patients who participated in these studies expressed their preference for nifedipine because it produced fewer side effects.
3. The importance of giving adequate doses of oral nitrates is evidenced by Curfman's work [61]. When ISDN was administered at a dosis sufficient to obtain the same hemodynamic effects as IVNTG, ISDN only offered modest therapeutic advantages over oral nitrates.
4. The main disadvantage is the frequency of adverse effects, fundamentally headache, at the dosage required to control angina at rest. On the other hand, although hemodynamic and antianginal effects generally do not reappear within 4–5 hours after taking the drug, when it is taken at night it does not always succeed in preventing the spasms that often occur in the first hours of the morning [66].

Nitroglycerin ointment (nitroglycerin gel)

This form of administration is particularly useful in patients with severe angina at rest who are confined to bed or chair [16], because it has been demonstrated to be effective up to 6 hours after administration [16, 66–68]. NTG gel has proved effective in vasospastic angina at rest [67]. In a randomized crossover study in this type of angina [67], nitroglycerin gel significantly reduced the number of anginal episodes, producing complete abolition of angina in 70% of cases. The only adverse effect was headache, which did not require drug withdrawal.

References

1. Cohn PF, Gorlin R: Physiologic and clinical actions of nitroglycerin. Med Clin North Am 1974; 58: 407–424.
2. Aronow WS: Clinical use of nitrates. I. Nitrates as antianginal drugs. Mod Conc Cardiovasc Dis 1979; 48: 31–35.
3. Triggle DI, Swamy VC: Pharmacology of agents that affect. Calcium agonist and antagonist. Chest (Suppl) 1980; 78: 174–179.
4. Salva JA: Nitratos orgánicos. Monografías cardiovasculares. Sociedad Castellana de Cardiología (Madrid) 1984; 4.
5. Needleman P, Johnsen EM, Jr.: Mechanism of tolerance development to organic nitrates. J Pharmacol Exp Ther 1973; 184: 709–715.
6. Ganz W, Marcus HS: Failure of intracoronary nitroglycerin to alleviate pacing-induced angina. Circulation 1972; 46: 880–891.
7. Brown BG, Bolson E, Petersen RB, Pierce CD, Doage HT: The mechanisms of nitroglycerin action. Stenosis vasodilation as a major component of the drug response. Circulation 1981; 64: 1089–1097.
8. McGregor M: The nitrates and myocardial ischemia. Circulation 1982; 66: 689–692.
9. Wyatt HL, Forrester JS, Tyberg JV, Golaner S, Sogan SE, Parmley WW, Swan HJC: Effect of graded reductions in regional coronary perfusion on regional and total cardiac function. Am J Cardiol 1975; 36: 185.
10. Holtz J, Bassenge E, Kinaaeter H, Kolin A: Vasomotion of coronary conductance and resistance vessels: interference of sympathetic constriction and nitroglycerin-induced vasodilation. In: Rafflenbeul W, Sichtlen PR, Balcon R (eds) Unstable angina pectoris. Georg Thieme, Stuttgart, 1981; 31–38.
11. Goldstein RE: Coronary vascular responses to vasodilator drugs. Prog Cardiovasc Dis 1982; 24: 419–36.
12. Kaverina NV, Chumbundze VB: Antianginal drugs. Pharmacol Therap 1979; 4: 109–122.
13. Florez J: Los nitratos: Sitios y mecanismos de acción. In: Pajarón A (ed) I jornadas cardiológicas cardiopatía isquémica. Servicio de Cardiología del Centro Médico Nacional Marqués de Valdecilla, Santander, 1981; 224–232.
14. Goldstein RE, Stinson EB, Scherer JL, Senigen RP, Grehl TM, Epstein SE: Intraoperative coronary collateral function in patients with coronary occlusive disease: Nitroglycerin responsiveness and angiographic correlations. Circulation 1974; 49: 298.
15. Abrams J: Nitroglycerin and long-acting nitrates. New Engl J Med 1980; 302: 1234–1237.

16. Cohn PF, Braunwald E: Chronic ischemic heart disease. In: Braunwald E (ed) Heart disease, a textbook of cardiovascular medicine. WB Saunders, Philadelphia, 1984; 1334–1383.

17. McAnulty JH, Hattenhaner MT, Rosche J, Kloster FE, Rahimtoola SH: Improvement in left ventricular wall motion following nitroglycerin. Circulation 1975; 51: 140.

18. Bonka VS, Bodenheimer MM, Helfant RM: Relation between progressive decrease in regional coronary perfusion and contractile abnormalities. Am J Cardiol 1977; 40: 200–211.

19. Bodenheimer MM, Bonka VS, Herman GA, Tront RG, Farder H, Helfant RH: Reversible asynergy: histopathologic and electrographic correlations in patients and coronary artery disease. Circulation 1976; 53: 792–799.

20. McEwan FM, Berman NA, March JE, Ferglin DM, McLanghlin PR: Effect of intravenous and intracoronary nitroglycerin on left ventricular wall motion and perfusion in patients with coronary artery disease. Am J Cardiol 1981; 47: 102–112.

21. Martin G, Gimeno JV, Ramirez A, Cosin J, Baguena J: Effects of high-frequency harmonics on cardiac relaxation indices. Am J Physiol 1981; 240: 669–675.

22. Needleman P, Blehm DJ, Rotskoff KJ: Relationship between glutathione-dependent denitration and the vasodilator effectiveness of organic nitrates. J Pharmacol Exp Ther 1968; 165: 286–289.

23. Glancy DL, Richter MA, Ellis EV, Johnson W: Effect of the swallowed isosorbide dinitrate on blood pressure, heart rate and exercise capacity in patients with coronary artery disease. Am J Med 1977; 62: 38–46.

24. Rafflenbeul W, Urthaler F, Russell RO, Lichtlen P, James TN: Dilation of coronary artery stenoses after isosorbide dinitrate in man. Br Heart J 1980; 43: 546–549.

25. Feldman RL, Pepine CJ, Conti R: Magnitude of dilation of large and small coronary arteries by nitroglycerin. Circulation 1984; 64: 324–333.

26. Chaitman WD, Dupras G, Theroux P, Mizgala H: Coronary artery spasm during exercise in patients with variant angina. Circulation 1979; 59: 580–585.

27. Fuller CM, Raizner AE, Chahine RA, Nahormek P, Ishimori T, Verani M, Nitishin A, Mokotoff D, Luchi RJ: Exercise-induced coronary artery spasm: angiographic demonstration, documentation of ischemia by myocardial scintigraphy and results of pharmacologic intervention. Am J Cardiol 1980; 46: 500–506.

28. Williams JF, Glick G, Braunwald E: Studies on cardiac dimensions in intact unanesthesized man. V. Effects of nitroglycerin. Circulation 1975; 32: 767–783.

29. Needleman P, Lange S, Johnson E: Organic nitrates: relationship between biotransformation and rational angina pectoris therapy. J Pharmacol Exp Ther 1972; 181: 489–497.

30. Dahany DT, Burwel DT, Aronow WS, Prakash R: Sustained hemodynamic and antianginal effect of high dose oral isosorbide dinitrate. Circulation 1977; 55: 381–187.

31. Abrams J: Usefulness of long-acting nitrates in cardiovascular disease. Am J Med 1978; 64: 183–186.

32. Dibianco R, Ronan JA, Donohue DJ, Lindgren KM: A new oral slow release form of isosorbide dinitrate. Effect on the hemodynamics and exercise capacity of patients with angina. Chest 1983; 84: 707–713.

33. Giles TA, Iteld BJ, Quiroz AC, Mautner RK: The prolonged effect of penthaerythritol tertranitrate on exercise capacity in stable effort angina pectoris. Chest 1981; 82: 142–145.

34. Bassan MB, Weiler-Ravell D: The additive antianginal action of oral isosorbide dinitrate in patients receiving propanolol. Magnitude and duration of effect. Chest 1983; 83: 233–240.

35. Markis JE, Gorling R, Mills RM, Williams RA, Scheitzer P, Ransil BJ: Sustained effects of orally administered isosorbide dinitrate on exercise performance of patients with angina pectoris. Am J Cardiol 1979; 43: 265–271.

36. Thadani U, Fung H, Darke C, Parker JO: Oral isosorbide dinitrate in angina pectoris: comparison of duration of action and dose-response relation during acute and sustained therapy. Am J Cardiol 1982; 49: 411–419.

37. Danahy DT, Aronow WS: Hemodynamics and antianginal effects of high dose oral isosorbide dinitrate after chronic use. Circulation 1977; 56: 205–212.
38. Stewart DD: Remarkable tolerance to nitroglycerin. Philadelphia Polyclinic 1888: 172.
39. Schellin JL, Lasagna L: A study of cross-tolerance to circulatory effects of organic nitrates. Clin Pharmacol Ther 1967; 8: 256–260.
40. Zelis R, Mason DT: Isosorbide dinitrate: Effect on the vasodilator response to nitroglycerin. JAMA 1975; 234: 166–170.
41. Lee G, Mason DT, De Maria AN: Effects of long-term oral administration of isosorbide dinitrate on the antianginal response to nitroglycerin: Absence of nitrate cross-tolerance and self-tolerance shown by exercise testing. Am J Cardiol 1978; 41: 82–87.
42. Parker JO, Fung H, Ruggirell D, Stone JA: Tolerance to isosorbide dinitrate: rate of development and reversal. Circulation 1983; 68: 1074–1080.
43. Bogaert MG, Rossell MT: Vascular effects of the dinitrate and mononitrate esters of isosorbide, isomannide and isoidide. Arch Pharmacol 1972; 275: 339–343.
44. Packer M, Meller J, Medina N, Yushak M, Gorlin R: Hemodynamic characterization of tolerance to long-term hydralazine therapy in severe chronic heart failure. N Engl J Med 1982; 306: 57–61.
45. Dalal JJ, Yad L, Parker JO: Nitrate tolerance. Influence of isosorbide dinitrate on the hemodynamic and antianginal effects of nitroglycerin. J Am Coll Cardiol 1983; 2–115.
46. Lange RL, Reid MS, Tresch DD, Keeland MH, Bernhard VM, Coolidge G: Nonatheromatous ischemic heart disease following withdrawal from chronic industrial nitroglycerin exposure. Circulation 1972; 46: 666–678.
47. Klock JC: Nonocclusive coronary disease after chronic industrial nitroglycerin exposure. Amer Heart J 1975; 89: 510–513.
48. Thompson RH: The clinical use of transdermal delivery devices with nitroglycerin. Cardiovasc Rev Rep 1983; 4: 91–99.
49. Abrams J: The brief saga of transdermal nitroglycerin discs: Paradise lost. Am J Cardiol 1984; 54: 220–224.
50. Chien YW: Pharmaceutical considerations of transdermal nitroglycerin delivery: The various approaches. Am Heart J 1984; 108: 207–216.
51. Thompson RH: Uso clinico de dispositivos de administración percutánea de nitroglicerina. Cardiovasc Rev Rep 1984; 5: 340–345.
52. Hollenberg M, Go M: Clinical studies with transdermal nitroglycerin. Am Heart J 1984; 108: 223–231.
53. Reicheck N, Priest CH, Zimzin D, Chandler Th: Antianginal effects of nitroglycerin patches. Am J Cardiol 1984; 54: 1–7.
54. Hurst JW, King SB, Walter PF, Friesienger GC, Edwards JE: Atherosclerotic coronary heart disease: angina pectoris, myocardial infarction and other manifestations of myocardial ischemia. In: Hurst JW (ed) The heart. McGraw-Hill, New York, 1982; 1009–1149.
55. Dauwe F, Affaki G, Waters DD, Theroux P, Mizgala HF: Intravenous nitroglycerin in refractory unstable angina (Abstract). Am J Cardiol 1979; 43: 416.
56. Distante A, Maseri A, Severi S, Biagini A, Chierchia S: Management of vasospastic angina at rest with continuous infusion of isosorbide dinitrate. Am J Cardiol 1979; 44: 533–539.
57. Mikolich JR, Nicoloff NB, Robinson PH, Logue RB: Relief of refractory angina with continuous intravenous infusion of nitroglycerin. Chest 1980; 375–379.
58. Hill NS, Antman EM, Green LH, Alpert JS: Intravenous nitroglycerin: a review of pharmacology, indications, therapeutic effects and complications. Chest 1981; 79: 69–76.
59. Page A, Gatean P, Ohayan J, Coupillaud J, Le Minh D, Besse P: Interet de la trinitrine intraveineuse dans l'angor instable. Arch Mal Coeur 1982; 75: 325–332.
60. Kaplan K, Davison R, Parker M, Przybylek J, Teagarden JR, Lesch M: Intravenous nitro-

glycerin for the treatment of angina at rest unresponsive to standard nitrate therapy. Am J Cardiol 1983; 51: 694–698.

61. Curfman GD, Heinsimer JA, Lozner EC: Intravenous nitroglycerin in the treatment of spontaneous angina pectoris: A prospective randomized trial. Circulation 1983; 67: 276–282.

62. Herling IM: Intravenous nitroglycerin: Clinical pharmacology and therapeutic considerations. Am Heart J 1984; 108: 141–149.

63. Sanz G: Utilidad clínica de los nitratos. In: Pajarón A (ed) I jornadas cardiológicas. Cardiopatía Isquémica. Centro Nacional Marqués de Valdecilla, Santander, 1981; 284–298.

64. Ginsburg R, Lamb JH, Schroeder JS, Hu M, Harrison DC: Randomized double-blind comparison of nifedipine and isosorbide dinitrate therapy in variant angina pectoris due to coronary artery spasm. Am Heart J 1982; 103: 44–48.

65. Hill JA, Feldman RL, Pepine CJ, Conti CR: Randomized double blind comparison of nifedipine and isosorbide dinitrate in patients with coronary arterial spasm. Am J Cardiol 1982; 49: 431–438.

66. Malpartida F, Alegría E, Barba J, De la Morena G, Perugachi C, Ancin R, Lorente D, Olmos L: Espasmo coronario. In: Sociedad Española de Cardiología (ed) Avances en cardiología. Editorial Científico Médica, Barcelona, 1983; 1–14.

67. Salerno JA, Previtali M, Medici A, Chimienti M, Bramucci E, Lepore R, Specchia G, Bobba P: Treatment of vasospastic angina pectoris at rest with nitroglycerin ointment. A short term controlled study in the coronary care unit. Am J Cardiol 1981; 47: 1128–1134.

68. Coma Canella I, López Sendón J: Efecto hemodinámico de la nitroglicerina gel en la insuficiencia cardiaca secundaria a infarto agudo de miocardio. Rev Esp Cardiol 1983; 36: 43–48.

10.4 Comparison of Four Calcium Antagonists with Placebo and Propranolol

V. BALA SUBRAMANIAN

Material and methods

Patients (Table 1)

Patients were 30 to 70-years-old and met the following criteria for inclusion:
1. Chronic and stable effort angina of at least 3 months duration.
2. Disappearance of pain with rest and/or sublingual nitrates.
3. Consumption of at least four tablets weekly of nitroglycerin.
4. Appearance of typical angina with treadmill exercise.
5. Appearance of at least 1 mm ST segment depression with a slope of less than 0.1 mv/sec in two bipolar leads of the monitor electrocardiogram.
6. Confirmed coronary disease evidenced by recent myocardial infarction, positive thallium imaging or arteriography.

Test design

All trials commenced with two weeks of simple-blind placebo. After this, patients were submitted to a randomized double-blind crossed drug study.

Table 1. Patients.

Drug	Dose (mg/day)	Trial	Type	Number of patients
Propranolol	240	Verapamil v. propranolol	Double blind	22
Diltiazem	360*	Diltiazem v. placebo	Simple blind	20
Nicardipine	60*	Nicardipine v. placebo	Simple blind	20
Nifedipine	30	Nifedipine v. placebo	Double blind	24
Nifedipine	60	Nifedipine v. verapamil	Double blind	28
Verapamil	360	Verapamil v. placebo	Double blind	28

* The most effective dose, previously determined by dosage trials.

Each trial consisted of giving the test drug three times a day for 2 to 4 weeks.

Evaluation

Placebo and drug effects were objectively assessed by comparing results of maximum treadwheel effort tests performed before admission to the study and at 2-week intervals while each medication was given, whether active or inactive. All effort tests were scheduled in the morning, at least 2 hours after a light breakfast and 90 to 180 minutes after the last drug dosis. Patients arrived at the exercise laboratory 30 minutes before testing and rested comfortably. They were instructed not to smoke or take nitroglycerin tablets on the morning of the test day.

The exercise test was performed on a Quinton type treadwheel linked to a microcomputer (Marquette Computer Assisted System for Exercise). The exercise test protocol is shown in Table 2. Speed and inclination were automatically controlled by the computer. The test was clocked using a digital device with a precision of 0.1 minutes. All tests were prolonged until the patient developed symptoms that forced interruption of exercise. Criteria for interruption were: angina (grade 2), leg pain, severe dyspnea or fatigue. We respected standard security measures and the legal requisites for exercise testing laboratories recommended by the American Heart Association. Two bipolar electrocardiographic leads (CM5 and CC5) were continuously monitored at rest, during exercise and for at least 5 minutes after concluding exercise. Systolic blood pressure was measured with a mercury sphygmomanometer.

The electrocardiographic leads monitored were CM5 (negative electrode in the sternal manubrium and exploring electrode in LV5) and CC5 (negative electrode in RV6 and exploring electrode in LV5). To monitor arrhythmias, a lead where the P waves were clearly visualized was controlled. The electrocar-

Table 2. Treadwheel protocol for all tests.

Stage	Time (min)	Speed		Gradient (%)
		(m/h)	(km/h)	
1	3	2	3.2	0
2	3	3	4.8	4
3	3	3	4.8	8
4	3	3	4.8	12
5	3	3	4.8	16
6	3	3	4.8	20
7	3	4.5	7.2	20

diogram at rest was fed into the computer. The computer calculated ST segment depression at point J with respect to the most horizontal part of the PR segment, expressing this depression in multiples of 0.1 mm. Mean ST segment depression, heart rate and the number of ectopic beats in both leads were automatically printed out every minute during and after exercise. During the examination, the electrocardiogram was continuously recorded at a paper speed of 1 mm/sec. Ectopic complexes were recorded in real time. At the end of the examination, the computer recorded exercise duration, maximum heart rate, maximum ST depression and the number of ectopic complexes. A continuous register of heart rate and ST depression was obtained with the three leads. Computer measurement circuits were calibrated every day.

Data collection

We obtained the following information from the continuous recordings:
a) heart rate and ST level at rest;
b) heart rate, ST level and number of ectopic beats per minute during and after exercise;
c) maximum heart rate;
d) maximum ST depression (in leads CM5 and CC5) and
e) duration of exercise.
The following variables were calculated:
a) increase in heart rate = heart rate − heart rate at rest;
b) 1 mm time = time required to produce a depression of 1 mm in the ST segment with respect to resting level;
c) maximum corrected ST depression (MST) = ST depression at the conclusion of exercise corrected for resting values;
d) maximum ST depression/exercise duration; and
e) increase in heart rate/exercise duration.
Statistical analysis was made with the Student t test for paired samples. All trials were approved by the hospital ethics committee.

Results

Duration of exercise (Table 3)

Exercise duration increased with propranolol treatment by 5.5 minutes after 4 weeks of treatment in comparison with placebo. This value was statistically significant ($p < 0.001$) and represented a 42% improvement in exercise tolerance. Eighteen per cent of the patients interrupted exercise for non-anginal motives, such as leg pain and fatigue.

Verapamil improved exercise tolerance from 6.6 to 11.2 minutes, an increment of 70% over placebo levels. In 70% of patients, angina did not appear and exercise was interrupted for non-anginal reasons.

Diltiazem increased exercise tolerance from 5.6 to 9.5 minutes, a 70% increment. Fifty per cent of the patients stopped exercise for angina and the rest for other reasons.

Treatment with low doses of nifedipine (30 mg per day) did not significantly increase exercise tolerance. Exercise duration was 6.8 ± 0.6 minutes with placebo and 6.9 ± 0.7 minutes with nifedipine. Only 5% of patients remained free of anginal pain.

Increasing the nifedipine dosis (20 mg three times daily) improved duration of exercise from 5.7 to 7.9 minutes, an increment of 39%. This was statistically significant ($p<0.001$). Twenty-nine per cent of these patients did not have angina during effort.

Nicardipine (15 and 30 mg per day) produced no improvement over placebo. A larger dosis of nicardipine improved exercise tolerance from 6.4 ± 0.5 to 7.8 ± 0.7 minutes ($p<0.001$), a 22% increment. Twenty-five per cent of these patients had no anginal pain during exercise.

Changes in the ST segment

The 1 mm time in CM5 is shown in Table 4. The exercise time required to produce a 1 mm descent in the ST segment in comparison with resting values was calculated by a computer program. In the propranolol trial, 3.3 ± 0.4 minutes of exercise were required to produce a change of 1 mm in ST segment level with placebo; 5.7 ± 0.5 minutes were needed with propranolol. This was statistically significant ($p<0.001$), representing a 73% increment. Diltiazem increased this time by 62%, verapamil by 64% and nifedipine (60 mg/day) by 49%. All these values were statistically significant when compared with the

Table 3. Time (in minutes) and percentage of patients who remained asymptomatic with treatment. All values expressed as mean ± SD.

Treatment (dosis in mg 3× daily)	Exercise time		Change (%)	p < value	Free of angina (%)
	Placebo	Drug			
Propranolol (80)	5.5 ± 0.4	7.8 ± 0.5	+ 42	0.001	18
Diltiazem (120)	5.6 ± 0.7	9.5 ± 0.9	+ 70	0.001	50
Nicardipine (20)	6.4 ± 0.5	7.8 ± 0.7	+ 22	0.001	25
Nifedipine (10)	6.8 ± 0.6	6.9 ± 0.7	+ 2	NS	5
Nifedipine (20)	5.7 ± 0.3	7.9 ± 0.5	+ 39	0.001	29
Verapamil (120)	6.6 ± 0.5	11.2 ± 0.8	+ 70	0.001	71

placebo (p<0.001). Nicardipine only produced a 17% increment, which was not statistically significant.

Maximum ST depression (MST) (Table 5)

In the propranolol trial, a mean MST depression of -2.4 ± 0.2 mm in the CM5 lead appeared when placebo was given. With propranolol, these values decreased by 29% (p<0.001). None of the calcium antagonists improved this variable. There was a small increase of 16% with diltiazem, but this was not statistically significant.

MST/exercise duration, CM5 (Table 6)

Propranolol treatment improved this variable by 50% (p<0.001). Diltiazem produced a 38% increment, verapamil 42%, nifedipine 32% and nicardipine 26%. All these values were statistically significant.

Table 4. One mm times (min) with trial drugs.

Treatment	1 mm times		Change (%)	p < value
	Placebo	Drug		
Propranolol	3.3 ± 0.4	5.7 ± 0.5	+ 73	0.001
Diltiazem	3.4 ± 0.4	5.5 ± 0.7	+ 62	0.001
Nicardipine	4.8 ± 0.5	5.6 ± 0.7	+ 17	NS
Nifedipine*	3.9 ± 0.3	5.8 ± 0.4	+ 49	0.001
Verapamil	4.4 ± 0.3	7.2 ± 0.5	+ 64	0.001

* 60 mg/day.

Table 5. Maximum S-T segment depression (mm) with different drugs.

Treatment	S-T depression		Change (%)	p < value
	Placebo	Drug		
Propranolol	− 2.4 ± 0.2	− 1.7 ± 0.1	− 29	0.001
Diltiazem	− 1.9 ± 0.1	− 2.2 ± 0.2	+ 16	NS
Nicardipine	− 1.8 ± 0.2	− 1.6 ± 0.2	− 12	NS
Nifedipine*	− 2.0 ± 0.2	− 2.0 ± 0.2	0	NS
Verapamil	− 2.0 ± 0.2	− 2.0 ± 0.2	0	NS

* 60 mg/day.

Heart rate

Heart rate at rest was significantly reduced, by 20 bpm, with propranolol, a reduction of 26% (Table 7). Diltiazem slowed heart rate by 11 bpm and verapamil by 9 bpm (−12%). The other two calcium antagonists, nifedipine and nicardipine, produced respective elevations of 3 and 8 bpm. The increase in heart rate with nicardipine was statistically significant ($p<0.001$). Maximum heart rate was not significantly influenced by any of the calcium antagonists (Table 8). Mean values showed a change of 3 to 6 bpm. On the other hand, propranolol produced a marked reduction of 35 bpm, a 23% decrease, which was statistically significant ($p<0.001$). Likewise, there was a 42% reduction in the exercise-induced increment in heart rate under propranolol treatment (Table 9). All the calcium antagonists significantly reduced this variable ($p<0.001$), diltiazem by 28%, verapamil 23%, nicardipine 21% and nifedipine 20%.

Table 6. MST/exercise times (minutes in CM5 lead) with the trial drugs.

Treatment	Exercise/MST times		Change (%)	p < value
	Placebo	Drug		
Propranolol	0.48 ± 0.06	0.24 ± 0.03	50	0.001
Diltiazem	0.48 ± 0.06	0.30 ± 0.05	38	NS
Nicardipine	0.31 ± 0.05	0.23 ± 0.32	26	0.02
Nifedipine*	0.39 ± 0.04	0.026 ± 0.03	32	0.001
Verapamil	0.34 ± 0.03	0.20 ± 0.02	41	0.001

* 60 mg/day.

Table 7. Heart rate (bpm) at rest with trial drugs.

Treatment	Heart rates		Change (%)	p < value
	Placebo	Drug		
Propranolol	76 ± 3	56 ± 2	− 26	0.001
Diltiazem	75 ± 3	64 ± 2	− 15	0.001
Nicardipine	71 ± 3	79 ± 4	+ 11	0.01
Nifedipine*	74 ± 2	77 ± 2	+ 4	NS
Verapamil	74 ± 3	65 ± 2	− 12	0.001

* 60 mg/day.

Table 8. Maximum heart rate (bpm) with trial drugs.

Treatment	S-T depression		Change (%)	p < value
	Placebo	Drug		
Propranolol	135 ± 3	104 ± 3	− 23	0.001
Diltiazem	123 ± 3	120 ± 4	− 2	NS
Nicardipine	123 ± 3	129 ± 3	+ 5	NS
Nifedipine*	125 ± 3	130 ± 2	+ 4	NS
Verapamil	120 ± 3	126 ± 3	+ 5	NS

* 60 mg/day.

Table 9. Increase in heart rate-exercise time ratio (IHR/exercise time) (bpm) with trial drugs.

Treatment	S-T depression		Change (%)	p < value
	Placebo	Drug		
Propranolol	10.7 ± 0.4	6.2 ± 0.3	− 42	0.001
Diltiazem	8.8 ± 0.3	5.9 ± 0.2	− 28	0.001
Nicardipine	8.1 ± 0.3	6.4 ± 0.2	− 21	0.001
Nifedipine*	9.0 ± 0.3	7.2 ± 0.2	− 20	0.001
Verapamil	7.0 ± 0.3	5.4 ± 0.2	− 23	0.001

* 60 mg/day.

Discussion

When new drugs are introduced, their effectiveness must be precisely contrasted with that of placebo. Standard doses should be used for the same disease. When oral diuretics were introduced at the beginning of the 50s, they were compared with the mercurials. The mercurials soon fell into disuse and all new oral diuretics were compared to the thiazides. Digitalis is still the standard inotropic agent with which all new drugs are compared. Propranolol was the first β-blocking agent for clinical use and it is still the drug most utilized in this group. A large body of literature is available on its safety, efficacy and dosis-response ratio in animals, normal volunteers and patients with angina and other cardiovascular diseases. It is therefore logical to use propranolol as a standard for comparison of the calcium antagonists.

The optimal situation would be to perform this type of trial in the same group of patients with a multiple randomized, crossed or parallel design. For us, the multiple crossed design was clearly impracticable. In the first place, not all the drugs were available at the same time. In the second place, most calcium antagonists attain maximum efficacy at 4 weeks of treatment; as such, to test 5 drugs, we would have needed at least 24 weeks per patient, including the placebo period. Third, it is well known that β-blocking agents can produce an acute suppression syndrome and calcium antagonists have a similar problem. Incorporation of drug-free phases would have prolonged the study period still more. Fourth, production of placebos of identical appearance to the trial drugs would have supposed unsurmountable logistic and technical problems. Fifth, the natural variation of the disease process would have become unpredictable over such long time periods, particularly after treatment with various cardio-active drugs.

A parallel study design would have required convoking simultaneously a large number of patients and it is difficult to find a large number of patients that satisfy inclusion and exclusion criteria. The next alternative is the multi-center study, which would not solve any of the above problems and would add other variables, such as differences in exercise protocols, data recopilation and observer variability.

We therefore decided to use the same methods, exercise protocols and criteria for inclusion and exclusion in all our patients. This allowed us to gradually accumulate data and, at the end of the program, assess the drugs tested with those already evaluated, slowly increasing the quantity of comparative data. Only recently, using modern computer techniques, has such a method been possible, but it is surely destined to receive wider acceptance and utilization.

Logically, the next question concerns the homogeneity of our group of patients. It is extremely difficult to obtain a completely homogeneous population in any angina study. Extension of the anatomic lesions varies and the severity of coronary artery obstruction does not always correspond to functional capacity. This motivated us to use the criterion of exercise capacity and develop a controlled standardized treadwheel effort test for angina, excluding asymptomatic individuals with ST depression. Mean exercise duration for all the tests suffered minimal variations, 5.5–6.8 minutes. The time needed to produce a 1 mm descent in ST varied from 3.3 to 4.8 minutes. Maximum ST depression was 1.8 to 2.4 mm. Heart rate at rest was 71–76 bpm and maximum heart rate was 120–135 bpm.

It would have been difficult, if not impossible, to obtain identical values, but our values were within acceptable limits of variability and were more favorable than those of numerous multicenter studies. We firmly believe that compiling such objective data with the same trial design and observations in leading centers, would be a coherent way to build a large data base for evaluating these drugs. We also think that this method is less subject to error than comparison of various trials realized with different designs and protocols.

One of the drawbacks of any trial that includes a large number of objective variables is that individual dosages cannot be established. Not all patients need the same dosage; some respond to higher doses and others to lower doses. It is likely that any drug will be effective if used in sufficient doses, but the so-called effective dose should be tolerable for patients. A very effective drug that has lethal or intolerable side effects cannot be used.

We solved this problem by making preliminary studies to determine the dosages that were both effective and well tolerated. We have made numerous studies with verapamil and consider 120 mg, 3 times daily, to be the most effective and safest dosis. This has been corroborated by many authors. Recently, Pine et al. compared the effects of 240, 360 and 480 mg of verapamil in 26 patients, finding that 360 mg a day is the most effective of the three. Treatment with 480 mg/day was slightly more effective, but the frequency of side effects increased [1].

The nifedipine dosis was determined by 2 separate trials. At first, we could not demonstrate that 30 mg nifedipine per day exercised significant antianginal effects in comparison with placebo. We were surprised by this negative result, but later communications and those of other institutions confirmed our results. Mueller and Chahine reported the provisional findings of American multicenter double-blind, placebo-controlled studies of nifedipine in chronic stable angina. They found that 30 mg/day did not increase the period before onset of angina in comparison with placebo [2]. Likewise, ST changes did not vary with this dosis. When the dosis was raised (mean of 51 mg/day), exercise duration increased from 241.9 to 351.2 seconds, an increment of 45%. The difference in the results of the higher and lower doses was statistically significant ($p < 0.001$). In 114 patients in placebo-controlled acute and long-term studies, exercise duration increased 38%. The authors observed more side effects and concluded that, compared with 10 mg, the 20 mg dosage prolongs exercise in stable angina without increasing side effects, such as headache and dizziness. This was unexpected and seemed contradictory, since the multicenter study did not demonstrate that the 10 mg dose had significant efficacy.

Katz et al. tested 60 mg/day of nifedipine in 21 patients treated with nitrates and propranolol [3]. Using an objective protocol and double blind, they found nifedipine to be ineffective. They had the impression that low doses were ineffective and that higher doses should be tested. This illustrates the existing controversy over adequate nifedipine dosage: the variations observed in dosis response could be due to genetic or ethnic differences in absorption. Brugmann et al. [4] communicated similar findings. Our results showed a 39% improvement in exercise duration with 60 mg nifedipine per day, accompanied by a fairly high incidence of side effects. Our findings thus concur with other data published using objective end points and long-term dosages.

We also studied diltiazem dosage. Low doses of diltiazem (60 and 90 mg, 3 times daily) were effective, but the best results were obtained with 360 mg/day.

This was confirmed in a later study comparing 180 and 360 mg/day of diltiazem with 240 mg/day of propranolol. The lower dosis of diltiazem produced less of an improvement in exercise tolerance in comparison with propranolol, while the higher dosis achieved equivalent results. Our data suggest that 180 mg/day of diltiazem may be sufficient for patients with mild angina, but larger doses are invariably needed for patients who present impaired exercise capacity. In the absence of data from other studies, we evaluated nicardipine by beginning with a very low dosis, 5 mg three times daily. Raised to 10 mg three times daily, nicardipine was still ineffective, but with 20 mg three times daily we observed a slight improvement. The 20 mg dosis presented no side effects and was well tolerated. Its efficacy was moderate and it was clear that we had not reached the most effective dosis levels. The next trial consisted in administering 30 and 40 mg three times daily. Forty milligrams produced an increment of 36.1% in exercise tolerance. Even at this dosage, the drug was well tolerated and few side effects were observed. It is possible that nicardipine absorption is different from nifedipine absorption and is associated with fewer side effects. The correct nicardipine dosis is approximately three times larger than that of nifedipine.

The calcium antagonists differ in chemical structure, effective dosage, form of absorption and first step metabolism. Their cardiovascular effects are well documented.

These drugs can be divided into two groups. Verapamil and diltiazem do not increase heart rate at rest, but produce mild bradycardia. This effect is attributed to a nonspecific sympathetic inhibition. The reduction of heart rate at rest is mild and equivalent to that produced by 20 mg propranolol three times a day. The effect continues for 24 hours, as confirmed by ambulatory monitoring. Mean heart rate per hour is significantly reduced. This is not surprising, because mean hourly heart rate controlled in an ambulatory patient represents a combination of cardiac activity at rest and in activity. Maximum rate at the end of exercise is unaltered by the calcium antagonists; this finding suggests the possibility of increasing heart rate during exercise, which can be interpreted as a true improvement in myocardial oxygen consumption. Verapamil and diltiazem both have an inhibitory effect on atrioventricular conduction and we have occasionally seen first and second degree atrial block with these drugs. Both are similarly effective and should be given at a dosage of 360 mg/day. There is a marginal difference between their side effects and there is no cross-resistance between them. Used as single therapeutic agents, they seem to be the drugs of choice for stable chronic angina because they combine a powerful calcium antagonist effect with nonspecific sympathetic inhibition. Nifedipine and nicardipine act in different ways. Neither of these drugs affects atrioventricular conduction or inhibits sympathetic tone, but they increase intrinsic negative inotropism. Nifedipine is a potent hypotensor that has been shown to reduce blood pressure at doses as low as 5 mg three times a day. Oral absorption is rapid: serum levels three times greater than therapeutic levels are reached 30 minutes after ingestion in some susceptible patients. Reduction of blood pressure and intrinsic negative inotropic effect can abruptly induce reflex sympathetic stimulation since nifedipine does not have an inhibitory effect on the sympathetic system. This may explain the increases in heart rate and appearance of angina after taking them.

It seems logical to assume that these drugs would produce better effects if combined with small doses of βωadrenergic blocking agents to counteract increases in sympathetic tone; it may also be necessary to add β-adrenergic blockers to avoid reflex tachycardia. The effect on heart rate may account for their limited efficacy, because this is one of the major factors in oxygen consumption. Physiologically, a greater than necessary heart rate is beneficial in maintaining adequate tissue perfusion. The calcium antagonists could be used as coadjuvants in patients with adequate β-blocking treatment who need additional therapy and in patients who can benefit from a reduction in after-load. Several authors have demonstrated that the effectiveness of nifedipine is much greater at larger doses, doses of more than 160 mg/day having been used. The larger dosis seems to be associated with an increase in side effects, a problem that does not seem to be eliminated by spacing doses throughout the day [4, 5]. During a recent symposium on nifedipine, this was extensively discussed in a round table [6]. Blesse, of Burgundy, mentioned that he never discontinues nifedipine treatment because of side effects. Gourgon, of Paris, dissented, affirming that there was a 20% incidence of side effects that lead to suspension of treatment in 12–15% of their patients. He also said that patients with severe unstable angina who were dependent on nifedipine treatment tolerated side effects better. These side effects always appeared 30 to 90 minutes after ingestion; if drug administration is spaced in 6 daily doses, side effects appear six times a day.

Hugenholtz, Kimura and Krikler observed no side effects in their patients. This is somewhat disconcerting because this American multicenter trial communicated a 20% incidence of side effects and Krikler, in a collaboration with Dargie, clearly enumerated several side effects [2, 7]. The recent introduction of nifedipine tablets may remedy this problem since they produce sustained serum levels without rapid absorption peaks.

In conclusion, calcium antagonists are all effective in increasing exercise tolerance in patients with chronic stable angina and can improve objective ischemia parameters. Their degree of efficacy compares favorably with that of propranolol, the standard β-blocking drug.

Summary

We tested the relative effectiveness of four slow calcium channel blocking agents in prolonging the time required to produce angina during treadwheel exercise in patients with chronic and stable effort angina. Identical exercise protocols were used. The electrocardiogram was monitored by an *on line* digital computer that calculated variations in the ST segment and heart rate. Diltiazem, nicardipine, nifedipine and verapamil were studied; all were compared with placebo and propranolol. Use of identical inclusion and exclusion criteria and the same analytic methods eliminated variability and observer bias. Propranolol (80 mg three times per day) prolonged exercise time before angina appeared by 2.3 minutes in comparison with placebo. Diltiazem (120 mg three times daily) increased exercise time by 2.2 minutes and verapamil (120 mg three times per day), by 4.6 minutes. Generally speaking, drugs that tend to reduce heart rate at rest have a more powerful antianginal effect than the dihydropyridine derivatives, which have little influence on this variable. Our results indicate that slow calcium channel blockers have a more powerful antianginal effect than placebo or propranolol and different effectiveness with doses acceptably tolerated. The mechanism of action of these substances differs from that of the β-blocking agent propranolol.

The pharmacological properties of calcium antagonists are markedly different from those of β-blocking agents. It is evident that there is now such a wide variety of drugs available that both physician and researcher need to know their effectiveness in comparison with a standard β-blocking agent. A single trial of all these substances in a large number of hospital patients is practically impossible for several reasons, such as availability of patients, manufacturers' cooperation and time requirements. Multicenter trials are an alternative, but equipment, protocols and prototypes vary from one hospital to another, and many methodologic and technical problems would be entailed in establishing accurate comparisons.

There seems to be no satisfactory solution to this problem, but we decided to begin by studying all the drugs with the same protocol. All our trials had a placebo phase and a 4-week treatment phase with the test drug. The same exercise protocol and computerized electrocardiographic monitoring system were used for all trials. Identical electrocardiographic leads were monitored, exercise end points coincided and the same variables were analyzed. We feel that within the limits imposed by the nonhomogeneous population, random variability and the effects of sequential factors, our results are useful for comparing relative efficacy of the different calcium antagonists. In this communication, the most important findings of all the trials were schematized to offer a global comparison of the antianginal efficacy of four calcium antagonists in our population (Table 1).

Patients were comparable in age, sex, exercise tolerance and severity of coronary disease. A total of 142 patients were objectively evaluated during this trial. To simplify, placebo values were assigned 100% value and variations were expressed as percentage changes compared with placebo values. The original data and probability values were tabulated using the Student t test.

References

1. Pine MB, Citron PD, Baily DJ, et al.: Verapamil versus placebo in relieving stable angina pectoris. Circulation 1982; 65: 17.
2. Mueller HS, Chahine RA: Interim report of multicenter double-blind, placebo controlled studies of nifedipine in chronic stable angina. Am J Med 1981; 71: 645.
3. Katz RI, Weintraule WS, Bodenheimer MM, et al.: Failure of low dose nifedipine to improve exercise in stable angina (Abstract). Am J Cardiol 1982; 49: 895.
4. Brugmann V, Dirchrsinger J, Blasini R, Rudolph R: Anti-ischemic efficacy of varying dosages of nifedipine. Herz 1982; 2,7: 235.
5. Deanfield J, Fox K, Wright C, Maseri A: Effects of increasing doses of nifedipine in angina (Abstract). Clin Sci Mol Med 1981; 61: 27.
6. Puech P: Round-table discussion. In: Puech P, Krebs R (eds) 4th International Adalat Symposium. New therapy of ischaemic heart disease. Excerpta Medica, Amsterdam, 1980; 278.
7. Dargie HJ, Lynch PG, Krikler DM, et al.: Nifedipine and propranolol: a beneficial drug interaction. Am J Med 1981; 71: 677.

10.5 Pathophysiology of Unstable Angina Pectoris: Clinical, Angiographic and Therapeutic Observations

PIERRE THÉROUX, XAVIER BOSCH, YVES TAEYMANS,
ALAIN MOISE and DAVID D. WATERS

Unstable angina: concepts and definition

The concept of unstable angina has emerged from clinical observations that patients experiencing acute myocardial infarction often report retrospectively a history of premonitory chest pain during the days, weeks or months preceeding the infaction [1–3]. This clinical concept was reinforced by further observations that when patients with the clinical pattern of increasing severity of angina were followed prospectively, a large proportion developed myocardial infarction [4–8]. The next logical step was to consider these patients as suffering a pre-infarction state. However, myocardial infarction does not occur in all patients and the term of unstable angina appears more appropriate.

Many clinical subsets of unstable angina patients are recognized and the definition has little changed over years except for more emphasis on the clinical form of unstable angina occurring early from 3 days to 3 months after acute myocardial infarction and the recognition of the Prinzmetal's variant form of angina [9] as a separate entity. The clinical patterns of unstable angina now widely accepted are:

1. Crescendo angina, meaning patients with anginal pain increasing in severity, duration and/or frequency. New onset angina is classified as crescendo angina if the progression pattern is observed; if not, it is considered as stable angina;
2. acute coronary insufficiency, i.e. prolonged chest pain poorly relieved by nitroglycerin and without the electrocardiographic or enzymatic criteria for an acute myocardial infarction; and
3. unstable angina following a myocardial infarction, defined by apparition of pain at rest or during minimal exercise following the infarction. Documentation of the site of ischemia on the electrocardiogram may help subdivide this form of ischemia between local ischemia and ischemia at a distance [10].

Although the clinical classification has little changed over years, our understanding of the pathophysiology of the disease and our clinical approach to management have evolved.

Pathophysiology of unstable angina

The exact cause of unstable angina remains unknown. The syndrome is clinically heterogenous and mixed mechanisms involving many factors to a various extent are likely to be operative in its pathogenesis. Many hypothesis have been formulated. Anatomical factors such as fixed lesion and vessel occlusion have been advocated as a cause [11, 12]. More recently functional mechanisms such as spasm [13, 14], abnormal coronary artery tone [15], platelet product activity [16], platelets deposits [17] and prostaglandins [18] have been proposed. Demonstration of the predominant role of coronary artery spasm in Prinzmetal's variant angina has made attractive and popular the hypothesis of an abnormal coronary artery tone and of a primary reduction of blood supply to explain unstable angina which shares with Prinzmetal's angina a similar pattern of pain occurring at rest. However, further observations on the clinical and angiographic features of unstable angina and on the responses to provocative testing and to medical treatment suggest that mechanisms other than spasm may be more important etiologic factors.

Clinical pattern of pain in unstable angina

Some of the patients hospitalized in the coronary care unit for unstable angina have vasospastic disease which is recognized at a later time when an electrocardiogram obtained during an episode of chest pain reveals transient ST segment elevation. The exact incidence is not known. In our experience, 3 to 5% of patients hospitalized in the coronary care unit have true Prinzmetal's variant angina, representing 15% of patients admitted for unstable angina [19]. These patients can be suspected clinically by the pattern of recurrent chest pain, often of very brief duration and rapidly relieved by sublingual nitroglycerin when more sustained. The circadian distribution of episodes of chest pain also differs between unstable angina and Prinzmetal's angina.

In this study, the 24-hour distribution of episodes of chest pain was compared in 28 consecutive patients with rest angina associated with ST segment elevation and in 37 patients also with rest angina but without ST segment elevation during episodes of chest pain. Patients with ST segment elevation suffered pain mainly between midnight and 8:00 A.M., the episodes of pain decreasing rapidly thereafter to be minimal in the evening. Conversely, patients with unstable angina had few episodes of pain between midnight and noon; the number of episodes increased thereafter to reach a maximum in the evening.

Coronary angiographic lesions in unstable angina

In Prinzmetal's angina, an angiographic marker exists in the presence of reversible coronary artery spasm. Such an angiographic marker does not exist for unstable angina. The coronary anatomy is usually considered as being similar to that seen in other forms of coronary artery disease [20, 21].

To try to get a better characterization of coronary artery lesions, we designed a study in which the coronary angiograms of 38 patients with unstable angina, who had undergone angiography in the past and who had not experienced intercurrent bypass surgery or myocardial infarction were compared with those of 38 patients with stable angina who also had two coronary angiograms [22]. The series of patients with unstable angina was consecutive. Patients with stable angina were selected from a pool of 140 patients to match the unstable angina patient exactly for the number of diseased vessels on the first angiogram and to the nearest available for age, time interval between the two angiograms, and presence of previous myocardial infarction or Q waves. The final analysis also showed that the two groups of patients were well matched for the presence of risk factors. The time elapsed between the two readings (first to second angiogram) was 40 months. Progression of disease was defined by the consensus of three observers on a 20% decrease in lumen diameter when the initial stenosis was 50% or greater, and on a 30% decrease when the initial obstruction was less than 50%.

Paired analysis of matched samples showed that progression of the disease had occurred in 29 of the 38 unstable patients, compared to only 12 of the 38 stable patients ($p < 0.005$). Multifocal progression (11 unstable versus 2 stable patients, $p < 0.01$), progression to a greater than 70% stenosis (21 unstable versus 5 stable patients, $p < 0.05$), and progression in the left main coronary artery and/or the proximal left anterior descending artery (9 unstable patients versus 1 stable patient, $p < 0.01$) were also more marked in the patients with unstable angina. Therefore, occurrence of unstable angina can be regarded as a clinical hallmark of progression of coronary artery disease, both in extent and in severity.

Provocative testing in unstable angina

Useful informations on the pathophysiology can also be gained from the results of provocative testing. Ninety-two consecutive unstable angina patients without ST segment elevation during pain were exercised on the treadmill 6 ± 3 days after admission after stabilization of the anginal syndrome. Twenty-nine patients with uncontrolled angina were excluded from the test. In contrast to the low sensitivity of exercise testing in Prinzmetal's angina [23], 80% of the unstable angina patients tested had positive findings for chest pain and ST segment depression. This result is particularly significant considering that the test was submaximal and limited to 5 Mets or to 70% of age-predicted maximal heart rate. Furthermore, no patients developed ST segment elevation during exercise. Angiography performed in all cases demonstrated 29 patients with high-risk multivessel disease defined by a stenosis of 50% or more of the left main artery (2 patients) or of 70% or more of the 3 coronary vessels (18 patients) or of 2 vessels when the proximal left anterior descending coronary artery was involved (9 patients). A good correlation was found between the presence of high-risk multivessel disease and the occurrence of angina during exercise (21 of 29 patients versus 20 of 63 without high-risk multivessel disease, $p<0.001$), exercise duration ($p<0.001$) and number of leads with ST segment depression during exercise ($p<0.001$).

Response to treatment in unstable angina

The important role of the fixed coronary artery obstruction in the etiology of unstable angina is further substantiated by the success of coronary artery bypass surgery and of percutaneous transluminal coronary angioplasty in controlling this disease [24]. However, other phenomena may be superimposed on the fixed obstructive lesion including spasm [14], abnormal tone [15], platelet deposits [16, 17] or inadequate collaterals. Studying the clinical response to various drugs may help identify some of these mechanisms. An example is the Veteran Administration Cooperative Study which has shown a protective effect of aspirin in men with unstable angina [25].

Table 1. Calcium antagonists in unstable angina. Potential beneficial effects.

Reduction in myocardial oxygen demand
– slowing of heart rate
– vasodilation and reduced afterload
– negative inotropic effect
Increase in myocardial oxygen supply
– prevention of coronary artery spasm
– decrease in coronary artery tone
– increase in collateral blood flow
Cardio-protective effect and delay in cell necrosis

Table 2. Use of calcium antagonists in unstable angina.

Authors	Year	Study design	Treatment group	No pts	No with ST elevation	Success rate All pts	Pts with ST elevation
Parodi et al.	1979	double-blind cross-over	– Verapamil vs placebo	12	8	75%	–
Moses et al.	1981	open	– Nifedipine + β-blocker	19	10	73%	60%
Hugenholtz et al.	1981	open	– Nifedipine + β-blocker	31	–	90%	–
Mehta et al.	1981	double-blind	– Verapamil vs placebo	15	4	86%	75%
Gerstenblith et al.	1982	double-blind	– Nifedipine + β-blocker – Placebo + β-blocker	138	52	56% vs 38%	64% vs 33%
André-Fouet et al.	1983	single-blind	– Diltiazem vs propranolol	70	29	62% vs 50%	67% vs 43%
Blaustein et al.	1983	open	– Nifedipine + β-blocker	47	13	47%	67%
Muller et al.	1983	double-blind	– Nifedipine + β-blocker in 50% – Propranolol-isosorbide dinitrate	126	45	70% vs 73%	–

Calcium antagonists have many effects on the heart which may be beneficial in unstable angina (Table 1). They reduce myocardial oxygen demand by their action on heart rate, blood pressure and the inotropic state; they also increase oxygen supply by preventing coronary artery spasm, decreasing coronary artery tone and promoting collateral blood flow; their protective effect against calcium overload during the ischemic state may also be beneficial [26]. On the other hand, β-blockers have the potential of provoking coronary artery spasm by leaving unopposed the α-adrenergic vasoconstrictor tone [27]. For this reason, many studies have been performed in recent years using a calcium antagonist in unstable angina (Table 2). Parodi et al. [28] studied 12 patients, 8 with ST segment elevation, and observed that verapamil decreased the number of episodes of chest pain by 75% compared to no improvement with placebo. Moses et al. [29], Hugenholtz et al. [30] and Blaustein et al. [31] added nifedipine to the conventional treatment with β-blockers and nitrates and found symptomatic improvement in most patients; these three studies also included a large proportion of patients with ST segment elevation during chest pain. Gerstenblith et al. [32] randomized 138 patients already treated with propranolol and nitrates to double blind administration of nifedipine or placebo and observed significantly less treatment failure during a follow-up of 4 months in the group receiving the calcium antagonist in addition to the usual treatment; in this study, the benefit of nifedipine was found exclusively in patients with ST segment elevation during pain whereas treatment failure in patients with ST segment depression was as frequent with nifedipine as with placebo. André-Fouet et al. [33] observed no difference in the clinical response of 70 patients, 29 with ST segment elevation, randomized to diltiazem or propranolol. In the larger, randomized, double-blind study published by Muller et al. [34], nifedipine alone was found equivalent to conventional therapy for controlling chest pain and for preventing myocardial infarction during a 14 day study period. In this study, pre-randomization propranolol was continued as a background therapy in more than half the patients while the others received nifedipine or propranolol; 45 of the 126 patients in this series had ST segment elevation during pain.

Diltiazem versus propranolol in unstable angina

All the studies aforementioned have included a large proportion of patients with ST segment elevation and most have used a combination of treatment. To avoid these two possible counfounding effects on the results, we designed a study using a β-blocker alone or a calcium antagonist alone for the study of patients with unstable angina excluding Prinzmetal's variant angina. The latter was diagnosed by performing a 12-lead ECG whenever the patients experienced an episode of chest pain. Randomization was performed 12 to 24 hours after admission to one of the two study drugs, propranolol 80 mg t.i.d. or diltiazem 120 mg t.i.d. Considered for the study were patients with crescendo angina, patients with acute coronary insufficiency and those with spontaneous angina occurring early after an acute myocardial infarction. Inclusion in the study required documentation of transient ST segment or T wave changes during an episode of chest pain. Of a total of 314 consecutive patients admitted with this diagnosis, 66 patients entered the trial. The others were excluded for various reasons defined in the original protocol, the most frequent reasons being age over 65 (11%), previous coronary artery bypass surgery (14%), documented variant angina (14%) and treatment with a β-blocker drug present at admission (18%).

After randomization and beginning of the study drug, the protocol was adjusted to the current management of unstable angina patients at our Institution. If the patient became pain free, he was progressively mobilized and coronary arteriography performed after 3 to 6 days. If the clinical condition remained unstable despite medication, the period of bed rest was prolonged and an intravenous infusion of nitroglycerin started; early coronary angiography was considered if chest pain persisted despite this treatment. Persistent chest pain was also an indication for coronary artery bypass surgery whenever possible. Surgery was also performed on asymptomatic patients for elective reasons based on the severity of the coronary obstructive lesions. Follow-up was obtained 1 month after randomization. The clinical characteristics of patients at entry were compared by an unpaired Student's t-test for continuous variables and by a chi-square for discrete variables.

Thirty-six patients were randomized to propranolol and 30 to diltiazem. Age, sex, family history of coronary artery disease, incidence of previous myocardial infarction and diabetes, smoking habits, cholesterol blood levels, extent of coronary artery disease and impairment of a ventricular function were similar in the two treatment groups. Four patients in the propranolol group had no ≥70% coronary artery stenosis and 1 patient in the diltiazem group. One-vessel disease was present in 11 patients in each groups and multivessel disease in respectively 19 and 17 patients. Arteriography was not performed in 3 patients because of early infarction or death.

The mean number of episodes of chest pain per day was 0.72 ± 0.2 per patient before randomization and decreased similarly with the two treatments, to 0.25 ± 0.014 with propranolol and 0.29 ± 0.18 with diltiazem. During the first month of follow-up, death occurred in 2 patients on propranolol and 1 on diltiazem; one patient on propranolol suffered a myocardial infarction and 3 on diltiazem. Coronary artery bypass surgery for persistent angina was performed in 3 patients on propranolol and 2 on diltiazem and for severity of coronary artery disease in respectively 10 and 11 patients (NS). After one month, 30 of the medically treated patients were symptom-free, 17 in the propranolol group and 13 in the diltiazem group. Angina was present in 3 propranolol patient and no diltiazem patient.

The results of this study show that the clinical benefit obtained with diltiazem and with propranolol are very comparable when patients with ST segment elevation are excluded. The design of our study however, does not eliminate the possibility of added benefit in some patients of the combined treatment nor does it document that treatment with an active drug is superior to treatment with placebo since the latter was not used. The fact that both a calcium antagonist and a β-blocker had similar clinical efficacy may suggest that coronary artery spasm is not the main factor involved in unstable angina when patients with ST segment elevation are excluded. This observation is in agreement with the clinical and angiographic observations previously discussed.

Summary

The syndrome of unstable angina is clinically heterogenous and was derived from clinical observations on patients with a changing pattern of angina. In some of these patients, a vasospastic disease can be documented. However, in the vast majority, the clinical manifestation is different with episodes of pain tending to occur at different time during the day. When these patients are re-catheterized during their episode of unstable angina, a significant increase in the extent and in the severity of the coronary obstructive lesions can be demonstrated. The treadmill test performed in 'stabilized' patients, usually remains positive for subendocardial ischemia with a response corrolating with the severity of coronary atherosclerosis.

Medical management oriented to the control of coronary artery spasm with calcium antagonists appears extremely useful in patients with ST segment elevation during their episodes of chest pain. However in the other patients no clear benefits of calcium antagonists over the β-blockers seem to exist. Missing the exact pathophysiological mechanism, the optimal treatment remains multifactorial with a place for β-blockers, long-acting nitrates, calcium antagonists and platelet-active drugs.

References

1. Sampson JJ, Eliaser M: The diagnosis of impending acute coronary artery occlusion. Am Heart J 1973; 13: 676.
2. Feil H: Preliminary pain in coronary thrombosis. Am J Med Sci 1937; 193: 42.
3. Master AM, Dack S, Jaffe HL: Premonitory symptoms of acute coronary occlusion; a study of 260 cases. Ann Int Med 1941; 14: 115.
4. Levy H: The natural history of changing patterns of langina pectoris. Ann Int Med 1956; 44, 1123.

5. Vakil RJ: Intermediate coronary syndrome. Circulation 1961; 24: 557.

6. Beamish RE, Storrie VM: Impending myocardial infarction. Recognition and management. Circulation 1960; 21: 1107.

7. Wood P: Acute and subacute coronary insufficiency. Br Med J 1961; 1: 1779.

8. Prinzmetal M, Kennamer R, Merliss R, Wada T, Bor N: Angina pectoris 1. A variant form of angina pectoris. Am J Med 1959; 27: 3275–3388.

10. Schuster EH, Bulkley GH: Early post-infarction angina. Ischemia at a distance and ischemia in the infarct zone. N Engl J Med 1981; 305: 1101–1105.

11. Alison HW, Russell RO, Mantle JA, Kouchoukos NT, Moraski RE, Rackley Ch E: Coronary anatomy and arteriography in patients with unstable angina pectoris. Am J Cardiol 1978; 41: 204–209.

12. Holmer DR, Hartzer GO, Smith HC, Fuster V: Coronary artery thrombosis in patients with unstable angina. Br Heart J 1981; 45: 411–416.

13. Biagini A, Mazzel MG, Carpeggiani C et al.: Vasospastic ischemic mechanism of frequent asymtomatic transient ST-T changes during continuous electrocardiographic monitoring in selected unstable angina patients. Am Heart J 1982; 103: 13–10.

14. Maseri A, Severi S, Denes M, L'Abbate A, Chierchia S, Marzilli M, Ballestra AM, Parodi O, Biagini A, Distante A: Variant angina: one aspect of a continuous spectrum of vasospastic myocardial ischemia. Pathogenetic mechanisms, estimated incidence and clinical and coronary arteriographic findings in 138 patients. Am J Cardiol 1978; 42: 1019.

15. Epstein STE, Talbot Th L: Dynamic coronary tone in precipitation, exacerbation and relief of angina pectoris. Am J Cardiol 1981; 48: 797–803.

16. Sobel M, Salzman EW, Davies GC et al.: Circulating platelet products in unstable angina pectoris. Circulation 1981; 63: 300–306.

17. Folts JT, Crowell EB, Rowe GG: Platelet aggregation in partially obstructed vessels and their elimination with aspirin. Circulation 1976; 54: 365.

18. Serneri GG, Masotti G, Poggesi L, Galanti G, Morettini A, Scarti L: Reduced prostacyclin production in patients with different manifestations of ischemia heart disease. Am J Cardiol 1982; 49: 1146–1151.

19. Théroux P, Waters DD: Acute therapy for Prinzmetal angina in the coronary care unit. In: Rafflenbeul W, Lichtlen PR, Balcon R (eds) Unstable angina pectoris. New York, Thieme-Stratton Inc 1981; 160–166.

20. Balcon R, Brooks N, Warnes C, Cattell M: Clinical spectrum of unstable angina. In: Rafflenbeul L, Lichtlen PR, Balcon R (eds) Unstable angina pectoris. New York, Thieme Stratton Inc 1981; 42–44.

21. Rackley Ch E, Russel RO, Rogers WJ, Mantle JA, Papapietro SE: Unstable angina pectoris: Is it time to change our approach? Am Heart J 1983; 103: 154–156.

22. Moise A, Théroux P, Taeymans Y et al.: Unstable angina and progression of coronary atherosclerosis. N Engl J Med 1983; 309: 685–689.

23. Waters DD, Szlachcic J, Bourassa MG, Scholl JM, Théroux P: Exercise testing in patients with variant angina results, correlation with Clinical and angiographic features, and prognostic significance. Circulation 1982; 65: 265–274.

24. Rahimtoola S: Coronary bypass surgery for unstable angina. Circulation 1984; 69: 842–848.

25. Lewis HD, Davis JW, Archibald DG et al.: Protective effects of aspirin against acute myocardial infarction and death in men with unstable angina. N Engl J Med 1983; 309: 396–403.

26. Théroux P, Taeymens Y, Waters DD: Calcium antagonists. Clinical use in the treatment of angina. Drugs 1983; 25: 178–195.

27. Robertson RM, Wood AJJ, Vaughn WK, Robertson D: Exacerbation of vasotonic angina pectoris by propranolol. Circulation 1982; 65: 281–285.

28. Parodi O, Maseri A, Simonetti I: Management of unstable angina al rest by verapamil. A double-blind, cross-over study in coronary care unit. Br Heart 1979; 41: 167–174.
29. Moses JW, Wertheimer JH, Bodenheimer MM, Banka VS, Feldman M, Helfant RH: Efficacy of nifedipine in rest angina refractory to propranolol and nitrates in patients with obstructive coronary artery disease. Ann Intern Med 1981; 94: 425–429.
30. Hugenholtz PG, Michels HF, Serruys PW, Brower RW: Nifedipine in the treatment of unstable angina, coronary spasm and myocardial ischemia. Am J Cardiol 1981; 47: 163–173.
31. Blaustein AS, Heller GV, Kilman BS: Adjunctive nifedipine therapy in high-risk, medically refractory, unstable angina pectoris. Am J Cardiol 1983; 52: 950–954.
32. Gerstenblith G, Ouyang P, Achuff SC et al.: Nifedipine in unstable angina. A double-blind randomized trial. N Engl J Med 1982; 306: 885–889.
33. André-Fouet X, Usdin JP, Gayet CH et al.: Comparison of short-term efficacy of diltiazem and propranolol in unstable angina at rest. A randomized trial in 70 patients. Eur Heart J 1983; 4: 691–698.
34. Muller JE, Turi ZG, Pearle DL et al.: Nifedipine and conventional therapy for unstable angina pectoris: a randomized, double-blind comparison. Circulation, 1984; 69: 728–739.

10.6 Treatment of Primary Angina

J. CARLOS KASKI and A. MASERI

Effective treatment of a disease depends on knowledge of its causal mechanisms and availability of drugs or therapeutic procedures that can prevent or counteract these etiopathogenic mechanisms. Although in recent years the concept of 'primary' angina (angina not caused by increased myocardial oxygen demand, the ischemia mechanism being a reduction in coronary blood flow) has gained acceptance, knowledge of its etiopathogenesis is not sufficiently complete to contribute to the development of specific therapeutic measures.

The best known form of 'primary' angina is due to coronary artery spasm. This mechanism is responsible for Prinzmetal's angina and can be found associated with unstable angina, myocardial infarction, severe ventricular arrhythmias and sudden cardiac death [1–6].

There are other recognized forms of primary angina:
a) dynamic coronary stenosis,
b) coronary occlusion by blood components, and
c) inadequate coronary vasodilation ('X syndrome').

The coronary spasm phenomenon has been recognized and its clinical, electrocardiographic and angiographic aspects have been described in detail, but the processes that determine its genesis and capricious appearance have yet to be clarified. There is scant information on the natural history of this disorder [7]. In this communication, we propose to discuss the following points, which we consider relevant for rational management of 'primary' angina patients:
a) Coronary spasm and other forms of dynamic stenosis.
b) Treatment of primary angina due to dynamic stenosis (excluding coronary spasm).
c) Therapeutic possibilities in Prinzmetal angina.
d) Evaluation of the effectiveness of treatment.

Diagnosis of coronary spasm and other forms of dynamic coronary stenosis

Until a few years ago, the concept of a fixed stenosis that prevents coronary blood flow from increasing to compensate elevations in myocardial oxygen demand was the basic pathophysiologic concept of angina pectoris. This concept has been the key to therapeutic strategy of ischemic heart disease; reduction of myocardial oxygen consumption or stenosis bypass were the primordial therapeutic objectives [8, 9]. Recently, this mechanical approach has come under review and a growing number of researchers report that hemodynamic coronary circulatory events can produce ischemia, whether or not there are organic epicardial vascular lesions [2, 4, 10–18]. This modification of the prevalent idea behind the mechanisms responsible for transitory myocardial ischemia has made it easier to comprehend several clinical presentations of the disease that had been previously catalogued as 'apathic' by the traditional interpretation [12, 14, 16]. The clinical spectrum of these dynamic changes goes well beyond the concept of coronary spasm; for instance, variations in coronary arterial tone at the level of organic stenoses can be responsible for changes in ischemic threshold in patients with chronic stable angina and may account for the improvement observed in these patients with nitrites and calcium antagonists [12, 14–18].

At the present, three types of dynamic stenosis are recognized:

a) Physiological variations in arterial tone at the level of atheromas: more than 75% of coronary stenoses are excentric, the middle vascular layer retaining intact its potential for changing arterial diameter. Although physiologic changes (= 10%) in diameter do not produce appreciable resistance modifications in normal coronaries, these changes can be very important in the presence of subintimal plaques, because they modulate coronary reserve to the extent permitted by the severity and flexibility of the stenosis [12, 14–16, 19, 20]. These physiologic modifications in arterial tone cannot be considered to be spasms (mechanism responsible for Prinzmetal angina) in the sense of the definition of spasm we will give later.

b) Intravascular occlusion by blood components: various authors have postulated this mechanism, which may be a coherent explanation for certain cases of unstable angina [21].

c) Coronary spasm: this is a dynamic stenosis occasioned by inappropriate active, nonphysiological, focal or diffuse constriction of one or more epicardial arteries. It can be either an abnormal epicardial vessel response to physiological stimuli or a normal response to pathological stimuli. As such, the coronary spasm mechanism produces a complex interaction between arterial smooth muscle, with different degrees of reactivity that oscillate in cycles and unpredictably, and diverse endogenous stimuli of unknown nature. This entity differs from dynamic stenoses, which can be consistently reproduced by constrictor stimuli acting on the critical organic stenosis [19].

Practical implications of dynamic stenosis concept

Establishing whether the coronary reserve is fixed or variable in each patient, and eventually, the mechanisms determining this behavior, will allow us to rationally orient treatment and the prevention of transitory ischemic episodes. Depending on the relative weight of dynamic factors and organic lesions in producing angina, we can act on the components responsible for reducing blood flow and on the factors that increase myocardial oxygen demand.

Study of the angina patient's response to a maximum ergometric test, with and without vasodilators [18], enabled us to clinically characterize coronary reserve and confirm the relative degree of participation of fixed stenoses in the genesis of angina.

Treatment of angina due to dynamic stenoses

Patients with coronary spasm are not included in this section. Treatment of these subjects is detailed below.

Patients with low effort tolerance

In the patients in whom coronary atheromas *per se* determine the appearance of myocardial ischemia with a minimum workload during the exercise test (less than 3 Mets) and this response is unmodified or only minimally improved by vasodilators, coronary revascularization surgery may be the best option. In these cases, presence of an associated dynamic component has little clinical significance considering the minimal increments in myocardial oxygen demand.

Reduction of myocardial oxygen consumption using β-adrenergic receptor blockers is another beneficial therapeutic measure for this type of patients.

Patients with fixed coronary reserve

In patients with an intermediate or elevated ergometric capacity and fixed coronary reserve (response to exercise does not vary with vasodilators), whose transitory ischemic episodes are generally preceded by an increase in heart rate, β-adrenergic blockers are the treatment of choice, given the scant possibility that a dynamic vasospastic component is associated.

Patients with variable coronary reserve

With some frequency, we have seen that in patients with chronic effort angina and coronary atheroma, exercise tolerance varies with different normal daily activities and ergometric test results improve substantially with vasodilators (less ischemia in the face of greater oxygen demand). This suggests the presence of a dynamic component, possibly due to changes in coronary vasomotor tone (not necessarily spasm). This type of disorder occurring at the level of coronary stenoses can be angiographically demonstrated with vasoconstrictors (e.g. ergonovine) or vasodilators (nitrites and calcium antagonists). In our center, we usually prescribe a combination of verapamil (80–120 mg/6–8 hrs) and isosorbide dinitrate (20–40 mg/6–8 hrs) for these patients. We add β-blockers if we confirm that a combination of increased myocardial oxygen demand and primary flow changes is the origin of angina.

Mixed angina

Groups II and III may represent the two extremes of the spectrum of coronary disease. Between them are situated what is usually the majority of patients seen in daily practice. In these patients, fixed stenoses and dynamic factors are unpredictably conjugated, leading to a clinical expression with an enormous symptomatic variability (day to day, week to week), angina at rest and dramatic changes in exercise tolerance within time periods so short that they generally cannot be attributed to an advance in the atherosclerotic process. In these patients, we must evaluate the degree in which fixed stenoses are responsible for the ischemic episodes and how much dynamic factors contribute to angina.

We make this assessment by determining coronary reserve with maximum ergometric tests before and after giving vasodilators. In patients with a relatively fixed reserve and minimal dynamic component, we use drugs that reduce oxygen consumption. On the contrary, in patients in whom the critical factor is the vasomotor component, the calcium antagonists and nitrites are our first line medications.

The introduction of drugs with β-adrenergic blocking effects and vasodilator properties may offer the possibility of a rational single-drug treatment for patients who need both a reduction in myocardial demand and increased flow [22].

Treatment of Prinzmetal angina

We studied patients in whom the diagnosis of coronary spasm had been confirmed, but adequate therapeutic regimen had still not been established.

512

Definition and individualization of the problem

In conjunction with a meticulous clinical history accurately describing the features of the patient's angina attacks, continuous ambulatory ECG facilitates determination of the prevalence of ischemic episodes, the percentage of asymptomatic episodes, spontaneous variability and the temporal distribution of episodes. It also serves to detect ventricular arrhythmias accompanying ischemic ECG modifications.

Treatment of the acute episode

When ischemic ST segment changes are frequent – symptomatic or not – prolonged, refractory to treatment with sublingual nitrites or associated with malignant ventricular arrhythmias, the patient should be hospitalized and given intravenous isosorbide dinitrate or nitroglycerin to curb the acute episode [23, 24].

We do not think a 'fixed' dosis should be prescribed: nitrites can be given until the desired effect is obtained, as long as they do not produce an excessive reduction in blood pressure. When an episode takes place in the catheterization laboratory, intracoronary administration of these drugs is usually very effective. A valid alternative for treating acute episodes is sublingual nitrites (0.5–0.6 mg nitroglycerin or 5–10 mg isosorbide dinitrate), which usually reverse the picture in less than 2 minutes. If there is no evidence of clinical or ECG improvement in this time, the next step is to give these drugs intravenously.

Prevention of recurrent attacks

Once the patient's condition has stabilized, coronary reserve can be assessed with an effort test; low tolerance suggests the need for additional therapeutic measures. Coronariography should be done to determine if there are severe lesions that require specific measures.

Response to spasm provocation tests and their reproducibility should be explored if we intend to use these tests to control the efficacy of treatment.

Medical treatment

Nitrites

These were the first drugs available for treating Prinzmental angina. They were so effective in regulating acute attacks that their use in preventing recurrent attacks was a logical consequence. However, in view of the short half life of sublingual preparations, oral long-acting drugs should be used. A dosage of 20–40 mg isosorbide dinitrate every 6 hours has an efficacy comparable to that of nifedipine [25, 26], although we usually combine nitrites and calcium antagonists.

Calcium antagonists

Numerous studies have corroborated the efficacy of these agents in preventing recurrent episodes of Prinzmetal angina [28–33]. Nifedipine, verapamil and diltiazem are presently the drugs most used. These three compounds have a similar efficacy when used at adequate dosages.

In our experience, the dosages that control recurrence of coronary spasm in most patients are: 10–30 mg/6–8 hrs of nifedipine, 80–160 mg/6–8 hrs verapamil and 60–90 mg/6 hrs diltiazem. We occasionally prescribe an additional dosis for the time of day when ischemic episodes are most prevalent, as determined clinically or by continuous ECG.

Effectiveness and tolerance should be considered for each patient individually. Failure of one calcium antagonist does not necessarily mean the others will be ineffective. There are new calcium antagonists presently being studied.

β-adrenergic blockers

The results of Guazzi et al. [35], not confirmed by other authors or general consensus, indicate that these agents produce little benefit and may be harmful in many cases of vasospastic angina [36].

Other therapeutic agents

Various attempts have been made in our center to orient therapy toward the mechanisms that may be involved in producing coronary spasm, but results have been negative. Prostacycline (PGI_2) [37], ketanserine (serotonergic receptor blocker) [38], phentolamine [39], and thromboxane A_2 blockade [40] have been found to be incapable of preventing variant angina episodes. Likewise, use of prazosin was ineffective in the study of Winniford et al. [41]

Amiodarone, a potent antiarrhythmic with antianginal properties [42], was useful in the treatment and prevention of ergonovine-induced ischemia in patients with coronary spasm [43].

Evaluation of therapy

Available information on the therapeutic efficacy of diverse drugs for treating

Prinzmetal angina is fundamentally based on analysis of patient symptoms and nitroglycerin consumption, undoubtedly valuable clinical parameters. In any case, we think that a more objective evaluation of the problem would serve as a basis for rational management of these patients, in view of the finding that an elevated percentage of episodes is completely asymptomatic [2, 11] and the form of presentation of attacks is spontaneously variable, with phases of relative quiescence and sometimes, remissions not due to any measure [7]. Continuous ambulatory recording of the ECG (24–96 hrs) helps us make an objective analysis of these factors, which should be taken into account when considering the effects of antianginal drugs.

In spite of the initial enthusiasm of various authors for using coronary spasm induction tests to evaluate the response of vasospastic angina to treatment [44, 45], a disturbing absence of correlation between disease activity and ergonovine response has been reported [46]. It is apparent that provocation tests are only valid for appraisal of treatment in highly selected groups.

Surgical treatment

Myocardial revascularization

In an elevated percentage of patients, spasm occurs at the level of coronary atheromas [2]. When these obstructions *per se* determine myocardial ischemia and condition low effort tolerance without coronary spasm intervening, revascularization surgery should be considered. This decision always entails individual patient analysis and there are no 'formulas of proven effectiveness'.

Results of surgery in these patients are promising [47], in contrast with those obtained in patients with Prinzmetal angina and minimal lesions [47, 48]. In the latter group, the percentage of venous bypass occlusions is high and symptoms return with relative frequency [49].

Surgical treatment of coronary spasm

The association of revascularization surgery and sympathetic denervation was proposed as an option in patients with spasm refractary to medical treatment. Bertrand et al. in 1980 [50] and Betriu et al. in 1983 [49] reported good results with this technique.

Autotransplant, for complete denervation, has been used in a limited number of patients [51] and the conclusions that can be drawn from use of this technique are still scarce.

References

1. Maseri A, Mimmo R, Chierchia S, Marchesi C, Pesola A, L'Abbate A: Coronary spasm as a cause of acute myocardial ischaemia in man. Chest 1975; 68: 625–633.
2. Maseri A, Severi S, De Nes M, L'Abbate A, Chierchia S, Marzilli M, Ballestra A, Parodi O, Biagini A, Distante A: 'Variant' angina: One aspect of a continuous spectrum of vasospastic myocardial ischemia. Pathogenetic mechanisms, estimated incidence, clinical and coronarographic findings in 138 patients. Am J Cardiol 1987; 42: 1019–1035.
3. Maseri A, L'Abatte A, Pesola A, Ballestra AM, Marzilli M, Maltinti G, Severi S, De Nes DM, Parodi O, Biagini A: Coronary vasospasm in angina pectoris. Lancet 1977; 1: 713–717.
4. Maseri A, Chierchia S: Coronary vasospasm in ischaemic heart disease. Chest 1978; 78: 210–215.
5. Maseri A, Severi S, Marzullo P: Role of coronary arterial spasm in sudden coronary ischemic death. Ann NY Acad Sci 1982; 204–217.
6. Maseri A, L'Abatte A, Baroldi G, Chierchia S, Marzilli M, Ballestra AM, Severi S, Parodi O, Baigini A, Distante A, Pesola A: Coronary vasospasm as a possible cause of myocardial infarction: A conclusion derived from the study of 'preinfarction' angina. N Engl J Med, 1978; 299: 1271–1277.
7. Bott-Silverman C, Heupler FA: Natural history of pure coronary arterial spasm in patients treated medically. J Am Coll Cardiol 1983; 2: 200–205.
8. Friedberg CK: Diseases of the heart, 3rd ed. Saunders, New York, 1966.
9. Braunwald E: Control of myocardial oxygen consumption. Physiological and clinical consideration. Am J Cardiol 1971; 27: 416–432.
10. Chierchia S, Brunelli C, Simonetti I, Lazzari M, Maseri A: Sequence of events in angina at rest: Primary reduction in coronary flow. Circulation 1980; 61: 759–768.
11. Chierchia S, Lazzari M, Simonetti I, Maseris A: Haemodynamic monitoring in angina at rest. Herz 1980; 5: 189–198.
12. Epstein SE, Talbot TL: Dynamic coronary tone in precipitation, exacerbation and relief of angina pectoris. Am J Cardiol 1981; 69: 797–803.
13. Brown BG, Bolson E, Petersen RB, Riever CD, Dodge HT: The mechanisms of nitroglycerin action: Stenosis vasodilation as a major component of the drug response. Circulation 1981; 69: 1089–1097.
14. Gorlin R: Dynamic vascular factors in the genesis of myocardial ischemia. J Am Coll Cardiol 1983; 163: 897–906.
15. Maseri A: Pathogenetic mechanisms of angina pectoris: Expanding views. Br Heart J 1980; 43: 648–660.
16. Maseri A, Chierchia S, Davies GJ, Fox KM: Variable susceptibility to dynamic coronary obstruction: An elusive link between coronary atherosclerosis and angina pectoris. Am J Cardiol 1983; 52: 46–51.
17. Brown BG: Coronary vasospasm: Observations linking the clinical spectrum of ischemic heart disease to the dynamic pathology of coronary atherosclerosis. Arch Int Med 1981; 141: 716–722.
18. Kaski JC, Freedman B, Shahrom M, Crea F, Bugiardini R, Maseri A: Clinical assessment of variable coronary flow reserve in anginal patients (Abstract). Eur Heart J 1984; 5: 68.
19. Crea F, Davies GJ, Romeo F, Chierchia S, Bugiardini R, Kaski JC, Freedman B, Maseri A: Myocardial ischemia during ergonovine testing: Different susceptibility to coronary vasoconstriction in patients with exertional and variant angina. Circulation 1984; 69: 690–695.
20. McAlpin RN: Contribution of dynamic vascular wall thickening to luminal narrowing during coronary arterial constriction. Circulation 1980; 61: 296–301.
21. Folts JD, Crowell EB, Rowe GG: Platelet aggregation in partially obstructed vessels and its elimination with aspirin. Circulation 1976; 54: 365–370.

22. Kaski JC, Rodriguez-Plaza L, Crea F, Freedman B, Maseri A: Treatment of exercise-induced ischemia with BM 14.190 Carvedilol. a new B-blocker with vasodilating activity (Abstract). Eur Heart J 1984; 5: 271.

23. Hillis D, Braunwald E: Coronary artery spasm. N Engl J Med 1978; 299: 695–702.

24. Distante A, Maseri A, Severi S, Biagini A, Chierchia S: Management of vasospastic angina at rest with continuous infusion of isosorbide dinitrate: A double cross-over study in a coronary care unit. Am J Cardiol 1979; 44: 533–539.

25. Hill JA, Feldman RL, Conti CR: Randomised double-blind comparison of nifedipine and isosorbide dinitrate in patients with coronary arterial spasm. Am J Cardiol 1982; 49: 431–438.

26. Ginsburg R, Lamb IH, Schroeder JS, Hu M, Harrison DC: Randomised double-blind comparison of nifedipine and isosorbide dinitrate therapy in variant angina pectoris due to coronary artery spasm. Am Heart J 1982; 103: 44–48.

27. Crean PA, Ribeiro P, Crea F, Davies GJ, Ratcliffe D, Maseri A: Failure of transdermal nitroglycerin to improve chronic stable angina: A randomized, placebo controlled, double-blind, double crossover trial. Circulation 1983; 68: III–405.

28. Heupler FA Jr, Proudfit WL: Nifedipine therapy for refractory coronary artery spasm. Am J Cardiol 1979; 44: 798–803.

29. Goldberg S, Reichek N, Wilson J, Hirschfield JW, Muller J, Kastor JA: Nifedipine in the treatment of Prinzmetal's (variant) angina. Am J Cardiol 1979; 44: 804–810.

30. Antman E, Muller J, Goldberg S, MacAlpin R, Rubenfire M, Tabatznik B, Liang CS, Heupler F, Achuff S, Reichek N, Geltman E, Kerin NZ, Neff RK, Braunwald E: Nifedipine therapy for coronary artery spasm. N Engl J Med 1980; 302: 1269–1273.

31. Serveri S, Davies GJ, Maseri A, Marzullo P, L'Abatte A: Long-term prognosis of 'variant' angina with medical treatment. Am J Cardiol 1980; 46: 226–232.

32. Johnson SM, Mauritson DR, Willerson JT, Hillis LD: A controlled trial of verapamil for Prinzmetal's variant angina. N Engl J Med 1981; 304: 862–866.

33. Pepine CJ, Feldman RL, Whittle J, Curry C, Conti R: Effects of the calcium antagonist diltiazem in patients with variant angina: A randomized double-blind trial. Am Heart J 1981; 101: 719–725.

34. Kaski JC, Rodriguez-Plaza L, Maseri A: Nisoldipine: A new calcium antagonist effective in the prevention of coronary artery spasm. Clin Sci 1984; 67: 57.

35. Guazzi M, Fiorentini C, Polese A, Magrini F, Olivari MT: Treatment of spontaneous angina pectoris with β-blocking agents: A clinical, electrocardiographic and haemodynamic appraisal. Br Heart J 1975; 37: 1235–1245.

36. Robertson RM, Wood AJ, Vaughn WK, Robertson D: Exacerbation of vasotonic angina pectoris by propranolol. Circulation 1982; 65: 281–289.

37. Chierchia S, Patrono C, Crea F, Ciabattoni G, DeCaterina R, Cinotti GA, Distante A, Maseri A: Effects of intravenous prostacyclin in variant angina. Circulation 1982; 65: 470–476.

38. Freedman SB, Chierchia S, Rodriguez-Plaza L, Bugiardini R, Smith G, Maseri A: Ergonovine-induced myocardial ischemia: No role for serotonergic receptors? Circulation 1984; 70: 178–183.

39. Chierchia S, Cavies GJ, Berkenboom G, Crea F, Crean P, Maseri A: Adrenergic receptors and coronary spasm: An elusive link. Circulation 1982; 66: 702–705.

40. Chierchia S, DeCaterina R, Crea F, Patrono C, Maseri A: Failure of Thomboxane A2 blockade to prevent attacks of vasospastic angina. Circulation 1982; 66:702–705.

41. Winniford MD, Filipchuk N, Hillis LD: α-adrenergic blockade for variant angina: A long-term, double-blind, randomized trial. Circulation 1983; 67: 1185–1188.

42. Kaski JC, Girotti LA, Elizari MV, Lazzari JO, Goldberg A, Tambussi A, Rosenbaum MB: Efficacy of amiodarone during long-term treatment of potentially dangerous ventricular

arrhythmias in patients with chronic stable ischemic heart disease. Am Heart J 1984; 107: 648–655.

43. Rutitzky B, Girotti AL, Rosenbaum MB: Efficacy of chronic amiodarone therapy in patients with variant angina pectoris and inhibition of ergonovine coronary constriction. Am Heart J 1982; 103: 38–43.

44. Theroux P, Waters DD, Affaki GS, Crittin J, Bonan R, Mizgala HF: Provocative testing with ergonovine to evaluate the efficacy of treatment with calcium antagonists in variant angina. Circulation 1979; 60: 504–510.

45. Girotti LA, Crosatto JR, Messuti H, Kaski JC, Dyszel E, Rivas CA, Araujo LI, Vetulli HD, Rosenbaum MB: The hyperventilation test as a method for developing successful therapy in Prinzmetal's angina. Am J Cardiol 1982; 49: 834–841.

46. Winniford MD, Johnson SM, Mauritson DR, Hillis LD: Ergonovine provocation to assess efficacy of long-term therapy with calcium antagonists in Prinzmetal's variant angina. Am J Cardiol 1983; 51: 684–688.

47. Raizner AE, Chahine RA: The treatment of Prinzmetal's variant angina with coronary bypass surgery. In: Hurst JW (ed) The heart, update II, McGraw-Hill, New York, 1980; 85.

48. Gaasch WH, Lufschanowski R, Leachman RD, Alexander JK: Surgical management of Prinzmetal's variant angina. Chest 1974; 66: 614–621.

49. Betriu A, Pomar JL, Bourassa MG, Grondin CM: Influence of partial denervation on the results of myocardial revascularization in variant angina. Am J Cardiol 1983; 51: 661–667.

50. Bertrand ME, Lablanche JM Rousseau MG, Warembourg H, Stankowtak C, Soots G: Surgical treatment of variant angina: Use of plexectomy with aorto-coronary bypass. Circulation 1980; 51: 877–882.

51. Betriu A, Pomar JL, Bourassa MG, Grondin CM: Influence of partial sympathetic denervation on the results of myocardial revascularization in variant angina. Am J Cardiol 1983; 51: 661–667.

10.7 Conclusions

A. BETRIU

To conclude this chapter, we can reaffirm the efficacy of medications now available for treating angina pectoris. A major point is the role of the nitrites, which continue to stay in spite of β-adrenergic blockers, which are a useful complement to the nitrites, and the more recent introduction of the calcium antagonists. In practice, each patient can benefit from the appropriate therapeutic regimen, which should be adjusted to the form of presentation of angina, its timing and severity. Thus, not only is selection of a drug (or combination of drugs) important, but also the dosage and times of administration.

There is no doubt that therapeutic efficacy also derives from better knowledge of the pathophysiological mechanisms of angina. The importance of obstructive dynamic factors and variations in coronary vasomotor tone, including spasm, should be particularly emphasized, as our speakers have done. There is a large field for future investigation, for instance, the idea of a reversible platelet thrombus as the cause of a sudden reduction in coronary flow is an attractive hypothesis.

11. Angina Pectoris (II) Instrumental Procedures

11.1 Introduction

A. CORTINA

Instrumental procedures, like any other skill, require a learning period with around 100 cases for angioplasty. Aside from this technical apprendiceship, another fundamental aspect of these procedures is establishing their indications and contraindications, which must be done on the basis of experience with use of the techniques.

Experience requires knowledge of the *natural history* and long-term results of the *clinical history modified* by medical treatment, angioplasty and/or surgery for coronary disease. On the other hand, because of the introduction of new drugs and technological advances, the *unnatural or modified history* of coronary disease can experience important changes, making it more difficult to select one treatment or another. The decision-making process involves compiling national and international data to obtain sufficient objective information on which to base selection. Unfortunately, these data records often present problems of lack of uniformity, inclusion of small series, poor results of early series, etc. A critical analysis of the problems must be made; an example is the results of the Coronary Artery Surgery Study. To begin with, these results produced a reduction of more than 25% in coronary surgery in the United States. In these cases, the personal contributions of experts can be fundamental.

Each group also has to be pragmatic in extrapolating findings from the literature to other localities, weighing and evaluating personal experience and local results to provide the most appropriate treatment for each patient.

For these reasons, decision making is not easy. In certain respects, Hippocrates' aphorism is still applicable: 'Art is long, life is short, opportunities are brief and experience subject to error, therefore, judgements are difficult'.

11.2 Current Status of Coronary Angioplasty in Spain

J.L. DELCAN and L. MARTINEZ ELBAL

Ever since the first percutaneous transluminal coronary angioplasty (PTCA) took place in this country [1], experience has been slowly gained in this field, and some 3,500 patients are estimated to have treated by this procedure.

In an attempt to establish the current status of PTCA in Spain, we submitted a simple questionnaire to 20 Spanish hospitals where this procedure is applied. The questionnaire referred to the number of procedures, the rate of success, the vessels involved, the number of single or multiple dilatations, the reasons for the indication and major complications. The questionnaire was answered by 12 of the 20 centres. The obtained data were used to elaborate the present communication.

Results

Number of angioplasties

Until April 1987, PTCA had been undergone by 1845 patients and a total of 2279 vessels had been involved. Five of the 12 hospitals had had less than 100 cases; 3 had had between 100 and 200; another 3, between 200 and 300; and only one had had more than 400.

Indications

In 1337 (72.4%) cases, PTCA had been indicated as a result of angina pectoris, which in 778 cases was stable, while in 674 it was defined as unstable (resting angina, progressive angina, post-infarction angina, variant angina or new onset angina). Thus, the indication was stable angina in 42% of the patients, and unstable angina in 36% (Fig. 1). In 292 cases (16%), PTCA was undergone in the context of an acute myocardial infarction (AMI), either as an immediate deblocking therapy in the hyperacute stage (whether or not associated with

INDICATION OF PTCA

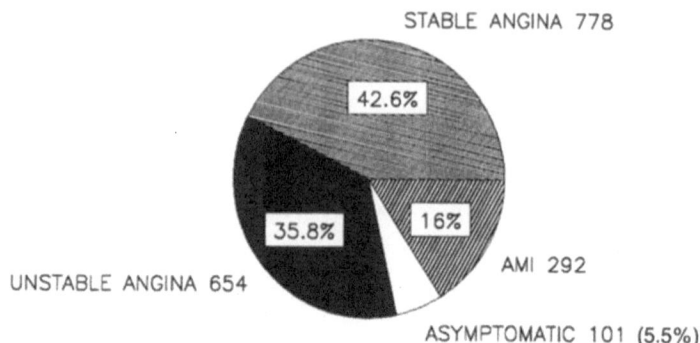

STABLE ANGINA 778

Fig. 1. Indication of PTCA. Note a high proportion of patients with unstable angina.

intracoronary fibrinolysis) or in the course of the hospitalisation, as an optional therapy and often to complement systemic fibrinolysis. In 101 cases (6%), PTCA was performed on asymptomatic patients for purely anatomical considerations when the myocardium was considered to be at risk.

Anatomy

PTCA involved only one vessel in 1586 patients (86%), and two or three vessels in 235 (14%). Most frequently, the procedure involved the anterior descending artery (1344 cases), which accounted for 59 per cent of all the

VESSELS ATTEMPTED

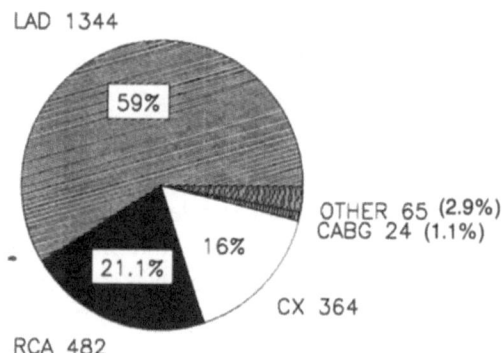

Fig. 2. Location of coronary lesions attempted by PTCA. LAD = left anterior descending, RCA = right coronary artery, Cx = circumflex artery, CABG = Safenous bypass grafts, OTHER includes diagonal, ramus medianus and septal braches (1 case).

524

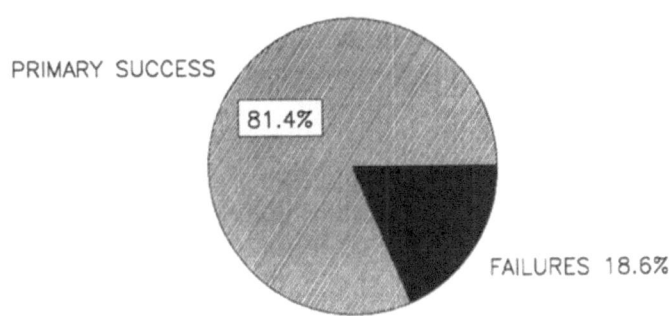

EARLY OVERALL RESULTS
(vessels attempted)
N = 2.279

PRIMARY SUCCESS

81.4%

FAILURES 18.6%

Fig. 3. Relative percentage of immediate angiographic success and failure.

attempted vessels. The percentage ranged from 47 to 78 per cent depending on the hospital, but it was the most frequent procedure in every case. The right coronary artery ranked second, and was involved 482 times (21%); the circumflex artery, in turn, was involved in 364 (16%) of the cases (Fig. 2). PTCA involved an aorto-coronary graft on 24 occasions (1%) and minor vessels, branches of the three main ones, in 65 (3%) of the cases. On 137 occasions, angioplasty was attempted under non-acute complete occlusion of the vessel.

Results

Of the 2279 vessels involved in PTCA procedures, immediate angiographic success (stenosis reduced by at least 40%, with residual stenosis below 50%) was obtained in 1845 (81.4%) of the cases, while failure was registered in 434 (18.6%) (Fig. 3).

Complications

Death, non-lethal AMI and the need for emergency aorto-coronary graft surgery were the major complications of the procedure. Each category was considered to be exclusive.

The rate of mortality directly associated with the procedure was 1.02% (19 patients). This figure does not include the patients who died after the operation. Non-lethal AMI was recorded in 81 patients (4.3%), and here again it does not include those who underwent surgery. Seventy four patients (4.1%) underwent emergency surgery, and the corresponding results were not given in the questionnaires (Fig. 4).

MAJOR COMPLICATIONS
(2019 PATIENTS)

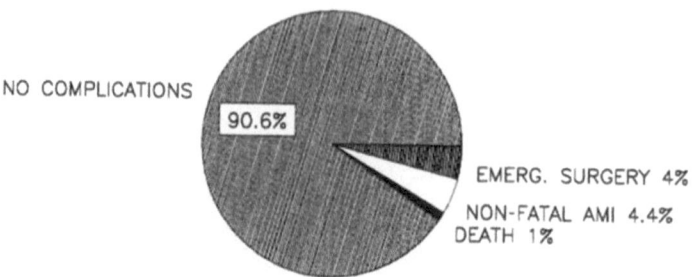

NO COMPLICATIONS

90.6%

EMERG. SURGERY 4%
NON-FATAL AMI 4.4%
DEATH 1%

Fig. 4. Major complications (death, non-fatal acute myocardial infarction and emergency surgery) in 2019 PTCA patients.

Discussion

The number of PTCA procedures performed in Spain to this date is very low in terms of the country's population and the local incidence of coronary disease. A report commissioned to an expert committee by the Health Department of the Catalonian Community [2] contends that if the right number of coronarygraphies were performed in the Community, a total of 600 coronary angioplasties would be performed each year. The extrapolation of these data to the total Spanish State indicates that the total number of procedures would be of approximately 4,000. This figure dramatically outdoes the 1986 value, which was of about 1,500.

If the number of angioplasties is to be increased and adapted to our requirements, the number of diagnostic coronarygraphies among patients with ischemic cardiopathies who currently do not have hospital treatment, must be raised. This can only be attained by improving primary cardiologic care to identify the candidates to an optional angiographic study.

The high percentage of PTCA indications due to unstable angina as shown in this study may reflect, in addition to an undoubtable ambiguous component in its definition, the type of pathology that is seen in our hospitals. The less than optimal structure of cardiological care outside the Spanish hospitals prevents the follow-up of patients with stable angina, who should be the leading candidates to PTCA.

The survey also shows a significant amount of angioplasties for AMI (16%). Almost half the cases, however, were recorded in two centres with programmes of angioplasty in the hyperacute stage. With some minor exceptions, the rest were procedures performed a few days after the infarction with

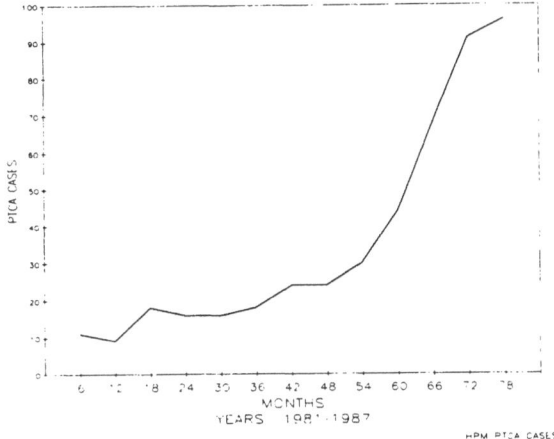

Fig. 5. Number of angioplasties performed over six-month periods from 1981 to 1987 in one of the participating hospitals. The marked increase that took place in the last three years (1984–1987) should be noted.

anatomical indication or due to post-infarction angina. Many of these patients were treated with intravenous fibrinolysis in the course of the early hours after the infarction.

The number of angioplasties performed in Spain has been increasing exponentially in recent years. Although this report refers to a survey of the last six years, it should be noted that the experience of most of the 12 hospitals does not date so far back. Only two hospitals in this country started to use this procedure in late 1980, and the number of cases was very small for three years (Fig. 5). The increase in the number of angioplasties as from 1983–1984 was the result not only of a major acceleration of the number of cases in the more experienced hospitals but also of the fact that most of the hospitals started to apply the technique in those years.

Nevertheless, PTCA experience is rather atomised. Of the 12 hospitals who participated in the survey, five have had less than 100 patients, and this proportion seems to be the same in all the Spanish hospitals where angioplasty is performed. Surprisingly, an analysis of the rate of success of each hospital shows relatively uniform results, and no improvement is evident with the increase in the number of procedures.

The high rate of immediate success with PTCA reflected in this study (81.4%) compares favourably with the NHLBI Registry where the rate of success went up from 61% when the cases of all the centres were considered jointly, to 85% when only hospitals with an experience of 100 cases or more were taken into account [3]. A factor that could influence the high rate of success is that a majority of the angioplasties under consideration were performed with steerable material, where the chances of reaching and dilating the stenosis are much greater than with conventional balloon catheters. Unlike the NHLBI experience, these have been used in a rather small number of cases in this country in the early days of the experience. The uniform results obtained by the different surveyed hospitals without regard to the number of cases is more difficult to account for, but it could be pinned down to different patient eligibility criteria, whose anatomic conditions (calcification, eccentricity, stenosis proximity, etc.) have not been detailed. Thus, there is a possibility that the least experienced groups may have chosen more easily dilatable lesions.

The small percentage of dilatation of multiple vessels (14% as compared to 29% in the French Cooperative Study) may reflect that the technique is in a relatively early stage of development in Spain. Only three of the hospitals have performed multiple angioplasties (21, 28 and 35 per cent, respectively).

The number of major complications shown by this study is also acceptable (1% mortality, 4% emergency surgery and slightly over 4% non-lethal AMI) and is similar to the report of the NHLBI Registry [4, 5].

From the simple data contained in this report, it can be concluded that:

1. PTCA procedures have increased quickly in the last three years, but they still have not reached a suitable quantitative level in terms of population and the incidence of coronary disease.
2. In general terms, experience is shared among too many centres which, in many cases, apply the procedure to a very small number of patients each year.
3. The results obtained to date with this technique in Spain are comparable to those reported in other studies. The same holds for the incidence of complications, but the experience in complex angioplasties in patients in whom multiple vessels are affected is still very limited.

Hospitals that have participated in the survey

Hospital Carlos Haya, Málaga – Dr J.L. Castillo, Dr F. Alvarez
Clínica Universitaria Navarra, Pamplona – Dr D. Martínez Caro, Dr E. Alegría, Dr J. Calabuig
Hospital Clínico S. Carlos, Madrid – Dr C. Macaya
Hospital Clínico Universitario, Zaragoza – Dr A. Peleato
Hospital General Gregorio Marañón, Madrid – Dr J.L. Delcán, Dr L. Martínez Elbal
Hospital La Paz, Madrid – Dr N. Sobrino, Dr L. Calvo
Hospital Marqués de Valdecilla, Santander – Dr J.L. Ubago, Dr T. Colman, Dr A. Figueroa
Hospital Nuestra Señora del Pino, Las Palmas – Dr A. Medina, Dr A. Betancour
Hospital Reina Sofía, Córdoba – Dr J. Suárez de Lezo
Hospital Universitario, Sevilla – Dr J. Cubero, Dr Calderón
Hospital Valle de Hebrón, Barcelona – Dr Angel, Dr Anivarro
Hospital Virgen de la Arrixaca, Murcia – Dr F. Picó, Dr J.A. Ruiz, Dr J.V. Campos

528

References

1. Ubago JLM, Pomar JL, Figueroa A, Colman T, Ruiz R, Lamelas L: Dilatación de estenosis coronaria mediante angioplastia transluminal percutánea. Rev Esp Cardiolog 1981; 34: 167–171.
2. Grupo de trabajo Comisión asesora de alta tecnología médica de la D.G. Planificación y Ordenación Sanitaria: ACTP, Informe especial para la Consellería de Sanitat de Catalunya. Unpublished data.
3. Detre KM, Myler RK, Kelsey F, Van Raden M, To T, Mitchell H: Baseline characteristics of patients in the NHLBI PTCA registry. Am J Cardiol 1984; 53: 7c–11c.
4. Mock MB: Acute and chronic outcome of percutaneous transluminal coronary angioplasty. Am J Cardiol 1984; 53: 67c–68c.
5. Cowley MJ, Dorros G, Kelsey SF, Van Raden M, Detre KM: Acute coronary events associated with percutaneous transluminal coronary angioplasty. Am J Cardiol 1984; 53: 12c–16c.

11.3 Coronary Angioplasty: A New Way to Revascularization of the Heart

A. ORIOL, C. CREXELLS and J.M. AUGÉ

Since its introduction by Grüntzig in 1977 [1] percutaneous transluminal coronary angioplasty (PTCA) has evolved as an accepted alternative to coronary bypass surgery, providing the anatomy of the disease is appropriate [2].

Rationale of the procedure

Whenever blood flow within the coronary arteries is reduced by a developing atheroma plaque, inflation of a balloon at the level of the obstructing lesion should reduce the degree of obstruction, thus relieving anginal pain and/or improving the response to exercise.

If the achieved reduction leaves an obstruction of more than 50% the procedure cannot be considered an initial success and the chances for restenosis or reappearance of symptoms increase considerably [3, 4]. Nevertheless, many consider that the possibility to delay surgery a few years is a considerable achievement. In fact, some now recommend simply dilating the lesion supposedly responsible for the angina [5]. The old surgical principle of 'complete revascularization' does not apply to PTCA, yet it is considered a form of revascularization.

Pathology of dilation

Inflation of the balloon almost invariably produces a rupture of the intima and sometimes that of the media itself at the edge of the atheroma plaque. This rupture takes the form of a split and sometimes a real dissection which is responsible for the enlargement of the arterial lumen. Sometimes, though not often, the balloon produces an aneurism of the facing normal wall at the point of the atheroma. This is especially frequent when lesions are calcified and eccentric. An even rarer situation would be that of the flattening out of a newly developed cholesterol plaque which is redistributed within the surrounding inner layers [6, 7, 8].

Indications for PTCA

Initially restricted to single vessels and single lesions [9, 10], experience and new catheter designs have extended indications to almost any lesion, provided that the acting team has ample experience and that the lesion may be reached by the catheter balloon. Multiple lesions, both in the same vessel and in different vessels, whether long, eccentric, calcified or distal, can all be attempted [2].

It is important to emphasize yet again that the majority of patients presently considered candidates for coronary bypass surgery might also be considered candidates for coronary angioplasty. Experience, skills and facilities are the only limiting factors.

Moreover, one should bear in mind that unlike cardiac surgery, angioplasty can easily be repeated.

On one end of the scale we therefore have the 'ideal' patient [1, 2] with recent onset of angina pectoris caused by a single, proximal, concentric, noncalcified, subtotal obstructive coronary stenosis, in the setting of normal left ventricular function and failed medical management. On the other end, the only serious and widely accepted counterindication to PTCA: a left main trunk lesion, the mortality of which has so far, repeatedly shown to be unacceptably high [11, 12]. Yet in such a situation it is still possible that PTCA be the best way out. This is the case of iatrogenic coronary stenosis of the left ostium. To attempt PTCA has a risk as high as a 10% mortality rate but reintervention may well be as high as 25% [13].

It is no longer reasonable to insist that angioplasty candidates should also be candidates for coronary bypass surgery, or that PTCA cannot be attempted if standby surgery is not available. It is not rare to see patients whom, because of advanced age [14] and/or compromised left ventricular function [15], have to be put into a PTCA program rather than go through high risk bypass surgery [2]. Dilation of selected lesions such as those in a non dominant isolated right coronary artery or a small diagonal or marginal branch can reasonably be attempted without commitment to operation, should acute obstruction occur [2].

Finally, PTCA indications should also include both percutaneous saphenous vein angioplasty [16] and internal mammary artery graft [17], as a way to avoid reoperative bypass surgery should obstructions appear.

Most common procedural aspects of coronary angioplasty

If PTCA is synonymous with breakage, major concern should be given to platelet reaction. Initially 'dicoumarinic' anticoagulation was used and maintained for several months. All patients are at present put on antiplatelet treatment two days before PTCA and this is continued for six months. What seems most effective, yet probably not sufficient, is a small dose of aspirin (250 mg) in association with dipyridamole (75 mg) [2, 18].

A second major concern is also a consequence of injury. Arterial spasm must be avoided. Intracoronary nitroglycerine, nitroglycerine ointment or intravenous drip are all used throughout. Calcium channel blockers are also administered routinely and 10,000 units of heparin should be given as soon as the sheath is introduced into the femoral artery.

The result of an exercise test done a few days after PTCA should be taken into consideration when determining long term medication.

Most cases will be discharged home with a calcium channel blocker and the above mentioned association of aspirin and dipyridamole. In a few multisegment or multilesion cases, there is need to continue with a β-blocker and long-acting nitrates in spite, perhaps, of a certain clinical improvement.

If one considers PTCA as a surgical-like intervention as we do, patients should be kept for 1–2 days in the intensive care unit until an exercise test is carried out and the patient can finally be discharged.

Immediately after PTCA the sheath should not be removed until spontaneous Heparin dissipation has taken place; that is, approximately within 4 hours. This practice will allow for a quick look in case a major complication should occur. Furthermore, in those cases in which arterial dissection is extensive or when the dilated zone appears disrupted and grossly irregular, we keep the sheath in place until the next morning for a new radiological control. This practice has given us some good results in a few cases in which a closing down artery could be reopened with longlasting success.

Immediate results and complications

The time has come to evaluate results with physiological criteria and not only from the anatomical point of view.

Success should be considered as that case in which symptoms disappear and there are no complications, together with a residual obstruction that does not exceed 50%. Furthermore, lesions with initial obstructions below 70% should not be attempted unless there is clear evidence for myocardial ischaemia. The benefit of dilation does not outweigh the potential hazard of an early restenosis [19].

ANGIOGRAPHIC AND CLINICAL PRIMARY SUCCESS
RATE AND CUMULATIVE EXPERIENCE IN PTCA

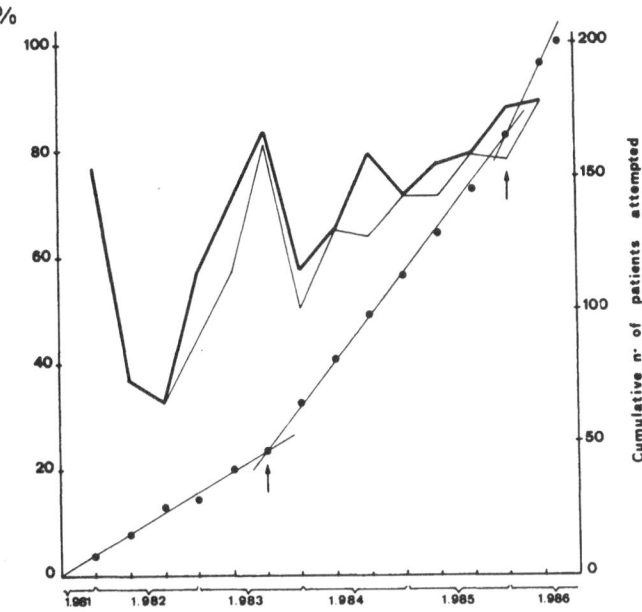

Fig. 1. In five years, both angiographic (heavy line) and clinical (thin line) success rate increased similarly and significantly. The dots show cumulative number of cases carried out. The best eye fit allows for two break points in the frequency of attempted PTCA. From an initial rate of 2 patients per month this goes up to 4 and finally 7 patients per month.

Good training, experience and an adequate turnover should guarantee good results when performing PTCA in a large hospital with highly skilled cardiac surgeons and appropriate equipment [20, 21, 22].

Minimum requirements were well defined long ago [21] and are still very much te same [23]. A reasonably well trained operator is one who after attending a special demonstration course performs 25 to 50 procedures under supervision and continues from there on with a minimum of 2 PTCA per week. This operator should previously also have complete training in cardiology and have performed more than 1,000 coronary angiographic procedures by himself. All of this should lead, in the first 200 cases, to a level of 90% primary success rate with less than 5% combined incidence of procedure-related infarction and need for urgent bypass surgery, with an overall mortality rate around 1%.

To achieve the above mentioned goal it is necessary to have a turnover of at least 8 PTCA a month [23].

In our Hospital, PTCA started late in 1981 and nearly 300 procedures have been carried out. In Fig. 1, the learning curve with the first 200 cases is shown

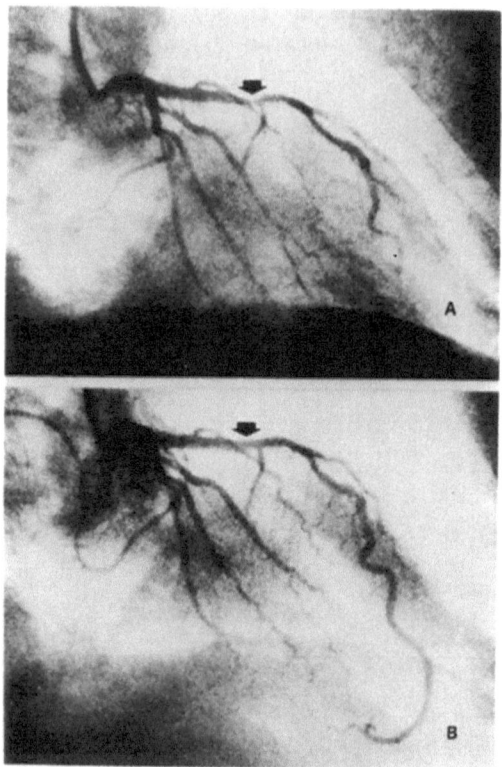

Fig. 2. Left coronary arteriography in the right anterior oblique position. A. Severe and concentric single lesion in the middle third of the anterior descending artery; just before a septal branch. B. Angiographic result immediately after PTCA.

both for angiographic and clinical success, that is, an angiographic success with no major complications.

The results obtained in our centre in the last 100 cases with an average rate of 5 PTCA per month show an 86% success which in the last 50 cases goes up to 89% when the average number of cases per month increases to 7. Again, considering solely the last 100 cases: two patients went to emergency surgery, one because of a dissection of the left stem produced by the guiding catheter and the other because of reocclusion of the dilated lesion.

Three patients developed myocardial infarction, two related to a secondary branch coming out from the dilated lesion and the third due to reocclusion of the dilated lesion six hours after PTCA.

The patient with dissection of the main trunk died 8 hours after operation, representing the only case of mortality associated to the procedure.

A few examples of dilated lesions are shown in Figs 2 to 6.

534

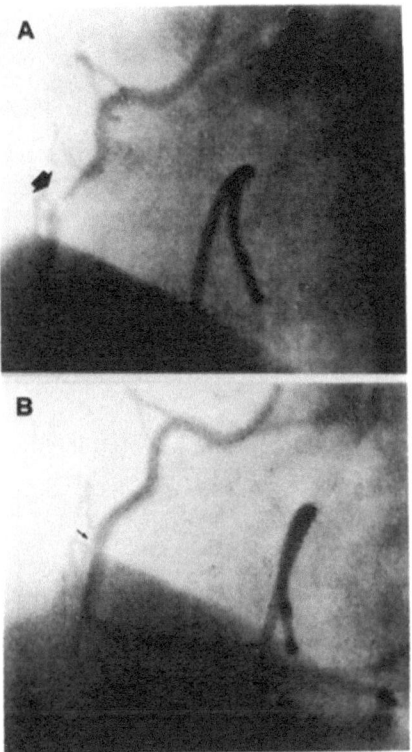

Fig. 3. Right coronary arteriogram in left anterior oblique position showing a severe narrowing in the middle third of the artery (A) which disappears with PTCA (B).

Restenosis in the long-term follow-up

Long-term clinical follow-up of patients submitted to PTCA has shown that symptoms may reappear due to restenosis of the dilated lesion [3, 4, 24]. Thus, recatheterization of such patients some time after the procedure has been advocated and is presently performed in the majority of centers. Early and recent studies have shown that if restenosis occurs it is most likely to do so in the first 4 to 6 months, so that re-evaluation of asymptomatic patients is usually done at this time. Reported rates of restenosis range from 17% to 47% [3, 24, 25] but several definitions of restenosis have been proposed. The NIH first defined restenosis as an increase in diameter of 30% or more [25]. Although this definition describes angiographic progression of a residual lesion, its clinical significance may not be the same from patient to patient. Thus, residual lesions of 20% or 50% may show similar degrees of restenosis but the clinical implications will probably differ.

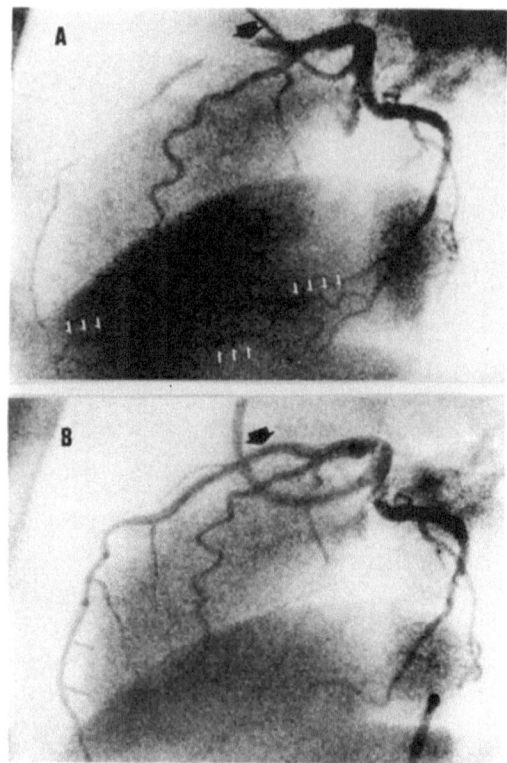

Fig. 4. Left coronary arteriogram in lateral view showing a complete and proximal obstruction of the anterior descending artery. Collateral circulation (white arrows) from the circumflex artery fills up the distal portion. At the bottom (B), the same case after successful PTCA. Notice that collateral circulation has disappeared.

Recently, definition of restenosis as an established percentage of reduction of vessel caliber has been proposed. Restenosis, defined as greater than 50% diameter stenosis at the time of follow-up angiography, has been shown to occur in 30.2% of patients with successful PTCA [3]. Our group considers that restenosis is present when reduction in lumen diameter is of 70%. By using this criterion, our figure of restenosis is of 30% with a 96% of follow-up [4].

Applying univariate and multivariate analysis, to different variables, factors related to restenosis may be isolated. There is now enough experience to sustain that good long term results are associated with the presence of some evidence of intimal disruption of the dilated lesion, a residual diameter stenosis of 30% or less (Fig. 7) and absence of unstable angina prior to PTCA. Excentricity of the dilated lesion and systemic hypertension also appear to increase the chance for restenosis. Future research is necessary to improve restenosis rate, the Achilles' heel of angioplasty.

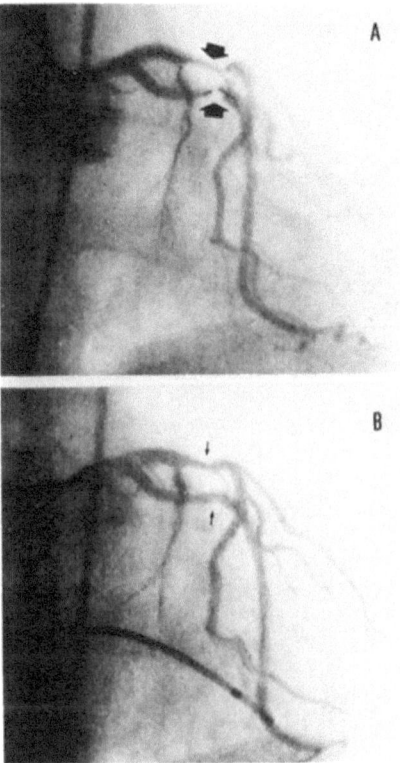

Fig. 5. Left coronary arteriogram in anteroposterior view. A. Large arrows point towards two lesions in the anterior descending artery and in the circumflex artery. The relatively proximal situation of both, allowed for successful PTCA. B. Result six months later.

Cost/effectiveness relationship

Costs of PTCA and CABG are determined by the following concepts:
a) Disposable material, notably catheters.
b) Duration of the procedures.
c) Hospital stay before and after the procedure.
d) Number of physicians and others involved in each procedure.
e) Surgical team stand-by time.
Although a detailed financial study is outside the scope of this chapter, some general considerations should be made.

The longer the PTCA procedure the higher the costs due to duration and surgical team stand-by time. Moreover, long, difficult cases imply the use of many expensive different type and sizes of disposable dilation catheters. If the procedure is not successful, CABG will ensue with all additional costs related

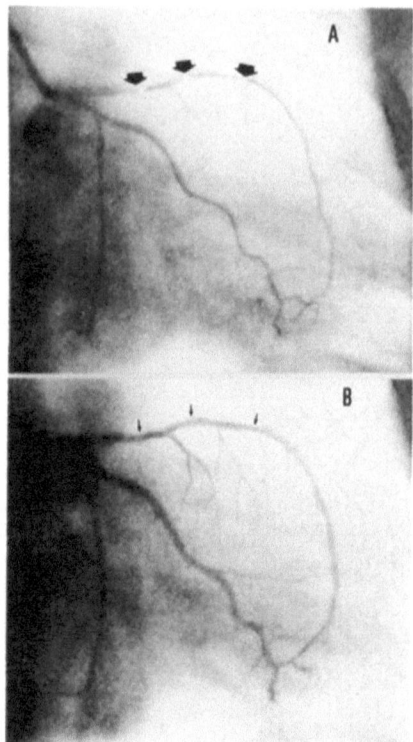

Fig. 6. Left coronary arteriogram showing three consecutive lesions (tandem) in the first and middle third of the anterior descending artery (A). A pull out triple PTCA left the artery without narrowings and the patient free of symptoms (B).

to the procedure itself as well as to the longer hospital stay. On the other hand, short successful cases which require few catheters, are definetely less expensive. Patients are discharged home earlier and hospital stay and surgical team stand by times are shorter.

Results from a multicenter study show that PTCA is less expensive than CABG although the margin of cost advantage for PTCA is limited. If primary success rate of PTCA decreases, PTCA to CABG cost ratio will also decrease until both costs equalize. It is presently considered that for PTCA to be worthwile economically the mean success rate of the team performing the procedure should be above 70% [27, 28].

Finally, hospital policies also determine the cost effectivenes ratio of PTCA. Everything that contributes to reducing duration of the procedure and length of stay will lower the cost of PTCA. Hospital administration should increase facilities and personnel in order to improve coordination between the surgical

538

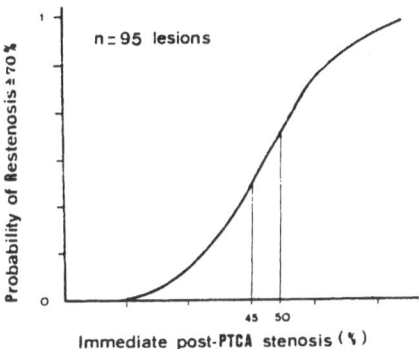

Fig. 7. Logistic curve relating residual stenosis after successful PTCA to probability of angiographic restenosis [4].

and the PTCA teams. It is assumed that if PTCA could take place during the initial diagnostic cardiac catheterization procedure, costs would be substantially reduced [29, 30]. A minimum number of cases should also be done to achieve a good cost per unit relationship. The price to be paid for underuse has been well stablished in peripheral vascular disease [31] and there is nothing to consider this will not apply to coronary angioplasty. Thus, paradoxically, PTCA requires from hospital officials both increased facilities and a greater turnover if a cost containment policy has to be implemented.

Related future developments: laser

As in other fields of therapeutics, PTCA has eased the practice of techniques otherwise not fully developed.

Although laser had already been shown to eliminate atherosclerotic plaques in vitro and in vivo [32–36], the feasibility of its application to coronary patients remained problematic. Yet, the attractiveness of this technique lies in the fact that while PTCA remodels the atherosclerotic plaque and eliminates the obstruction, laser fully eliminates the plaque.

The dangers involved with laser, however, still prevent its wide application. Vessel wall perforation is the main problem to solve although accumulation of toxic byproducts of vaporisation, distal embolisation and long term results of vessel wall damage are considered potential dangers of laser angioplasty [37].

Although several modification of laser technology aimed at destroying atheromatous plaques without harming healthy arterial wall are under investigation [38–39] the problem is not fully solved.

Percutaneous clinical work has been performed however in the peripheral circulation [40–41] but the angioscopes used in this field are still too large to be used in the coronary circulation, and the danger of coronary artery perforation is still considerable.

Another approach to the problem consisting of using a metal-tipped fibre which results in lower perforation rate in animal experiments has just been introduced in coronary patients [42–43] following successful peripheral vascular experience [41].

This consists of creating a lumen through total obstructions. Once the lumen is obtained, the stenosis is opened up with the standard balloon angioplasty technique.

These associated procedures may probably improve the results of PTCA and increase the number of patients who would benefit from non-surgical revascularization. Meanwhile, laser technology will certainly improve, so that in the future the benefits of laser in eliminating atherosclerotic plaques will be applied in usual clinical practice.

References

1. Grüntzig AR: Transluminal dilatation of coronary artery stenosis. Lancet 1978; 1: 263–265.
2. Hartzler GO: Coronary angioplasty: indications and results. In: Speer Schroeder J (ed) Invasive cardiology. Cardiovascular Clinics 15/1. FA Davis, Philadelphia, 1985; 97–107.
3. Leimgruber PP, Roubin GS, Hollman J et al.: Restenosis after successful coronary angioplasty in patients with single-vessel disease. Circulation 1986; 73: 710–717.
4. Guiteras P, Augé JM, Masotti M, Peraza C, Crexells C, Oriol A: Determinants of restenosis after coronary angioplasty. In: Unger F (ed) Coronary artery surgery in the nineties. Springer-Verlag, Berlin, in press.
5. DeFeyter PJ, Serruys PW, Arnold A et al.: Coronary angioplasty of the unstable angina related vessel in patients with multivessel disease. Eur Heart J 1986; 7: 460–467.
6. Block PC, Myler RK, Stertzer S, Fallon JT: Morphology after transluminal angioplasty in human beings. N Engl J Med 1981; 7: 382–385.
7. Block PC: Mechanism of transluminal angioplasty. Am J Cardiol 1984; 53: 69C–71C.
8. Sanburn TA, Faxon DP, Haudenschild C, Gottsman SB, Ryan TJ: The mechanism of angioplasty: evidence for aneurysm formation in experimental atherosclerosis. Circulation 1983; 68: 1136–1140.
9. Grüntzig A, Senning A, Siegenthaler WE: Nonoperative dilatation of coronary artery stenosis: Percutaneous transluminal coronary angioplasty. N Engl J Med 1979; 301: 61–68.
10. Berger SM, Gornfinkle HJ: Candidates for transluminal coronary angioplasty. Am J Cardiol 1981; 48: 810.
11. Grüntzig AR: Percutaneous transluminal dilatation of chronic coronary artery stenosis. In: Mason DT (ed) Advances in heart disease. Grune & Stratton, New York, 1980; 65–80.
12. Ford WD, Wholey MH, Zikria EA, Miller WH, Sadamani SR, Koimatur AG, Sullivan ME: Percutaneous transluminal angioplasty in the management of occlusive disease involving the coronary arteries and saphenous vein bypass grafts. J Thorac Cardiovasc Surg 1980; 79: 1–11.
13. Crexells C, Caralps JM, Oriol A: Coronary angioplasty in iatrogenic coronary artery stenosis. J Thorac Cardiovasc Surg 1983; 85: 634–637.

540

14. Dorros G, Janke L: Percutaneous transluminal coronary angioplasty in patients over the age of 70 years. Cath Cardiovasc Diagn 1986; 12: 223–229.
15. Sowton E: Coronary angioplasty as a salvage procedure. In: Vecht RJ (ed) Angioplasty. Pitman, London, 1984.
16. Jones EL, Douglas JS, Gruentzig AR et al.: Percutaneous saphenous vein angioplasty to avoid reoperative bypass surgery. Ann Thorac Surg 1983; 36: 389–395.
17. Dorros G, Lewin RF: The brachial artery method of transluminal internal mammary artery angioplasty. In: International Symposium on Interventional Cardiology (Abstracts). Texas Heart Institute, Houston, 1986; 23.
18. Chesebro JH, Clements IP, Fuster V et al.: A platelet-inhibitor-drug trial in coronary artery bypass operations. Benefit of peri-operative dipyridamole and aspirin therapy on early postoperative vein-graft patency. N Engl J Med 1982; 307: 73–78.
19. Ischinger TI, Gruentzig AR, Hollman J et al.: Should coronary arteries with less than 60% diameter stenosis be treated by angioplasty? Circulation 1983; 68: 148–154.
20. Mathur VS, Massumi A, Hall RJ: Percutaneous transluminal coronary angioplasty: how important is stand-by surgery? Texas Heart Inst 1984; 11: 110–111.
21. Williams DO, Grüntzig A, Kent KM et al.: Guidelines for the performance of percutaneous transluminal coronary angioplasty. Circulation 1982; 66: 693–694.
22. Health and Public Policy Committee. American College of Physicians; Philadelphia, Pennsylvania: Percutaneous transluminal angioplasty. Ann Intern Med 1983; 99: 864–869.
23. Hartzler GO: Percutaneous transluminal coronary angioplasty: view of a single relatively high frequency operator. Am J Cardiol 1986; 57: 869–872.
24. Kaltenbach M, Kober G, Scherer D, Vallbracht C: Recurrence rate after successful coronary angioplasty. Eur Heart J 1985; 6: 276–281.
25. Holmes DR, Vlietstra RE, Smith HC et al.: Restenosis after percutaneous transluminal coronary angioplasty (PTCA): a report from the PTCA Registry of the National Heart, Lung, and Blood Institute. Am J Cardiol 1984; 53: 77C.
26. Jang GC, Block PC, Cowley MJ et al.: Relative cost of coronary angioplasty and bypass surgery in a one vessel disease model. Am J Cardiol 1984; 53: 526–556.
27. Bresco S, Oriol A, Garcia J, Augé JM, Crexells C: Coste de la ACTP en un hospital terciario de nuestro medio. Rev Esp Cardiol 1985; 38: 79–82.
28. Reeder GS, Krishan I, Nobrega FT et al.: Is percutaneous coronary angioplasty less expensive than bypass surgery? N Engl J Med 1984; 311: 1157–1162.
29. Myler RK, Stertzer SH, Clark DA et al.: Coronary angioplasty at the time of initial cardiac catheterization: 'ad hoc' angioplasty possibilities and challenges. Cathet Cardiovasc Diagn 1986; 12: 213–214.
30. Feldman RL, Macdonald RG, Hill JA et al.: Coronary angioplasty at the time of initial cardiac catheterization. Cathet Cardiovasc Diagn 1986; 12: 219–222.
31. Doubilet P, Abrams HL: The cost of underutilization. Percutaneous transluminal angioplasty for peripheral vascular disease. N Engl J Med 1984; 310: 95–102.
32. Lee G, Ikeda RM, Kozina J, Mason DT: Laser dissolution of coronary atherosclerotic obstruction. Am Heart J 1981; 102: 1074–1075.
33. Gerrity RG, Loop FD, Golding LAR, Ehrhart LA, Argenyi ZB: Arterial response to laser operation for removal of atherosclerotic plaques. Cardiovasc Surg 1983; 85: 409–421.
34. Eldar M, Battler A, Neufeld HN et al.: Transluminal carbon dioxide-laser catheter angioplasty for dissolution of atherosclerotic plaques. J Am Coll Cardiol 1984; 3: 135–137.
35. Abela GS, Normann SJ, Cohen DM et al.: Laser recanalization of occluded atherosclerotic arteries in vivo and in vitro. Circulation 1985; 71: 403–411.
36. Ginsburg R, Kim DS, Guthamer D, Toth J, Mitchell RS: Salvage of an ischemic limb by laser angioplasty: description of a new technique. Clin Cardiol 1984; 7: 54–58.

37. Murphy-Chutorian D, Kosek J, Mok W, Quay S, Huestis W, Mehigan J, Profitt D, Ginsberg R: Selective absorption of ultraviolet laser energy by human atherosclerotic plaque treated with tetracycline. Am J Cardiol 1985; 55: 1293–1297.
38. Boulnois JL: Photophysical processes in recent medical laser developments. Las Med Sci 1986; 1: 47–66.
39. Medical applications of the excimer laser (Editorial): Lancet 1986; ii: 82–83.
40. Ginsberg R, Wexler L, Mitchell RS, Profitt D: Percutaneous transluminal laser angioplasty for treatment of peripheral vascular disease. Radiology 1985; 156: 619–624.
41. Cumberland DC, Sanborn TA, Tayler DI, Moore DJ, Welsh CL, Greenfield AJ, Guben JK, Ryan TJ: Percutaneous laser thermal angioplasty: initial clinical results with a laser probe in total peripheral artery occlusions. Lancet 1986; i: 1457–1459.
42. Cumberland DC, Starkey IR, Oakley GDG, Fleming JS, Smith GH, Goiti JJ, Tayler DI, Davis J: Percutaneous laser-assisted coronary angioplasty (Letter). Lancet 1986; ii: 214.
43. Crea F, Davies G, McKenna W, Pashazade M, Taylor K, Maseri A: Percutaneous laser recanalisation of coronary arteries (Letter). Lancet 1986; ii: 214–215.

11.4 Long-term Results of Coronary Artery Bypass Graft Surgery: Experience of the Montreal Heart Institute

LUCIEN CAMPEAU, MARC ENJALBERT, CLAUDE M. GRONDIN, JACQUES LESPÉRANCE and MARTIAL G. BOURASSA

Introduction

The first successful aortocoronary saphenous vein bypass was performed in 1964 by Garret and associates [1], and it was subsequently popularized by Favoloro and Effler [2]. Kolessov reported the first internal mammary artery-to-coronary artery anatomosis in 1966 [3]. It seems appropriate to review the results of direct revascularization of the myocardium twenty years later. We have evaluated the long term results in patients who received saphenous vein grafts in our institution more than 10 years ago. Long term improvement of angina and late survival were related to preoperative variables, graft patency and to changes in the grafts as well as in native coronary arteries.

Material and methods

At the time of our latest study, 500 patients had a minimum follow-up of 10 years. These patients received saphenous vein grafts between September 1969 and August 1972. Excluded were 29 patients who had associated surgery, and 36 who died during the first month (early hospital mortality of 7.6%). Of these 435 patients, the majority had effort angina. Their age ranged from 37 to 68 years (mean: 48 ± 18), 84% were male subjects, 68% had 2 to 3 vessel disease and 78% had optimal left ventricular contraction. They received 1 to 4 grafts (mean: 1.8 ± 0.7). A graft was defined as a segment of vein whose distal end was connected to a coronary artery, its proximal end being anastomosed to one of the following structures: another vein (two coronary anatomoses-y-graft, natural or constructed), to another coronary artery by side-to-side anastomosis (multiple sequential coronary anastomoses) or to the aorta (single coronary anastomosis parallel graft), or as the first segment of a sequential multiple coronary anatomoses bypass. Sixty-eight per cent were single coronary anastomosis-grafts, 14.6% were of the y type grafts and 17.4% were sequential multiple coronary anastomoses-grafts.

Control angiographic examinations were carried out at four post-operative intervals (Table 1). Most of these patients were unselected, derived from 2 series of consecutive patients who were asked to have sequential angiographic examinations as part of a prospective study on the natural history of saphenous vein grafts [4–7]. Series 1 comprises patients among our first 138 and series 2 are from patients 379 to 478 who were operated upon after 2 years of experience and modifications of surgical techniques, as described in details elsewhere. Of the eligible candidates (at least 1 patent graft at previous examination, no reoperation and still alive) 93% were examined within 1 month 85% near 1 year, 68% between 5 and 7 years and 51% between 10 and 12 years. One hundred and ninety five patients who were not part of these 2 series, had early examination as a routine procedure and 40 were examined between 6 and 18 months because of symptoms. All patients who had an examination near 1 year, either as part of the prospective study or because of symptoms, were offered the subsequent examinations at 5 to 7 years and at 10 to 12 years and were thus unselected at these two latest studies. At the latest examination, there were 82 unselected patients, having 147 grafts inserted at surgery. Of the 148 potential candidates, 41 were judged unsuitable because they were either too old (above 75 years), to ill, or lived too far. Of the 107 suitable subjects, 77% accepted. No significant difference existed between the patients who were studied and those who were not. For example, the age was similar (48 and 51), graft patency at 1 year was 90 and 91%, the proportion of patients with angina at 10–12 years were 46% and 41% respectively. The study group thus appeared fairly representative of the total series.

Occlusion of a graft was recognized by selective opacification of its remaining stump or lack of its visualization following a 50 ml bolus injection of

Table 1. Angiographic examinations after CABG.

Time after surgery	Series 1	Series 2	Others	Total
Within 1 month				
No of patients (pts)	124	83	195	402
No of grafts (gts)	182	184	355	721
Between 6 and 18 months				
No of pts	96	66	40	202
No of gts	154	152	60	366
Between 5 and 7 years				
No of pts	45	37	18	100
No of gts	41	83	29	153
Between 10 and 12 years				
No of pts	40	20	22	82
No of gts	75	33	39	147

radiopaque substance into the ascending aorta. Graft obstruction was identified as diffuse when more than 2/3 of the graft's length was involved, and as segmental or localized when the modification was less extensive. Narrowing at anastomotic sites, believed related to inappropriate suture techniques, was usually observed within the first month [4–5]. On the other hand localized narrowing on the body of the graft as well as diffuse narrowing, attributed to fibrous hyperplasia of the intima were observed during the first year. Changes developing after the first year were attributed to atherosclerosis [6–7], except for total obstruction which was most likely also caused by this disease in most cases. Measurement of the internal graft diameter sites were obtained with a vernier caliper, the catheter being used as a reference for correction of magnification differences whenever grafts cineangiograms were compared to those of previous studies.

Survival was recorded in the 435 patients who had pure bypass surgery and the course of effort angina was studied in the 427 who had this symptom prior to the operation. Deaths from all causes were included. Angina was considered improved when decreased by at least one grade (Canadian Cardiovascular Society classification [8]), or when relieved completely. Less than 10% of angina free patients and the majority of partially improved patients had associated medical therapy. The postoperative course of angina and survival were related to age, sex, classical risk factors for atherosclerosis, severity and duration of angina, resting EKG, left ventricular contraction, the number of arteries having an obstruction of at least 70% and graft patency one year after surgery. Survival curves and annual improvement rates were calculated by the life table method of Cutler and Ederer [9]. The significance of differences was determined by the method described by Mantel [10].

Recurrence of angina was then studied with respect to changes in grafts and to progression of atherosclerosis in unbypassed vessels 10–12 years after surgery. Progression of atherosclerosis in the native coronary arteries was considered significant in the following situations:
a) new stenosis of at least 50%;
b) an increased narrowing of at least 20–30% in preexisting lesions; and
c) development of total obstruction [11].
Left ventricular contraction was estimated from a right anterior oblique view, cine-ventriculogram and considered optimal when the point score was below 6 (sum of wall motion status of five equal length segments graded as follows: akinesis and severe hypokinesis 3, moderate hypokinesis 2, light hypokinesis 1, and normal 0).

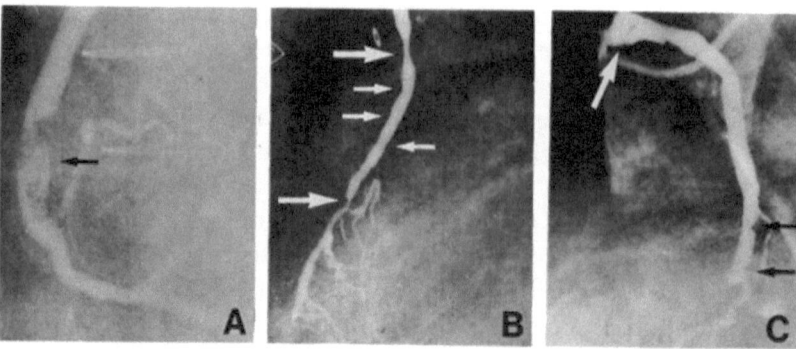

Fig. 1. Changes developing in saphenous vein grafts after the first year following bypass surgery, and attributed to atherosclerosis. A. Large cauliflower-like 'atheroma'. B. Small arrows showing wall irregularities and small 'plaques'. Large arrows showing stenoses, concentric (above) excentric (below). C. Diaphragm-like lesion (large arrow), spurs (small arrows).

Results

Changes in vein grafts

Changes in vein grafts are shown in Table 2. Sixty-three per cent of these grafts were patent at 10–12 years but only 18% were unchanged, others were either occluded (37%) or showed late modifications compatible with atherosclerosis (27%). Of these 'atherosclerotic' lesions, 70% reduced the graft lumen by at least 50%. These modifications consisted of wall irregularities, plaques, concentric or excentric stenoses having smooth or irregular contours, tubular narrowings, spurs and cauliflower like lesions (Fig. 1). Only 39.5% were

Table 2. Status of saphenous vein grafts after CABG.

Status of grafts	Near one year		At 10–12 years	
	No	%	No	%
Closed	88	24	54	37
Patent	278	76	93	63
Early stenosis*	72	20	10	7.5
Diffuse narrowing	186	51	14	9.5
Atherosclerosis*	–	–	43	27
Unchanged	20	55	26	18
Satisfactory				
(includes narrowing < 50%)	240	66	58	39.5

* With or without diffuse narrowing.

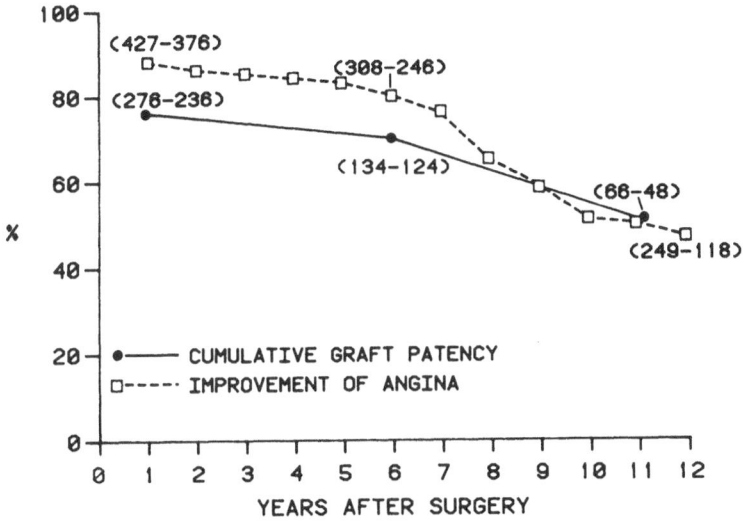

Fig. 2. Improvement of angina and cumulative graft patency of combined prospective series.

considered to have a satisfactory hemodynamic status; i.e. without narrowing $\geq 50\%$. The cumulative graft patency in the prospective series was 89% at 2 weeks, 76% at one year, 70% at 5 to 7 years, and 51% between 10–12 years (Fig. 2).

Changes in the native coronary circulation

Progression of atherosclerosis at 10 to 12 years after surgery in arteries with preexisting lesions in the baseline preoperative coronary angiograms is summarized in Table 3. The stenosis in the proximal segments of grafted arteries almost always progressed to total obstruction. New stenoses were found in only 7% of unbypassed arteries and in 14% of grafted vessels, usually near the graft-coronary anastomosis.

Table 3. Progression of preexisting lesions in native coronary arteries without total obstruction before surgery in 82 patients studied at 10–12 years after CABG.

Coronary arteries	No of arteries studied	Arteries with progression	
		No	%
Ungrafted	53	25	47%
With patent graft	46	28	61%
With closed graft	45	42	94%
Total	144	95	66%

Improvement of angina

Improvement of angina by at least 1 grade was observed in 88% at one year, 80% at 6 years and in only 47% at 12 years (Fig. 2). Complete relief was recorded in 69% at 1 year, 63% at 6 years and in only 36% at 12 years. Thus about half of the survivors are still improved and 1/3 are angina free 12 years after surgery. The improvement is fairly sustained during the first six years, but loss of partial improvement as well as recurrence of angina are 3 to 4 times more frequent between 6 and 12 years after surgery. Improvement of angina parallels the patency rate as shown in Fig. 2.

Factors influencing improvement of angina

Improvement of angina was not influenced by age, sex, classical risk factors for atherosclerosis and resting EKG. It correlated well with the severity of angina before surgery, chronic heart failure, status of left ventricular contraction and graft patency 1 year after surgery (Table 4).

Recurrence of angina related to changes in grafts and in nonbypassed arteries

Of the 82 patients who had angiographic examinations at 10–12 years 59 were angina free at 1 year, 10 were partially improved and 13 were unimproved. Of

Table 4. Factors influencing improvement of angina following CABG.

	No of pts before surgery	Proportion of improved pts among survivors	
		At 1 yr	At 10 yrs
Severity of preoperative angina			
– grade 1–2	121	96%[a]	61%[a]
– grade 3–4	315	78%	40%
Chronic heart failure			
– absent	381	94%[b]	61%[b]
– present	54	61%	19%
Left ventricular contraction			
– score <6	338	93%[a]	63%[b]
– score ≥6	97	78%	34%
At one year			
– at least one patent graft	162	88%[b]	54%[b]
– no patent graft	40	58%	30%

[a] $p < 0.05$
[b] $p < 0.01$

the 59 angina free patients, 29 remained unchanged and 30 experienced recurrence of angina between 1 and 12 years. Of the 10 partially improved patients, only 3 remained unchanged. Eighty-three per cent who experienced recurrence of angina developed important modifications in at least one of their grafts, or showed significant progression of atherosclerosis in their native circulation whereas this was observed in only 45% of the patients in whom improvement persisted (Table 5).

Determinants of late survival

Late survival at 10 years was 69% (excluding early hospital mortality of 7.6%). Late survival was not influenced by sex, classical risk factors for atherosclerosis, severity and duration of angina, and the resting EKG. It appeared related to the age, heart failure, status of left ventricular contraction and graft patency at 1 year (Table 6).

Discussion

In spite of the imperfect technology of this pioneer era, long term improvement of angina is gratifying. Patients with apparently less severe disease, having grade 1 or 2 angina only, free of heart failure and whose left ventricular contraction was fairly normal, improved more frequently and longer. Brymer et al. [12], however have not found early relief of angina related to the extent of coronary artery disease nor to left ventricular dysfunction. In our experience, improvement of angina was also influenced by myocardial revascularization documented one year after surgery. Jones et al. [13] reported that 70% of patients having complete correction at the time of surgery were angina free five years later, as compared to 58% of patients in whom correction had been incomplete. Others have found good correlation between exercise testing

Table 5. Fate of improvement of angina after CABG related to changes in grafts or coronary arteries.

Changes in grafts or coronary arteries	Improvement of angina	
	Continued No 29	Lost (recurrence) No 30
Present	13 (45%)	25 (83%
Absent	16	5
	$p < 0.05$	

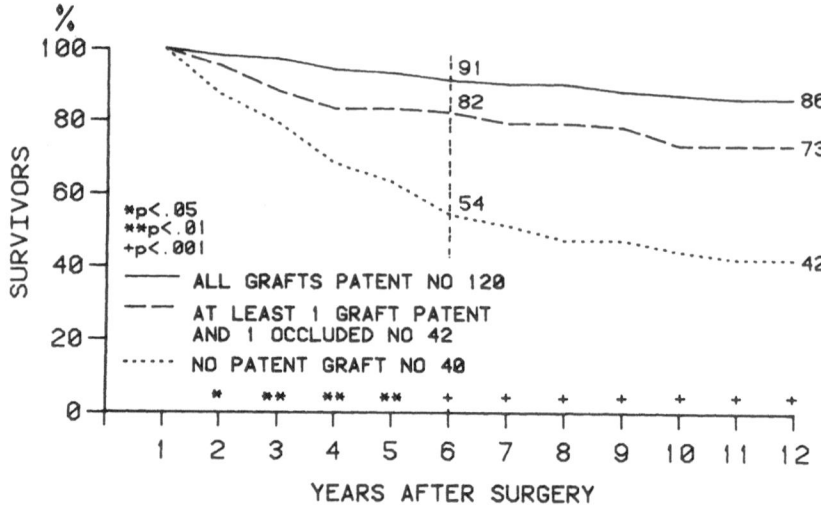

Fig. 3. Survival related to graft patency one year after surgery.

results and the degree of surgical correction at control angiography up to 5 years after surgery [14, 15]. It is likely that our more severely diseased patients would have improved equally well had the surgical correction been more complete.

Table 6. Factors influencing late survival after CABG (excluding early deaths).

	No of pts before surgery	Proportion of pts alive	
		At 1 yr	At 10 yrs
Age			
< 50 yrs	205	99%	78%[b]
≥ 50 yrs	230	98%	59%
Heart failure			
absent	381	99%[a]	76%[c]
present	54	89%	14%
L.V. contraction			
score < 6	338	99%	77%[b]
score ≥ 6	97	95%	47%
At one year			
at least one patent graft	162	–	85%[c]
no patent graft	40	–	44%

[a] $p < 0.05$
[b] $p < 0.01$
[c] $p < 0.001$

Decreased improvement of angina has been variously reported at a mean yearly rate of 1.8% to 9.6% during the first 3 to 4 years [14, 16, 17]. In our experience the improvement rate decreases by approximately 1.5% per year during the first six years, and at a much greater mean yearly rate of 5.5% during the subsequent six years. This greater attrition in later years coincides with a higher graft occlusion rate and the more frequent development of graft atherosclerosis during that period, as compared to the initial first six years [7].

It thus appears that improvement of angina, both early and late after surgery as well as its recurrence are closely related to graft patency, degree of revascularization, and development of atherosclerosis in grafts and in the native coronary arteries. These correlations suggest that improvement of angina is related to direct myocardial revascularization. However, improvement in patients having no patent graft whatsoever remains unexplained. In this series, 26 of the 40 patients without a patent graft improved, 9 of whom had total relief. Improvement was still observed 12 years after surgery in 29% of survivors (5/17). Numerous mechanisms have been considered, including combined medical therapy and changes in lifestyle, fibrosis following intra- or postoperative myocardial infarction replacing the ischemic myocardium, interruption of the pericoronary efferent nerve pathways, and a pain-denial placebo phenomenon [18–21]. We accept that improvement of angina after bypass surgery is related to direct revascularization of the myocardium in most cases, but other mechanisms, related or not to the surgery, may also be involved.

As expected, survival is significantly better in patients below 50 years of age. It is also influenced by left ventricular function: over 75% of patients without heart failure or with an optimal left ventricular contraction score were still alive 10 years following surgery, as compared to less than 50% in patients without these characteristics. Early survival has from the onset been thought related to left ventricular function [12, 22–26]. Although Jones et al. [13] concluded that the early and five year survival appeared to be mediated primarily through improved revascularization rather than through differences in left ventricular function, in our series, 85% were still alive 10 years after surgery when revascularization was documented at the one year control angiographic examination, as compared to only 44% when it was not. Cosgrove et al. [25] and Lawrie and associates [26] have stressed the importance of complete revascularization in achieving longer late survival.

Other variables, such as ventricular arrhythmias on the resting EKG, heart murmur, left main stenosis ≥50%, and the use of diuretics were also found predictive of 3 to 4 year survival [24]. We had also found in 807 patients who had pure saphenous vein graft surgery among our first 1000 patients operated between October 1969 to June 1974, that the six year late survival (excluding early mortality) was also influenced by abnormal resting EKG [27]. Randomized trials have clearly shown the influence on survival of left main stenosis, as well as triple vessel disease in patients having moderately severe angina [28, 29]. Indeed, in these two situations, surgery, as compared to medical therapy, appears to prolong life.

It is reasonable to assume that late results in patients operated in the pioneering era of bypass surgery shall be markedly improved. Surgical teams have already documented considerable improvement in five year follow-up of patients operated in the mid to late seventies as compared to those of the late sixties [25]. The percentage of asymptomatic patients increased from 66% to 74%; survival passed from 89% to 92%. These improvements are attributable to greater technical experience, better technologies and patient management. The subsequent course however, after the first 5 years, appears influenced rather by the development of atherosclerosis in the grafts and in the native coronary arteries. It is hoped that a better control of the classical risk factors for atherosclerosis, particularly smoking and serum lipid abnormalities, will slow down these processes. Several teams have observed that internal mammary artery grafts remain patent much longer and seldom develops atherosclerosis, suggesting that it should be used when possible instead of saphenous vein grafts [30–34].

Summary

The course of effort angina and survival were studied 1 to 12 years after aortocoronary bypass surgery in our first 500 patients operated between September 1969 and August 1972. Control angiographic examinations were obtained in 202 patients at one year and in 82 at 10–12 years. Complete relief of angina was observed in 63% at one year and in 36% at 12 years. Improvement of angina was related to its severity before surgery, left ventricular function and graft patency. Both relief and recurrence of angina were related to myocardial revascularization. Its relief correlated well with graft patency whereas its recurrence coincided with obstructive changes in grafts or in native ungrafted coronary arteries. At 10–12 years, 63% of the grafts were patent, 27% had focal narrowings attributed primarily to atherosclerosis and only 18% were unchanged. Progression of the disease was found in 47% of ungrafted arteries. Late survival was related to age at surgery, left ventricular function and graft patency. Eighty-five per cent of patients who had at least one patent graft at one year were still alive at 10 years.

552

Acknowledgment

This study was supported in part by the Research Funds from the Jean-Louis Lévesque foundation.

References

1. Garrett HE, Dennis EW, De Bakey ME: Aortocoronary bypass with saphenous vein graft. JAMA 1973; 223: 792–794.
2. Favaloro RG: Saphenous vein autograft replacement of severe segmental coronary artery occlusion. Ann Thorac Surg 1968; 5: 334–339.
3. Kolessov VI: Mammary artery-coronary artery anastomosis as method of treatment for angina pectoris. J Thorac Cardiovasc Surg 1967; 54: 535–544.
4. Bourassa MG, Lespérance J, Campeau L, Simard P: Factors influencing patency of aortocoronary vein grafts. Circulation 1972; 45 (Suppl 1): 79.
5. Campeau L, Crochet D, Lespérance J, Bourassa MG, Grondin CM: Post-operative changes in aortocoronary saphenous vein grafts revisited: angiographic studies at two weeks and at one year in two series of consecutive patients. Circulation 1975; 52: 369–377.
6. Campeau L, Lespérance J, Corbara F, Hermann J, Grondin CM, Bourassa MG: Aortocoronary saphenous vein bypass graft changes 5 to 7 years after surgery. Circulation 1978; 58 (Suppl 1): 170.
7. Campeau L, Enjalbert M, Lespérance J, Vaislic C, Grondin CM, Bourassa MG: Atherosclerosis and late closure of aortocoronary saphenous vein grafts: sequential angiographic studies at 2 weeks, 1 year, 5 to 7 years, and 10 to 12 years after surgery. Circulation 1983; 68 (Suppl 2): 1–7.
8. Campeau L: Granding of angina pectoris. Circulation 1976; 54: 522.
9. Cutler SJ, Ederer F: Maximum utilization of the life table method in analyzing survival. J Chron Dis 1958; 8: 699.
10. Mantel N: Evaluation of survival data and two new rank order statistics arising in its consideration. Cancer Chermothes Rep 1966; 50: 163.
11. Bourassa MG, Enjalbert M, Campeau L, Lespérance J: Progression of coronary artery disease between 10 and 12 years after coronary artery bypass graft surgery. In: Prognosis of coronary heart disease – Progression of coronary arteriosclerosis; edited by H. Roskamm, Springer-Verlag, Berlin, 1983; 258–273.
12. Brymer JF, Hannah H III, Pugh DM, Dunn M, Reis RL: Left ventricular function and coronary obstruction as predictors of survival following aorta-coronary bypass. J Thorac Cardiovasc Surg 1976; 72: 73–79.
13. Jones EL, Craver JM, Guyton RA, Bone DK, Hatcher CR, Reichwald N: Importance of complete revascularization in performance of the coronary bypass operation. Am J Cardiol 1983; 51: 7–12.
14. Frick MH, Harjola PT, Valle M: Persistent improvement after coronary bypass surgery: Ergometric and angiographic correlations at 5 years. Circulation 1983; 67: 491–496.
15. Lawrie GM, Morris GC Jr, Howell JF, Ogura JW, Spencer WH III, Cashion WR, Winters WL, Beazley HL, Chapman DW, Peterson PK, Lie JT: Results of coronary bypass more than 5 years after operation in 434 patients. Am J Cardiol 1977; 40: 665–672.
16. Adam M, Mitchel BF, Lambert CJ, Geisler GF: Long-term results with aorta-to-coronary artery bypass grafts. Ann Thorac Surg 1972; 14: 1.

17. Anderson RP, Rahimtoola SH, Bowchek LI, Starr A: The prognosis of patients with coronary artery disease after coronary bypass operations. Time related progress of 532 patients with disabling angina pectoris. Circulation 1974; 50: 274.

18. Benchimol A, Dos Santos A, Desser KB: Relief of angina pectoris in patients with occluded coronary bypass grafts. Am J Med 1976; 60: 339–343.

19. Achuff SC, Griffith LSC, Conti CR, Humphries JO, Brawley RK, Gott VL, Ross RS: The 'angina-producing' myocardial segment: an approach to the interpretation of results of coronary bypass surgery. Am J Cardiol 1975; 36: 723–733.

20. Campeau L, Heitz A, Crochet D, Lespérance J: Long-term improvement of effort angina following aorto-coronary saphenous vein bypass graft surgery: increased myocardial blood flow or pain denial placebo effect. Am J Cardiol 1976; 37: 126.

21. Mnayer M, Chahine RA, Raizner AE: Mechanisms of angina relief in patients after coronary artery surgery. Br Heart J 1977; 39: 605–609.

22. Collins JJ Jr, Cohn LH, Sonnenblick EH, Herman MV, Cohn PF, Gorlin R: Determinants of survival after coronary artery bypass surgery. Circulation 1973; 47 and 48 (Suppl 3): 132.

23. Chaitman BR, Bourassa MG, Heitz A, Campeau L: Influence of left ventricular function and other parameters on early and late mortality following coronary bypass surgery. Can J Surg 1977; 20: 119–126.

24. Hammermeister KE, DeRouen TA, Dodge HT: Variables predictive of survival in patients with coronary disease. Selection by univariate and multivariate analyses from the clinical, electrocardiographic, exercise, arteriographic, and quantitative angiographic evaluations. Circulation 1979; 59: 421–428.

25. Cosgrove DM, Loop FD, Sheldon WC: Results of myocardial revascularization: a 12-year experience. Circulation 1982; 65 (Suppl 2): 37–43.

26. Lawrie GM, Morris GC, Silvers A, Wagner WF, Baron AE, Beltangady SS, Glaeser DH, Chapman DW: The influence of residual disease after coronary bypass on the 5-year survival rate of 1274 men with coronary artery disease. Circulation 1982; 66: 717–723.

27. Campeau L: Survival following aortocoronary bypass surgery. Cleveland Clin Quartely 1978; 45: 160.

28. Takaro T, Hultgren HN, Lipton MJ and participants in the study group: The VA cooperative randomized study of surgery for coronary arterial occlusive disease. II. Subgroup with significant left main lesions. Circulation 1976; 54 (Suppl 3): 107.

29. European Coronary Surgery Study Group: Prospective randomized study of coronary artery bypass surgery in stable angina pectoris: a progress report on survival. Circulation 1982; 65 (Suppl 2): II–67–71.

30. Lytle BW, Loop FD, Cosgrove DM, Easley K, Taylor PC: Long-term (5–12 years) sequential studies of internal mammary artery and saphenous vein coronary bypass grafts. Circulation 1983; 68 (Suppl 3): 114.

31. Okies JE, Page US, Bigelow JC, Krause AH, Salomon NW: The left internal mammary artery: the graft of choice. Circulation 1983; 68 (Suppl 3): 21.

32. Tector AJ, Schmal TM, Janson B, Rallies JR, Johnson G: The internal mammary artery graft: its longevity after coronary bypass. Ann Thorac Surg 1981; 34: 408.

33. Singh RN, Sosa JA, GE: Long-term fate of the internal mammary artery and saphenous vein grafts. J Cardiovasc Surg 1983; 86: 359.

34. Grondin CM, Campeau L, Lespérance J, Enjalbert M, Bourassa MG: Comparison of late changes in internal mammary artery and saphenous vein grafts in two consecutive series of patients 10 years after operation. Circulation 1984; 70 (Suppl 1): 208–212.

11.5 The Netherlands Coronary Surgery Study (N.C.S.): Coronary Bypass Surgery in Patients with Mild Angina Pectoris

G.T. MEESTER, R.W. BROWER and H.J. TEN KATE

Introduction

On January 1, 1976 four University Hospitals in The Netherlands started a cooperative study to evaluate the effects of coronary bypass surgery on left ventricular function. This study, *The Netherlands Coronary Surgery Study (N.C.S.)* is supported by the Dutch Government and is carried out within the framework of The Netherlands Interuniversity Cardiology Institute. The main goal is the analysis of cardiac function after coronary bypass surgery in patients with coronary artery disease. Various other aspects of coronary bypass surgery (mortality, morbidity, complication rates and subjective results) are also evaluated.

In the past decade several large cooperative studies have been carried out (Table 1) [1–7]. The Veterans Administration Study and the Coronary Artery Surgery Study (C.A.S.S.) are both randomized studies, where medical therapy is compared to surgical therapy with an emphasis on survival and validity. A third, the European Multicenter C.A.B.G. Trial, is especially dedicated to the question of whether coronary bypass surgery improves survival in patients with angina pectoris. Assessment of cardiac function before and after bypass surgery in these trials is only scarcely available.

Table 1. Summary of major cooperative studies on coronary bypass surgery.

Study	Number of centers	Number of patients	Begin year	Follow-up (years)	Randomiz. med./surg.	Study aim
V.A.	13	1000	1972	5	yes	life expectancy
C.A.S.S.	15	2000	1975	7	yes	life expectancy
E.C.S.	12	768	1973	5	yes	life expectancy
N.C.S.	4	848	1976	1 + 3	no	cardiac function

Methods

The Netherlands Coronary Surgery Study required that, after the coronary bypass operation, each patient agreed to undergo two repeat catheterizations, the first at 1 year and another at 3 years after surgery. The databank design allowed for a total of 1,000 patients. New patients were entered into the databank over a period of 3 years. Follow-up information was collected over the next 3 postoperative years.

Data acquisition in the four centers was standardized, not only for history and physical examination and other diagnostic interventions, but also for the cardiac catheterization procedure and quantification of ventricular function. Data analysis during cardiac catheterization was carried out in an identical manner by means of a catheterization computer system, identical in all four centers [8, 9]. Patients with overt forms of heart disease were excluded from the study. The different categories of patient data in The Netherlands Coronary Surgery Study are summarized in Table 2. Each of these categories consists of a number of defined questions. All information was coded on forms. A page of the study protocol describing the coronary angiogram is shown in Fig. 1.

For every patient approximately 1,000 different data were collected per follow-up study. For data storage and data processing, a dedicated information system was designed and implemented [8].

Mild angina pectoris: within the total study group the following (retrospective) inclusion criteria were applied to define a patient as mildly symptomatic at entry in the study:

*Table 2.*N.C.S.: categories of patient data followed up preoperatively and 1 and 3 years after operation.

N.C.S.: Patient forms:	
1.	Administrative information and dates of clinical events
2.	History, symptoms, associated conditions
3.	Medical therapy, diet
4.	Physical examination
5.	Electrocardiogram
6.	Biochemical data
7.	Hemodynamic information
8.	Atrial pacing stress test
9.	Quantitative LV angiogram
10.	Coronary angiogram
11.	Bypass angiogram
12–13	Surgical information
14–16	Mortality and autopsy
17.	Other, special events

ASSESSMENT OF CARDIAC FUNCTION
PROJECT OF THE INTERUNIVERSITY CARDIOLOGY INSTITUTE

NAME:	DATE
	FOLLOW UP NO.

CORONARY ARTERIOGRAM

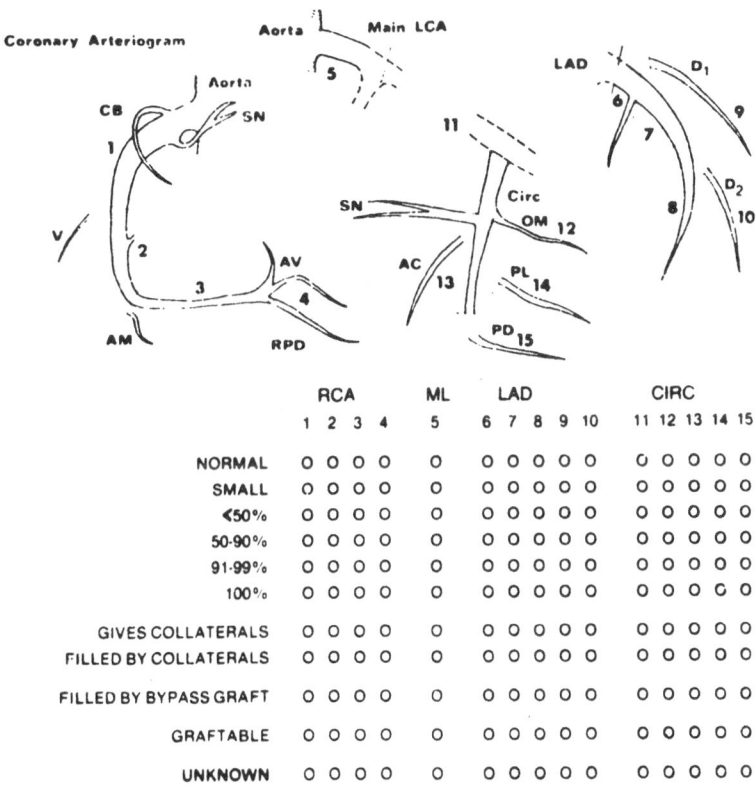

	RCA				ML	LAD					CIRC				
	1	2	3	4	5	6	7	8	9	10	11	12	13	14	15
NORMAL	o	o	o	o	o	o	o	o	o	o	o	o	o	o	o
SMALL	o	o	o	o	o	o	o	o	o	o	o	o	o	o	o
<50%	o	o	o	o	o	o	o	o	o	o	o	o	o	o	o
50-90%	o	o	o	o	o	o	o	o	o	o	o	o	o	o	o
91-99%	o	o	o	o	o	o	o	o	o	o	o	o	o	o	o
100%	o	o	o	o	o	o	o	o	o	o	o	o	o	o	o
GIVES COLLATERALS	o	o	o	o	o	o	o	o	o	o	o	o	o	o	o
FILLED BY COLLATERALS	o	o	o	o	o	o	o	o	o	o	o	o	o	o	o
FILLED BY BYPASS GRAFT	o	o	o	o	o	o	o	o	o	o	o	o	o	o	o
GRAFTABLE	o	o	o	o	o	o	o	o	o	o	o	o	o	o	o
UNKNOWN	o	o	o	o	o	o	o	o	o	o	o	o	o	o	o

Fig. 1. N.C.S.: page of study protocol used for coding coronary angiogram. From these data the coronary score in calculated.

1. N.Y.H.A. class 1 or 2;
2. no angina at rest, no unstable angina pectoris;
3. normal or nearly normal physical activity pattern.

In order to more nearly match the comparable study group of the C.A.S.S. study we excluded patients over 65 years of age and those with main stem disease of 50% or more narrowing.

Because all patients in the study group underwent coronary bypass surgery,

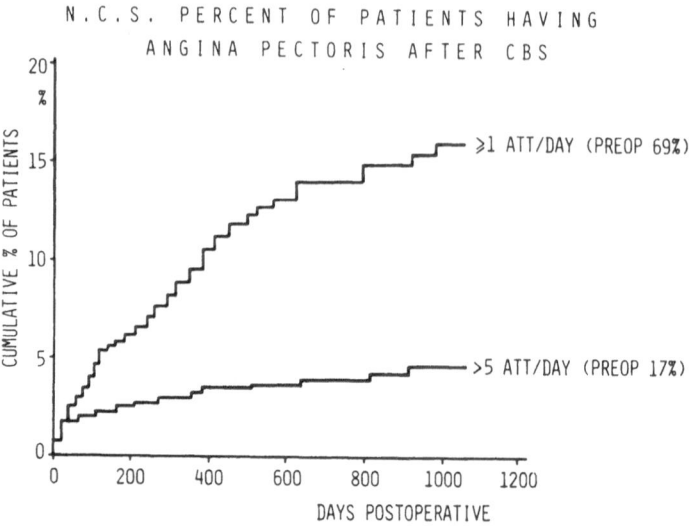

Fig. 2. N.C.S.: angina pectoris after bypass surgery, recurrence over follow-up period.

these criteria result in a study group consisting of patients with angiographic coronary artery disease and either a previous myocardial infarct or mild angina pectoris without physical limitations or both. According to these definitions 199 (24%) out of the total group of 848 patients can be regarded as mildly or non-symptomatic. Data on these 199 patients are presented here.

Overall results

At this moment the total database contains 848 operated patients. Follow-up data, including catheterization and coronary angiography are available in 550 patients one year after their surgery, and in 398 patients three years post-operatively. Part of the non-invasive data are summarized in Table 3.

Overall mortality. Hospital mortality was approximately 1% (10 of 848 patients). In the first year postoperative an additional 4 patients died and 14 others in the following 2 years.

Bypass patency (see Table 4). These 848 patients received in total 2332 bypasses, an average of 2.7 per patient. The patency rate after one year was 80%, after 3 years 78%.

Angina pectoris. After 3 years more than 80% of the patients is still free of symptoms or considerably improved (Fig. 2). There is, however, a partial recurrence of angina over this period of three years. At the end of the study period approximately 15% of the patients have once more symptoms of angina pectoris.

Incidence of myocardial infarctions (see Fig. 3). In the total group of 848 patients 53% experienced one or more myocardial infarcts before surgery. During the operation and also in the years thereafter, new infarcts occurred:

Table 3. N.C.S.: summary of non-invasive medical data. In all patients values expressed as mean with standard deviation or in % of total group.

	Surgery	1 yr after surgery	3 yrs after surgery
Number of patients	848	550	398
Men	91%	93%	94%
Women	9%	7%	6%
Age (yrs)			
Total population: mean ± S.D.	52 ± 7	53 ± 7	55 ± 7
range	28 – 69	29 – 71	32 – 72
Weight (kg)			
Total population: mean ± S.D.	74 ± 9	75 ± 9	75 ± 10
Overweight	18%	22%	24%
Cholesterol AO 7.2 mmol/l	41%	36%	32%
Potential hyperchol. (< 7.2)			
+ medical therapy or diet	22%	12%	15%
Hypertension			
≥ 160/95 mm Hg	35%	23%	25%
Potential hypertension	12%	21%	19%
No hypertension	53%	56%	56%
Smokers	50%	37%	39%
Ex-smokers or non-smokers	50%	63%	61%
Angina pectoris	99%	34%	43%
> 1 attack/day	69%	8%	11%
NYHA function			
Class I	3%	64%	49%
II	43%	30%	41%
III	41%	5%	8%
IV	13%	1%	2%
Physical activity (%)			
None or almost none	47%	6%	8%
Medium	48%	42%	44%
Regular + heavy	5%	52%	48%

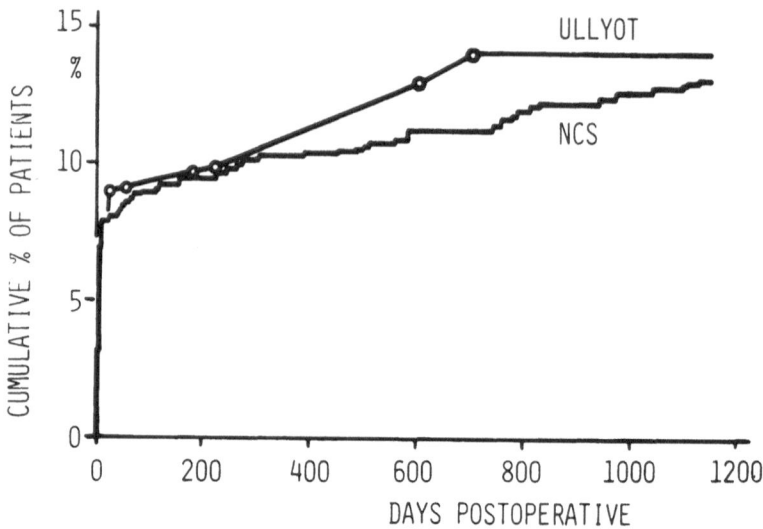

Fig. 3. Myocardial infarcts after bypass surgery over observation period. Results plotted of N.C.S. and of Ullyot c.s. [10].

Table 4. N.C.S.: summary of invasive medical data. Coronary score summation of lesions in coronary angiogram (0) is no lesions – to circa 50 for extremely severe disease. See text.

	Surgery	1 yr after surgery	3 yrs after surgery
Number of patients	848	550	398
Number of bypasses	2332	1453	1005
Patency rate (%)	–	80.1	78.0
Coronary score	14.3	6.1	7.9
Ejection fraction (%) mean ± S.D.	0.62 ± 0.13	0.61 ± 0.14	0.60 ± 0.13
EDV (m^1/m^2) mean ± S.D.	75 ± 22	79 ± 25	77 ± 25
Wall mass (g/m^2) mean ± S.D.	112 ± 39	110 ± 35	105 ± 29
Wall thickness (cm) mean ± S.D.	0.90 ± 0.23	0.90 ± 0.20	0.87 ± 0.17
Cardiac index (1/min/m^2) mean ± S.D.	3.2 ± 1.0	3.4 ± 0.9	3.2 ± 0.8
LVEDP (mm Hg) mean ± S.D.	13.2 ± 6.7	15.2 ± 7.3	16.0 ± 7.2
Regional wall motion			
All 5 RAO segm. normal (%)	37	33	32
1 or more segm. hypo/akin. (%)	55	60	60
1 or more segm. dyskin. (%)	8	7	7

the incidence of perioperative infarcts was 7.5%, while during the first post-operative year 3% of the patients had a new infarct, in the following two years another 4%. After a coronary bypass operation, therefore, the incidence of myocardial infarction can be summarized as occurring in 2–3% of the patients per year. This is approximately similar to the infarct incidence of 3.8% per year (14% over 43 months) as reported by Ullyot [10], also in surgically treated patients. In the Norwegian Multicenter Study Group [11] a somewhat higher infarct incidence was mentioned of 5% per year. However, this study concerned a group of medically treated patients all with a previous myocardial infarct.

Results for the mildly symptomatic group (see Table 5)

Mortality in the mildly symptomatic group was equal to the mortality in the total group: one year mortality was 2.5% (5 out of 199), three year mortality 4.5% (9/199). In the mildly symptomatic group 46% had a myocardial infarct before operation (91/199), while perioperative infarcts occurred in 5.5%. A

Table 5. N.C.S.: comparison of results in mildly symptomatic patients compared to rest of study group. For selection criteria of mildly symptomatic patients see text, section 'Methods'. n.s.: no significant difference (χ^2-test).

	Mild symptoms		Non-mild symptoms		
	Mean ± S.D.	n	Mean ± S.D.	n	
Age	51.5 ± 6.1	199	52.2 ± 7.1	571	
NYHA					
Class I	15 (8%)		10 (2%)		
II	184 (92%)	199	153 (27%)	571	
III	–		309 (54%)		
IV	–		99 (17%)		
Angina at rest	–		336 (59%)		
Physical activity					
None/almost none	–		365/570 (64%)		
Moderate/heavy	199/199 (100%)		204/570 (35.8%)		
Infarcts					
Preop.	108/199 (46%)		251/570 (56%)		n.s.
at 3 year postop.	8/199 (4%)		33/571 (6%)		n.s.
periop.	11/199 (5.5%)		49/571 (9%)		n.s.
Graft patency rate					
1 year	233/304 (76.6%)		782/1024 (76.4%)		n.s.
3 year	156/201 (77.6%)		559/690 (81%)		n.s.

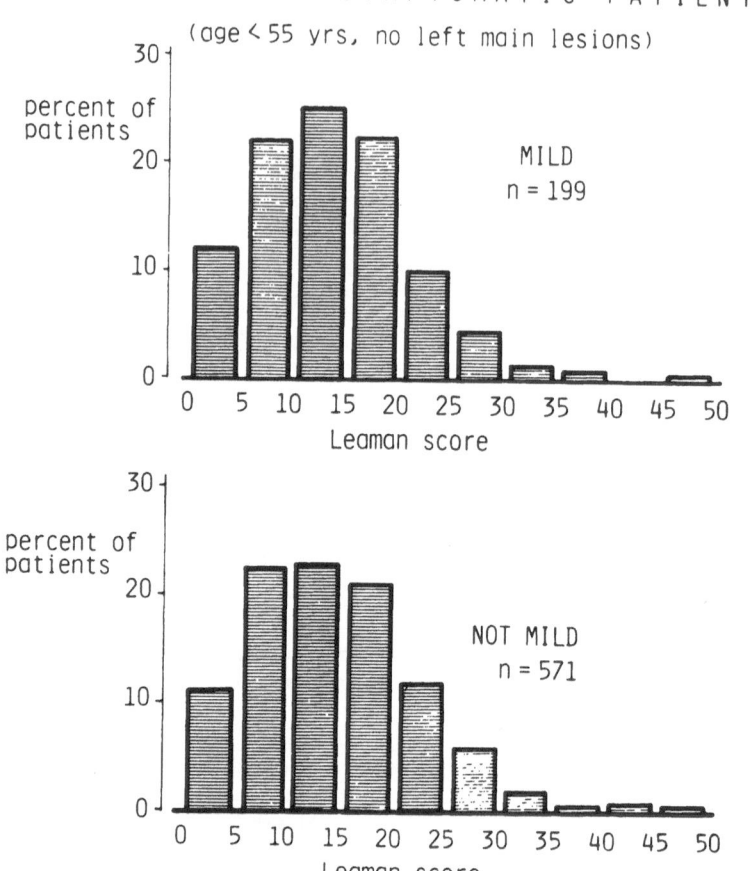

Fig. 4. Coronary score as calculated from coronary angiograms compared for mildly and non-mildly symptomatic patients.

new infarct after surgery during the three year observation period occurred in 8 patients (4%).

The infarct rate both before and after operation therefore was somewhat lower in the group of mildly symptomatic patients then in the patients with non-mild symptoms. Preoperative infarcts were present in 46% of these patients, as opposed to 56% in the non-mild group. The postoperative infarct incidence was 1.5% per year in the mild group and 2%–3% in the non-mild patients. The difference is not statistically significant. The angiographic severity of the disease was assessed from coronary angiograms both before operation as well as 1 and 3 years later. All angiograms were coded in group

562

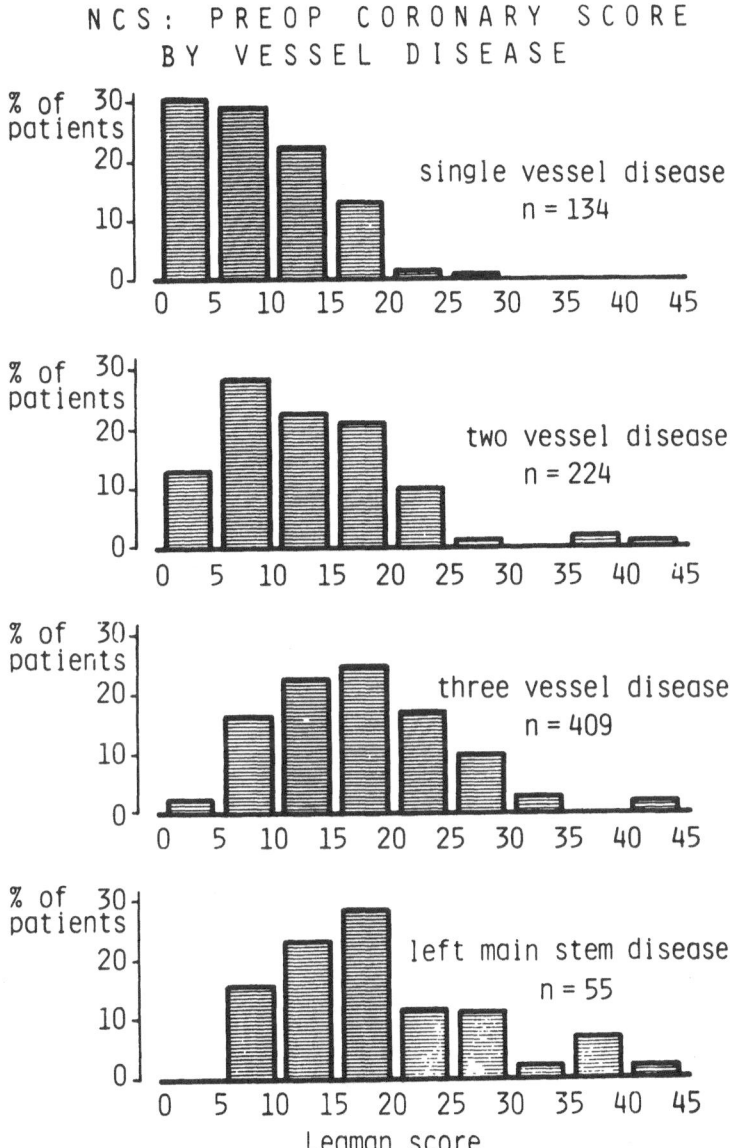

NCS: PREOP CORONARY SCORE BY VESSEL DISEASE

single vessel disease
n = 134

two vessel disease
n = 224

three vessel disease
n = 409

left main stem disease
n = 55

Leaman score

Fig. 5. N.C.S.: coronary score in groups of patients divided according to the number of diseased vessel, on the coronary angiogram. For calculation, see Leaman c.s. [12].

sessions by experienced angiographers. Results were expressed in a scoring system [12], ranging from 0 to 50 between normal and multiple obstructions in many branches. A bypassed lesion corrected the score for that lesion. In general the coronary angiographic score for mild symptomatic patients did not differ from the score of the other, non-mild patients (Fig. 4). Thus, a systematic difference in the angiographic severity of the coronary artery disease in these two groups could not be demonstrated.

The coronary score was also compared to the usual description of one, two and three vessel disease, often used to separate patient groups (Fig. 5). As expected, patients with one vessel disease tend to have a lower score than the two and three vessel disease groups. There was, however, considerable overlap. A medium severe coronary score in the range of 15 to 20 could be found in 13% of patients with one vessel disease, in 21% of patients with two vessel disease, in 25% for three vessel disease and in 29% of patients with left main disease. We consider therefore a description of the severity of coronary artery disease by counting the number of diseased vessels of no practical value. For the purpose of studies such as these, a coronary angiographic scoring system is absolutely essential for comparing patients to each other and to themselves.

This scoring system also demonstrates the progression of angiographic disease between the first and the third year follow-up studies. The mean score for the complete group of patients was seen to go up from 6.1 to 7.9 (Table 4). Extrapolating this in a linear fashion indicates that approximately 8 years after operation the coronary score is again at its preoperative level.

Left ventricular function

The results for the two follow-up studies compared to the preoperative situation are shown in Table 6. From this table can be seen that left ventricular enddiastolic pressure, ejection fraction and enddiastolic volume do not show a systematic difference between the mild and the non-mild patients. The difference in cardiac index (measured by thermodilution) is small and only significant before operation. The differences in wall thickness and mass are also small and have a direction contrary to expectations. These results must probably be attributed to chance.

There is, however, a significant trend within the mild group, enddiastolic volume declines over the observation period from 77 to 70 ml/cm². Also left ventricular wall thickness, and with it wall mass, decrease between the preoperative and the 3 year measurements. The differences, however, are small and it is doubtful whether they are of any practical significance, even more so because these values are within the normal range (EDV 70 ± 20 ml/m² and wall thickness 0.8–1.0 cm).

Table 6. N.C.S.: comparison of indicators of cardiac function in patients with mild symptoms versus non-mild patients. n.s.: not significant (χ^2-test); P: level of significance.

		Mild symptoms		Non-mild symptoms		
		Mean ± S.D.	n	Mean ± S.D.	n	
E.D.P. (mm Hg)	preop.	13.3 ± 6.3	197	13.1 ± 7.0	557	n.s.
	1 year	15.4 ± 6.9	119	15.2 ± 7.4	374	n.s.
	3 year	15.7 ± 6.6	83	16.2 ± 7.5	275	n.s.
C.I. (l/m²)	preop.	3.20 ± 0.66	189	3.00 ± 0.72	539	P<0.01
	1 year	3.10 ± 0.66	74	2.97 ± 0.75	300	n.s.
	3 year	2.82 ± 0.82	31	2.78 ± 0.82	163	n.s.
E.F.	preop.	0.62 ± 0.12	179	0.62 ± 0.13	517	n.s.
	1 year	0.62 ± 0.12	105	0.61 ± 0.15	350	n.s.
	3 year	0.63 ± 0.10	71	0.60 ± 0.14	253	n.s.
E.D.V. (ml/m²)	preop.	77 ± 20	184	74 ± 22	541	n.s.
	1 year	74 ± 23	113	78 ± 26	364	n.s.
	3 year	70 ± 22	74	77 ± 26	261	n.s.
L.V. wall thickness (cm)	preop.	0.94 ± 0.22	134	0.89 ± 0.22	347	P<0.01
	1 year	0.87 ± 0.17	101	0.91 ± 0.21	251	n.s.
	3 year	0.84 ± 0.19	52	0.87 ± 0.16	161	n.s.
L.V. wall mass (ml/m²)	preop.	118 ± 39	132	110 ± 38	343	P<0.05
	1 year	103 ± 29	100	114 ± 38	251	n.s.
	3 year	97 ± 34	52	106 ± 29	159	n.s.

Summary and conclusions

Results are presented from a cooperative study in The Netherlands on the effects of coronary bypass surgery on left ventricular function. In 199 mildly symptomatic patients, two follow-up catheterizations were carried out over a period of 3 years after their coronary bypass operation. These 'mild' patients are compared to a group of 571 patients with more severe disease. Infarcts before and after operation occurred somewhat less in the mild group, the difference was, however, not statistically significant.

Coronary angiograms did not show a systematic difference between the mild and the non-mild patients. The subjective severity of angina pectoris as expressed by the symptoms of the patient therefore was not related to the status of the coronary angiogram.

Graft patency and several postoperative cardiac function parameters such as left ventricular enddiastolic pressure, cardiac index, ejection fraction and enddiastolic volume were practically identical in both groups of patients. The mildly symptomatic group did show a significant decrease in enddiastolic volume and left ventricular wall thickness over the observation period. This is in contrast to the more severe group, where these variables remained unchanged. Initial preoperative values did not show any differences between groups.

These data show that the mildly symptomatic patient with angina pectoris will have just as severe lesions on the coronary angiogram as the more severely disabled patient. Also, these mild patients have to expect a similar surgical and late mortality and also the same incidence of myocardial infarct after operation.

In view of these similarities it is felt that the subjective severity of angina pectoris cannot be used as a basis for judging the underlying severity of disease nor for clinical decisions on the management of these patients.

References

1. Read C, Murphy ML, Hultgren HN, Takaro T: Survival of men treated for chronic stable angina pectoris. J Thorac Cardiovasc Surg 1978; 75: 1–16.
2. Hultgren HN, Detre KM, Takaro T, Murpshy ML, Thomsen JH: The VA cooperative study of coronary arterial surgery: baseline characteristics of study population and survival in subgroups with medical versus surgical treatment. In: Yu PN, Goodwin JF (eds) Progress in cardiology. Lea & Febiger, Philadelphia, 1977; 67–79.
3. Detre K, Murphy ML, Hultgren H: Effect of coronary bypass surgery on longevity in high and low risk patients. Lancet 1977; 2: 1243–1245.
4. Alderman EL, Fisher L, Maynard C et al.: Determinants of coronary surgery in a consecutive patient series from geographically dispersed medical centers. Circulation 1982; 66 (Suppl 1): 6–15.
5. Mock MB, Ringqvist I, Fisher LD et al.: Survival of medically treated patient in the coronary artery surgery study (CASS) registry. Circulation 1982; 66: 562–568.
6. Varnauskas E: Prospective randomised study of coronary artery bypass surgery in stable angina pectoris. Lancet 1980; 1: 491–495.
7. Varnauskas E, Olsson SB: The European multicenter CABG trial. In: Yu PN, Goodwin JF (eds) Progress in cardiology. Lea & Febiger, Philadelphia, 1977; 83–89.
8. Brower RW, Katen HJ ten, Meester GT: Interim data processing in The Netherlands. Study on coronary artery bypass graft surgery. Comput Biomed Res 1980; 13: 87–101.
9. Meester GT, Bernard N, Zeelenberg C, Brower RW, Hugenholtz PG: A computer system for real time analysis of cardiac catheterization data. Cath Cardiovasc Diagn 1975; 1: 113–132.
10. Ullyot DJ, Wisneski J, Sullivan RW, Gertz EW, Ryan C: The impact of coronary artery bypass on late myocardial infarction. J Thorac Cardiovasc Surg 1977; 73: 165–175.
11. Norwegian Multicenter Study Group: Timolol-induced reduction in mortality and reinfarction in patients surviving acute myocardial infarction. N Eng J Med 1981; 304: 801–807.
12. Leaman DM, Brower RW, Meester GT: Coronary artery bypass surgery. A stimulus to modify existing risk factors? Chest 1982; 81: 16–19.

11.6 Laser Treatment of Coronary Artery Disease

GARRETT LEE, MING C. CHAN, MARSHALL H. LEE,
RICHARD M. IKEDA, JOHN L. RINK, WILLIAM J. BOMMER,
ROBERT L. REIS, ELIAS S. HANNA, and DEAN T. MASON

Extension of the principle of microwave amplification by stimulated emission of radiation (maser) [1] afforded the development of laser (light amplification by stimulated emission of radiation) from devices that emit energized light within the visible spectrum [2]. Initial medical application of such photoradiation included retinal coagulation [3], tumor ablation [4], dermal surgery [5], and gastric hemostasis [6]. These advances have led to progress in the dissolution of obstructive atherosclerotic vascular disease with laser radiation [7]. In experiments carried out in our laboratories in the late 1970s performing balloon angioplasty in human cadaver coronary arteries [8], we found that balloon catheters could not traverse many subtotal coronary stenoses. Our initial concept of using lasers was to create a large enough channel through the obstructive lesion to allow the passage of a balloon catheter for coronary angioplasty. The application of laser as it has evolved during the past few years into the clinical treatment of coronary artery disease is described in the present report.

Laser physics

The typical laser is composed of a column of active material (lasing medium) bounded at both ends by parallel mirrors forming a resonator [9]. At one end, the mirror is fully reflecting. At the other end, the mirror is partially transparent, reflecting most of the confined energy while permitting laser emission that is then modified for its target application. The atoms in the active material can be primed to an excited state electrically, chemically, or by means of high-intensity light pulses. A photon (a quantum of electromagnetic radiation) is spontaneously emitted when an atom in an excited state reverts to a lower energy state [9]. When a photon interacts with another atom in an excited state, the resulting emission is stimulated, producing two photons of equal wavelength that are coordinated in time and space [9]. Thus, the presence of other identical atoms stimulated in this way results in a cascading production of photons of equal wavelength, coordinated in time and space, as reflected photons travel back and forth within the lasing medium. The laser generates photons analogous to the way in which a light bulb emits light energy. However, the laser generates photons with a narrow band of wavelengths specific to the lasing medium (monochromatic) that are coordinated in phase with one another in time and space (coherent), and that travel parallel to one another (collimated) in one direction [9]. On the other hand, ordinary light consists of photons with a wide spectrum of wavelengths that are not synchronized in time and space, and that travel in random directions. These physical properties of laser emission make it possible to produce and focus light into a precise beam of prodigious energy capable of destroying atherosclerotic plaque.

Instrumentation

The most frequently used laser instruments in medicine possess power outputs from milliwatts to about 100 watts. Certain of these lasers are small solid-state devices [9]. Ruby lasers emit a red light with a wavelength of 0.694 μm, while neodymium-doped ytrrium aluminum garnet (Nd-YAG) lasers produce a near-infrared beam with a wavelength of 1.06 μm. The Nd-YAG laser can be operated either in the continuous wave mode (steady beam), or in the pulsed mode, delivering a set of equally spaced pulses by a passively mode-locked laser. There are also gas lasers with lasing media such as argon and carbon dioxide, which are usually operated in the continuous wave mode [9]. The argon beam lies within the blue-green portion of the visible light spectrum (peak wavelengths of 0.488 and 0.514 μm), while carbon dioxide emits a mid-infrared beam (10.6 μm). Since the infrared beams are invisible, it is necessary to provide a second visible aiming laser beam of low power in order to achieve precise placement during surgical manipulations.

Optical fibers

The development of flexible optical fibers has made it possible to propagate light internally into body cavities, and coincidentally to transmit images formed by optical fiber bundles within internal organs back to the viewer without open surgical exposure [9]. A laser light beam is confined internally to the optical fiber due to refractive properties of the fiber, and incident energy can be conducted to its target with very little energy loss.

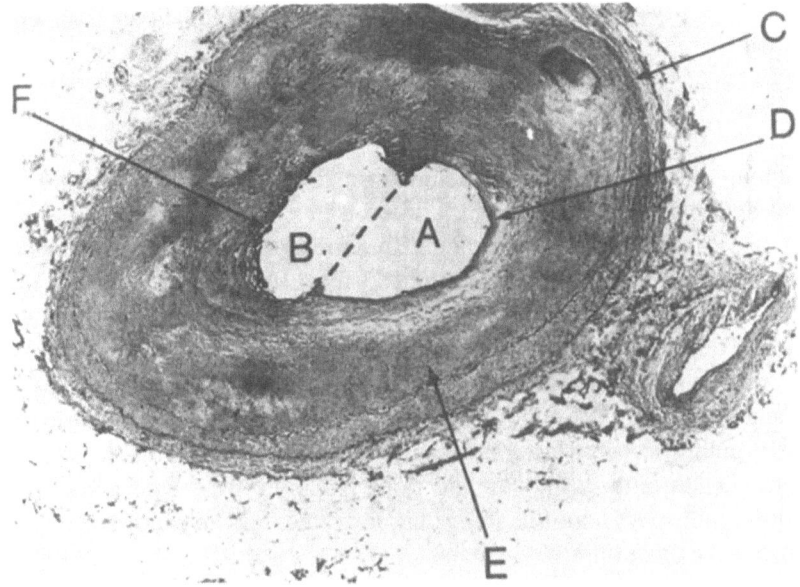

Fig. 1. Cross-section of obstructed human epicardial coronary artery. Following laser vaporization of hyalinized fibrous obstructing plaque (B), there was relief of stenotic lumen (A) with consequent twofold widening of vessel patency. C = coronary artery smooth muscle wall; D = endothelial stenotic lining; E = circumferential atherosclerotic hyaline plaque; F = remnants of fibrous collagen charred by laser radiation. (Original magnification × 63). (From [7].)

Experimental studies

Acute effects on atherosclerotic disease

Several studies have documented the immediate effects of laser radiation on human cadaver atherosclerotic coronary disease [7, 10]. The atherosclerotic plaque is primarily composed of mixtures of lipoid, hyalinized and calcified materials in order of their increasing densities. When diseased vessels are exposed to laser radiation, a vaporized area or crater is produced. Around the vaporized area is a charred lining. When the laser beam is transmitted through an optical fiber, it can be directed coaxially as close as possible along the central axis of the blood vessel, dissolving plaque adjacent to the stenotic lumen and thereby extending the diameter of the existing channel (Fig. 1). Rapid vaporization can be achieved with plaque containing materials of lower densities such as lipid-laden deposits [7, 10]. Laser penetration is retarded by high density deposits such as heavily calcified plaque. Moreover, greater extent of charred remnants may be found in the laser-induced channel of calcified plaque than in hyalinized plaque obstruction. In lipid-laden plaque occluded coronary artery, no charred debris is found in its laser-treated passageway.

Chronic effects on atherosclerotic disease

The long-term effects of laser radiation on atherosclerotic disease were demonstrated by inducing aortic atherosclerosis in swine fed a hyperlipidemic diet [11]. The aorta was surgically opened and the diseased intima was exposed to CO_2 laser beam with a spot diameter of 0.9 mm utilizing energies of less than 10 joules. The vaporized craters measured approximately 2 mm in diameter and 1 mm in depth. Two days following laser treatment, the crater was covered with platelet-fibrin thrombi. By two weeks the crater was still depressed but the surface had rapidly endothelialized with some fibrin and platelets remaining. By eight weeks the lased site was still visible as a re-endothelialized crater. Moreover, thrombogenic complications did not occur under these experimental conditions. Thus this study demonstrated that the vaporized crater had a chronic lasting effect.

Effects on thrombotic obstruction

Since vascular thrombosis often accompanies atherosclerotic disease, the effect of laser radiation on human thrombus has been studied [12]. Blood was obtained from normal human volunteers and allowed to clot. The clotted samples were cut to fixed lengths of 3 to 11 mm. The argon laser energy required to penetrate greater depths of thrombus increased in a linear dose fashion. The longer the red blood clot, the higher was the energy necessary to canalize the clot. The spectrophotometric scan of freshly formed thrombus demonstrated a typical absorption curve for hemoglobin pigments (with major absorbent peaks between wavelengths 400–600 nm) [12]. Argon energies have wavelengths between 488–514 nm and are easily absorbed by red blood clots.

Complications

The exciting potential of lasers to vaporize atherosclerotic disease is countered by certain dangers of this procedure. Vascular perforation is one of the major risks and use of high laser energies for long durations to vaporize plaque tends to increase this hazard. Thus far, a laser beam wavelength that is absorbed by plaque but spares the normal vascular wall has not been found. In in-vivo dog experiments to determine the feasibility of laser catheter intervention into the coronary artery, a coronary guiding catheter was inserted into the right internal carotid artery and the distal tip of the catheter was positioned at the left coronary orifice under fluoroscopic guidance [13]. A flexible 200 to 400 μm central core quartz fiber was advanced through the coronary catheter and into the proximal left coronary artery without untoward effects. Laser energies approximating those used to vaporize plaque were transmitted into the coronary lumen from an argon laser source. The resulting laser burns perforated the coronary artery thereby causing cardiac tamponade.

Another complication of laser phototherapy has been observed in rabbits fed an atherogenic diet and allowed to develop atherosclerotic lesions. Low level laser energies from an argon laser were applied via flexible $400 \mu m$ diameter core quartz fiber to vaporize the plaque lesions [14]. In animals examined immediately after laser treatment, a vaporized crater was produced within the atherosclerotic plaque at the endothelial surface; in others the medial layer was also injured. Importantly, in half of the animals that were followed and had their aortas studied one to 14 days following the procedure, aortic aneurysms with muscular wall damage had resulted. These problems may be avoidable by applying catheter laser angioplasty while visualizing specific plaque target sites and/or using safe dose increments of laser energies.

The vaporization of human plaque by laser produces gas; analysis of the gaseous products of laser irradiated plaque reveals water vapor, carbon dioxide, nitrogen, hydrogen and light hydrocarbon fragments consistent with a process of incomplete combustion [15]. Laser vaporization also produces minute particles that can effluoresce from the focal point of the concentrated beam. Phototherapy of calcified obstructions may also result in dislodged debris in the vascular channel [7, 10]. Further, the transmission of argon energies into blood exposes human red cells to intense heat. Consequently, there was lysis of erythrocytes as reflected by a fall in hematocrit and a rise in plasma hemoglobin [16].

Fiberoptic laser catheter

Vaporizing an atherosclerotic lesion in a blood vessel necessitates the precise placement of the laser fiber. Our fiberoptic laser catheter was first conceived in 1977 incorporating features of the balloon angioplasty catheter and fiberoptic laser systems being applied in medicine at that time [17, 18]. Experimental studies using prototype catheters have shown the feasibility of simultaneously visualizing and vaporizing atherosclerotic plaques implanted in living animals [19, 20]. By viewing the obstructed area, the laser light can be directed to the diseased target for controlled thermal therapy (Fig. 2). Complications such as vascular perforation and aneurysm formation may be avoided. Further, plaque and thrombus obstructions may be differentiated. The latter distinction may be noteworthy, since differing energy densities may be necessary for laser penetration.

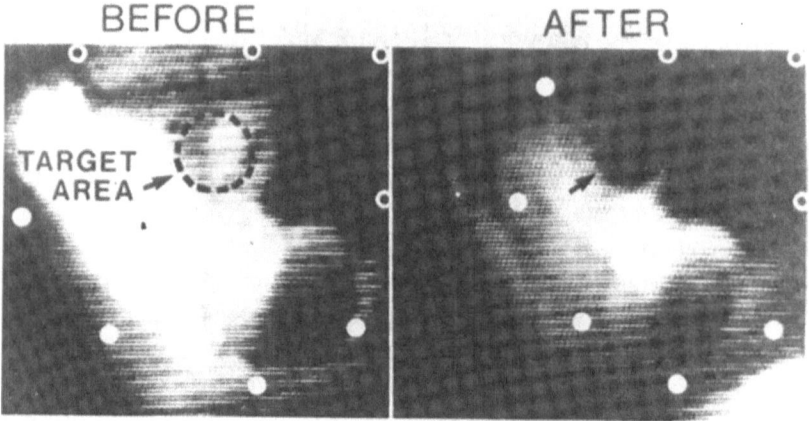

BEFORE　　　　AFTER

Fig. 2. Left panel: image obtained by fiberoptic visualization of an atherosclerotic diseased human cadaver iliac artery in which the lumen shows subtotal obstruction by fatty fibrous plaque material. The region adjacent to the vascular lumen (black dashed circle) has been targeted for laser irradiation (circumferential dots depict the vascular lumen; open dots indicate vascular lumen beyond the illustration). *Right panel:* following laser phototherapy, the target area is vaporized (arrow), thus expanding the patency of the vascular lumen (circumferential dots show the vascular lumen), (From [20].)

A laser catheter designed for use in peripheral vessels was tested in living dogs [21]. The catheter prototype (outer diameter 3 mm, length 100 cm) is coupled to a viewing handpiece which is connected to a television monitor. Thus the fiberoptic bundle can transmit and record a picture of the blood vessel's interior lumen in real time (Fig. 3). The device has three hollow passageways extending from the handpiece to the catheter tip. These include channels for viewing the obstruction, housing the laser fiber and suctioning/ flushing capabilities (removal of gas, blood, particulate debris, and injection of contrast dye or perfluorocarbon blood substitutes). A balloon around the distal catheter tip can also be inflated to momentarily halt the flow of blood. Similar but smaller laser catheter systems need to be developed and tested in the coronary arteries.

Laser-heated metal cautery cap

A laser-heated metal cautery cap mounted at the distal fiberoptic tip was developed in our laboratories and studies have been conducted in human cadaver atherosclerotic vessels [22] and in living animal vessels. The device avoids the inherent problems of direct free laser beam inadvertently straying from the target area causing vascular perforations and aneurysms. It also

572

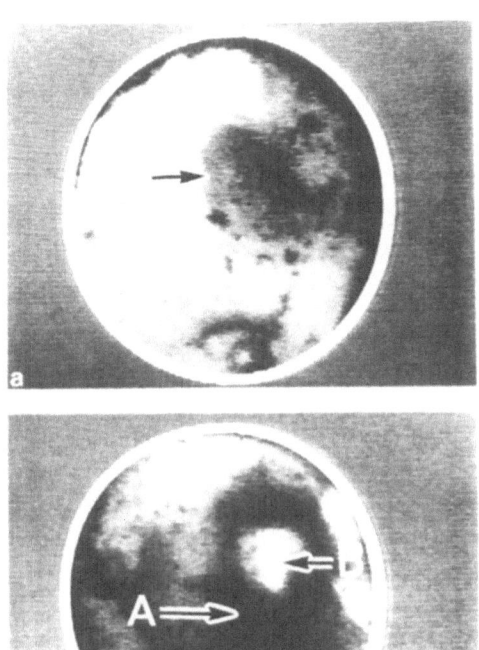

Fig. 3. Panel A: this picture obtained via the viewing channel of the fiber-optic laser catheter demonstrates an implanted atherosclerotic plaque obstruction (arrow). The implanted plaque is surrounded by the normal and smooth vascular wall lining. *Panel B:* this picture taken via the viewing channel shows the implanted atherosclerotic obstruction (arrow A) and the vaporized hole (arrow B) within the blockage following argon-ion laser irradiation. (From [21].)

minimizes hazards to patients and possible operator retinal damage. Studies on human cadaver atherosclerotic vessels showed that the metal cautery cap was capable of instantaneously dissolving these lesions upon physical contact (Fig. 4). The depth of penetration varied with contact duration and the physical characteristics of the obstructive material. Despite these advantages, certain limitations of the cautery cap have been recognized. Vascular wall dessication can occur around the heated metallic side wall, and particulate matter can cling onto the metal cautery cap following prolonged tissue exposure. Thus, while technical improvements are needed prior to clinical application, the laser-heated metal cautery cap delivery system possesses important advantages over bare-tipped fibers in terms of efficacy and safety during recanalization of atherosclerotic vascular obstructive disease.

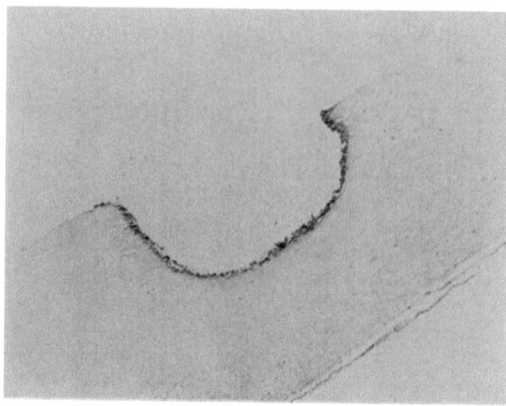

Fig. 4. Hyalinized atherosclerotic plaque showing punched out debris-free crater where collagen has been totally vaporized by the fiberoptic laser-heated metal cautery cap. Rim of crater demonstrates coagulated charred material. (Original magnification × 40). (From [22].)

Acknowledgments

We thank the San Francisco Laser Center for its support and Ms Leslie Silvernail for technical assistance.

References

1. Schawlow AL, Townes CH; Infrared and optical masers. Phys Rev 1958; 112: 1940–1949.
2. Maiman TH: Stimulated optical radiation in ruby. Nature 1960; 187: 493–494.
3. Kapany NS, Peppers NA, Zweng HC, Flocks M: Retinal photocoagulation by laser. Nature 1963; 199: 146–149.
4. Bellina JH: Carbon dioxide laser in gynecology. Obstet Gyn Ann 1977; 6: 371–391.
5. Apfelberg DB, Maser MR, Lash H, Rivers J: The argon laser for cutaneous lesions. JAMA 1975; 231: 486–489.
6. Dwyer RM, Yellin AE, Craig J: Gastric hemostasis by laser phototherapy in man. JAMA 1976; 236: 1383–1384.
7. Lee G, Ikeda RM, Kozina J, Mason DT: Laser dissolution of coronary atherosclerotic obstruction. Am Heart J 1981; 102: 1074–1075.
8. Lee G, Ikeda RM, Joye JA, Mason DT: Evaluation of transluminal angioplasty of chronic artery stenosis. Value and limitations assessed in fresh human cadaver hearts. Circulation 1980; 61: 77–83.
9. Lee G, Ikeda RM, Chan MC, Mason DT: Current and potential uses of lasers in the treatment of atherosclerotic disease. Chest 1984; 85: 429–434.
10. Lee G, Ikeda R, Herman I, Mason DT: The qualitative effects of laser irradiation on human arteriosclerotic disease. Am Heart J 1983; 105: 885–889.
11. Gerrity RG, Loop FD, Golding LAR: Arterial response to laser operation for removal of atherosclerotic plaques. J Thorac Cardiovasc Surg 1983; 85: 409–421.

574

12. Lee G, Ikeda RM, Stobbe D, Mason DT: Effect of laser radiation on human thrombus: Demonstration of a linear dissolution dose relationship between clot length and energy density. Am J Cardiol 1983; 52: 876–877.

13. Lee G, Seckinger D, Chan MC, Mason DT: Potential complications of coronary laser angioplasty. Am Heart J 1984; 107: 394–395.

14. Lee G, Ikeda RM, Theis JH, Mason DT: Acute and chronic complications of laser angioplasty: Vascular wall damage and formation of aneurysms in the atherosclerotic rabbit. Am J Cardiol 1984; 53: 290–293.

15. Clarke RH, Donaldson RF, Isner JM: Identification of photoproducts liberated by in vitro laser irradiation of atherosclerotic plaque, calcified valves, and myocardium. Lasers Surg Med 1984; 3: 358.

16. Theis JH, Lee G, Ikeda RM, Mason DT: Effects of laser irradiation on human erythrocytes; Considerations concerning clinical laser angioplasty. Clin Cardiol 1983; 6: 396–398.

17. Dwyer R, Haverback BJ, Bass M: Laser induced hemostasis in the canine stomach: Use of fiberoptic delivery system. JAMA 1975; 231: 486–489.

18. Gruntzig AR, Myler RK, Hanna ES: Coronary transluminal angioplasty. Circulation 1977; 56: 84.

19. Lee G, Ikeda RM, Dwyer RM, Mason DT: Feasibility of intravascular laser irradiation for in vivo visualization and therapy of cardiocirculatory diseases. Am Heart J 1982; 103: 1076–1077.

20. Lee G, Ikeda RM, Stobbe D, Mason DT: Laser irradiation of human atherosclerotic obstructive disease: Simultaneous visualization and vaporization achieved by a dual fiberoptic catheter. Am Heart J 1983; 105: 163–164.

21. Lee G, Ikeda RM, Stobbe D, Mason DT: Intraoperative use of dual fiberoptic catheter for simultaneous in vivo visualization and laser vaporization of peripheral atherosclerotic obstructive disease. Cathet Cardiovasc Diagn 1984; 10: 11–16.

22. Lee G, Ikeda RM, Chan MC, Mason DT: Dissolution of human atherosclerotic disease by fiberoptic laserheated metal cautery cap. Am Heart J 1984; 107: 777–778.

11.7 Conclusions

J. CALDERON MONTERO

Dr Oriol summarizes in an up to date fashion the indications, contraindications and complications of angioplasty, a technique that after ten years of experience has become indispensable in modern cardiology.

Dr Delcán describes the present status of transluminal angioplasty in Spain. He summarized the experience of diverse groups, which although not very large in comparison with that of other countries, is still enough to draw our own conclusions.

Dr Campeau described the long-term results of coronary surgery. The choice of medical or surgical treatment has been extremely debated. Only long-term follow-up of patients treated with one or another method in similar randomly selected groups can resolve this controversy. On the other part, if it is now evident that surgery improves the quality of life of the anginal patient, who may become symptom-free after the operation, it is less likely that it significantly prolongs life expectancy. Nonetheless, for major left main coronary artery disease, this now seems to be perfectly demonstrated. As for disease in other locations, opinions vary although they tend to confirm that surgery produces a longer survival in certain patient groups. In subjects under 65 with group I or II angina and more than 76% stenosis, there is no difference between medical and surgical treatment. It would therefore be advisable to opt for medical treatment, except in patients with important three-vessel disease and low ejection fraction, in whom surgical treatment prolongs survival. In patients with group III or IV angina and three-vessel disease, long-term results are clearly better with surgical treatment, especially if the ejection fraction is less than 50%. In main left trunk disease of 70% or more, surgical survival is superior to that obtained with medical treatment. Nonetheless, the conduct to follow can be determined by the type of dominance and impairment of left ventricular function.

Dr Meester described his experience with revascularization surgery in a group of highly selected patients, those with mild angina but with often severe disease. Results cannot be assessed by the patient's symptomatic improvement since there were previously few symptoms, but by evolution and survival. From the data provided, it can be deduced that the evolution of patients of this type is better with surgery.

Finally, Dr Mason described the role of laser in the treatment of coronary lesions. This treatment is still in an experimental phase, but initial results show promise. Research in this field should continue before the technique is applied to human clinical practice.

12. Myocardial Infarction (I)

12.1 Introduction

A. PAJARON LOPEZ

The creation of Coronary Units, or Cardiologic Intensive Care Units (a more modern term that better defines their function) in the early 60s served to fundamentally reduce the mortality rate of myocardial infarction by recuperating patients with primary ventricular fibrillation. The units were effective and, as a consequence of the large number of patients with coronary problems, they were soon popular throughout the civilized world. Later, mainly as a result of the creation of these Cardiologic Intensive Care Units, the complications of myocardial necrosis in the acute phase of infarction were studied more intensively and causes of mortality were found to be cardiogenic shock and ventricular wall rupture. These two causes are so fundamental that the mortality rate cannot be further reduced without treating them.

Years later, once the complications of myocardial infarction were known and had been successfully treated, the efforts of researchers working in Coronary Units were divided into attempts to save as much cardiac muscle as possible by drug treatment (β-blockers, nitrites, calcium antagonists, etc.) or to act on the recent thrombus with parenteral or intracoronary fibrinolytics. The following chapters will deal with these problems.

12.2 Recanalization of Coronary Arteries by Thrombolytic Agents in Acute Myocardial Infarction

K. PETER RENTROP, MARC COHEN and SUSAN T. HOSAT

Fletcher et al. were the first to demonstrate the feasibility of intravenous thrombolytic therapy in acute myocardial infarctions [1]. Subsequently, at least twenty controlled trials were performed to assess the efficacy of intravenous thrombolysis in acute myocardial infarction using mortality as the primary end point [2–20]. Of the seven trials which showed statistically significant improvement of survival with intravenous thrombolytic therapy, six excluded patients with more than 12 hours of chest pain [2, 4, 5, 7, 8, 10]. The Third European trial demonstrated improved survival in patients with increased risk of mortality, as assessed prospectively on the basis of simple clinical criteria prior to randomization [10].

Whereas Fletcher et al. employed streptokinase in order to reestablish antegrade flow, subsequent investigators felt that clot lysis in the main vessel would occur too late to result in myocardial salvage [21, 22]. It was hypothesized that systemic effects could explain the benefits of thrombolytic therapy. The breakdown of fibrinogen results in a reduction of blood viscosity, causing a decrease in afterload [23]. In addition, it was suggested that blood flow to the infarct area via collaterals might be improved due to a reduction in viscosity as well as dissolution of microthrombi in collateral vessels [21, 22].

The evolution of coronary angiography into a safe technique, encouraged us to study the coronary artery morphology in patients during the first hours of myocardial infarction [24]. In addition, the coronary catheter provided a tool which enabled selective delivery of streptokinase directly to the site of obstruction. This resulted in a much higher concentration of the drug at the clot than could be achieved by intravenous infusion of a comparable dose [25, 26]. Finally, during the infusion, the coronary catheter allowed periodic assessment of the effects of thrombolytic therapy [25, 26].

Thus intracoronary Streptokinase infusion represents a new therapeutic concept; simultaneously, it can serve as an important research tool. However, several disadvantages are apparent. The necessity for acute angiography restricts application of this procedure to institutions where angiographic facilities and trained personnel are available. In addition to the bleeding risk associated with thrombolysis and subsequent anticoagulation, the danger of angiography in the setting of acute infarction must be considered. Therefore any trials, which examine the risk/benefit ratio of intracoronary thrombolytic infusion should ideally have two control groups: a conventionally treated group in which acute angiography is performed and a second group in which acute angiography is performed but thrombolytic therapy is not administered. Such a randomized trial has been performed at Mount Sinai Hospital, Elmhurst Hospital, and New York University-Bellevue Hospital in New York City. One hundred and twenty-four patients were randomly allocated to one of four study groups: one received an infusion of intracoronary streptokinase (2,000 units per minute); another received an infusion of both intracoronary streptokinase and intracoronary nitroglycerin (0.01 mg/min); the third received an infusion of intracoronary nitroglycerin alone; the fourth group was treated medically, and not subjected to acute angiography [27].

Complete coronary obstruction was acutely recanalized in 12/19 patients treated with streptokinase only, and in 19/23 patients treated with streptokinase and nitroglycerin (p = n.s.). These recanalization rates are within the range of 60–90% reported in the literature [28, 29]. The acute recanalization rate of 6% (1/18 patients) in the group treated with nitroglycerin only was significantly lower than that of the two streptokinase groups. In the nitroglycerin group, repeat angiography on day 10–14, revealed patency of 77% (10/13) of initially completely obstructed vessels, none of which had acutely recanalized. There were no differences among treatment groups, indicating gradual, endogenous thrombolysis in patients not treated with streptokinase.

Time from onset of infarction to peak CK was significantly shorter in patients in whom complete coronary obstruction was acutely recanalized (15.9 ± 7.1 hrs) than in patients in whom complete obstruction was not acutely recanalized (21.5 ± 6.1 hrs; $p < 0.05$). However, early peaking of the CK curve is not a specific marker of reperfusion since the time required to reach peak CK was not significantly different in patients with incomplete coronary obstruction at baseline angiography (14.6 ± 5.0 hrs) than in patients in whom complete obstruction was acutely recanalized.

Mortality data in various small randomized trials have been conflicting [27, 30]. Pooling the data from eight randomized trials, Furberg calculated a mortality of 11% in patients treated with intracoronary streptokinase (n = 42/382), and 12.4% in the control group (n = 45/364) [31]. In view of this small difference, it would take a very large sample size to prove a treatment effect.

A considerably smaller sample would be necessary to demonstrate a treatment effect on ejection fraction, which is known to correlate with mortality [32]. Therefore, ejection fraction data was extracted from the Registry of the

European Society of Cardiology [33]. Paired data was available in 125 patients who had contrast left ventriculograms prior to streptokinase infusion and before hospital discharge. Improvement of ejection fraction was found to correlate with incomplete obstruction of the infarct vessel at the time of preintervention angiography, presence of angiographically demonstrable collaterals to the infarct area and recanalization of complete coronary obstruction. The largest increase of ejection fraction occurred when preintervention ejection fraction was low. In patients with complete coronary obstruction, the duration of symptoms prior to recanalization correlated with extent of functional improvement. Increase of ejection fraction became negligible at three hours after the onset of pain. However, patients with incomplete coronary obstruction or well developed collaterals, may benefit from reperfusion beyond these narrow time constraints.

Intracoronary streptokinase infusion may be associated with several patient management problems. Hemodynamically unstable patients may not tolerate dye injection; further, they may be unable to maintain a recumbent position on the catheterization table. These factors, as well as the potential need for resuscitative efforts, may interfere with the efficacy of this procedure. We have found the use of intraaortic balloon counterpulsation in patients with severely depressed left ventricular function, but not yet in frank shock, to be useful in preventing these problems.

Reocclusion after successful recanalization is associated with a high risk of fatal reinfarction [34], necessitating anticoagulation with Heparin for at least 4 days following reperfusion. There is a risk of significant bleeding due to thrombolytic therapy and subsequent anticoagulation [34], necessitating exclusion of all patients susceptible to life threatening bleeding complications.

Recent investigations have assessed acute recanalization rates associated with intravenous infusion of higher doses of streptokinase than were utilized in the aforementioned randomized trials. Our data support the contention that acute recanalization rates cannot be determined reliably on the sole basis of late patency rates and CK curves. Emplyoing acute angiography prior to and during IV streptokinase infusion, recanalization rates between 10% and 62% have been reported [29, 35, 36]. Randomized studies comparing intracoronary vs. intravenous streptokinase infusion revealed uniformly higher acute recanalization rates with intracoronary infusion, although the differences were not statistically significant in all studies [29, 35, 36]. The effects of high dose intravenous Streptokinase infusion on mortality and left ventricular function, and the complication rates of this treatment have not been adequately studied.

Summary

Intracoronary infusion of streptokinase is associated with acute recanalization rates of 60 to 90%. Mortality data in the published trials are conflicting. Improvement of ejection fraction was found to correlate with imcomplete coronary obstruction prior to angiography, presence of collaterals to the infarct area and recanalization of complete obstruction. CK showed a significantly earlier peak in patients in whom complete coronary obstruction is recanalized acutely than in those in whom recanalization is not achieved. However, early peaking of the CK curve is not a specific marker of reperfusion, since it also occurs in patients with incomplete coronary obstruction at baseline angiography. Intravenous infusion of conventional doses of streptokinase was found to be associated with improved survival in some trials in which therapy commenced within 12 hours after onset of infarction. Acute recanalization rates in patients who received high doses of intravenous streptokinase were lower than recanalization rates associated with intracoronary Streptokinase infusion. The risks and benefits of high dose intravenous streptokinase must still be assessed.

References

1. Fletcher AP, Sherry S, Alkjaersig N, et al.: The maintenance of a sustained thrombolytic state in man II. Clinical observations on patients with myocardial infarction and other thromboembolic disorders. J Invest 1959; 38: 1111.
2. Schmutzler R, Heckner F, Koertge P, et al.: Zur thrombolytischen Therapie der frischen Herzinfarktes. I. Einfuehrung, Behandlungsplaene. Allgemeine klinische Ergebnisse. Dtsch Med Wochenschr 1966; 91: 581.
3. Dioguardi N, Mannucci PM, Lotto A, et al.: Controlled trial of streptokinase and heparin in acute myocardial infarction. Lancet 1971; 2: 891.
4. Schmutzler R, Fritze E, Gebauer D, et al.: Fibrinolytic therapy in acute myocardial infarction, Throm Diath Haemorrh 1971; (Suppl) 47: 211.
5. Breddin K, Ehrly HM, Fechler L, et al.: Die Kurzzeitbrinolyse beim akuten Myocardinfarkt. Dtsch Med Wochenschr 1973; 98: 861.
6. European Collaborative Study: Controlled trial of urokinase in myocardial infarction. Lancet 1975; 2: 624.
7. Brochier M, Raynaud R, Planoil T, et al.: Le traitement par l'urokinase des infarctus du myocarde et syndromes de menace. Etude randomisée de 120 cas. Arch Mal Coeur 1975; 68: 563.
8. Haider M, Ambrosch L, Groll-Knapp E, et al.: Ergebnisse der Oestereichischen Herzinfarkstudie, in Sailer S (ed): Die Fibrinolyse-Behandlung des akuten Myokard-Infarktes. Wien, Verlag Brueder Hollinek 1976; 45.
9. Klein W, Pavek P, Brandt D, et al.: Resultate einer Doppelblindstudie beim Myokardinfarkt, in Sailer S (ed): Die Fibrinolyse-Behandlung des akuten Myokard-Infarktes. Wien, Verlag Brueder Hollinek 1976; 65.
10. European Cooperative Study Group for Streptokinase Treatment in Acute Myocardial

Infarction: Streptokinase in acute myocardial infarction. N Engl J Med 1979; 301: 797.

11. Lippschuts EJ, Ambrus JL, Ambrus CM, et al.: Controlled study on the treatment of coronary occlusion with urokinase-activated human plasmin. Am J Cardiol 1965; 16: 93.

12. Amery A, Roeber G, Vermeulen HJ, et al.: Single-blind randomized multicentre trial comparing heparin and streptokinase treatment in recent myocardial infarction. Acta Med Scand 1969; 187 (Suppl 505): 5.

13. Richter IH, Epstein S, Cliffton E: An evaluation of fibronolysis therapy in acute myocardial infarction. Angiology 1969; 20: 95.

14. Heikinheimo R, Ahrenberg P, Honkapohja H, et al.: Fibrinolytic treatment in myocardial infarction. Acta Med Scand 1971; 189: 7.

15. European Working Party: Streptokinase in recent myocardial infarction: A controlled multicentre trial. Br Med J 1971; 3: 325.

16. Gormsen J: Biochemical evaluation of standard treatment with streptokinase in acute myocardial infarction. Acta Med Scand 1972; 191: 77.

17. Bett JHN, Biggs JC, Castaldi PA, et al.: Australian multicentre trial of streptokinase in acute myocardial infarction. Lancet 1973; 1: 57.

18. Gormsen J, Tidstrom B, Feddersen C, et al.: Biochemical evaluation of low dose of urokinase in acute myocardial infarction: A double blind study. Acta Med Scand 1973; 194: 191.

19. Ness PM, Simon TL, Cole C, et al.: A pilot study of streptokinase study in acute myocardial infarction; observations on complications and relation to trial design. Am Heart J 1974; 88: 705.

20. Aber CP, Bass NM, Berry CL, et al.: Streptokinase in acute myocardial infarction: A controlled multicentre study in the United Kingdom. Br Med 1976; 12: 1100.

21. Bouvier CA, Ruegsegger P, Nydick I: Etude histologique de l'effet d'enzymes fibrinolytiques sur l'evolution d'un infarctus experimental chez le chien. Helv Med Acta 1960; 516: 656.

22. Ruegsegger P, Nydick I, Abarquez R: Effect of fibrinolytic (plasmin) therapy on the physiopathology of myocardial infarction. Amer J Cardiol 1960; 519.

23. Neuhof H, Hey D, Glasser E, et al.: Hemodynamic reactions induced by streptokinase therapy in patients with acute myocardial infarction. Eur J Int Care Med 1975; 1: 27.

24. Rentrop P, Blanke H, Karsch KR: Koronarmorphologie und linksventrikulaere Pumpfunktion im akuten Infarkstadium und ihre Aenderung im chronischen Stadium. Z Kardiol 1979; 68: 335.

25. Rentrop P, Blanke H, Karsch KR, et al.: Acute myocardial infarction: Intracoronary application of nitroglycerin and streptokinase in combination with transluminal recanalization. Clin Cardiol 1979; 2: 354.

26. Rentrop P, Blanke H, Karsch KR, et al.: Selective intracoronary thrombolysis in acute myocardial infarction and unstable angina pectoris. Circulation 1981; 63: 307.

27. Rentrop P, Feit F, Blanke H, et al.: The First Mt. Sinai – New York University randomized reperfusion trial: Effects of Intracoronary Streptokinase and Intracoronary Nitroglycerin Infusion on Coronary Angiographic Patterns and Mortality in Patients with Acute Myocardial Infarction. N Engl J Med in press.

28. Khaja F, Walton Jr J, Brymer J, et al.: Intracoronary fibrinolytic therapy in acute myocardial infarction. N Engl Med 1983; 303: 22.

29. Saltups A, Boxal J, Ho B, et al.: Intracoronary vs. intravenous streptokinase in acute myocardial infarction. Circulation 1983; 68: 111, 119.

30. Kennedy JW, Ritchie JL, Davis KB, et al.: Western Washington randomized trial of intracoronary streptokinase in acute myocardial infarction. N Engl J Med 1983; 309: 1477.

31. Furberg CD: Clinical value of intracoronary streptokinase. Am J Cardiol 1984; 53: 626.

32. Shah PK, Pichler M, Berman DS, et al.: Left ventricular ejection fraction determined by radionuclide ventriculography in early stages of first transmural infarction. Relation to short-term prognosis. Am J Cardiol 1980; 45: 542.

33. Rentrop P, Smith H, Painter L, Holt J: Changes in left ventricular ejection fraction after intracoronary thrombolytic therapy. Results of the Registry of the European Society of Cardiology. Circulation 1983; 68 (Suppl 3): 55–60.
34. Merx W, Doerr R, Rentrop P, et al: Intracoronary infusion of streptokinase in acute myocardial infarction. Postacute management and hospital course in 204 patients. Am Heart J 102: 1181, 181.
35. Rogers WJ, Baxley WA, Hood WP, et al.: Prospective randomized trial of intravenous vs. intracoronary streptokinase in myocardial infarction. J Am Coll Cardiol 1983; 2: 629.
36. Alderman EL, Jutzy KR, Berte LE, et al.: Randomized comparison of intravenous vs. intracoronary streptokinase for myocardial infarction. Am J Cardiol 1984; 54: 14–19.

12.3 Rupture of the Free Ventricular Wall during the Acute Phase of Myocardial Infarction: Diagnosis and Treatment

J. LÓPEZ-SENDÓN and I. COMA CANELLA

Introduction

Rupture of the free ventricular wall is one of the most serious complications of acute myocardial infarction, constituting the second cause of death after cardiogenic shock [1, 2]. Its incidence ranges between 15 and 70% in postmortem studies, and probably reaches 3–4% of all patients admitted to a coronary unit with the diagnosis of acute myocardial infarction. In spite of its elevated incidence, which represents 20.000 deaths per year in the United States alone [3], it is surprising to find that free ventricular wall rupture has always been considered a necessarily lethal complication of infarction, and little attention has been paid to possible diagnostic and therapeutic measures. Nonetheless, death from cardiac rupture is due to tamponade, and if early diagnosed it is, in principle, a treatable condition.

Natural course of rupture

In broad terms, rupture of the free ventricular wall can take three possible courses.

Instantaneous death

Rupture of the ventricular wall produces hemorrhage into the pericardial cavity. In most cases, acute hemorrhage is of sufficient volume to originate acute cardiac tamponade and death of the patient in a few minutes [1, 2, 4, 5], as far present knowledge of the pathophysiology of this complication has been able to determine. Postmortem studies disclose that the pericardial sac is distended by blood, which is characteristically partially coagulated and not adhered to pericardium or ventricular epicardium [2, 5] (Fig. 1).

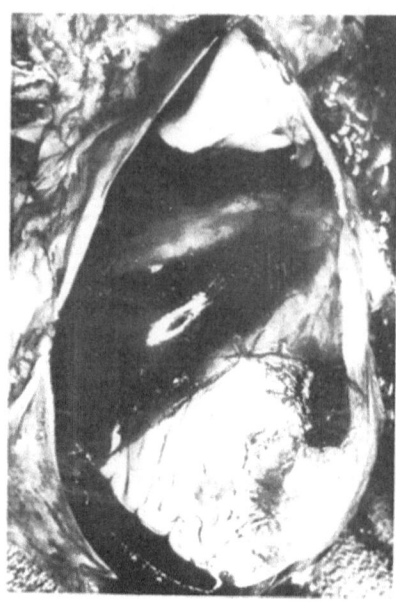

Fig. 1. Rupture of the left ventricle after acute myocardial infarction. Sudden death. The pericardial cavity is occupied by a fresh clot, not adhered to the epicardial or pericardial surfaces.

Subacute rupture

In a certain number of cases, death is not instantaneous [2, 5–25]. Patients present clinical signs of cardiac tamponade before dying and postmortem studies reveal coagulated blood in the pericardial cavity, the clot being more or less organized and adhered to the pericardium. This indicates that the myocardial tear and hemorrhage took place hours or even days before the patient's death [2, 10] (Fig. 2). The fact that a patient does not die immediately after cardiac rupture is undoubtedly due to the existence of a less severe tamponade, which can be attributed to diverse factors: pericardial adhesions or intrapericardial clots in the area of the rupture or intraventricular thrombi over the torn area can prevent massive escape of blood into the pericardial cavity [7, 9, 10]. Probably the most important and common factor that determines the subacute nature of a rupture not followed by massive acute cardiac tamponade and instantaneous death is the progressive nature of the rupture [1, 7, 8, 10]. Dislaceration of the ventricular wall is often not abrupt; the ventricular myocardium tears gradually, sometimes producing an irregular and anfractuous wound [26]. The initial orifice communicating the ventricular and pericardial cavities can be very small or virtual [1, 4, 7, 10, 20], not allowing passage of a voluminous hemorrhage capable of producing instant death.

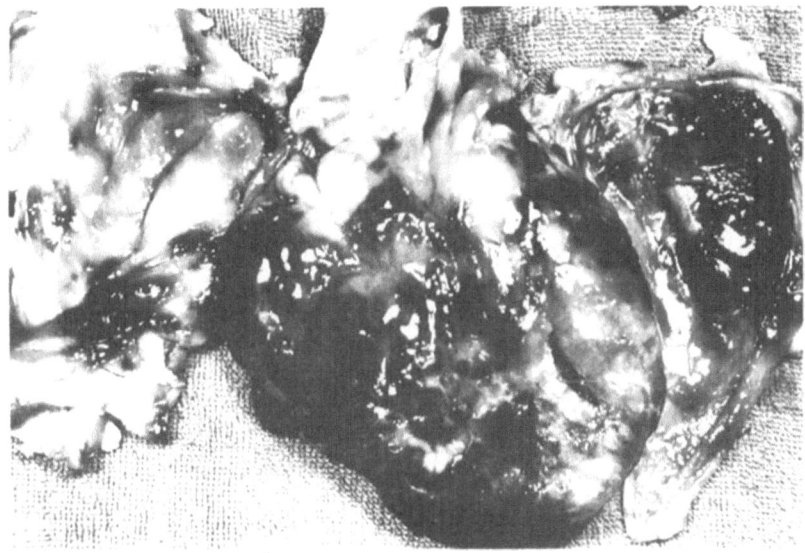

Fig. 2. Subacute rupture of the left ventricle. The intrapericardial clots are organized and adhered to the epicardial and pericardial surface, indicating that the hemorrhage took place several hours before the patient's death.

Progressive or abrupt enlargement of the tear would be the cause of death [1, 2, 9, 10]. The concept of gradual rupture is extraordinarily important because it allows time for making the correct diagnosis and attempting surgical repair [9–25].

Pseudoaneurysm

In a few cases, pericardial adhesions impede massive hemorrhage after ventricular rupture. The blood remains localized in part of the pericardial cavity, encapsulated by walls formed by pericardium and clots and communicating with the ventricular cavity through the tear [7, 27–30]. In turn, the pseudoaneurysm evolves toward rupture, although the patient may survive for months.

Diagnosis

Diagnosis of cardiac rupture is generally based on indirect clinical, hemodynamic or echocardiographic findings demonstrative of hematic pericardial effusion or cardiac tamponade. Direct demonstration of a rupture can only be done by angiography [21] and it is debatable if this diagnostic method is appropriate. Since diagnosis of free ventricular wall rupture necessarily entails surgery in a high risk patient (acute myocardial infarction), diagnostic criteria should be highly efficient and with maximum specificity, even at the cost of loss of diagnostic sensitivity. On the other part, since these surgical decisions are always urgent, cardiological teams should establish their own diagnostic criteria for surgery without delay, which often motivates conflicts between clinicians and surgeons. These conflicts are generally handled by observation of the patient's clinical evolution, but subacute cardiac rupture leads to death, almost always suddenly.

Clinical manifestations

Cardiac rupture is traditionally described as a picture of intense precordial pain followed by loss of consciousness, respiratory arrest, jugular ingurgitation, cyanosis, bradycardia with loss of pulse (electromechanical dissociation) and death in a few minutes [1, 2, 4, 10, 27]. Unfortunately, one of the most specific criteria is sudden death, in which case the diagnosis has merely academic value, at least at present. Moreover, similar pictures can correspond to propagation of infarction, pulmonary embolism, etc. On the other hand, in subacute rupture, the clinical picture is usually less marked: rarely does the patient lose consciousness; there is almost never electromechanical dissociation or arrhythmias and rupture may even have begun before hospital admission [9]. Aside from this, possible clinical signs of tamponade, such as jugular ingurgitation and hypotension, are similar to those of ischemic right ventricular function [11]. For these reasons, clinical manifestations are suggestive but rupture cannot be diagnosed on the basis of clinical data alone.

Electrocardiogram

There is no electrocardiographic alteration that is diagnostic of rupture. Electrocardiographic alterations induced by abrupt pericardial distension (e.g. sinus bradycardia followed by AV junctional rhythm, or AV block with recuperation of normal sinus rhythm in a few minutes, or even tachycardia [1, 2, 4, 6, 32, 34]) are infrequent in subacute rupture, although their presence should make us suspect this complication. The same occurs with other electrocardiographic alterations considered indicative of rupture: M-shaped QRS complexes [2, 24] or tall peaked T waves [35]. However, diagnosis cannot be based on these electrocardiographic findings.

Hemodynamic alterations

The study of simple hemodynamic parameters by right heart catheterization with a Swan-Ganz catheter provides a precise diagnosis of cardiac tamponade

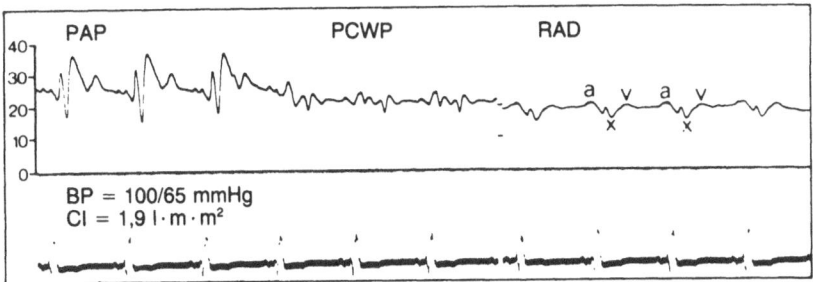

Fig. 3. Hemodynamic pattern of cardiac tamponade secondary to rupture of the free left ventricular wall. Right atrial pressure (RAP) attains levels similar to pulmonary capillary pressure (PCP). Characteristically, the 'y' sinus is erased in the RAP curve. PAP: pulmonary artery pressure.

and differential diagnosis with other entities that can produce similar clinical situations, such as ischemic right ventricular dysfunction or pulmonary embolism.

The most important hemodynamic alterations in cardiac tamponade are the following [8, 36, 37] (Fig. 3):

1. More than 10 mm Hg of right atrial pressure, reaching levels similar to those of pulmonary capillary pressure.
2. Morphology of the right atrial pressure curve. The contour of the right atrial pressure curve shows a very characteristic pattern. In cardiac tamponade, the 'x' sinus is sharp and deep and the 'y' sinus is practically erased. This typical right atrial pressure curve is of extraordinary importance in the differential diagnosis of cardiac tamponade and right ventricular infarction [38]. In the latter situation, right atrial and pulmonary capillary pressures may equalize, but the 'y' sinus is never erased, being normal or deeper than the 'x' sinus [33]. It is interesting that when a patient with right ventricular infarction and right ventricular ischemic dysfunction suffers cardiac rupture and tamponade, the predominant pattern is that of tamponade [9]. Alterations in the atrial pressure curve constitute the most important element in the differential diagnosis of this disorder, and therefore it is extremely important to obtain good quality recordings.
3. Fall in blood pressure. Blood pressure always declines in rupture, but not always to a great extent; in hypertensive patients, blood pressure may remain at normal levels. Arterial hypertension is a risk factor for rupture [2, 27], but a patient with high blood pressure is unlikely to have cardiac rupture with hemopericardium.
4. Paradoxical pulse. In many cases paradoxical pulse is observed as a result of a decrease in systolic blood pressure of more than 10 mm Hg during inspiration [9, 36, 37]. This sign is not specific of tamponade and can be found in any situation with low minute volume.

5. Reduction in cardiac output. In most cases of cardiac tamponade, cardiac output is markedly decreased. However, this finding is of little diagnostic interest because levels are not always abnormal and reduced cardiac output is not specific of rupture or tamponade.

Hemodynamic tamponade criteria

Hemodynamic tamponade criteria, basically increased right atrial pressure, which can reach levels similar to pulmonary capillary pressure, and alterations in the right atrial pressure curve are probably the most reliable indirect data presently available. Of a total of 21 patients with acute myocardial infarction accompanied by hemodynamic criteria of tamponade, in 20 hemopericardium secondary to rupture of the free left or right ventricular wall was confirmed by autopsy or during surgery. In the remaining patient, tamponade was secondary to serous effusion. These findings show that the tamponade criteria mentioned are very specific for cardiac rupture in AMI patients. Nonetheless, diagnostic sensitivity cannot be calculated because it is probable that there are cases of rupture in which the hemorrhage into the pericardial cavity, at least initially, is not sufficiently voluminous to produce the hemodynamic alterations characteristic of cardiac tamponade.

Pericardiocentesis

Until now, pericardiocentesis has been considered important for diagnosis and treatment of cardiac rupture [11]. However, it is a dangerous technique and there may be false positives if the ventricular cavity is reached or false negatives if the exploratory puncture is incorrect or the hemopericardium is loculated by pericardial adhesions [9, 21]. It may still be useful in cases of acute rupture in which, theoretically, immediate evacuation of part of the pericardial contents may be the only measure that will save the patient's life.

Angiography

Demonstration of the escape of contrast from the ventricular into the pericardial cavity is a direct criterion for cardiac rupture. Nonetheless, as a diagnostic method angiography has two serious disadvantages: it is a risky examination in this situation and the rupture can be located in the left or right ventricular wall [23] or in the atria [39]. To make a complete study, various angiographic injections would be necessary. Finally, angiography can be negative because hemorrhage is not continuous. Were this not the case, cardiac tamponade would be massive in a few minutes. For these reasons, angiography is not useful as a routine diagnostic method.

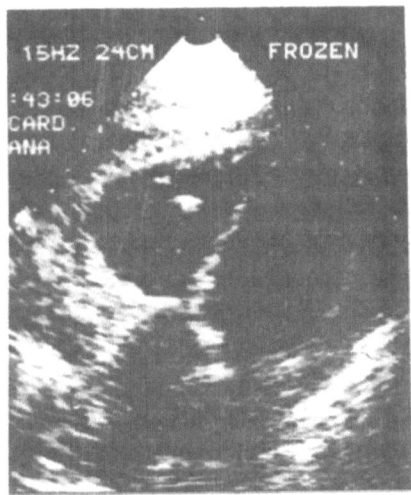 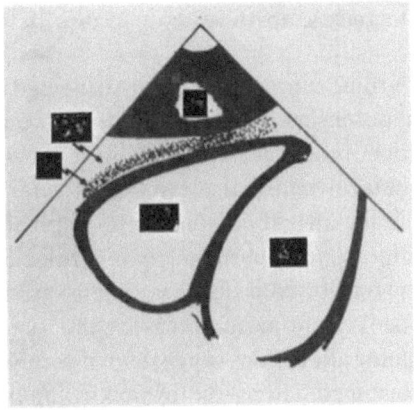

Fig. 4. Pericardial effusion in a patient with rupture of the left ventricular wall. The intraper-icardial image is suggestive of the presence of a clot (C). PC: pericardial cavity. L: liver. RV: right ventricle. LV: left ventricle (transverse subcostal plane).

Echocardiography

Demonstration of pericardial effusion in a patient with acute myocardial infarction and clinical signs of cardiac rupture is highly suggestive of this complication. Nonetheless, echocardiography also has limitations. Pericardial effusion is frequent in patients with acute myocardial infarction, especially in patients with heart failure [40]. Useful images cannot always be obtained and sometimes the coagulated blood has a density similar to that of myocardium [41], making it difficult to identify effusion with M mode echocardiography. This technique may serve to differentiate hemopericardium with clots, typical of cardiac rupture, from other types of effusion [23, 24, 42] (Fig. 4). In these cases, bidimensional echocardiography could be a very important diagnostic technique if the criteria for intrapericardial clots could be defined with a specificity approaching 100%. Our present experience, still limited, showed that in the acute phase of infarction high density acoustic images partially occupying the pericardial cavity were very specific of coagulated blood, but are not always observed because the blood may not be coagulated or may be totally coagulated, since there will either be no echoes in the pericardial cavity or the echoes will be indistinguishable from myocardium.

Diagnostic attitude

Cardiac rupture should be suspected in any patient who presents an episode of hypotension, low cardiac output, elevation of central venous pressure, syncope, bradycardia or postinfarctional angina with intense pain in the course of acute myocardial infarction. Under these circumstances, it is important to obtain an echocardiogram, if possible bidimensional, and it is still more important to perform right cardiac catheterization. Echocardiographic findings can be considered very sensitive because occasionally (twice in our experience), hemopericardium secondary to cardiac rupture exists without hemodynamic alterations suggestive of cardiac tamponade. However, there are still no very specific criteria for making an accurate diagnosis (in our series, one of 8 patients who met criteria for hemopericardium in the bidimensional echocardiographic images did not have rupture). A prospective study in a large series of patients with acute myocardial infarction is necessary to determine the specificity of echocardiographic criteria for hemopericardium. In contrast, hemodynamic criteria for cardiac tamponade, fundamentally an elevation of more than 10 mm Hg in right atrial pressure and disappearance of the 'y' sinus, are very specific. Of 22 patients with this hemodynamic pattern, 3 had rupture of the right ventricular free wall and 18 of the left ventricular free wall; in only one was no cardiac rupture found in surgery, a patient with abundant serous effusion. Nonetheless, hemodynamic criteria are relatively insensitive and bidimensional echocardiography has demonstrated that some patients with cardiac rupture do not immediately suffer tamponade. We can conclude that the hemodynamic alterations are specific enough to establish the surgical indication and that echocardiographic findings of hemopericardium are very suggestive of rupture and more sensitive than hemodynamic criteria, but cannot be used alone as the basis for indicating surgery.

Evolution

The natural evolution of subacute cardiac rupture is to death, except for the rare cases of pseudoaneurysm. Four patients were diagnosed as subacute rupture and refused surgery; all died within 3 to 72 hours. Only occasionally did a patient survive for weeks or months without surgery, thanks to formation of a pseudoaneurysm. In these patients, the risk of sudden death by rupture of the pseudoaneurysm is very high. For these reasons, once cardiac rupture is diagnosed, surgical repair must be attempted.

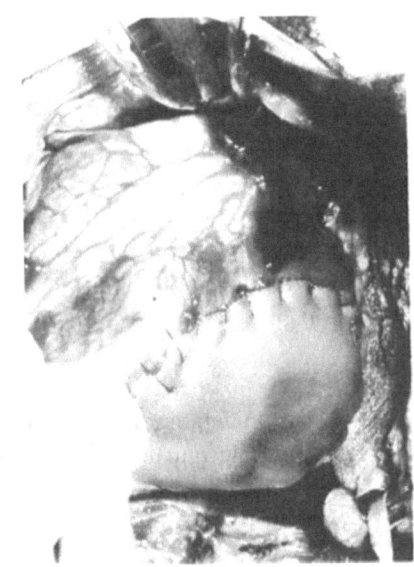

Fig. 5. Teflon patch sutured to the left ventricular wall in a patient with cardiac rupture.

Treatment

Once the diagnosis is made, the hemodynamic situation can be maintained or slightly improved by fluid administration, positive inotropic agents or removal of part of the pericardial effusion. Under no circumstances can this type of treatment be considered definitive. Surgery is the only therapeutic measure that provides an acceptable survival rate. Until now, at least 20 cases have been described in which the patient did not die during surgery [9–25, 43] and long-term survival has been attained in sporadic cases [25].

Surgical repair of the ruptured area of the free ventricular wall can be technically simple or extremely complex [3, 9, 11]. The difficulty of repair and selection of surgical technique are determined by the size of the myocardial tear and the condition of the tissue around the zone of rupture. If the tear is small and the surrounding myocardium is not brittle, it can be closed by sutures supported by teflon strips, or better, by a teflon patch over the infarcted zone (Fig. 5). The stitches should be placed as far as possible from the tear, in healthy tissue if possible. Although not indispensable, surgery should be done with extracorporeal circulation and without aortic clamping and cardioplegy because of the risk of hemorrhage if the myocardial tear is enlarged by manipulation. In general terms, small ruptures in the anterior wall of the left ventricle can be operated on without extracorporeal circulation, but those situated in the diaphragmatic wall require assisted circulation because the heart has to be moved to access the tear, and this is usually accompanied by poor hemodynamic tolerance. If the myocardium is fragile, the infarcted area may have to be resected. Theoretically at least, this would be ideal because it would avoid the possibility of new myocardial tears. The difficulty in these cases lies in the lack of a precise definition of the limits of the infarcted area, which can be very extensive and makes ample resection impossible.

Postsurgical evolution

Although surgery is the only effective treatment for rupture of the free ventricular wall, mortality is high.

Of a total of 19 patients operated on in Ciudad Sanitaria La Paz, 3 died during surgery and only 6 were still alive 6 months after surgery. The causes of death in the immediate or late postoperative period were varied; renal failure, heart failure and peripheral embolism were among the main ones. New surgical techniques must be developed that will produce a more prolonged survival.

Summary

Rupture of the free ventricular wall is one of the main causes of death during the acute phase of myocardial infarction. Although it is considered an untreatable complication, it is often not followed by sudden death, providing an opportunity for correctly diagnosing it and attempting surgical repair. The present article comments on the experience of the cardiology team of the Ciudad Sanitaria La Paz with diagnosis and treatment of subacute heart rupture, a total of 23 patients having been operated on.

The hemodynamic criteria for cardiac tamponade (more than 10 mm Hg rise in right atrial pressure, attaining levels similar to those of pulmonary capillary pressure; deep 'x' sinus and disappearance of the 'y' sinus) are very specific of rupture, since we found only one false positive. In contrast, these criteria are probably not very sensitive, because rupture was confirmed during surgery in two patients without tamponade.

Suture of a teflon patch over the myocardial tear can prolong the patient's life, although the elevated mortality in the first weeks after surgery requires more agressive surgical techniques in the future.

Acknowledgement

We would like to thank all the members of the Departments of Cardiac Surgery, Coronary Diseases, Cardiology and Experimental Surgery of the Ciudad Sanitaria La Paz, without whose help and coordinated efforts it would have been impossible to establish the diagnostic criteria and surgical indications for ventricular rupture in acute myocardial infarction.

References

1. Cordeiro A, Ravara LP, Almeida MO, Corjao Clara J: Les dilacérations myocardiques mortelles au cours de l'infarctus aigu. Arch Mal Coeur 1972; 63: 1003.
2. López-Sendón J, Calderon Montero J, Moreno Yanguela M, Sarrion Guzman M, Novo Valledor L, Eizaguirre J: La rotura de la pared libre del ventriculo izquierdo en el infarto agudo de miocardio. Su predicción y patogenia. Rev Esp Cardiolog 1978; 31: 401.
3. Rivera R: Tratamiento de las complicaciones quirúrgicas del infarto de miocardio. In: Martín Jadraque L, Coma Canella I, González I, López Sendón J (eds) Cardiopatía isquémica. Norma, Madrid, 1981; 721.
4. Dissman W, Srurren RP, Buschman HJ: Die klinische diagnose der herzrupture. Z Kreislauf 1967; 56: 1067.
5. Lewis AJ, Burchell HB, Titus JL: Clinical and pathologic features of postinfarction cardiac rupture. Am J Cardiol 1969; 23: 43.
6. Haiat R, Halphen CH, Chiche P: Les ruptures pariétales du coeur à la phase aigue de l'infarctus du myocarde; diagnostic précoce et approche thérapeutique actuelle. Arch Mal Coeur 1974; 67: 1457.
7. Van Tassel RA, Edwards JE: Rupture of the heart complicating myocardial infarction. Analysis of 40 cases including nine examples of left ventricular false aneurysm. Chest 1972; 61: 104.
8. Lautsch EV, Lanks KW: Pathogenesis of cardiac rupture. Arch Path 1967; 84: 264.
9. Coma Canella I, López Sendón J, Nunez L, Ferrufino O: Subacute left ventricular free wall rupture following acute myocardial infarction. Bedside hemodynamics, differential diagnosis and treatment. Am Heart J 1983; 106: 278.
10. López Sendón J, Coma Canella I, Nunez L: Taponamiento cardiaco por rotura de la pared libre ventricular en el infarto agudo de miocardio. Rev Portug Cardiolog 1982; 1: 229.
11. Bates RJ, Bentler S, Resnekov L, Agnastopoulos CE: Cardiac rupture. Challenge in diagnosis and management. Am J Cardiol 1977; 40: 429.
12. Calic A, Kerth W, Barbour D, Cohn K: Successful surgical therapy of ruptured myocardium. Chest 1974; 66: 188.
13. Fitzgibbon GM, Hooper GD, Heggtveit HA: Successful treatment of post infarction external cardiac rupture. J Thorac Cardiovasc Surg 1972; 63: 622.
14. Montegut FJ: Left ventricular rupture secondary to myocardial infarction. Report of survival with surgical repair. Ann Thorac Surg 1972; 14: 75.
15. Cobbs BW, Hatcher ChR, Robinson PH: Cardiac rupture: Three operations with two long-term survivals. JAMA 1973; 223: 532.
16. O'Rourke MF: Subacute heart rupture following myocardial infarction. Clinical features of a correctable condition. Lancet 1973; 2: 124.
17. Anagnostopoulos E, Beutler S, Levett JM, Lawrence JM, Lin ChY, Replogle RL: Myocar-

dial rupture. Major left ventricular infarct rupture treated by infarctectomy. JAMA 1977; 238: 271.

18. Kendall RW, Dewood HA: Postinfarction cardiac rupture – Surgical success and review of the literature. Ann Thorac Surg 1978; 25: 311.

19. Eisenmann B, Bareiss P, Pacifico AD, Jeanblanc B, Kretz JG, Baehrel B, Warter J, Kieny R: Anatomic, clinical and therapeutic features of acute cardiac rupture. Successful clinical management fourteen hours after myocardial infarction. J Thorac Cardiovasc Surg 1978; 76: 78.

20. Nunez L, De la Llana R, López Sendón J, Coma Canella I, Gil Aguado M, Larrea JL: Diagnosis and treatment of subacute free wall ventricular rupture after infarction. Ann Thorac Surg 1983; 35: 525.

21. Windsor HM, Chang VP, Shanahan MX: Postinfarction cardiac rupture. J Thorac Cardiovasc Surg 1982; 84: 755.

22. Pifarre R, Sullivan HJ, Griego J, et al.: Management of left ventricular rupture complicating myocardial infarction. J Thorac Cardiovasc Surg 1983; 86: 441.

23. Gonzalez Maqueda I, López Sendón JL, Iglesias A, Pabon Osuna C, Martin Luengo E, Martin Jadraque L: Rotura de la pared libre de ventrículo derecho postinfarto agudo de miocardio. Presentación de un caso. Rev Esp Cardiolog 1984; 37: 72.

24. López Sendón J, Calvo Orbe L, Cabrera A, Oliver J, Larrea JL, Martin Jadraque L: Utilidad de la ecocardiografía 2D en el diagnóstico de rotura cardiaca. Presentación de un caso. Rev Esp Cardiolog 1984; 37: 70.

25. Mestres CA, Murtra M, Igual A, Martinez Gutierrez F, Batalla J, Petit M: Siete años de seguimiento de una roture postinfarto de ventrículo izquierdo tratada guirúrgicamente con éxito. Rev Esp Cardiolog 1984; 37: 67.

26. Coma Canella I, Gamallo C, López Sendón J, Cuevas Santos J: Rotura cardiaca atípica sin necrosis electrocardiográfica. Rev Clin Esp 1980; 158: 235.

27. Davidson KH, Parisi AF, Harrington JJ, Barsamian EM, Fishbein MC: Pseudoaneurysm of the left ventricle: an unusual echocardiographic presentation. Review of the literature. Ann Intern Med 1977; 86: 430.

28. Roelandt J, Van den Brand, Veltter WB, Nauta J, Hugenholtz PG: Echocardiographic diagnosis of pseudoaneurysm of the left ventricle. Circulation 1975; 52: 466–472.

29. Chatherwood E, Mintz GS, Kotler M, Parry W, Segal BL: Two dimensional echocardiographic recognition of left ventricular pseudoaneurysm. Circulation 1980; 62: 294–303.

30. Ballester Rodes M, López Sendón J, McDonald L: Rotura de la pared libre de ventriculo izquierdo identificada mediante ecocardiografia bidimensional. Presentación de un caso de seudoaneurisma ventricular tras resección de un aneurisma apical. Rev Esp Cardiolog 1984; 37: 75.

31. Coma Canella I, López Sendón J, Gamallo C: Low output syndrome in right ventricular infarction. Am Heart J 1979; 98: 613.

32. Calderon Montero J, Salces Blesa A: El electrocardiograma en el taponamiento cardiaco. Estudio experimental. Rev Esp Cardiol 1955; 9: 192.

33. Meurs AAH, Vos AK, Verhey JB, Gerbrandy J: Electrocardiogram during cardiac rupture by myocardial infarction. Br Heart J 1970; 32: 232.

34. Mir MA: Prognostic value of the M complex. An electrocardiographic sign of impending cardiac rupture following myocardial infarction. Scot Med J 1972; 17: 319.

35. London RE, London SB: Rupture of the heart. A critical analysis of 47 consecutive autopsy cases. Circulation 1965; 31: 202.

36. Shabetai R, Fowler NO, Guntheroth WG: The hemodynamics of cardiac tamponade and constrictive pericarditis. Am J Cardiol 1970; 26: 480.

37. López Sendón J, Coma Canella I: Valoración de la función ventricular en la unidad coronaria.

Monitorización hemodinámica. In: Martín Jadraque L, Coma Canella I, López Sendón J, González Maqueda, I (eds) Cardiopatia isquémica. Norma, Madrid, 1981; 431.

38. López Sendón J, Coma Canella I, Gamallo C: Sensitivity and specificity in the hemodynamic diagnosis of acute right ventricular infarction. Circulation 1981; 64: 515.

39. Hellerstein HK, Van Kyke AE: Atrial myocardial infarction. A contemporary view. In: Hurst JW (ed) The heart, Update IV McGraw-Hill, New York, 1979; 43.

40. Galve E, Evangelista A, Garcia Castillo H, et al.: Derrame pericárdico en el curso del infarto agudo de miocardio. Estudio ecocardiográfico. Rev Esp Cardiolog 1983; 26 (Suppl 2): 52.

41. López Sendón J, Garcia Fernandez MA, Coma Canella I, Silvestre J, DeMiguel E, Martin Jadraque L: Identification of blood in the pericardial cavity in dogs by two dimensional echocardiography. Am J Cardiol 1984; 53: 1194.

42. Garcia Fernandez MA, Moreno M, Rossi PN, López Sendón J, Banuelos F: Echocardiographic features of hemopericardium. Am Heart J 1984; 107: 1035–1036.

43. Lofstrom B, Mogensen L, Nyquist O, Orinius E, Sjogren A, Werner B: Studies of myocardial rupture with cardiac tamponade in acute myocardial infarction III. Attempts at emergency surgical treatment. Chest 1972; 61: 10.

12.4 Myocardial Revascularization with Acute Myocardial Infarction

MARCUS A. DEWOOD, J. PAUL SHIELDS, RALPH BERG JR and ROBERT N. NOTSKE

Introduction

Careful monitoring and treatment of rhythm disturbances have resulted in reduction in the incidence of hospital mortality after myocardial infarction. Since the 1970's, the majority of mortality due to myocardial infarction occurs secondary to extensive left ventricular dysfunction [1]. Clinical, pathologic and experimental observations suggest that acute myocardial infarction frequently evolves over a period of time [2, 3]. In the clinical setting, because the extent of acute and chronic damage is correlated with short- and long-term mortality [4], two strategies for therapy have evolved over the past several years. The first has involved efforts to limit acute myocardial damage. The second has included strategies aimed at secondary measures offering protection from further coronary related events such as reinfarction or sudden death in the months to years after myocardial infarction.

Animal studies [5] have amply demonstrated that early restoration of blood flow frequently resolves many of the contractile abnormalities observed during acute coronary occlusion. Since it is now known that most patients suffering transmural myocardial infarction demonstrate complete absence of antegrade coronary flow in the vessel leading to the infarcted area [6], limitation of myocardial damage by restoration of blood flow has been extensively investigated. Since acute myocardial infarction reflects the culmination of events resulting from acute, insufficient coronary perfusion, clinical interventions have focused on the concept of restoration of adequate myocardial perfusion soon after the onset of acute myocardial infarction. This concept of 'reperfusion' has been enthusiastically embraced because of the perception that the progressive nature of myocardial damage can be favorably modified by resolution of the coronary obstruction. Various methods of reperfusion have been employed because experimental studies have generally demonstrated beneficial results with early reperfusion. The major vehicles for restoration of coronary blood flow have been surgical revascularization as well as thrombolytic therapy [7] with and without mechanical methods [8].

If the goals of therapy in acute myocardial infarction include restoration of adequate blood flow in order to limit myocardial damage as well as offer long-term protection to the patient, early surgical reperfusion may be helpful. Support for this concept has occurred largely because early bypass grafting may not only limit the extent of the acute event but may provide protection from postinfarction ischemia and thereby reduce the frequency of future coronary related events. This may be so because of the ability to bypass the acutely occluded vessel as well as offer early and definitive therapy to patients with major residual stenosis or multi-vessel disease. This article will examine results derived from clinical studies that have investigated short- and long-term effects of surgical reperfusion on mortality.

Surgical revascularization during myocardial infarction

Many pilot studies [9, 10] have indicated that surgical revascularization soon after infarction was associated with low mortality. Following these observations, Berg and coworkers [11] reported the first large experience with surgical reperfusion for acute myocardial infarction. Mortality in this series was 5.2% (5 of 96). Importantly, the major cause of mortality in the patients who died was advanced presurgical cardiogenic shock. This study was also important because it was the first series wherein reperfusion was performed as part of an organized and planned approach to acute myocardial infarction.

Following this, Phillips and coworkers [12] reported their results in 75 patients undergoing emergency myocardial revascularization. The majority of patients in this series were suffering anterior wall myocardial infarction. The electrocardiographic findings on discharge from the hospital were quite variable but indicate that 39 patients demonstrated transmural infarction while 30 patients had electrocardiographic findings consistent with nontransmural infarction and 13 patients demonstrated only nonspecific electrocardiographic abnormalities. The study of Phillips and coworkers confirmed the low mortality reported by previous investigators as there was only one hospital death in the 75 patients (1.2%). Likewise, the mortality in the follow-up period (mean follow-up 18 months) was remarkably low (2.8%) as well. Second, this study supported the findings of earlier work [13] describing the presence of intracoronary thrombus often found during surgical treatment of myocardial infarction.

Conventional and surgical treatment of acute myocardial infarction

Work from our medical centers was designed to compare results of surgical reperfusion with a conventionally managed group comprised of a similar population [13]. We followed two concurrently managed groups in a 387 patient study. From the middle of 1972 to the end of 1976, 200 patients 65-years or younger were admitted to our hospitals and treated with conventional therapy. The short- and long-term fate of the conventional therapy group was compared to 187 patients who were treated by early surgical coronary reperfusion. Patients having distal coronary disease, insignificant coronary disease, leukemia, chronic diseases or those considered 'too ill' by the attending physician were excluded from both groups retrospectively. Patients were given conventional therapy for transmural infarction because:

1. it was the practice of the physician attending the case;
2. the patient was not present in the hospital during the early phase of infarction (the definition of 'early' was variable, and was left to the cardiologist's judgement);
3. the time from onset of symptoms was unclear, or the patient refused cardiac catheterization or surgical reperfusion.

Both the conventionally managed patients and the surgical treatment group were similar in standard clinical descriptors as is demonstrated in Table 1. These characteristics include the average age of each group, the incidence of previous myocardial infarction, total creatine kinase activity on study entry as well as the area of infarction which was defined by the initial electrocardiogram when the patient was evaluated. The anterior wall was affected in approximately half of each group as was the inferior or inferoposterior wall. Likewise, the number of patients with 1, 2, or 3 vessel disease as defined by arteriography or autopsy examination was insignificant between groups when coronary anatomy was known. There was a higher number of patients with cardiogenic shock in the surgically treated group. This occurred because patients who were considered too ill to survive any therapy were removed from the conventional therapy group. It was felt that inclusion of these patients would provide unfair bias against the medical therapy group.

The hospital mortality of these patients who were removed from medical therapy was 81% (17 of 21). The hospital mortality in the two groups approached statistical significance. The medical therapy group overall demonstrated an 11.5% (23 of 200) mortality and the surgically treated group experienced a 5.8% (11 of 187) mortality ($p<0.08$). Although the overall hospital mortality favored the surgical reperfusion group, it was observed that the mortality difference widened even further if the subset of patients with cardiogenic shock were excluded from analysis. For example, the hospital mortality *in the absence of cardiogenic shock* was 1.2% (2 of 169) in the surgically treated group, but was 9.3% (18 of 193) (p<0.01) in the conventional treatment group.

In this study [13] two points were clarified. First the major differences in short- and long-term mortality between the two groups occurred because of the exceptionally low mortality of the surgically treated cohort that was treated early (i.e. within 4 to 6 hours from symptom onset) (Fig. 1). Secondly it was observed that anterior transmural infarction was associated with a much higher mortality in patients treated with either conventional or surgical reperfusion. As is shown in Fig. 1, the hospital mortality was 2% (2 of 100) in the group treated by surgical revascularization within 6 hours from symptoms onset. This was significantly lower than the 11.5% (23 of 200) hospital mortality of the conventionally treated group. In the follow-up period (mean follow-up 36 months) the mortality difference widened between the two groups. Total mortality of the surgical group rose to 6% (6 of 100) but the mortality in the conventional treatment group rose to 20.5% (41 of 200) (p<0.001). These data suggest that early reperfusion (i.e. within 6 hours) resulted in significantly lower hospital and long-term mortality than conventional therapy.

Table 1. Clinical characteristics of groups I and II on entry into study.

	Group I (N = 200)	Group II (N = 187)
Age (yr) (mean ± SD)	53.2 ± 8.1	52.7 ± 9.1
Incidence of previous MI	28 (14%)	30 (16%)
Patients with abnormal (>90 IU) elevation of total CK activity in initial sampling	119 (59.5%)	110 (58.8%)
Area of infarction (ECG)		
Anterior[a]	73 (36.5%)	88 (47.0%)
Anterolateral[a]	29 (14.5%)	14 (7.5%)
Inferior	74 (37.0%)	72 (38.5%)
Inferoposterior	11 (5.5%)	8 (4.3%)
Lateral	6 (3.0%)	2 (1.1%)
Uncertain	7 (3.5%)	3 (1.6%)
No of vessels with CAD[b]		
1	38 (27.4%)	59 (31.5%)
2	57 (41.0%)	67 (35.8%)
3	44 (3.5%)	61 (32.6%)
Clinical Class (Killip)		
I	123 (61.5%)	112 (59.9%)
II	60 (30.0%)	48 (25.6%)
III	10 (5.0%)	9 (4.8%)
IV[a]	7 (3.5%)	18 (9.6%)

[a] Probability value p<0.05 in comparing groups I and II.
[b] CAD = coronary artery disease (coronary anatomy available in 139 patients (69.5%) of group I.

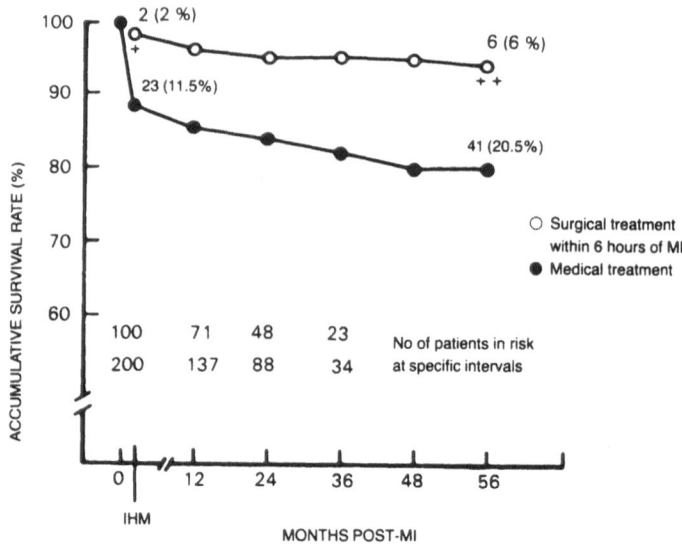

Fig. 1. In-hospital mortality and survival curves of patients undergoing reperfusion within 6 hours (open circles) and patients treated with conventional medical therapy (closed circles). + = $p<0.01$; ++ = $p<0.001$; pts = patients. (By permission of the authors and the American College of Cardiology.)

Ten year experience with surgical treatment of acute myocardial infarction

Although many centers have presented results characterizing experience with the surgical treatment with acute myocardial infarction, few have presented long-term follow-up studies. Accordingly we presented our ten year experience with the surgical treatment of acute myocardial infarction [14]. Clinical characteristics of the group with transmural myocardial infarction are listed in Table 2. As is shown in Fig. 2, of the 440 patients who underwent surgical reperfusion, 291 patients were placed on cardiopulmonary bypass within 6 hours of symptom onset. One-hundred forty nine patients were placed on bypass longer than 6 hours from the onset of chest pain. The average time from symptom onset to therapy in the early group was 4.5 hours, while the average interval from symptom onset to treatment in the late reperfusion group was 9 hours. As is shown in Fig. 2, there was a significantly lower mortality when patients were treated earlier. The hospital mortality was 3.8% (11 of 291) in the early reperfusion group while the mortality of the late reperfusion group in the hospital was 8% (12 of 149) (p = 0.05). In long-term follow-up, the outlook was less favorable in the patient group receiving late reperfusion. The total mortality for the early treatment group was 8.2% (24 of 291), while the late therapy group demonstrated a 21% total mortality (31 of 149) (p<0.01).

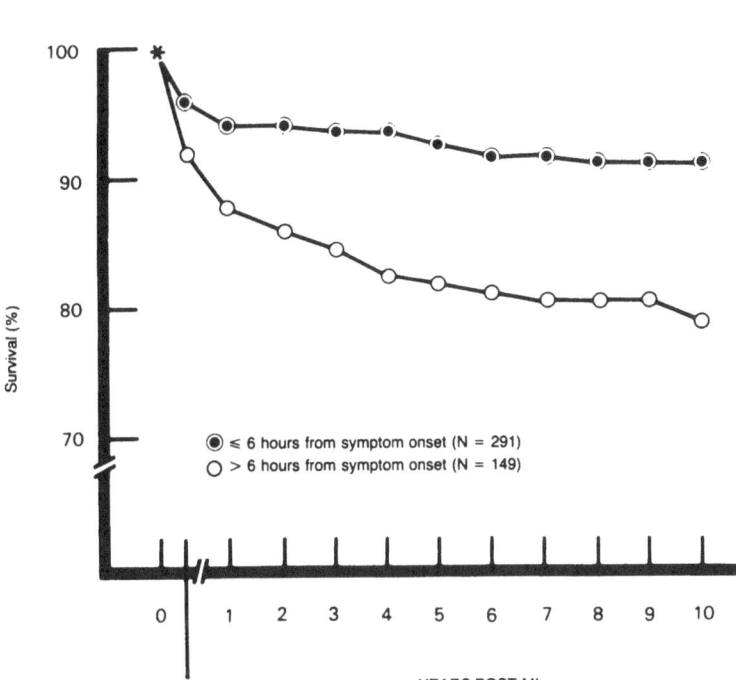

Fig. 2. In-hospital and long-term mortality for patients undergoing early versus late reperfusion. The in-hospital mortality (IHM) was significantly lower in the early treatment group. The difference widened over the follow-up period of 10 years. IHM = in-hospital mortality; MI = myocardial infarction. (From DeWood et al. [14] by permission of the American Heart Association, Inc.)

The long-term follow-up was 5.3 years. Although the mortality differences in the two groups were significantly different, it is unclear whether the mortality difference is a reflection of a larger and fixed contractile deficit or that it correlates with the time interval from occlusion to reperfusion. *If* a longer period of occlusion in patients results in larger infarction, a more benign clinical course might be expected in the early treatment group. This appeared to be the case in the patient population we studied and implies that early intervention is more likely to result in a long-term favorable outcome. It should be recognized however, the duration of myocardial infarction in man is unknown and it is not possible to prove that lower mortality is a direct reflection of smaller infarction due to earlier reperfusion and protection of myocardium distant from the point of occlusion. Thus the mechanisms associated with lower mortality in the early treatment group cannot be clarified presently, although early restoration of blood flow is an attractive explanation.

Multi-vessel disease in transmural myocardial infarction

Patients suffering angina pectoris in the presence of multi-vessel disease frequently demonstrate decreased survival. An important predictor of early and late mortality in patients sustaining a transmural infarction has been poorly defined because baseline coronary arteriography and appropriate follow-up has not been performed to examine the effects of multi-vessel disease. The impact of surgical reperfusion in the presence of multi-vessel disease and transmural myocardial infarction has been analyzed by our group [14]. As is shown in Table 2, the presence of significant 1, 2, or 3 vessel disease was 29%, 41% and 30% respectively. The hospital mortality was 2.3%, 4.4% and 9.0% for 1, 2, and 3 vessel disease treated surgically (see Fig. 3). Importantly, the patients who demonstrated triple-vessel coronary disease were oftentimes the same patients who had experienced cardiogenic shock at the time they underwent coronary bypass surgery. Mortality in the absence of presurgical shock was 2.8% (11 of 397). Half of the patients with cardiogenic shock also had suffered previous myocardial infarction and demonstrated extensive left ventricular dysfunction.

As is shown in Fig. 3, the long-term follow-up demonstrated higher mortality with multi-vessel disease. As is shown, the mortality was 8%, 12%, and 17.4% in the patient groups with 1, 2, or 3 vessel disease respectively. Thus the presence of multi-vessel disease especially in the presence of previous infarction or cardiogenic shock was found to be an important determinant of

Table 2. Population characteristics: transmural infarction.

No of patients	440
Age (mean ± SD)	54 ± 8.2 yr
(range)	32–80 yr
Gender (% male)	348 (79.0%)
Previous MI	69 (15.7%)
Area of infarct	
Anterior	228
Inferior	212
Vessels with CAD (≥ 50%)	
1 vessel	127 (28.8%)
2 vessel	181 (41.2%)
3 vessel	132 (30.0%)
Clinical Class (Killip & Kimball)	
I	260 (59.1%)
II	110 (25.0%)
III	27 (6.1%)
IV	43 (9.7%)

MI = myocardial infarction; CAD = coronary artery disease.

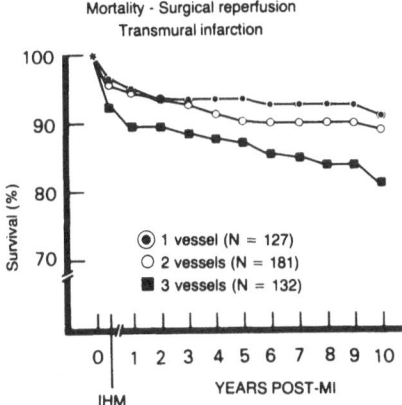

Fig. 3. In-hospital and late mortality for the transmural myocardial infarction group analyzed by the number of coronary arteries diseased. Patients with one and two vessel disease demonstrated low mortality, while three vessel disease was associated with the highest mortality. (From DeWood et al. [14] by permission of the American Heart Association, Inc.)

short- and long-term mortality. Mortality curves in all groups appeared to be more favorable than results with conventional therapy [13, 15, 16]. Whether these data support the concept that complete revascularization at the time of acute myocardial infarction is helpful in preventing future coronary related events cannot be proven. Nevertheless, protection from these events may account for the relatively low incidence of sudden death and reinfarction that has been reported following bypass surgery for evolving infarction [17].

Surgical treatment of nontransmural myocardial infarction

Surgical reperfusion can be used as effective therapy for patients suffering nontransmural myocardial infarction [14]. As is shown in Fig. 4, we followed 261 patients who underwent coronary arteriography and surgical revascularization for nontransmural myocardial infarction from 1973 to mid 1981. This study comprised an eight year experience with the surgical treatment of nontransmural infarction (the patient population is described in Table 3).

We found a much lower prevalence of triple-vessel disease in the nontransmural group as compared to the transmural infarction group as is shown in Tables 2 and 3. Nevertheless, despite the higher frequency of multi-vessel disease in this patient population, the mortality for the group was lower than the transmural group with triple-vessel disease. In this study, the mortality in the hospital was 3% (8 of 261). The average follow-up for the group was 4.3 years (range 1 to 8 years). The long-term mortality of the group rose to 6.5%

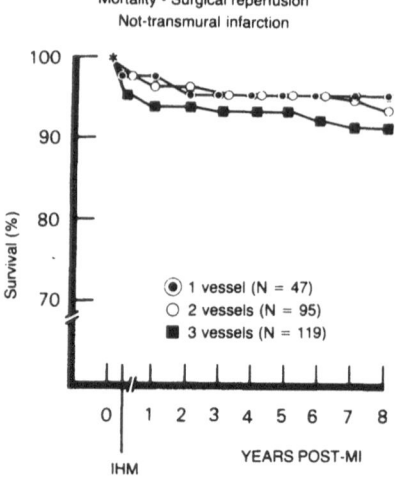

Fig. 4. Mortality of the nontransmural myocardial infarction group treated by early surgical reperfusion. The hospital and late mortality was low in patients with one and two vessel disease and was highest with three vessel disease. (From DeWood et al. [14] by permission of the American Heart Association, Inc.)

(17 of 261) as there were an additional 9 deaths in the long-term follow-up period.

Effects of multi-vessel disease in nontransmural myocardial infarction treated by surgical reperfusion

As is demonstrated in Fig. 4, the in-hospital and long-term mortality of the nontransmural group described in Table 3 was evaluated according to the

Table 3. Population characteristics: nontransmural infarction.

No of patients	261
Age (mean ± SD)	58.4 ± 9 yr
(range)	34–77 yr
Gender (% male)	203 (78.0%)
Previous MI	51 (19.5%)
Left main CAD	30 (11.5%)
CAD distribution	
1 vessel	47 (18.0%)
2 vessel	95 (36.0%)
3 vessel	119 (46.0%)

MI = myocardial infarction; CAD = coronary artery disease.

presence of 1, 2, or 3 vessel disease. The mortality for 1 and 2 vessel disease was 2.1%. Triple vessel disease was frequently associated with previous myocardial infarction and this group experienced a 4.2% mortality (5 of 119). Despite the higher mortality in these patients, the long-term outlook appeared favorable for all groups that had undergone early revascularization. As is shown in Fig. 4, the total mortality for 1, 2, or 3 vessel disease was 4.2%, 6.3%, and 8.4% respectively over the 8 year follow-up period.

Inspection of Fig. 4 indicates that the survival curves were stable regardless of the number of vessels involved even though three-vessel disease was associated with the highest mortality. This was an unexpected finding but may indicate factors other than the number of vessels diseased (such as ejection fraction at the time of acute infarction) are important determinates of survival following surgical treatment of nontransmural infarction. Likewise these data suggest that bypass surgery in the presence of multi-vessel disease may offer some protection from fatal long-term cardiac events.

As with the transmural group, mortality associated with the nontransmural infarction group treated with surgical reperfusion was lower than reports which have examined early and late mortality subsequent to conventional therapy for nontransmural infarction [15, 16]. The low mortality associated with surgical reperfusion for this type of acute ischemic syndrome clearly suggests that surgical reperfusion is a potentially acceptable alternative to conventional therapy. This may be especially important when considering the frequent presence of multi-vessel disease in the presence of evolving necrosis.

World wide experience with surgical revascularization during acute myocardial infarction

Most centers have reserved surgical revascularization for complicated myocardial infarction. Many attempts at surgical revascularization for acute myocardial infarction occurred in patients already hospitalized for elective surgery with known coronary anatomy, as therapy for preinfarction angina that evolved to early infarction, as a result of a cardiac catheterization mishaps, or was offered to the patient because of extension of established infarction with continued or recurrent chest pain. We reviewed studies from 16 centers in which this technique has been applied as therapy for acute evolving infarction (Table 4). As is shown the overall mortality with surgical reperfusion for acute myocardial infarction was 4.9% (52 of 1052 patients). The studies demonstrating mortality in excess of 5% usually involve patients who are experiencing various stages of cardiogenic shock, in whom other interventions have failed (and therefore involved some time delay to surgical revascularization), or who have undergone multiple defibrillations for severe rhythm disturbances.

Table 4. Worldwide results with surgical reperfusion for acute myocardial infarction.

Authors	Time interval between chest pain and operation (hr)	Number of patients	Hospital number	Mortality (%)
1. Mundth et al. [18]	24	1	0	0
2. Pifarre et al. [19]	12	3	0	0
3. Cohn et al. [20]	8	6	0	0
4. Sustaita et al. [21]	8	4	0	0
5. Cheanvechai et al. [22]	10	24	2	8.3
6. Keon et al. [23]	24	31	2	6.4
7. Dawson et al. [29]	12	11	4[a]	36.3
8. Guss et al. [24]	3	2	0	0
9. Mills et al. [25]	24	18	2[b]	11.1
10. Bolooki et al. [26]	8	25	2	8.0
11. Isch et al. [27]	4	3	0	0
12. Richmond et al. [28]	12	4	0	0
13. Nunley et al. [30]	24	17	1	5.9
14. Phillips et al. [32]	36	181	10[c]	5.5
15. Jones et al. [31]	24	21	0	0
16. DeWood et al. [14]	24	440[TM]	23[d]	5.2
		261[NTM]	8	3.1
Totals		1052	52	4.9

[a] All cardiac arrest preop.

[b] Left main occlusion.

[c] All mortalities in cardiogenic shock; 8 were failures after PTCA or thrombolysis for myocardial infarction.

[d] Includes 12 patients with advanced cardiogenic shock.

[TM] Transmural myocardial infarction.

[NTM] Nontransmural myocardial infarction.

The number of patients in each series varies, but most of the more recent work confirms this form of therapy can be delivered safely. In our center we attempt to treat patients prior to the onset of the complications associated with myocardial infarction. Even large anterior transmural infarctions are usually not supported by intraaortic balloon counterpulsation unless advanced shock is in evidence or there may be an unusual delay in transfer of the patient to the operating room. As an adjunct to surgical revascularization, we frequently use intraaortic balloon counterpulsation in the postoperative period for a short period of support. With this approach, patients suffering infarction who have demonstrated extensive contractile impairment of the left ventricle prior to surgery have also experienced low complication rates as well as low mortality.

610

Summary

This article has reviewed data comparing the medical and surgical treatment of acute myocardial infarction. Furthermore the experience in Spokane, Washington has been presented as well as results of surgical revascularization performed at multiple centers. For the most part, these centers have demonstrated that surgery can be performed with exceptionally low mortality. It would be simplistic to imagine that the pathophysiology of the various forms of myocardial infarction has been defined and therefore the best therapy or combinations of therapy have been determined.

A new era has clearly evolved with advances in thrombolytic therapy with and without subsequent percutaneous transluminal balloon angioplasty. Potentially these therapies represent an alternative method of reperfusion. Determining which therapy should be applied as well as the most appropriate combination of therapies that might result in low mortality and morbidity remains a major challenge for the future.

Which patients will do well when assessed by clinical parameters in the first several minutes to hours of acute myocardial infarction? Since coronary anatomy cannot be defined without arteriography and because patients in our center are rarely turned down for surgery because of multi-vessel disease, it is unlikely that a favorable bias has been introduced into our studies. Many centers are now entering into the area of reperfusion. Which is the best method of reperfusion is presently unknown. Surgical revascularization in conjuction with thrombolysis or following acute coronary angioplasty may prove to be an appropriate method and the procedures may become complimentary. Regardless of the outcome of these future studies, it is unlikely that any of these aggressive therapies can be measurably effective unless they are applied before profound hemodynamic deterioration due to extensive left ventricular damage occurs.

Acknowledgements

This study was supported in part by the Sacred Heart Medical Center and Deaconess Medical Center Foundations for Research, the Max Baer Heart Fund of the Eagles, and the Inland Empire Heart Research Foundation.

References

1. Page DL, Caulfield JB, Kastor JA, et al.: Myocardial changes associated with cardiogenic shock. N Engl J Med 1971; 285: 133–137.

2. Harnaryan C, Bennett MA, Pentecost BL, et al.: Quantitative study of infarcted myocardium in cardiogenic shock. Br Heart J 1970; 32: 728–732.

3. Gillespie TA, Sobel BE: A rationale for therapy of acute myocardial infarction. Limitation of infarct size. Adv Intern Med 1976; 22: 319–330.

4. Gelman EM, Ehsani AA, Campbell MK, et al.: The influence of location and extent of myocardial infarction on long-term ventricular dysrhythmia and mortality. Circulation 1979; 60: 805–814.

5. Costantini C, Corday E, Lang T, et al.: Revascularization after 3 hours of coronary arterial occlusion. Effects on regional cardiac metabolic function and infarct size. Am J Cardiol 1975; 36: 368–384.

6. DeWood MA, Spores J, Notske R, et al.: Prevalence of total coronary occlusion during the early hours of transmural myocardial infarction. N Engl J Med 1980; 303: 897–902.

7. Rentrop P, Blanke H, Karsch KR, et al.: Selective intracoronary thrombolysis in acute myocardial infarction and unstable angina pectoris. Circulation 1981; 63: 307–317.

8. Meyer J, Merx W, Schmitz H, et al.: Percutaneous transluminal coronary angioplasty immediately after intracoronary streptolysis of transmural myocardial infarction. Circulation 1982; 66: 905–913.

9. Scanlon PJ, Nemickas R, Tobin JR Jr, et al.: Myocardial revascularization during acute phase of myocardial infarction. JAMA 1971; 218: 207–212.

10. Loop ED, Cheanvechai C, Sheldon WC, et al.: Early myocardial revascularization during acute myocardial infarction. Chest 1974; 66: 478.

11. Berg R Jr, Kendall RW, Duvoisin GE, et al.: Acute myocardial infarction: A surgical emergency. J Thorac Cardiovasc Surg 1975; 70: 432–439.

12. Phillips S, Kungtahworn C, Zeff R, et al.: Emergency coronary artery revascularization: A possible therapy for acute myocardial infarction. Circulation 1979; 60: 241–246.

13. DeWood MA, Spores J, Notske RN, et al.: Medical and surgical management of myocardial infarction. Am J Cardiol 1979; 44: 1356–1363.

14. DeWood MA, Spores J, Berg R Jr, et al.: Acute myocardial infarction: A decade of experience with surgical reperfusion in 701 patients. Circulation 1983; 68 (Suppl 2): 8–16.

15. Cannom DS, Levy W, Cohen LS: The short- and long-term prognosis of patients with transmural and nontransmural myocardial infarction. Am J Med 1976; 61: 452–458.

16. Hutter AM Jr, DeSanctis RW, Flynn T, et al.: Nontransmural myocardial infarction: A comparison of hospital and late clinical course of patients with that of matched patients with transmural anterior and transmural inferior myocardial infarction. Am J Cardiol 1981; 48: 595–602.

17. DeWood MA, Berg R Jr: Coronary artery bypass surgery: 13 years experience with chronic stable angina pectoris, unstable angina pectoris and acute myocardial infarction. In: Hurst W (ed): Clinical essays on the heart, vol. 2. New York, McGraw-Hill, 1983; 159–170.

18. Mundth E, Hurchack P, Buckley M, et al.: Circulatory assistance and emergency direct coronary artery surgery for shock complicating acute myocardial infarction. N Engl J Med 1970; 283: 1382–1384.

19. Pifarre R, Spinozzola A, Nemickas R, et al.: Emergency aortocoronary bypass for acute myocardial infarction. Arch Surg 1971; 103: 525–528.

20. Cohn L, Gorlin R, Herman M, et al.: Aortocoronary bypass for acute coronary occlusion. J Thorac Cardiovasc Surg 1972; 64: 503–513.

21. Sustaita H, Chatterjee K, Matloff J, et al.: Emergency bypass surgery in impending and complicated acute myocardial infarction. Arch Surg 1972; 105: 30–35.

22. Cheanvechai C, Effler D, Loop F, et al.: Aortocoronary artery graft during early and late phase of acute myocardial infarction. Ann Thorac Surg 1973; 16: 249–260.

23. Keon WJ: Surgery for acute myocardial infarction and cardiogenic shock. Cardiovasc Rev Rep 1981; 2: 1120–1142.

24. Guss S, Zir L, Garrison H, et al.: Coronary occlusion during coronary angiography. Circulation 1975; 52: 1063–1068.
25. Mills N, Ochsner J, Bower P, et al.: Coronary artery bypass for acute myocardial infarction. South Med J 1975; 68: 1475–1480.
26. Bolooki H: Myocardial revascularization after acute myocardial infarction. Arch Surg 1976; 3: 1216–1224.
27. Isch J, Jolly W, Shumacker H Jr: Myocardial revascularization in acute myocardial infarction. J Indiana Med Assoc 1977; 70: 65–69.
28. Richmond D, Baird E: Coronary bypass grafting in the early stages of acute myocardial infarction. Med J Aust 1979; 1: 203–206.
29. Dawson J, Hall R, Hallman G, et al.: Mortality in patients undergoing coronary artery bypass surgery after myocardial infarction. Am J Cardiol 1974; 33: 483–486.
30. Nunley D, Grunkemeir G, Teply J, et al.: Coronary bypass operation following acute complicated myocardial infarction. J Thorac Cardiovasc Surg 1980; 85: 485–491.
31. Jones EL, Michalick R: Personal communication, 1983.
32. Phillips S, Kungtahworn C, Skinner JR: Emergency coronary artery reperfusion: A choice therapy for evolving myocardial infarction. Results in 339 patients. J Thorac Cardiovasc Surg 1983; 86: 679–688.

12.5 Twenty-five Years of Coronary Units: Perspectives for the Future

V. VALLE TUDELA

Introduction

Since this international symposium deals with the Coronary Unit (CU), we should first mention that the title of the communication is inexact, since I have taken the liberty of rounding out the figure. It has really been 26 years since the first CUs in the world were inaugurated. These coronary care units were initially established in North America, the first of them in the Toronto General Hospital, promoted by Brown and McMillan [1]. A few months later, the unit of Hughes Day in the Bethany Hospital of Kansas City [2] and that of Lawrence E. Meltzer in the Presbyterian University Medical Center of Pennsylvania [3] followed. In 1987 we celebrated the first 25 years of myocardial infarction care systematized in specific areas of the hospital with specialized and trained medical and nursing personnel and equipped with the technical means for treating possible complications of acute myocardial infarct (AMI). As we will see, the economic and human efforts involved have not been unrewarded. The intensive, sometimes aggressive therapeutic approach to AMI and ischemic heart disease has opened up new avenues of research and lead to substantial improvements in the diagnostic and therapeutic means available, which were unimaginable at the beginning of the sixties.

In this communication, we will briefly examine some ideas on the evolution of CU care and the achievements and future perspectives of these units. We will describe the present status of the CU in Spain and the results of a survey made by the Section of Ischemic Heart Disease and Coronary Units of the Spanish Cardiology Society, which obtained data from 42 CU throughout the country. The following sections will be developed:

a) Evolution in the concept of the CU and care provided.
b) Effectiveness of care and criteria for creation and equipment.
c) Present status of the CU in Spain: results of a 42-unit survey. Comparison with CUs in EEC countries.
d) Achievements of the CU: contributions to global hospital cardiologic activities.

e) Future perspectives and CU needs for Spain in the nineties.

Evolution in the concept of the CU and care provided

Medical progress and advances in care are rarely circumstantial. Installation of the first CU was preceded by the acquisition of knowledge and incorporation of cardiologic advances directly related to CU use and care. We should emphasize: the electrostimulation techniques (pacemaker) developed by Zoll since 1954 [4]; perfection of the closed-chest cardiac massage technique as it is now used, developed by Kouwenhoven, Jude and Knickerbocker in 1960 [5], and improvement of closed-chest continuous current defibrillation, studied by Lown and described by this author in 1962 [6]. Which is to say that when the first CUs were established, the most immediate and definitive techniques for treatment of cardiac arrest had been developed and their efficacy demonstrated. They only had to be put into systematic practice in diseases in which cardiac arrest is a frequent complication. The most common and appropriate disease requiring this treatment was AMI, thus arose the general idea that CUs were conceived for treating cardiac arrest [7].

The first three CUs, mentioned above, were created as the result of development of three lines of cardiologic research. In the Toronto General Hospital, research was being done in the incidence of arrhythmia in AMI using continuous ECG recording [1]. In Kansas City they were attempting to concentrate patients, personnel and technical means in a program for treating cardiac arrest. They had already confirmed the inefficiency of treating cardiac arrest with a mobile team that moved throughout the hospital to the patient's bedside at the sound of an alarm [2]. Care generally arrived too late. They therefore decided to group the patients at the greatest risk of suffering cardiac arrest and ended up by accumulating AMI patients. The Pennsylvania unit [3] was making a controlled evaluation of the efficacy of anticoagulant treatment in AMI and discovered a high incidence of serious arrhythmias in these patients, for whom they recommended close control and treatment.

In Spain, the first three units were created in 1969 in Barcelona (Hospital de la Santa Cruz y San Pablo) and in Madrid (Hospital Central de la Cruz Roja and Hospital General La Paz).

Since the first CU in 1962 to the present, the concept of the care provided and the population requiring attention in these units has evolved. The first generation CUs (1962–1964) [1–3, 7] emerged to offer cardiac arrest care. Between 1965 and 1968, as a result of studies originating in CUs created in the United States and Europe, the high incidence of arrhythmias as a cause of early mortality in AMI and the benefits of energetic treatment [8] became well established concepts. In 1968, under the auspices of the National Institutes of

Health (NIH), the so-called MIRU (Myocardial Infarction Research Unit) was created in the United States with clearly defined objectives of furthering research in the field of arrhythmias and cardiac arrest. Great progress was made in cardiac arrest thanks to the introduction of invasive methods for measuring hemodynamic parameters and the demonstration that they could be used with very low risk for the patient [9]. In 1969, the WHO proposed the CU as an 'area of continuous vigilance and treatment of arrhythmias and other complications of AMI' [11]. In 1971, the American Heart Association declared that the purpose of CU is the 'vigilance and treatment of AMI, unstable angina and other heart diseases' [12]. Between 1975 and 1980, the designation 'Intensive Cardiologic Care Unit' was proposed in Spain by members of the Section of Ischemic Heart Disease of the Spanish Cardiology Society, and its objective was defined as 'vigilance and treatment of acute, serious and recuperable heart diseases' [13, 14]. In 1979, the WHO established in a new document that 'hospitals should have specialized cardiologic equipment for treating acute heart disease' [15]. In 1982, the American Heart Associations emitted a new report in which the 'Cardiologic Care Unit offers assistance to patients with AMI, unstable angina, potentially lethal arrhythmias, severe heart failure and other unstable circulatory states' [16]. In the 1983 meeting of the Spanish Cardiac Society, the Section of Ischemic Heart Disease and Coronary Units published 'Coronary Units in Spain' [17], which concluded, after collecting the experience of 36 CUs throughout the nation, that Intensive Cardiologic Care Units should meet some general conceptual and functional prerequisites:

a) A CU should not be planned as an isolated unit, but integrated within the framework of a general hospital.
b) There should be an organic, functional and hierarchical integration into Cardiology departments.
c) Integration of the CU into the General Intensive Care Unit will be contemplated when less than four beds are required for daily care of acute heart diseases.
d) The CU should always be directed by a cardiologist.

To summarize this evolution in concepts, we could say that from the seventies to the eighties, the CU has become the Intensive Cardiologic Care Unit (ICCU) to optimize use of medical resources, extending the benefits of continuous vigilance and assistance to all types of patients with progressive heart diseases of potentially reversible gravity [17].

Effectiveness of CU care; criteria for creation and equipment

Hospital mortality for AMI has declined by 50% since the installation of CUs [18]. In 1967, Meltzer published a comparative study of the mortality due to

AMI in patients treated in conventional hospital rooms and in CU, finding a 30.8% mortality in the control group and 19.9% in the CU [8]. Later Norris communicated the results of two series: one with 757 patients treated from 1966–67, prior to creation of the CU, and the other with 574 patients treated in 1977–1979 in the CU. Mortality was 26% in the first series and 14% in the second [19]. Since CUs were established, we have had evidence that mortality has been declining within narrower margens. As such, in two Spanish series treated in the CU, 2,082 in 1974 and 7,342 in 1982, mortality declined from 16.4% in the first series to 13.9% in the second, 2.5% in 8 years, which is statistically significant [17]. To simplify, the efforts of the last 22 years have crystallized in a reduction of AMI hospital mortality to levels of 10 to 14% [20], unquestionably a therapeutic feat.

As for the delay in admitting AMI patients to the CU, in our environment [17] this time lapse is still too long. As is already known, delay in admission is a determinant factor of mortality [21] and it reflects the efficiency of a CU in its surroundings. Moreover, as regards the CU function of reducing mortality due to ventricular arrhythmias, early admission of AMI patients has the additional advantage of making thrombolysis viable. This technique has fully demonstrated its ability to produce early recanalization of the vessel responsible for the infarcted zone and is considered the most effective means available for limiting the infarction area [22–24], as long as the procedure is performed within the first four hours of AMI. To calculate the number of possible candidates for thombolytic therapy in our environment, we can use the data compiled by Froufe [17] in 1974 and 1982: 43% and 48.1% of AMI, respectively, were admitted to hospital with a delay of 4 hours or less. This means that a minimum of 3,500 to 5,000 AMI could benefit annually from thrombolysis. In spite of this, the average delay in admission is still very long, about 11 hours. As a result, many cases are admitted to our CU with late complications, which discloses the need for health campaigns among the general public, patients at risk for AMI and physicians who attend patients with early symptoms of the disease. These campaings have proved their effectiveness in population trials [25].

Criteria for CU creation: these criteria are mainly based on demographic information for each health zone and on the incidence of ischemic heart disease in a country. The criteria established by the WHO in 1969 and 1979 [10, 15], still not modified, consider that the needs for care of ischemic heart disease and complications in industrialized countries can be covered with one 8–10 bed CU for each population nucleus of 250,000 inhabitants (approximately equivalent to the health zones proposed by the future Spanish Ley de Sanidad). From a practical point of view, it is accepted that 'in provincial hospitals where a minimum of 100 annual AMI admissions is accredited, planning and creation of a CU is fully justified' [17].

Following the recommendations of the Coronary Research Group of the European Economic Community countries [12] and the NIH in their Consensus Development Conference on Critical Care Medicine [26], at least two categories or levels of CU should be projected: *type A or research CU and type B or care CU*. The *type A* CU fulfill care, education and research functions. They are reference units for other centers and should be installed in regional hospitals or heads of sanitary areas at a density of one per nucleus of 500,000 inhabitants or more. According to the structure of the Cardiology Service or Section where it would function and the number of annual infarctions attended, the CU can be planned as a physically independent unit or an annex to the General Intensive Care Unit [17]. Cost of installation and equipment of a 6-bed *type B* CU is estimated at 13 million pesetas and that of a *type A* unit is approximately three times as much [17].

Present status of the CU in Spain: results of a questionnaire completed by 42 units; comparison with CUs in other EEC countries

Throughout 1983, the Ischemic Heart Disease and CU Section of the Spanish Cardiac Society compiled information from a questionnaire on general functional conditions of CUs in Spain. Personal contact was established with a member of each unit's medical team, who was requested to answer the questionnaire. By means of these contacts, some centers were localized that had more sporadic contacts with the Section. We estimate that the questionnaire collected information from practically 95% of the CUs in Spain and from all those that regularly collaborate with the Spanish Cardiac Society. The questionnaire consisted of 37 questions distributed in the following sections:
a) general characteristics of the hospital: 3 questions;
b) characteristics of the CU: 8 questions;
c) medical personnel: 14 questions;
d) auxiliary personnel: 4 questions; and
e) equipment: 8 questions.
In the analysis of responses to each section, the number of CUs that completed the responses is indicated in parentheses. The units that answered the questionnaire are listed in the annex.

Figs 1 and 2 list numerical data for the CUs in Spain in 17 autonomic communities in the last trimester of 1983. In Fig. 1, the numbers in circles correspond to the number of CUs in the public network of the corresponding autonomic community. The numbers in squares indicate the total number of beds for acute patients in the CUs of the autonomous community. The numbers next to points representing cities, generally provincial capitals, reflect the CUs functioning in these cities. In the upper right hand part of Fig. 1 is shown

618

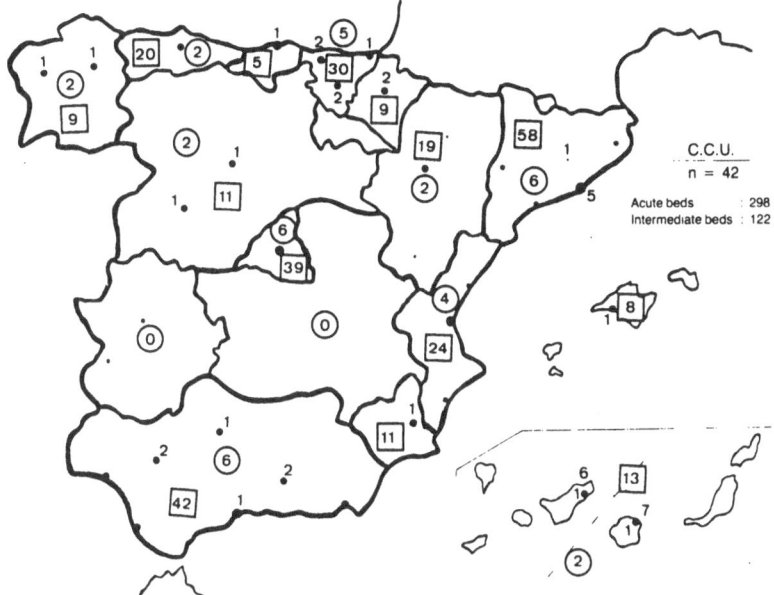

Fig. 1. Distribution of CUs in Spain. In each autonomic community, the number of CUs is indicated in the city or cities where they are located. The figure in the circle indicates the total number of CU and the figure in the square the total number of beds for acute patients.

the total number of acute beds (298) and intermediate care beds (122) available in the public network. The scarcity of intermediate care beds, which only reach 40% of the number of acute beds, should be emphasized. The distribution of CUs in provincial capitals is also striking, these units generally being concentrated in tertiary type hospitals, while large geographical areas, such as the two Castillian communities and Extremadura, have practically no CU. These communities may be affected by the generally good sanitary installations of the community of Madrid, where we have concrete references of 6 units, but we know of the activity of at least 3 or 4 more. Fig. 2 shows the degree of collaboration these CUs have with the Ischemic Heart Disease Section and the Spanish Cardiology Society. The numbers in parenthesis correspond to the CUs in each autonomous community and the underlined numbers to those that collaborate with the Spanish Cardiology Society. Not counting all the centers, but possibly only those with the greatest affinity, the degree of collaboration is about 70%, reflecting the competition between cardiology and intensive care for these units.

Table 1 lists the administrative features of the CUs. It is noteworthy that although there is a cardiology service in the hospital in 80% of cases, only 50% of the CUs are vinculated to this service. When an analysis is made of the Social Security units, the results are still less promising because in 76% of cases

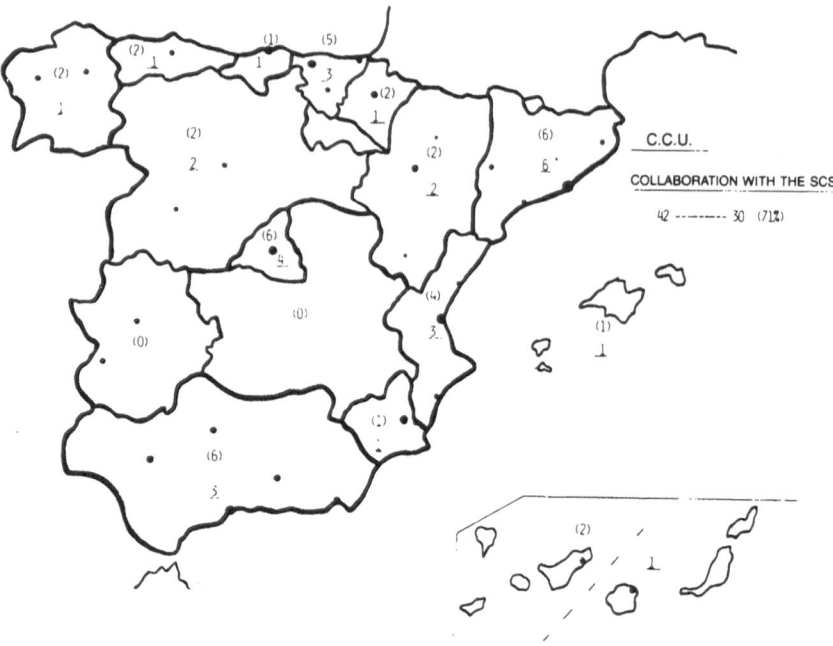

Fig. 2. Degree of collaboration of the CU with the activities of the Ischemic Heart Disease and Coronary Unit Section of the Spanish Cardiology Society. The number in parenthesis corresponds to the CUs in each community and the number underlined to that of CUs that collaborate with the Spanish Cardiology Society.

Table 1. Coronary unit questionnaire (N = 42).

Administrative characteristics:	
Existence of a cardiology service:	
Yes	34
No	8
Administrative dependence:	
Cardiology Service	21
Intensive Care Service	18
Others	3
Type of hospital:	
Social Security	21 (Depend. IC-76%)
Univerity hospital	10 (Depend. IC-20%)
Provincial hospital	5
Private hospital	3
Others	3

IC: intensive care.

the CUs depend on the Intensive Medicine Service. Table 2 shows general data and the annual patient volume. The small number of intermediate care beds must be underlined, since this number should at least be doubled [16]. The average CU size is about 7 beds, which is adequate. The type of patients admitted to the CU is interesting since at least 50% are AMI, the majority of admissions being for other forms of acute heart disease. The average stay of 5.5 days could be reduced by one day if there were more intermediate or conventional hospital beds. Table 3 lists the data on medical personnel. The number of physicians per unit is excessive and this medical personnel is of advanced age to be working in a shock area of the hospital. We should also consider the ramifications of the fact that 25% of the physicians dedicated to these tasks are not cardiologists, a tendency that has intensified in the last two years. In this same analysis of the specialization of the doctors working in CUs and examining the immediate perspectives, we could qualify the situation as alarming because almost 60% of the resident doctors undergoing formation in the CU do not intend to be cardiologists. Table 4 offers data on available technical means. In this table, aside from listing the percentages of CUs with various types of equipment, a contrasted evaluation is made of the scientific use made of this equipment and classfied as good (G), very poor (VP), poor (P) and insufficient. Noteworthy are the very low use made of electrophysiology units and intraaortic counterpulsation devices and the still limited benefits of cardiac surgery, especially myocardial revascularization surgery in relation with CU care. Table 5 compares average values for technical equipment between 45 CU in 7 European Economic Community countries [12] and 30 CU

Table 2. Coronary unit questionnaire (N = 42).

General characteristics	
Number of beds	298
Average	7.0 ± 2.5
Intermediate beds	100
CCU/Coronary beds	
Intermediate	2.98
(N = 39)	
General hospital beds	30,899
CCU beds	272
General coronary beds	
CCU	114
(N = 42)	
Annual patient volume	
Total admissions	19,550
AMI	8,313 (42.5%)
Average stay	5.5 days

Table 3. Coronary unit questionnaire (N = 42).

Medical personnel		
Full time	Part time	Total
152	119	271
X = 3.8 ± 2.1	3.0 ± 3.6	6–7 MD/CCU

Ages (N = 26 CCU, 173 MDs ... 64%)

29 – 55; X = 36.5 + 4.7

Professional qualifications of full-time physicians (N = 152)

Cardiologists	115 (75%)
Intensive care specialists	37 (25%)
Resident physicians	(N = 40 CCU, 66 MDs)
Average:	1.65 ± 1.4
Specializing in cardiology	27 (40%)
Specializing in intensive care	28 (43%)
Specializing in internal medicine	11 (16.6%)

Table 4. Technical equipment of the coronary unit (N = 30).

	Percentage	Output
'Bedside' HMDC	100	Good
Intensifier	73	Good
PCM	100	Good
Electrophysiology	63	Very Poor (VP)
Counterpulsation	53	Very Poor (VP)
Cardiac surgery	60	Poor
Intermediate beds	45	Insufficient

Table 5. Technical equipment as compared with EEC units.

Means	EEC 7 countries (45 CU, 1981)	Spain (30 CU, 1982)
Beds	9.6 ± 4.8	7.0 ± 2.5
Intermediate beds	64%	45%
Intensifier	80%	73%
Pulmonary artery pressure monitoring	91%	100%
Cardiac surgery	73%	60%
Physicians (FT + PT)	145	271
Average delay	7.4 ± 6.5 hrs	11 hrs
Research equipment		
Computerized arrhythmia monitoring	42%	0
Computerized hemodynamic measurements	32%	0
Isotopes	14%	0
Unstable angina	58%	13%

FT: full time. PT: part time.

in Spain. Fundamental differences between Spanish and EEC units are clearly appreciated in:

a) Less technical equipment in the Spanish CU, especially intermediate care equipment, cardiac surgery and the most recent technology, which is practically inexistent: computerized control of arrhythmias and hemodynamic parameters, isotope applications, etc.

b) More physcians dedicated to the tasks of the CU.

c) Longer average delay in patient admission.

d) Less research activity (as evaluated by the number of publications on a subject intensively studied, like unstable angina).

Achievements of the CU: its contributions to hospital cardiology activities

Aside from the main achievement of reducing AMI mortality by 50%, already emphasized, in its two decades of existence the CU has contributed decisively to research, testing and clinical applications in diverse fields, such as use of enzymes in cardiology, bedside hemodynamic studies and study of the natural history of unstable angina and coronary spasm [27–30]. Study of all the complications of AMI, its natural history and therapeutic approaches to the disease has been the main task of these units and has produced innumerable publications [31]. As for therapy, the CU has been a testing ground for assessing the therapeutic effectiveness of almost all the cardiovascular drugs and instrumental procedures introduced in the last 20 years [32–34]. The most interesting experimental studies motivated by the daily activities of the CU may be the methods for limiting the area of infarction, although their clinical application has been restricted [35, 36]. In the last three years, they have again moved to the forefront with the opportunities offered by thrombolytic therapy [23, 24]. The result of these achievements and others not mentioned has been an exponential increment in medical and technical information in the last 20 years, meaning that the present approach to AMI and ischemic heart disease is less passive and that the mental attitude of the physician is more physiopathologic, dynamic and aggressive. On the other hand, better knowledge of the natural history of the disease and prognostic factors obliges us to intervene earlier with therapy and to seek out the patients at highest risk to modify the disease's course with every available therapeutic resource, including surgery.

How do we assess the work of the CU within the context of hospital cardiologic activities? The available data, obtained from various technical reports elaborated by accredited international institutions dedicated to health organization and planning, indicate the following:

a) The European Union of Medical Specialties, an organization dependent on the EEC countries, reported on the formation of cardiology specialists [37] and referred to the CU saying: 'It should have a minimum of 6 beds and cardiology residents should be completely incorporated into its tasks for at least 6 months'.

b) The regional WHO office for Europe, in a technical report on the development of coronary care in the community [15], establishes and clearly accepts the sociosanitary benefits and cost-effectiveness of these units, specifying that: 'The CU also has an important role in many hospitals in treating acute cardiac problems not due to coronary attack, among which are left or right acute heart failure, severe arrhythmias, conduction disorders, cardiogenic shock, etc.'. The CU is where acute cardiology is practiced in the hospital.

c) The NIH report in 1983 on Critical Care Medicine [26] in relation to the CU emphasizes 'their contribution to the study and knowledge of the natural history of ischemic heart disease and their work in risk stratification of the cardiologic patient, as well as their protagonism in the application and development of new therapeutic cardiology means'.

As for the educational tasks of the CU in postgraduate cardiology specialization programs, it is opportune to review the results of a survey made in 1984 among 50 cardiologists of the state of Florida with 2–5 years of clinical practice. The survey was analyzed by C.R. Conti and titled: 'What is a clinical cardiologist in 1984' [38]. From this author's conclusions, we would like to underline the following opinions:

a) 98% of the specialists surveyed judged CU training of cardiology residents to be indispensable;

b) in a 24-month residency, 8 months should be destined to CU training; and

c) CU training is the heart of cardiology.

Contrasting with these opinions, which reflect the interest North American cardiologists have in the training acquired in the CU, is what we consider the irrational, troubling, unjust and biased situation of Spanish cardiology. In Spain:

a) 50% of the CU have no organic relationship with cardiology services;

b) 25% of the physicians in CUs are not cardiologists (this has occurred mainly since 1981); and

c) 60% of the resident physicians in the CU do not intend to be cardiologists.

In view of the discouraging reality of CU organization in Spain, it is urgent that we attempt to reorient the concept of the CU and integration of its functions and services into the hospital's cardiologic activities. If we do not act, Spanish cardiologists will be completely displaced from the 'heart of cardiology', possibly within a decade, and the CU will continue to form resident physicians for other specialties.

Future perspectives and equipment needs for the nineties in Spain

In the section on future perspectives, an optimistic view is usually given of the subject under study. However, we would like to base our opinions on the reality of our scientific progress and indicate the possible direction to follow until the next century. There are various cardiologic aspects and topics involved in which CUs will find their future projection, among them:

a) Incorporation of new technologies will improve the possibilities of diagnosis and control of arrhythmias and heart failure, and facilitate hemodynamic evaluation, coronary flow measurements, etc.

b) A closer relationship and degree of collaboration with cardiac surgery should be expected, in view of the increase in coronary surgery anticipated in Spain.

c) Cardiac catheterization laboratories will also be more active, because of the increment in the number of therapeutic procedures realized in them.

d) The CU will continue to be a 'lifesaver' for cardiologists, hemodynamics specialists and surgeons since Cardiological Intensive Care Units have their future assured.

In the educational field, CU activities will extend to:

a) resident physicians in cardiology and other specialties, in subjects such as arrhythmias, cardiovascular pharmacology, unstable angina, instrumental applications (pacemakers, bedside hemodynamic evaluation, percutaneous counterpulsation, etc.), heart failure, AMI complications, cardiovascular emergencies, etc.

b) Nursing, in areas similar to those indicated in *a*.

c) The population attended, through health information programs mainly related to ischemic heart disease.

Clinical investigation of ischemic heart disease in the CU should increase our knowledge of:

a) prophylaxis and treatment of arrhythmias in AMI;

b) electromechanical dissociation and cardiac rupture and general measures of cardiac protection and containment of the area of infarction;

c) pathophysiology of angina at rest and its therapy;

d) criteria for early release and risk stratification of patients; and

e) diagnostic application of new nonivasive methods.

To terminate, we will briefly discuss the theoretical needs for creation of new CUs in Spain in the nineties. By this time, the Spanish population, more socioeconomically developed, will have similar life styles and coronary risk factors as other industrial populations. We can calculate that the incidence of new cases of ischemic heart disease will at least approximate that attained in an epidemiological study in Manresa [39] of about 10% annually, which would lead to a growing demand for care. We have calculated future necessities by

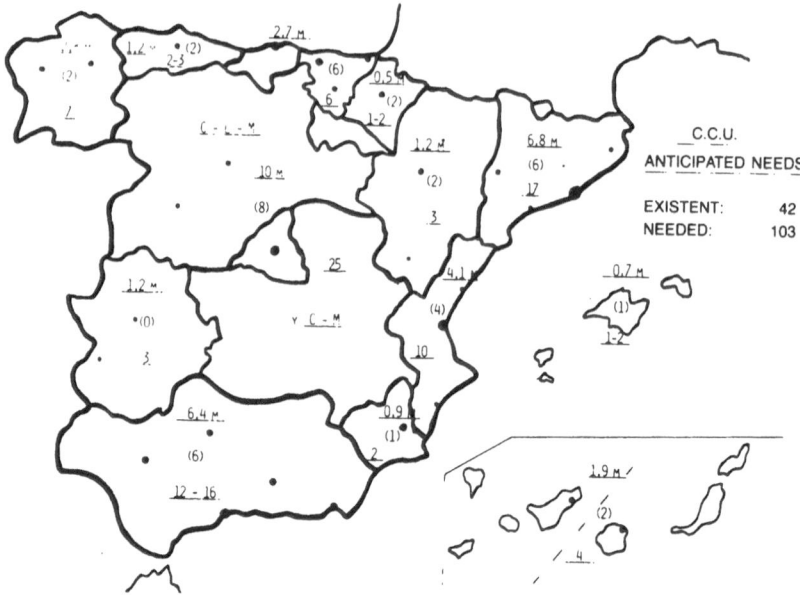

Fig. 3. Anticipated CU needs for 1990–1995. This calculation was made on the basis of 1 CU per 400,000 inhabitants. The numbers underlined and accompanied by M indicate millions of inhabitants in each autonomous community. The figures in parenthesis show the present number of CU. The number underlined is total required. The difference between these last two figures indicates the number of CU that have to be created. The value corresponding to Basque Country and Santander are grouped.

applying a looser criterion than that of the WHO [10], establishing a CU for each population nucleus of 400,000 inhabitants. Fig. 3 shows the Spanish population distribution expected for 1990–1995 in the different autonomous communities [40]. For each community, the population calculated in millions (M) is underlined and the present number of CU functioning is in parentheses. The other number underlined indicates the CU that will be needed if expectations are met as far as the incidence of ischemic heart disease. In the upper right hand part of the figure are shown the existing CU and anticipated necessities, which means that in the next 15 years the number of CU in Spain should double to provide adequate regional care for acute heart diseases. In view of this map, it is evident that the autonomous communities of Castille, Extremadura, Catalonia, Andalusia, Valencia and Galicia are those with the greatest need for new CU.

626

Summary

Since its creation in 1962, the concept of the Coronary Unit (CU) has evolved, presently being understood as the Cardiologic Intensive Care Unit. The effectiveness of the CU has been sufficiently confirmed by the 50% reduction in hospital mortality from acute myocardial infarct (AMI) that has been attained, the present rate being 10–14%. In our environment, 48% of infarctions are admitted within 4 hours of evolution, which represents 3,500 to 5,000 cases per year of patients who could be treated by thrombolysis. We present the results of a questionnaire completed by 42 CU in Spain and compared with those of 7 countries in the European Economic Community. It should be underlined that our CU have:
a) fewer technical means and intermediate care beds;
b) more physicians;
c) a longer average delay in admission; and
d) less research activity.
The present status of CU in Spain is described with due attention given to their troubling situation, which results from the following:
a) 50% have no organic relation with cardiology services;
b) 25% of the physicians are not cardiologists; and
c) 60% of the medical residents are not training to be cardiologists.
We comment on the future perspectives of the CU and cardiologic needs that can be anticipated in the next 10 years on the basis of population growth and estimating a need for one CU per 400,000-inhabitant population nucleus. The Spanish autonomous communities that need to create new CUs are: both Castillian communities, Extremadura, Catalonia, Andalusia, Valencia and Galicia.

Annex

1. Hospital Clínico y Provincial, Barcelona.
2. Centro Quirúrgico San Jorge, Barcelona.
3. Hospital de la Santa Cruz y San Pablo, Barcelona.
4. Hospital General Vall d'Hebrón, Barcelona.
5. Hospital Bellvitge-Princeps d'Espanya; L'Hospitalet de Llobregat, Barcelona.
6. Centro de Reanimación Cardíaca, Manresa, Barcelona.
7. Ciudad Sanitaria de Cruces, Bilbao.
8. Hospital Civil de Basurto (Fundación Vizcaya Pro-Cardíacos), Bilbao.
9. Residencia Sanitaria Reina Sofía, Córdoba.
10. Hospital Clínico, Granada.
11. Ciudad Sanitaria Virgen de las Nieves, Granada.
12. Hospital General Nuestra Señora del Pino, Las Palmas de Gran Canaria.
13. Hospital General, Lugo.

14. Ciudad Sanitaria La Paz, Madrid.
15. Clínica Puerta de Hierro, Madrid.
16. Escuela Nacional de Enfermedades del Tórax, Madrid.
17. Hospital Central de la Cruz Roja, Madrid.
18. Hospital General Ramón y Cajal, Madrid.
19. Sanitario Sear, Madrid.
20. Hospital General Carlos Haya, Málaga.
21. Hospital General Virgen del Lluch, Mallorca.
22. Hospital General Virgen de la Arrixaca, Murcia.
23. Hospital General de Asturias, Oviedo.
24. Hospital General Nuestra Señora de Covadonga, Oviedo.
25. Clínica Universitaria, Pamplona.
26. Hospital Provincial de Navarra, Pamplona.
27. Hospital Clínico de Salamanca, Salamanca.
28. Centro Médico Marqués de Valdecilla, Santander.
29. Hospital General de Galicia, Santiago de Compostela.
30. Hospital General Nuestra Señora de Aránzazu, San Sebastián.
31. Hospital Clínico de Sevilla, Sevilla.
32. Hospital General Virgen del Rocío, Sevilla.
33. Hospital General y Clínico de Tenerife, Tenerife.
34. Hospital General La Fe, Valencia.
35. Hospital Clínico, Valencia.
36. Hospital General, Valencia.
37. Hospital General Dr Peset, Valencia.
38. Hospital Clínico, Valladolid.
39. Hospital General Ortiz de Zárate. Vitoria.
40. Hospital General Santiago Apóstol, Vitoria.
41. Hospital Clínico de Zaragoza, Zaragoza.
42. Hospital General Miguel Servet, Zaragoza.

References

1. Brown KWG, MacMillan RL, Forbath N, Mel Grano F, Scott JW: Coronary Unit. An intensive care center for acute myocardial infarction. Lancet 1963; 2: 349.
2. Day HW: An intensive coronary care area. Dis Chest 1963; 44: 423.
3. Meltzer LE: Concepts and systems for intensive coronary care. Acad Med New Jersey Bull 1964; 10: 304.
4. Zoll PM: Treatment of Stokes Adams disease by external stimulation of the heart. Circulation 1954; 9: 482.
5. Kouwenhoven WB, Jude JR, Knickerbocker GG: Closed-chest cardiac massage. JAMA 1960; 178: 1074.
6. Lown B, Amarasinham R, Neuman J: New method for terminating cardiac arrhythmias – Use of synchronized capacitator discharge. JAMA 1962; 182: 548.
7. Grace WJ, Keyloun V: The coronary care unit. Butterworths, London, 1970.
8. Julian DG, Oliver MF: Acute myocardial infarction. E & Livingstone, Edinburgh, London, 1968.
9. Frommer PL: The myocardial infarction research program of the National Heart Institute. Am J Cardiol 1968; 22: 108.

10. WHO: The organization of coronary care units. Copenhagen, 1969.
11. Paul NYu, Bielsky MT, Edwards A: Resources for the optimal care of patients with acute myocardial infarction. Circulation 1971; 43: A-171.
12. Maseri A, Marchesi C, Chierchia S, Trivella MG: Coronary care units. (Sponsored by the Commission of the European Communities.) Martinus Nijhoff, Dordrecht, 1981.
13. Eizaguirre Perez AJ, Novo Valledor L: Valoración de las unidades de cuidados intensivos de cardiologia. Rev Esp Cardiolog 1975; 28: 37.
14. Malpartida F, Alegria E: Unidad coronaria. Ediciones Universidad, Navarra, 1979.
15. The development of coronary care in the community. Report on a WHO working group. Brussels, 1979.
16. Paul NYu, Conti CR, Jones P: Optimal resources for the care of patients with acute myocardial infarction and chronic coronary heart disease. Circulation 1982; 65: 654B.
17. Unidades Coronarias en España. Informe de la Sección de Cardiopatia Isquémica y Unidades Coronarias de la Sociedad Española de Cardiología. Rev Esp Cardiolog 1984; 37 (Suppl 3): 3.
18. Levy RI: Causes of the decrease in cardiovascular mortality. Am J Cardiol 1984; 54: 7C.
19. Norris RM, Sammel NL: Predictores de la muerte hospitalaria en el infarto agudo de miocardio. Progres Enf Cardiovasc 1981; 21: 146.
20. Hugenholtz PG, Laird-Meeter K, Balakumaran K, Ritsema HJ, Hagemeijer F: Intensive care of acute myocardial infarction: reflections on current coronary care. Intens Care Med 1978; 4: 1.
21. Pantridge JF, Adgey AAJ, Geddes JS, Webb SW: The acute coronary attack. Grune & Stratton, New York, 1975.
22. Braunwald E: Thirty-five years of progress in cardiovascular research. Circulation 1984; 70: III-8.
23. Laffel GL, Braunwald E: Thrombolytic therapy. A new strategy for the treatment of acute myocardial infarction. N Engl J Med 1984; 311: 770.
24. Passamani ER (ed): Limitation of infarct size with thrombolytic agents. Circulation 1983; 68 (Suppl 1): I-1.
25. Rowley JM, Hill JD: Early reporting of myocardial infarction: impact of an experiment in patient education. Br Med J 1982; 284: 1741.
26. Critical care medicine. Consensus Development Conference. National Institute of Health, 1983; 4: no 6.
27. Roark SF, Wagner GS, Izlar HL, Roe CR: Diagnosis of acute myocardial infarction in a community hospital. Significance of CPK-MB determination. Circulation 1976; 53: 965.
28. Swan HJC, Ganz W, Forrester J, Marcus H, Diamond G, Chonetter D: Catheterization of the heart in man with use of a flow-directed balloon-tipped catheter. N Engl J Med 1970; 283: 447.
29. Bruno FP, Cobb FR, Rivas F, Goodrich JK: Evaluation of 99m technetium stannous pyrophosphate as an imaging agent in acute myocardial infarction. Circulation 1976; 54: 71.
30. Unstable Angina Pectoris Study Group: National Cooperative Study to Compare Surgical and Medical Therapy. II. In-hospital experience and initial follow-up in patients with one, two and three vessel disease. Am J Cardiol 1978; 42: 839.
31. Karliner JS, Gregoratos G: Coronary care. Churchill & Livingstone, New York, 1981.
32. Wyman MG, Hammersmith L: Comprehensive treatment plan for the prevention of primary ventricular fibrillation in acute myocardial infarction. Am J Cardiol 1974; 33: 661.
33. Willerson JT, Curry GC, Watson JT, Leshin SJ, Mullins CB: Intraaortic balloon counter pulsation in patients with cardiogenic shock, medically refractory left ventricular failure, and/or recurrent ventricular tachycardia. Am J Med 1975; 58: 183.
34. Forrester JS, Diamond GA, Swan HJC: Medical therapy of acute myocardial infarctions by the application of hemodynamic subsets. Am J Cardiol 1977; 39: 137.

35. Maroko PR, Kjekhus JK, Sobel BE, Watanabe T, Covell JW, Ross J Jr, Braunwald E: Factors influencing infarct size following experimental coronary artery occlusion. Circulation 1971; 43: 67.
36. Gold HK, Leinbach RC, Maroko PR: Reduction of myocardial injury in patients with acute infarction by propanolol. Circulation 1971; 43: 67.
37. Hugenholtz PG, Boyadijan N: Report to the European Union of Medical Specialists by the subspecialty cardiology, 1980. Brussels.
38. Conti CR: What is a clinical cardiologist in 1984? Am J Cardiol 1984; 54: 229.
39. Tomas Abadal L, Balaguer Vintro I, Bernades Bernat E: Factores de riesgo e incidencia de nuevos casos en el estudio prospectivo de la cardiopatía isquémica de Manresa. Rev Esp Cardiolog 1976; 29: 127.
40. Anuario Banesto del Mercado Español 1984. Sucesores de Rivadeneyra SA, pp 99. Madrid.

12.6 Thrombolysis in Acute Myocardial Infarction

A. BETRIU, M. HERAS and G. SANZ

In the past few years we have learned that myocardial infarction is a relatively gradual process that can be influenced by several interventions [1]. In this regard, reduction of infarct size has been a major clinical issue, since the amount of preserved myocardium will definitely influence the outcome of patients with myocardial infarction [2–5]. Among all the interventions aimed at reducing infarct size, recanalization of the occluded vessel with thrombolytic agents has generated an increasing interest. Early trials began 25 years ago and dealt mainly with intravenous streptokinase (SK) [6, 7]. It is Rentrop, however, who deserves credit for his remarkable work with the use of intracoronary SK [8,9], a route of administration first applied by Chazov [10] and potentiated later by the angiographic documentation of coronary artery thrombosis as the cause of acute occlusion [11]. We have now gained a great deal of experience in the treatment of acute myocardial infarction with thrombolytic agents by using either the intravenous or the intracoronary route [12]. Nevertheless, several questions regarding this therapy in evolving myocardial infarction remain unsettled. In particular, the influence of coronary thrombolysis on both acute and long-term mortality, the critical time interval for the intervention to be initiated, the best drug, its optimal dose and the route of administration, and the management of the residual stenosis remain unknown. We need to answer all these questions before recommending the application of this therapeutic approach to the whole community.

The effect on mortality

The available series dealing with intravenous SK in acute myocardial infarction are not homogeneous, as they differ with respect to the number of patients entered, the time elapsed since the onset of pain to treatment, and the doses administered. Only five out of 22 controlled randomized trials with i.v. SK [6, 7, 13–32] showed a beneficial effect on prognosis. The Italian multicentric study (GISSI) [31] that includes 11806 patients admitted within the first twelve hours after the onset of symptoms, is the largest trial. In that study, 5860 patients were given 1500000 IU i.v. SK in an hour while the remaining 5852 were treated routinely. In-hospital mortality rates at day 21 were 10.7% and 13%, respectively; this accounts for an 18% global reduction in the risk of death with the active treatment (p = 0.0002). Patients presenting with recent onset of pain (less than 3 hours) and no previous myocardial infarction, and those aged 65 years or less and showing an anterior wall infarction seem to benefit the most. The multicentric ISAM study [32], of similar design, failed to show any demonstrable effect on survival at 3 weeks; a possible explanation for this may be the sample size as well as the low mortality rate in the control group, due perhaps to the routine use of i.v. nitroglycerine.

Results obtained with intravenous urokinase (UK) are similar to those with SK. Only one out of four controlled studies showed a beneficial effect on prognosis [33–36].

Series using the intracoronary route are more homogeneous, but the study populations are, in general, small [34–45]. In the Western Washington Study [42, 43] mortality rate at 30 days was 3.7% in the treated group (134 patients) and 11.2% in the control group (116 patients) (p<0.02); this difference lost its statistical significance at the end of the first year of follow-up (8.2% vs 14.7%). However, patients with adequate recanalization of their vessels had significantly lower mortality (2.5%) than patients with poor recanalization (23.1%) or those whose arteries remained occluded (19.6%). Since the one month mortality was so low, the weight assigned to each case appears to be exceedingly high. Authors reported a significant difference in in-hospital mortality between the two groups (p<0.02), a difference that was still present at 1 month. Yet, calculations made using data from figure 1 showed a p value <0.1 (NS) at 2 weeks, implying that the benefit of the first week vanishes in the second week to reappear at 30 days. A type I error may reasonably explain this paradox.

The multicentre Dutch study [44] entered 533 patients; of them, 269 were given intracoronary SK while the remaining 264 were controls. Forty-day mortality was 5.2% in the first group and 9.8% in the second (p<0.05); one year mortality rates were, respectively 8.5% and 15.9% (p<0.01). Criticisms of this trial concern changes introduced in the protocol when the study was already running. The last 117 patients in the treatment group received intravenous SK on arrival, while waiting for coronary angiography. Besides, the number of patients who underwent either coronary artery bypass grafts or angioplasty during the follow-up was higher in the SK group (23% vs 16%; p<0.01). It is obvious that the association of these procedures may have a major impact on prognosis. Finally, it is relevant to comment that the prevalence of ventricular fibrillation in the control group (23%) suggests that patients in this group were by chance at high risk.

Which is the maximal time interval after onset of symptoms to treatment?

On theoretical grounds, the benefit of thrombolysis should be confined to patients who are treated early [46, 47]. The first European Study [13], that analyses separately the outcome of patients treated before and after 12 hours from onset of symptoms, suggests that the beneficial effects of thrombolysis are limited to the former group. In the Italian trial [31] relative risk of death at 3 weeks was 0.74, 0.80, 0.87 and 1.19 for time intervals of 0–3 hours, 3–6 hours, 6–9 hours and 9–12 hours, respectively, since the onset of pain until treatment began. Reduction of mortality within the first three hours was 23%, and that of the first hour, 50%. In keeping with these data, Mathey [48] found the regional wall motion in the infarcted areas to be preserved in 82% of patients treated within the first two hours; this percentage decreased to 46% when treatment was instituted between 2 and 5 hours. Similarly, Koren [49], who treated 53 patients in the early phase (1.7 ± 0.8 hours), showed that preservation of myocardial function was time-dependent; thus, patients treated within the first 90 minutes had better global ejection fraction (56 ± 15 vs $47 \pm 14\%$, $p<0.05$), regional ejection fraction (51 ± 19 vs 34 ± 20, $p<0.01$) and lower QRS score than patients treated between 90 minutes and 4 hours. Davis [50] gave i.v. SK to 8 patients (11 interventions) within 45–120 minutes after onset of pain; none of these patients but one (who curiously had his reperfusion achieved within 60 minutes), developed a myocardial infarction. Moreover, it is important to know that myocardial infarction can still be prevented within the first two hours after the onset of symptoms, a time interval longer than that suggested by experimental coronary artery ligation.

Although time is not the only determinant of infarct following coronary occlusion, the role played by other factors, such as collaterals or intermittent restablishment of flow, is difficult to assess. Therefore, the duration of pain, which can be precisely determined in most patients, is the only variable on which we may rely to make the decision in favor of thrombolytic therapy. Although the ideal candidate is the patient admitted within the first hour after the onset of pain, the benefits of treatment may well be extended to patients arriving within three hours. With longer delays the unsefulness of coronary thrombolysis is doubtful, despite isolated observations [51]. In any case, indications must be settled on an individual basis. For example, we can still consider this treatment in patients with chest pain exceeding 3 hours and absent Q waves on ECG.

Which is the best drug, its optimal dose and the best route of administration?

The ideal drug must have a high thrombolytic power, be selective and easy to administer. Because of its logistic complexity, the future of the coronary route is very limited. Recent trials with intravenous SK have used high doses (700000 to 1500000 IU) [52, 53], which are usually delivered in a short time (1 hour). Although a high patency rate has been reported with this regime (up to 90% in some studies) [54], the few randomized trials comparing intracoronary and intravenous SK have shown the thrombolytic effect of the latter to be weaker [55–57]. Since the angiographic assessment of the coronary circulation is in general delayed (at 1 or 2 weeks) when the venous route is used, a substantial number of occluded vessels that recanalize spontaneously is falsely ascribed to a successful therapy. Results of treatment with i.v. UK are comparable to those achieved with SK, as shown by Tennant et al. [58] in a study that includes 143 patients randomized to UK or SK. Thus, it is hard to justify the use of UK on the basis of its higher costs.

Among selective fibrinolytic drugs, the tissue type fibrinogen activator (t-PA) has recently been obtained by recombinant DNA technology (rt-PA) [60]. At variance with the 'first generation', thrombolytic agents whose effect is based on the activation of circulating plasminogen, rt-PA selectively activates plasminogen in the presence of fibrin, that is, at the surface of the thrombus. Since a generalized lytic state is prevented, the risk of bleeding is considerably reduced. There are two trials, the American [61] and the European [62] studies, comparing the effects of SK and rt-PA given intravenously. Both studies used the same doses, but differed in their design. In the American protocol coronary angiography was performed before treatment administration while in the European study treatment was instituted prior to angiography; thus, the time interval to drug administration was different (almost 5 hours in the American trial and less than 3 in the European). In the former study, 60% of occluded vessels were recanalized by rt-PA and 35% by SK while, in the latter, the corresponding figures were 70% and 55% (in fact, the percentages given by the European workers are an estimate since the state of coronary anatomy prior to treatment was unknown). The rt-PA is a very interesting drug because its effectiveness when administered intravenously is comparable to that of intracoronary SK. However, bleeding complications may occur during catheterization, though they are enhanced by the combined use of heparin.

Prourokinase (pro-UK) (urokinase precursor) is another selective fibrinolytic agent whose half-life is longer than that of rt-PA [63]. Ongoing trials should demonstrate its effectiveness. APSAC (previously known as BRL 26.921) is an acylated derivative of SK, with selective thrombolytic action, that can be delivered in a short time (10–15 minutes). Been et al. [64], in a recent study, have analyzed the results of a series of 32 patients randomly allocated to the drug or placebo. At 90 minutes all the vessels in the treatment group were patent while only 2 coronary arteries of the placebo group were patent.

Despite the fact that this is a small group of patients, and previous catheterization was not performed, these excellent results are encouraging. Preliminary results of a French multicenter study including 50 patients have shown a higher percent of recanalization with APSAC than with SK (76% vs 64% respectively, at 90 minutes) [65].

Should we treat the residual stenosis?

Obstructive lesions complicated with thrombosis are usually severe, ranging from 60% to 95% of the luminal diameter [66]. Two approaches have been proposed to deal with the residual lesion, aortocoronary bypass and angioplasty. An aggressive treatment may be justified if one takes into account the high rate of reocclusion (13% to 25%) [67] after successful thrombolysis. In addition, reinfarction seems to be prevalent among patients in whom recanalization was achieved, as shown by the Dutch trial (at one year follow-up, 36 patients, or 13%, in the treated group and 16 patients, or 6% in the control group had a reinfarction; p<0.01) [44]. Similarly, the Italian trial found a different reinfarction rate between their two groups at 3 months (3.9% vs 2.1%, respectively) [31].

Although revascularization by means of an aortocoronary bypass operation in acute myocardial infarction can be performed with a surprisingly low risk, with or without previous thrombolysis [68, 69], controlled studies are lacking. As far as angioplasty is concerned, the preliminary results reported by Meyer [70] are of great interest. This trial includes 162 patients randomized to intracoronary thrombolysis alone (79 patients) or to intracoronary thrombolysis associated with angioplasty (83 patients); at 3 weeks, the mean residual stenosis of the first group was 73%, and 29% in the second group, whereas reocclusion rates were 18% and 12% and reinfarction rates 11% and 5%, respectively. Thrombolysis combined with acute angioplasty poses a logistic problem that a better knowledge of the natural history of reocclusion may allow us to circumvent. In this regard, it is interesting to note that 28 patients with total coronary occlusion receiving thrombolytic therapy and having had sequential angiographic evaluation showed reocclusion rates of 8.3% and 18% at one and ten days, respectively [71]. If low reocclusion rates within the first 24 hours after thrombolysis are confirmed, angioplasty could be delayed, thus facilitating widespread use of this procedure.

Conclusion

From this review of previous trials we conclude that thrombolytic therapy in acute myocardial infarction could now be extended to the community, provided that treatment is delivered within the first few hours after onset of chest pain in patients with no contraindications. Any delay should be avoided and this particularly applies to time wasted in-hospital. Until second generation drugs become commercially available, intravenous SK seems an adequate agent. Further investigation is still required to assess the benefits of combined procedures.

References

1. Braunwald E, Maroko PR: The reduction of infarct size – an idea whose time (for testing) has come. Circulation 1974; 50: 206–209.
2. Taylor GJ, Humphries JO, Mellits ED et al.: Predictors of clinical course, coronary anatomy and left ventricular function after recovery from acute myocardial infarction. Circulation 1980; 62: 960–970.
3. Hammermeister KE, De Rouen TA, Dodge HT: Survival analysis in medically and surgically treated patients with coronary disease: a critical review and experience in Seattle Heart Watch, a nonrandomized series. In: Hurst JW (ed) The heart. Update II. McGraw-Hill, New York, 1980; 239–253.
4. Sanz G, Castañer A, Betriu A et al.: Determinants of prognosis in survivors of myocardial infarction. A prospective clinical angiographic study. N Engl J Med 1982; 306: 1065–1070.
5. De Feyter PJ, Van Eenge MJ, Dighton DM et al.: Prognostic value of exercise testing, coronary angiography and left ventriculography 6–8 weeks after myocardial infarction. Circulation 1982; 66: 527–536.
6. Fletcher AP, Sherry S, Alkjaersig N, Smyrniotis FE, Jick S: The maintenance of a sustained thrombolytic state in man. II Clinical observations on patients with myocardial infarction and other thromboembolic disorders. J Clin Invest 1959; 38: 1111–1119.
7. Dewar HA, Stephenson P, Horler AR et al.: Fibrinolytic therapy of coronary thrombosis. Controlled trial of 75 cases. Br Med J 1963; 1: 915–920.
8. Rentrop KP, Blanke H, Karsh KR et al.: Acute myocardial infarction intracoronary application of nitroglycerin and streptokinase. Clin Cardiol 1979; 2: 354–363.
9. Rentrop KP, Blanke H, Karsh KR, Kaiser H, Köstering H, Leitz K: Selective intracoronary thrombolysis in acute myocardial infarction and unstable angina pectoris. Circulation 1981; 63: 307–317.
10. Chazov EI, Matveeva LS, Mazaev KV, Sargin KE, Sadovskaya GV, Ruda MY: Intracoronary administration of fibrinolysis in acute myocardial infarction. Ter Arkh 1976; 48: 8–9.
11. De Wood MA, Spores J, Notske R et al.: Prevalence of total coronary occlusion during the early hours of transmural myocardial infarction. Ann Intern Med 1982; 96: 115.
12. Yusuf J, Collins R, Peto R, et al.: Intravenous and intracoronary fibrinolytic therapy in acute myocardial infarction. Overview of results on mortality, reinfarction and side-effects from 33 randomized controlled trials. Eur Heart J 1985; 6: 556–585.
13. Amery A, Roeberg G, Vermenlen HJ, Verstraete M: Single-blind randomized multicentre trial comparing heparin and streptokinase treatment in recent myocardial infarction. Acta Med Scand Suppl 1969; 505: 5–35.
14. Heikenheimo R, Ahrenberg P, Honkapohja H, et al.: Fibrinolytic treatment in acute myocardial infarction. Acta Med Scand 1971; 189: 7–13.
15. Diognardi N, Mannucci PM, Lotto A, et al.: Controlled trial of streptokinase and heparin in acute myocardial infarction. Lancet 1971; 11: 891–895.

16. European Working Party: Streptokinase in recent myocardial infarction: a controlled multi-centric trial. Br Med J 1971; 11: 325–331.

17. Breddin K, Ehrby AM, Fecheer L, et al.: Die kurzzeit Fibrinolyse beim akuten Myokardin-farkt. Dtsch Med Wochenschr 1973; 98: 325–331.

18. Australian Multicenter Trial of Streptokinase in Acute Myocardial Infarction. Med J Aust 1977; 1: 553.

19. Ness PM, Simon TL, Cole C, Walston A: A pilot study of streptokinase therapy in acute myocardial infarction: observations on complications and relation to trial design. Am Heart J 1974; 88: 705–712.

20. Frank (Zielinski) B: Traitement de l'infarctus du myocarde par la streptokinase. Thèse pour le Doctorat en Medecine. Faculté de Medecine, Bichat-Beaujon, Université Paris, 1975.

21. Valere PE, Guerot C, Castielo-Ferroy A, et al.: L'infarctus myocardique. Traitement par la streptoquinase. La Nouvelle Presse Medicale 1975; 4: 192.

22. Aber CP, Bass NM, Beni CL, et al.: Streptokinase in acute myocardial infarction: a con-trolled multicenter study in the United Kingdom. Br Med J 1976; 2: 1100–1104.

23. Klein W, Pavek P, Brandt D et al.: Resultate einer doppelblind studie beim myokardinfarkt. En: Siler S (ed) Die Fibrinolysebehaudbrung des akuten Myokardinfarktes. Verlag Bruder Hollinek, Viena, 1976; 65–73.

24. Poliwoda H, Scheider B, Averanins HJ. Untersuch ungen zum Klinischen Verlant des akuten myokard infarktes. Gemeinschaftsstudie an 26 krankenhausern in Nord Deutschland. Med Klin 1977; 72: 451–458.

25. Benda V, Haider M, Ambrosch P: Ergebnisse der Osterreickischen Herzinfarkstudie mit streptokinase. Resultados del estudio austríaco sobre el efecto de la estreptoquinasa en el infarto de miocardio. Wien Klin Wochenschr 1977; 89: 779–783.

26. Witchitz S, Kolsky H, Moisson P, Chiché P: Streptokinase et infarctus du myocarde aigu. La fibrinolyse peût-elle limiter la necrose? Ann Cardiol Angiol 1977; 26: 53–56.

27. Lasierra C, Vilades J, Fernández C, et al.: Estreptoquinasa en el infarto agudo de miocardio. Revista Clínica Española 1977; 144: 251–257.

28. The European Co-operative Study Group: Streptokinase in acute myocardial infarction. Extended report of the European Co-operative trial. Acta Med Scand Suppl 1981; 648: 7–57.

29. Olson HG, Lyons KP, Butmar J, et al.: A randomized controlled trial of intravenous streptokinase in acute myocardial infarction. Circulation 1984; 70 (Suppl II): 155 (Abstract).

30. Schreiber TL, Miller DH, Borer JS, et al.: Efficacy of intravenous heparin versus streptoki-nase in acute myocardial infarction (Abstract). Circulation 1984; 70 (Suppl 2): 27.

31. GISSI: Effectiveness of intravenous thrombolytic treatment in acute myocardial infarction. Lancet 1986; 8478: 397–401.

32. The ISAM Study Group: A prospective trial of intravenous streptokinase in acute myocardial infarction: Mortality, morbidity and infarct size at 21 days. New Engl J Med 1986; 314: 1465–1471.

33. Lippschrutz EJ, Ambrus JC, Ambrus CM, et al.: Controlled study on the treatment of coronary occlusion with urokinase-activated human plasmin. Am J Cardiol 1965; 16: 93–98.

34. Gormsen J, Tidstrom B, Feddersen C, Plong J: Biochemical evaluation of low dose of urokinase in acute myocardial infarction. A double blind study. Acta Med Scand 1973; 194: 191–198.

35. Brochier M, Raynand R, Planiol T, et al.: Le traitement par l'urokinase des infarctus du myocarde et syndromes de menace. Etude randomisée de 120 cas. Arch Mal Coeur 1975; 68: 563.

36. European Collaborative Study: Controlled trial of urokinase in myocardial infarction. Lancet 1975; 11: 624–626.

37. Khaja F, Walson JA, Brymar JF, et al.: Intracoronary fibrinolytic therapy in acute myocardial infarction. N Engl J Med 1983; 303: 1304.

38. Anderson JL, Marshall HW, Bray BE, et al.: A randomized trial of intracoronary streptokinase in the treatment of acute myocardial infarction. N Engl J Med 1983; 303: 1312.

39. Leiboff RH, Katz RJ, Wasserman AG, et al.: A randomized angiographically controlled trial of intracoronary streptokinase in acute myocardial infarction. Am J Cardiol 1984; 53: 404.

40. Rentrop KP, Feit F, Blanke H, et al.: Effects of intracoronary streptokinase and intracoronary nitroglycerine infusion on coronary angiographic patterns and mortality in patients with acute myocardial infarction. N Engl J Med 1984; 311: 1464.

41. Raizner AE, Tortoledo FA, Verani MS, et al.: Intracoronary thrombolytic therapy in acute myocardial infarction. A prospective randomized controlled trial. Am J Cardiol 1985; 55: 301–308.

42. Kennedy JW, Ritchie JL, Davis KB, et al.: The Western Washington randomized trial of intracoronary streptokinase in acute myocardial infarction. A 12 month follow-up report. N Engl J Med; 1985; 312: 1073–1078.

43. Kennedy JW, Ritchie JL, Davis KB, Fritz JK: Western Washington randomized trial of intracoronary streptokinase in acute myocardial infarction. N Engl J Med 1983; 309: 1477–1482.

44. Simoons ML, Brand M, Zwaan C, et al.: Improved survival after early thrombolysis in acute myocardial infarction. Lancet 1985; 11: 578–581.

45. Anderson JL, Mc Ilvaine PM, Marshall HW: Long-term follow-up after intracoronary streptokinase for myocardial infarction. A randomized, controlled study. Am Heart J 1984; 108: 1402–1408.

46. Théroux P, Ross J, Franklin D, Kemper WS, Sasayaura S: Coronary arterial reperfusion. III Early and late effects on regional myocardial function and dimensions in conscious dogs. Am J Cardiol 1976; 38: 599–610.

47. Maroko PR, Libby P, Ginks W: Coronary artery reperfusion. I Early effects on local myocardial function and extent of myocardial necrosis. J Clin Invest 1972; 51: 2710.

48. Mathey DG, Sheehan FM, Shofer J, Dodge HT. Time from onset of symptoms to thrombolytic therapy: A major determinant of myocardial salvage in patients with acute transmural infarction. JACC 1985; 6: 518–525.

49. Koren G, Weiss AT, Hasin Y: Prevention of myocardial damage in acute myocardial ischemia by early treatment with intravenous streptokinase. N Engl J Med 1985; 313: 1384–1389.

50. Davies GJ, Chierchia S. Maseri A: Prevention of myocardial infarction by very early treatment with intracoronary streptokinase. N Engl J Med 1984; 311: 1488–1492.

51. Smalling RW, Fuentes F, Freund GC, et al.: Beneficial effects of intracoronary thrombolysis up to eighteen hours after onset of pain in evolving myocardial infarction. Am Heart J 1982; 104: 912–920.

52. Schröder R, Biamino G, Leitner ER, et al.: Intravenous short-term infusion of streptokinase in acute myocardial infarction. Circulation 1983; 67: 536–548.

53. Neuhaus KL, Tebbe U, Saner G, Kreuzer H, Köstering H: High dose intravenous streptokinase in acute myocardial infarction. Clin Cardiol 1983; 6: 426–434.

54. Ganz W, Buchbinder N, Marcus H, et al.: Intracoronary thrombolysis in evolving myocardial infarction. Am Heart J 1981; 101: 4–10.

55. Saltups A, Boxal J, Ho B: Intracoronary versus intravenous streptokinase in acute myocardial infarction. Circulation 1983; 68 (Suppl 3): 111–119.

56. Rogers WJ, Mantle JA, Hood WP Jr, Baxley WA, Whitlow PL, Reeves RC, Soto B: Prospective randomized trial of intravenous and intracoronary streptokinase in acute myocardial infarction. Circulation 1983; 68: 1051.

57. Blunda M, Meister SG, Schechter JA, Pickerning NJ, Wolf NH: Intravenous versus intracoronary streptokinase for acute transmural myocardial infarction. Catheter and cardiovasc Diag 1984; 10: 319–327.

638

58. Tennant SN, Dixon J, Venable TC, et al.: Intracoronary thrombolysis in patients with acute myocardial infarction: comparison of the efficacy of urokinase with streptokinase. Circulation 1984; 69: 756–760.

59. Van de Werf F, Ludhook PA, Bergmann SR, et al.: Coronary thrombolysis with tissue-type plasminogen activator in patients with evolving myocardial infarction. N Engl J Med 1984; 310: 609–613.

60. Van de Werf F, Bergmann SR, Fox KAA, et al.: Coronary thrombolysis with intravenously administered human tissue-type plasminogen activator produced by recombinant DNA technology. Circulation 1984; 69: 605–610.

61. The TIMI Study Group: The thrombolysis in myocardial infarction (TIMI) trial. Phase I findings. N Engl J Med 1985; 312: 932–936.

62. Verstraete M, Bory M, Colle D, et al.: Randomized trial of intravenous recombinant tissue-type plasminogen activator versus intravenous streptokinase in acute myocardial infarction. Report from the European Cooperative Study Group for recombinant tissue-type plasminogen activator. Lancet 1985; 1: 842–847.

63. Golasmith MF: Pro-UK. Another entry in the thrombolytic arena. JAMA 1985; 253: 1694–1695.

64. Been M, De Bono DP, Muir AL, et al.: Coronary thrombolysis with intravenous anisolated plasminogen streptokinase complex. BRL. Br Heart J 1985; 53: 253–259.

65. Brochier M, Garnier LF: Multicenter European trial with intravenous acylated SK (BRL 26921) versus heparin. Personal communication on the international symposium. Facts and hopes in thrombolysis in acute MI. Aachen, 1985.

66. Marx W, Dorr R, Rentrop P: Evaluation of the effectiveness of intracoronary streptokinase infusion in acute myocardial infarction. Post-procedure management and hospital course in 204 patients. Am Heart J 1981; 102: 1181.

67. Rutsch W, Scharti M, Moffy D, et al.: Percutaneous trans luminal coronary recanalization: procedure results and acute complications. Am Heart J 1981; 102: 1178.

68. De Wood MA, Spores J, Notske R et al.: Medical and surgical management of myocardial infarction. Am J Cardiol 1979; 44: 1356.

69. Phillips SJ, Zeff RH, Kongtawon C: Surgical therapy for evolving myocardial infarction: results in 138 patients. Herz 1981; 6: 55.

70. Meyer J: Early PTCA after thrombolysis. Heart and Circulation 1986; 1 (Suppl 1): 10–11.

71. Chesebro JH, Smith HC, Holmes DR, et al.: Reoclussion and clot lysis between 90 minutes, 1 day and 10 days after thrombolytic therapy for myocardial infarction (Abstract). Circulation 1985; 72 (Suppl 3): 55.

12.7 Conclusions

C. CREXELLS

Department of Nymodynamics, Hospital de la Santa Creu i Sant Pau, Barcelona, Spain

The experience of Dr Rentrop indicates that there is no difference in vessel patency 15 days after infarction between patients treated with streptokinase and those treated with nitroglycerin. Only patients with low ejection fraction had a mild improvement of this variable in the stroptokinase group. In this experiment, all the patients were treated within three hours of the onset of clinical symptoms. The methodologic rigor of this study and its results oblige us to continue to plan absolutely controlled experiments in this field to obtain as much information as possible in each case. For this reason, Dr Rentrop is of the opinion that intravenous treatment and determination of results by indirect methods are unreliable.

The introduction of new thrombolytic agents as tissue-type plasminogen activator will probably modify the short and long term results of thrombolysis.

At the same time that fibrinolytic therapy was being introduced early surgical reperfusion in acute myocardial infarction was also started. Doctor M.A. de Wood has shown us his experience in this field and has reviewed the most important series published up to now. The good results obtained in early surgical revascularization justify according to this author this attitude even in uncomplicated cases.

When both thrombolytic therapy and early surgical treatment of acute myocardial infarction were being developped coronary angioplasty appeared and has already been used in the treatment of residual lesion after thrombolysis. This approach will have to be validated and its results compared with that of surgical revascularization and of medical treatment alone.

Dr López-Sendón contributed an extensive experience in postinfarctional cardiac rupture, a complication associated with sudden death. In Dr López-Sendón's experience, some cases of subacute rupture followed by pseudoaneurysm due to pericardial apposition are susceptible to surgical patch treatment. From this observation can be deduced the importance of early diagnosis in which not only hemodynamic monitoring but the alertness and knowledge of the cardiologist are indispensable. This chapter cannot be considered concluded and new research is needed to ascertain early diagnostic signs, although it is difficult because of the relative rarity of this complication.

Finally, Dr Vicente Valle contributed a very interesting experience with the type and function of coronary units, and Dr A. Betriu reviewed the problems of thrombolysis in acute myocardial infarction.

The coronary unit of the future should establish a much more intense relationship with the Cardiac Surgery and Hemodynamics units. The studies by Rentrop, De Wood and López-Sendón, with the perspectives they open up, can only be continued within the framework of a narrow collaboration between these three units.

13. Myocardial Infarction (II)
Primary and secondary prevention

13.1 Introduction

F. NAVARRO LOPEZ

The second chapter dedicated to myocardial infarction will concentrate mainly on topics concerning primary and secondary prevention, presently an object of preferential attention in the literature.

In the first place, Dr I. Balaguer, of the Epidemiology Department of the Hospital de San Pablo, will review the state of treatment for hyperlipidemias. This subject has never lost validity and we now view it with different eyes since recent experimental and clinical research have been found to support the suspicion, as yet unconfirmed, that atherosclerosis is reversible, that is, that atheroma plaques can thin with cholesterol-reducing treatment. The results of a primary prevention study by the *Lipid Research Clinics* (LRC-CPPT), published in 1984, have conclusively demonstrated for the first time that reduction of cholesterol levels in blood can prevent myocardial infarction.

For the last decades, the association of cholesterol and coronary risk has been speculated on, although none of the numerous trials so far realized have been able to definitely confirm the efficacy of treatment to reduce lipemia. It suffices to recall the famous trials of the Coronary Drug Project and the Veterans Administration Cooperative Study. Finally, this 10-year clinical trial, one of largest in scope and most expensive in the history of medicine has demonstrated that administration of cholestiramine or placebo to more than 3,800 individuals with cholesterol levels over 256 mg/dl (selected from almost half a million possible candidates) can reduce cholesterolemia by an average of 8.5%, the incidence of infarction by 19% and cardiac mortality by 25%.

After this study, primary prevention of infarction has probably attained a previously inexistent clinical dimension. It poses the need that the physician prescribe and supervise long-term drug treatment in circumstances that until now did not seem to justify it.

Another controversial problem is that of long-term preventive treatment of patients who have had myocardial infarction. Today we know the natural history of these patients in detail and we know the risk they have of suffering coronary complications or premature death, although we are still not convinced that the prognosis can be favorably influenced. Among other reasons for this attitude, in the fact that the principal long-term determinant factors are: the degree of residual ventricular dysfunction, as reflected in percentage ejection fraction, and the number and severity of coronary lesions, in large measure predetermined at the time of infarction and apparently not very susceptible to modification.

Therapeutic measures proposed to prevent the disease's progress or palliate the consequences of ischemia are varied, but they have changed little since the 70s. Exercise, control of atherogenic risk factors, use of anticoagulants or antiarrhythmics and coronary revascularization surgery have been recommended. They have been recently received sharp criticism because none has passed the test of a controlled clinical trial.

At the beginning of the 80s, two new treatments seemed to destined to assume an important role in the prophylaxis of these patients: β-blocking agents and platelet antiaggregants. While platelet antiaggregants have still not offered any guarantee of effectiveness, the β-blocking agents have shown that they can reduce cardiac mortality by 20–25%, especially confirmed by Norwegian multicenter studies of timolol and 'BHAT'.

In view of these results, it seems difficult to continue with a *wait and see* attitude, withholding all prophylactic treatment, but it is not easy to accept the need for the *systematic administration* of β-blocking agents to every patient who has suffered a myocardial infarction, when we know that in an elevated percentage of cases an excellent prognosis is expected. It would be helpful if we knew the mechanisms of preventive action of these drugs to be able to detect the patient subgroups that might benefit from treatment. This would allow us to make *selective* preventive treatments, which presently seems impossible. Drs C. Permanyer, A. Castañer and G. Sanz will analyze the present situation of this problem in depth and orient us as to the most rational guidelines of therapeutic approaches in the light of present knowledge.

13.2 How, When and Whom to Treat for Dyslipemia

I. BALAGUER VINTRÓ

Clinical interest in the plasma lipid disorders continues to be centered on the contribution of hyperlipidemias to the risk of cardiovascular disease.

Advances in the study of dyslipemias, including the contributions of genetic biology, have shifted the focal point from the study of the plasma lipid components to the lipoproteins that transport them and their protein fractions. The classification of hyperlipoproteinemia phenotypes is still a valid basis for therapy [1]. Ninety-five per cent of the hyperlipemias observed are of exogenous origin and are therefore conditioned by dietetic habits. For individual control of patients with moderately increased plasma lipids, the key is diet. For severe forms (cholesterol above 350 mg and triglycerides over 500 mg in the index examination) and resistant moderate forms (cholesterol above 260 mg and triglycerides superior to 300 mg after several months of an adequate diet), drug treatment is indicated.

Quantitative and qualitative alterations in plasma lipids are termed dyslipemias. We will not consider here the diseases characterized by deposits of unaltered plasma lipid fractions (lipoidosis) [2, 3].

Quantitative determination of cholesterol and triglycerides (constituting, with the phospholipids, the principal plasma lipid components) is a good method for identifying and following-up hyperlipidemias [4].

Since the lipids are not soluble in plasma, they are transported in blood combined with proteins, forming compounds that are called lipoproteins. Since Fredrickson et al [1] classified the hyperlipoproteinemias in 1967, the various dyslipemias have been interpreted as lipoprotein, not lipid, abnormalities. There has been a progressive tendency to attribute the different hyperlipoproteinemias to alterations in the apolipoprotein or apoprotein fractions [5].

Although there are disorders due to the absence or reduction of certain lipoproteins or apoprotein fractions, the principal interest of clinicians lies in the hyperlipidemias because of their relationship with the risk of atherosclerotic complications and early onset of this disease. Other complications of hyperlipemias are the formation of deposits in skin and in extensor tendons, and gastrointestinal disorders due to alterations in triglyceride absorption [3].

Hyperlipemias as coronary risk indicators

These disorders are divided into endogenous and exogenous hyperlipemia. The most frequent cause of hyperlipemia is diet (exogenous hyperlipemia). Average cholesterol in a population correlates with fat consumption, especially saturated fats, as demonstrated by epidemiological studies such as that directed by Ancel Keys in 18 communities in 7 countries [6, 7]. Within each population, individual cholesterol levels also depend on congenital or acquired metabolic lipoprotein anomalies (primary or secondary endogenous hyperlipemias).

Total cholesterol concentration continues to be a good predictor for risk of coronary heart disease, although it was established in 1966 [8] that it loses predictive value with age. Most cholesterol is transported in plasma by low density lipoproteins and the rest almost exclusively by high density lipoproteins. The relationship between total cholesterol and coronary risk is directly determined by the low density lipoproteins and can be measured as LDL cholesterol. By contrast, the high density lipoproteins, measured as HDL cholesterol, correlate inversely with coronary risk according to observations first made in 1951.

The principal protein marker for identifying low density lipoproteins (LDL) is apo-B 100. The high density lipoprotein marker is apo-A-I, although the fraction that apparently correlates inversely with coronary risk is apo-A-II [10]. Although the cholesterol of this last lipoproteic fraction (HDL2 cholesterol) can be obtained by precipitation, the quantity involved is so small that minimal analytic errors produce important deviations in risk calculations. An attempt is being made to determine if apo-B or apo-A-I concentrations may be better indicators than LDL and HDL cholesterol. Some angiographic studies suggest this, but not definitively [11, 12].

Molecular biologists have begun to identify the genes of diverse apoproteins [5]. The first gene identified was that of apo-A-I, followed by that of apo-E, a protein fraction that serves as a marker for very low density lipoproteins. It is anticipated that the LDL receptor gene will be indentified in the future. The apo-B 100 gene is a more complex problem since it is a large protein.

The relationship between hyperlipemia and coronary risk has been confirmed in all the epidemiological studies, and it is considered to be one of the three principal coronary risk factors, together with hypertension and smoking. The elevated incidence and early onset of coronary heart disease in familial hypercholesterolemia make this endogenous hyperlipoproteinemia a clear-cut example of the relationship between cholesterol and atherosclerosis [13].

The epidemiological studies of primary prevention carried out in the seventies did not provide conclusions on the preventive efficacy of reducing cholesterol in the adult diet. In reality, only a modest reduction in cholesterol was achieved in the group studied [14]. However, in the study by the Lipid Research Clinics on primary prevention in cases of hyperlipemia, a significant correlation was found between changes in cholesterol concentration and attenuation of risk [15]. This confirms the findings by earlier studies in subgroups in which a larger decrease in cholesterol was achieved.

How can hyperlipemia be detected?

The simplest method for identifying most hyperlipemias is quantification of total serum cholesterol [6]. Although a cholesterol determination can be included in any routine analysis of the population, there are groups that may benefit more from analysis (Table 1).

Aside from serum cholesterol determination, if we examine the physical appearance of the serum under fasting conditions, we can detect significant hypertriglyceridemias. This simple test has a marked predictive value, as reported by Havel in 1970 [16]. Determination of triglycerides or their equivalent, the proportion of VLDL lipoproteins, serves to complete hyperlipemia detection.

The existence of qualitative dyslipemias can be suspected in the absence of increased cholesterol and/or triglycerides. Studies of average total cholesterol and HDL cholesterol, and the ratio between them in diverse populations, shows that there is a parallel between both values: populations with low total cholesterol concentrations also have low mean HDL cholesterol [17]. This

Table 1. When should a serum cholesterol study be requested?

1. In patients under 70 years of age with coronary heart disease, peripheral vascular obliteration or cerebrovascular disease
2. Children and siblings of all patients with coronary heart disease of onset before 50 years, or before 70 years if the patient had hypercholesterolemia
3. Individuals under 60 years if they are hypertensive and/or smoke more than 10 cigarettes a day
4. Children, siblings and other family members under 70 years of persons diagnosed as having hereditary hypercholesterolemia
5. Individuals with abnormal ECG at rest and/or positive effort test in the absence of clinical manifestations
6. Individuals with family history of premature death, coronary heart disease or diabetes
7. Before prescription of oral contraceptives
8. In candidates for pilot, railroad engineer and professionals who may endanger other persons

finding suggests that a reduction of HDL cholesterol in the presence of low total cholesterol may not reduce coronary risk.

Classification of the hyperlipoproteinemias

The classification of hyperlipoproteinemia phenotypes proposed by Fredrickson et al. in 1967 [1] is still valid. It includes some very infrequent forms, such as primary endogenous hyperlipemia (types I, III and V), as well as common forms. Among the latter are both primary and secondary disorders, such as exogenous hyperlipemias secondary to diet (types II and IV).

Exogenous hypertriglyceridemia (type I) is the only hyperlipemia not associated with ischemic heart disease. It is caused by a defect in lipase activity for fat clearance, which impedes intestinal triglyceride absorption. Type III was originally described as the presence of an abnormal lipoprotein (wide beta) and it is currently attributed to an error in apo-E [5]. It is clinically characterized by xanthomas in the palms of the hands and it is associated with ischemic heart disease and cerebral and peripheral atherosclerosis.

Type V corresponds to the sum of endogenous and exogenous hypertriglyceridemia and can present as a primary disorder in some phases of primary endogenous hypertriglyceridemia and in poorly controlled insulin-dependent diabetes.

The two most frequent types are those classified as II and IV by Fredrickson. Type II corresponds to either isolated hypercholesterolemia (type IIa) or hypercholesterolemia associated with hypertriglyceridemia (type IIb). What is characteristic of type II is the increase in LDL lipoproteins. Three endogenous forms were discovered: familial hypercholesterolemia, mixed familial hyperlipemia and polygenetic hypercholesterolemia [18].

Familial hypercholesterolemia is a stereotype of the relationship between the metabolic disorder and human arteriosclerosis. In the homozygotic form, there is clinical arteriosclerosis in the first two decades of life, often associated with valvular stenoses due to cholesterol deposits and polyarthritis, which can be erroneously diagnosed as rheumatic fever. Of the heterozygotes, half of the males present clinical heart disease before 50.

After the first clinical symptoms appear, coronary arteriography reveals severe, diffuse lesions of the three coronary trunks and their distal vessels, which makes the possibility of surgery remote [13]. Hereditary hypercholesterolemia is observed in 1 out of 200 to 500 adults. Endogamy favors the presentation of homozygotic forms. In contrast with other primary hyperlipemias, familial hypercholesterolemia can be diagnosed in umbilical cord blood, a measure that could be included in the studies for detecting other genetic anomalies.

Moderate forms of hypercholesterolemia not dependent on diet can correspond to frustrated forms of familial hypercholesterolemia or secondary forms. Of these, the most frequent are those observed in liver diseases, where they are accompanied by qualitative lipoprotein changes, and in slow-onset adult hypothyroidism, often diagnosed late.

Type IV corresponds to primary or secondary hypertriglyceridemias. The primary forms present with very high triglyceride levels and are rare. Secondary forms appear with moderate triglyceride increases related to diabetes or alcohol intake.

When and how should hypercholesterolemia be treated?

There are two prevalent postures with respect to the level at which a reduction in plasma cholesterol should be recommended. In comparisons of average cholesterol in populations in different countries, it has been found that the lower average cholesterol concentration, the lower is the coronary risk [6]. This would justify reducing individual cholesterol levels as much as possible. Nonetheless, various epidemiological studies have demonstrated that coronary risk does not decline below a certain cholesterol level, around 220 mg/dl [20]. Moreover, different prospective studies suggest that under 180 mg/dl the risk of death from cancer increases, especially intestinal cancer [21]. Although these findings have not been confirmed by other epidemiological studies, at the moment it would be advisable to limit cholesterol reduction to a minimum of 220 mg/dl. In practical terms, three serum cholesterol concentrations can be differentiated for purposes of control in the adult.

Cholesterol between 220 and 260 mg

A diet poor in saturated fats, refined sugars and total calories should be recommended. The objective is to avoid the increment in serum cholesterol that occurs with age. Control is more important in the presence of other main risk factors for coronary heart disease.

Cholesterol between 260 and 350 mg

Control should begin with diet. Most moderate hypercholesterolemias are exogenous and responsive to modifications in diet. Further analysis to determine more precisely the type of hyperlipemia are not necessary until we confirm that it is resistant to diet. However, in all moderate hypercholesterolemias, a complete clinical examination should be done to exclude secondary hypercholesterolemia (hypothyroidism, liver diseases, etc.).

Cholesterol over 350 mg or resistant to diet

The biochemical studies should include an examination of the physical aspect of the serum, triglyceride and cholesterol lipoprotein determinations, apoprotein analysis and simple electrophoresis, depending on laboratory facilities. The objective is to analyze the lipoprotein phenotype to correctly classify the type of hyperlipemia. A clinical examination for xanthomas and a study of family members should be made to exclude secondary forms.

Pharmacological hypercholesterolemia treatment

Drug treatment of hyperlipidemias should be reserved for primary endogenous forms and should be accompanied by diet and control of other risk factors, such as inactivity, obesity and diabetes. In other words, pharmacologic treatment is indicated in individuals under 60 with persistent levels of more than 260 mg [22].

There is no ideal drug for reducing serum cholesterol. None is sufficiently effective in all cases and the number of adverse reactions correlated more closely to the frequency and duration of the prescription than to the characteristics of the product.

Cholestyramine. This is a resin that chelates bile acids in the intestine, making them unabsorbable. Continued administration of bile acid chelating agents stimulates synthesis of cholesterol and fatty acids but the net result of the various metabolic interactions is a reduction in serum cholesterol and LDL cholesterol of 20–30% over initial levels. It does not seem to have a significant effect on triglycerides. It is recommended that cholestyramine be given in 8 g doses every 12 hours, preferably dissolved in skim milk. Cholestipol is another bile acid chelating resin used at doses of 20 g/day but it is not commercially available in Spain.

Clofibrate. This is the first of a large series of medications with similar effects. The reduction in cholesterol obtained with clofibrate is moderate, although it varies markedly from one case to another. The main indication for clofibrate is type III and IV hyperlipoproteinemias. The dose varies between 1.5 and 2 g/day.

Probucol. At a dose of 1 g/day, probucol produces a 13% decrease in total cholesterol without modifying HDL cholesterol or triglycerides [23]. Although its half-life is prolonged, no adverse effects have been seen during long-term administration.

Bezafibrate. This produces an effect on the lipids consisting in a sharp decline in LDL and triglycerides and a moderate reduction in total cholesterol with an increase in HDL cholesterol. It is used at a dosage of 450 to 600 mg/day [24].

Phenofibrate. This drug reduces both cholesterol and triglycerides. It is used at a dosage of 300 mg/day.

When and how should hypertriglyceridemia be treated?

There is no unanimity of opinion as to whether an isolated increase in triglycerides is a cardiovascular risk factor [25]. Most often, the increase in triglycerides is associated with other factors, such as diabetes and obesity, that are frequently admitted risks.

The practical course is to begin with diet in patients with triglyceride levels under 500 mg, or with drugs and diet in patients with higher levels. Physical exercise and control of obesity help to reduce triglycerides in individuals with moderate increases. In our environment, it should be remembered that alcohol intake is the most frequent cause of moderate symptomatic hypertriglyceridemia.

In the pharmacological treatment of hypertriglyceridemias, the drug most used is clofibrate, which produces a normalization of triglyceride levels in type III and IV endogenous forms. For type V, nicotinic acid is preferable.

Yatrogenic hyperlipemias

Utilization of plasma lipid reducing drugs that act only on certain fractions has led to studies of possible contradictory effects; for example, if LDL reduction is accompanied by a larger decrease in HDL or VLDL declines with the increase in LDL. Numerous studies demonstrate the existence of some of these effects, but the changes observed are generally slight. Another interesting iatrogenic aspect is the modification of the plasma lipid concentration with medications used on a long-term basis for other indications. This is very important when drugs are being given to prevent complications of other risk factors, as is the case with some of the most commonly used hypotensive medications, for instance β-blocking agents [26, 27]. Only a very objective assessment of the contribution of each risk factor will allow us to evaluate these interactions [28]. The diuretics can also increase low density lipoproteins and produce other metabolic effects on glycemia, uric acid and kaliemia.

652

References

1. Fredrickson DS, Levy RI, Lees RS: Fat transport ion lipoproteins: an integrated approach to mechanisms and disorders. *N Engl J Med* 1967; 276: 148–156.
2. Thannhauser SJ: *Lipoidosis.* Ed Científico-Médica, Barcelona, 1961.
3. Search RL: *Lipopathies.* Charles C Thomas, Springfield, 1971.
4. Balaguer Vintró I, Corominas Vilardell A: *Hiperlipidemias. Tratamiento dietético y farmacología.* JIMS, Barcelona, 1975.
5. Thompson G: Apoproteins: determinants of lipoprotein metabolism and indices of coronary risk. *Br Heart J,* 1984; 51: 585–588.
6. WHO: Prevención de la Cardiopatía Coronaria. Report of a Committee of Experts of the WHO. SIT, 678 WHO. Geneva, 1982.
7. Keys A: *Seven countries: a multivariate analysis of death and coronary heart disease.* Harvard Univ. Press, Cambridge (MA) London, 1980.
8. Gofman JN, Young W, Tandy R: Ischaemic heart disease, atherosclerosis and longevity. *Circulation,* 1966; 34: 679–697.
9. Barr DP, Russ EM, Eder A: Protein lipid relationship in human plasma in atherosclerosis and related conditions. *Am J Med,* 1951; 11: 480–493.
10. Kukita H, Hiwada K, Kokubu T: Serum apolipoprotein A I, A II and B levels and their discriminative values in relatives of patients with coronary aftery disease. *Atherosclerosis,* 1984; 51: 261–267.
11. Miller NE, Hammett F, Saltissi S, Rao S, Van Zeller A, Coltart J, Lewis B: Relation of angiographically defined coronary artery disease to plasma lipoprotein subfractions and apolipoproteins. *Br Med J,* 1981; 282: 1741–1744.
12. Wahyne TF, Alaupovic P, Curry MD, Lee ET, Anderson PS, Schcuter E: Plasma apolipoprotein B and VLDL, LDL and HDL cholesterol as a risk factor in the development of coronary artery disease in male patients examined by aniography. *Atherosclerosis,* 1981; 39: 411–424.
13. Balaguer Vintró L, Duarte Mantilla G: Familial hypercholesterolemia and coronary heart disease. *Cardiovasc Rev Rep,* 1982; 3: 1072–1078.
14. Balaguer Vintró I: Los resultados de los estudios epidemiológicos y el futuro de la prevención de la cardiopatía coronaria. *Med Clin (Barc),* 1983; 81: 572–575.
15. Lipid Research Clinics Program: The Lipid Research Clinics Coronary Primary Prevention Trial results II. The relationship of reduction in incidence of coronary heart disease to cholesterol lowering. *JAMA,* 1984; 251: 365–374.
16. Havel RJ: Typing of hyperlipoproteinemias. *Atherosclerosis,* 1970; 11: 3–6.
17. Knuiman JT, West CE, Burema J: Serum total and high density lipoprotein cholesterol concentrations and body mass index in adult men from 13 countries. *Amer J Epidemiology,* 1982; 116: 631–642.
18. Stone NJ: Primary type II hyperlipoproteinemia. In: Rifkind BM, Levy RI (eds) *Hyperlipidemia. Diagnosis and therapy.* Grune & Stratton, New York, 1977; 113–136.
19. De Gennes JL, Turpin G, Truffert J: Formes cutaneotendineuses de xanthomatose hypercholesterolemique. Etude clinique, biologique et génerative de 11 cas. *Atherosclerosis,* 1971; 13: 147–170.
20. The Pooling Project Research Group: Relationship of blood pressure, serum cholesterol, smoking habit, relative weight and ECG abnormalities to incidence of major coronary events. Final report of Pooling Project. *J Chron Dis,* 1978; 31: 201–272.
21. Williams RR, Sorlie PD, Feinleib M, McNamara PM, Kannel WB, Dawber ThR: Cancer incidence by levels of cholesterol. *JAMA,* 1981; 245: 247–252.
22. Carmena R: Hipercolesterolemia: Cuándo y cuánto hay que tratarla? *Med Clin (Barc),* 1983; 80: 261–262.

23. Miettinen TA, Huttunen JK, Kumlin T, Naukkarinen V, Mattila S, Ehnhol MC: High density lipoprotein levels during a five-year multifactorial intervention against coronary heart disease risk factors. In: Noseda G, Lewis B, Paoletti R (eds) *Diet and drugs in atherosclerosis.* Raven Press, New York, 1980: 184–194.

24. Olsson AG, Lang PD: One-year study of the effect of bezafibrate on serum lipoprotein concentrations in hyperlipoproteinemia. *Atherosclerosis,* 1978; 31: 421–428.

25. Hulley SB, Rosenman RH, Bawol RD, Brand RJ: Epidemiology as a guide to clinical decisions. The association between triglycerides and coronary artery disease. *N Engl J Med,* 1980; 302– 1383–1389.

26. Murphy S, Yasuhara H, Dollery T, Thompson GR: Effects of short term beta adrenoreceptor blockade on serum lipids and lipoproteins in patients with hypertension of coronary artery disease. *Br Heart J,* 1984; 51: 589–594.

27. Lehtonen A, Marniemi J: Effect of atenolol on plasma HDL cholesterol subfractions. *Atherosclerosis,* 1984; 51: 335–338.

28. Gotto AM, Wittels EH: Diet, serum cholesterol, lipoproteins and coronary heart disease. In: Kaplan NM, STamler J, (eds) *Prevention of coronary heart disease. Protocol management of the risk factors.* WB Saunders, Philadelphia, 1983; 33–50.

13.3 Prophylactic β-blocking Treatment after Myocardial Infarction

G. PERMANYER MIRALDA and E. GALVE BASILIO

Trial results

In recent years, random, double-blind, placebo controlled clinical trials have demonstrated a significant reduction in mortality (up to about 2 years) in patients given β-blocking agents from the 5th to 18th day after acute myocardial infarction (AMI) [1–7]. In some of these trials, a specific reduction in the rate of sudden death [1, 2] and reinfarction [1, 7] has been shown to exist.

The following analysis is a reflection on these findings from the viewpoint of a clinical cardiologist. We did not examine the multiple β-blocking agent trials made in the hyperacute phase of infarction [8], which have somewhat different objectives and still inconclusive results. Only trials of what is conventionally denominated 'late' onset treatment were considered, that is, those in which the β-blocking agent was given after the 5th day of evolution.

Likewise, our article will not analyze the methods of the clinical trials performed, which have been almost unconditionally accepted as being correct [9–12]. Table 1 summarizes features of the principal trials. In the first place, it is noteworthy that similar results were obtained with different β-blocking agents. In Fig. 1 is summarized the reduction in mortality attained with diverse β-blocking agents in six of the most important trials and the 95% confidence intervals for these results. Results were favorable for the drug in practically every trial. The two most rigorous and extensive trials were the BHAT ('β-blocker heart attack trial' [2], a North American multicenter propanolol trial (and the Norwegian timolol trial [1]. Their results had the narrowest confidence limits and in both cases the lower limit was clearly situated in the zone favorable to the drug, which confers great statistical reliability.

However, it should not be forgotten that the reduction in postinfarctional mortality with β-blockers has been demonstrated by the method of controlled clinical trials. These trials, although valuable, nonetheless constitute an experimental situation. What is analyzed in this situation is almost an artificial population, the result of a process of successive patient exclusions, parting

Table 1. Features of the principal clinical trials of β-blocker treatment after acute myocardial infarction.

Study	Dose, route	Date of onset after AMI	Duration of treatment	Age	Sex (% m)	Patients Eval.	Patients Rand-om.	Mortality Placebo n	Placebo %	Drug n	Drug %	Reduction p	Reduction %	Reinfarction Placebo n	Placebo %	Drug n	Drug %	Reduction p	Reduction %
Timolol	10 mg/ 12 hrs oral	6–8 days	12–33 mo	20–75	79	3,643	1,884 (52%)	113	21.9	58	13.3	<0.01	39	141	15.0	88	9.2	<0.001	38.7
BHAT (proprano-lol)	180–240 mg 24 hrs 3x oral	5–21 days	12–39 mo	30–69	84	16,400	3,837 (23%)	188	9.8	58	3.3	<0.005	26	–	–	–	–	–	–
Practolol	200 mg/ 12hrs oral	1–4 wks	14 mo	≤69	86	–	3,038	73	–	47	–	<0.02	–	89	–	69	–	NS	–
Metoprolol	15 mg i.v. followed by 100 mg/ 12hrs oral	i.v. on adm. (11h) 15' later	90 days	40–74	76	2,619	1,395 (53%)	62	8.9	40	5.7	<0.03	36	56	14.7	36	9.0	<0.046	34
Sotalol	320 mg/ 24 hrs oral	5–14 days	12 mo	30–69	80	3,234	1,456 (45%)	51	8.9	64	7.3	NS	18	33	5.7	29	3.3	<0.05	40
Oxprenolol	40 mg/ 12 hrs oral	1–90 mos	6–84 mo	36–65	100	–	1,103		76.6*		95.1*	<0.001	–	–	–	–	–	–	–
Pindolol	15 mg/ 24 hrs oral	1–21 days	2 yrs	≤69	–	2,500	529 (20%)		17.7		17.1	NS	3	41		37		NS	9

* Survival rate.

656

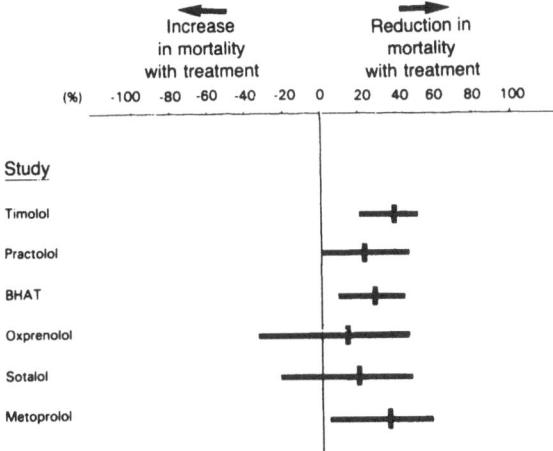

Fig. 1. Representation of the 95% confidence intervals corresponding to relative differences in global mortality between the placebo group and the group treated with β- blockers after infarction in the most important trials in the literature. In all of them, a result favorable to the drug is appreciated.

from a theoretically analyzable population until an appropriate group is obtained for analysis, which is then randomized. Fig. 2 illustrates what occurred with the Norwegian timolol trial, where it can be seen that the randomly distributed population included only 52% of the eligible candidates with confirmed infarction, who in turn were from a much larger group [1]. In the BHAT, the trial population was only 23% of the theoretically analyzable patients [2]. The rest were eliminated by successive exclusions (clinical contraindications and indications for β-blocker treatment, administrative reasons etc.). Extrapolation on the findings of these trials to the population at large can be done with a more or less elevated probability, according to subgroups, but it is always hypothetical.

On the basis of these trials, it can be stated that administration of β-blockers is effective in reducing late mortality after myocardial infarction. This assertion has historical value: this is the first group of drugs for which a consensus has been reached concerning its use in this type of ischemic heart disease. For the first time, the physician can count on a group of drugs known to influence the survival of infarction patients.

Criticism of clinical trial findings

There is undeniably a reduction in late postinfarctional mortality with β-

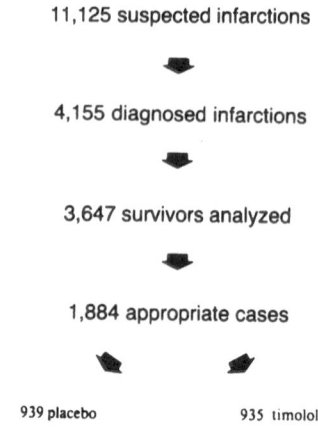

11,125 suspected infarctions

4,155 diagnosed infarctions

3,647 survivors analyzed

1,884 appropriate cases

939 placebo   935 timolol

Fig. 2. Representative scheme of the successive exclusions made in the course of the patient selection process in the timolol study[1]. Note the disproportion between the number of patients initially examined and those finally randomized.

blocking agents, but several critical considerations can be made relative to limitations in their value and methodologic problems. It may be more constructive to briefly review some of these problems and limitations, rather than make a simple value judgement on the use of these drugs. We will comment later on possible areas of investigation for future trials. We leave it to reader to form a personal opinion on the utility of these drugs.

1. The first drawback is that there is scant reduction in global mortality, taking into account how little spontaneous mortality the disease has in the groups studied. Without entering into the numerical findings of each study, a valid global estimation (that some authors consider optimistic) of the reduction in mortality would be 25% [13]. This means that if 8 of 100 patients die annually, only 6 would die with treatment [13]. Treatment would have benefited only two patients, having been apparently superfluous in 92. These figures may seem ridiculous, but it has been calculated that this would represent 2,500 more annual survivals in England. If we add to this the contribution of the β-blocking agents in preventing reinfarction (as well not documented), these figures acquire even greater value. However, it is still evident that they are not spectacular.

2. The second problem is that we do not know exactly how β-blocking agents exercise their protective effect, although there is a long list of possible actions [14]. We do not know if the protection they afford derives from their antiarrhythmic effect, antiischemic effect, eventual improvement of contractile function in ischemic patients or from a combination of all of them. The fact that the protective mechanism is unknown makes it difficult to

respond to questions such as: Do β-blocking agents simply delay death or reinfarction, or do they definitively act on a harmful mechanism, at least in some patients? The fact that this question remains unanswered contributes to our uncertainty as to whether the drug should be continued after one or two years.

3. There is a circumstantial, if not intrinsic, limitation in β-blocker use. This limitation is what we could describe as the provisional character of efficacy findings. It is evident that our attitude toward the management of ischemic heart disease is presently experiencing profound changes. It is likely that if the different β-blocker trials had been realized 10 years earlier, these drugs would now be firmly established in routine post myocardial infarction therapy. At the moment, we do not know what place they will occupy among local and systemic thrombolysis, angioplasty, antiarrhythmic drugs, elective surgery, platelet antiaggregants, etc., all of which are pending definitive evaluation.

4. The first objection any cardiologist would make to postinfarctional administration of a β-blocking agent is probably their adverse effects on rhythm, conduction or ventricular function. Surprisingly, in the different trials the number of patients who had to discontinue the drug because of these effects was small (less than 10%). What is more interesting, in many cases the proportion of patients excluded from drug treatment was similar to that found in the placebo group. Although the patients with a clear contraindication for treatment, such as refractory heart failure or bradyarrhythmias (about 20%), were excluded from treatment, theoretically they may be the patients who most need a measure of protection. Once more we run up against gaps in our knowledge: the reasons for exclusion in the different trials are not always defined by precise criteria. For example, what is understood by refractory heart failure is usually not specified. In a general population, we do not know what risk there is of these drugs having adverse effects in patients situated on the 'borderline', especially as concerns ventricular function. Making an overall evaluation of the diverse trials and considering that many of these patients have the most important spontaneous risk in their evolution and therefore have the greatest need for protection, the accepted tendency is to give these drugs with caution (except in the case of patients with clear contraindications – evident heart failure or persistent bradyarrhythmia). In 'borderline' cases, the risk of adverse effects is tolerable.

5. The studies made do not clarify if a particular β-blocker is better than the others. The general idea is that all of them exercise their preventive effects in a similar way, although there is an unproven theory that the drugs with intrinsic sympatheticomimetic activity (oxprenolol or pindolol) are less indicated [9]. Practically speaking, any β-blocking agent can be prescribed,

although it may be advisable to give drugs that have been experimented with and confirmed, such as timolol and propranolol [9]. Pharmacokinetic considerations can help in the choice; for example, it is probable that patient compliance is better with drugs that require fewer daily doses.

Which patients should be treated with β-blocking agents?

It has often been asserted that it is probably unnecessary to give β-blocking agents to all postinfarctional patients [15] because the spontaneous evolutive risk is so low in some of them that the improvement obtained with treatment would probably be unappreciable [16, 17]. What groups of patients benefit most from treatment? There is still no unequivocal response to this question. To begin with, we have to consider two apparent paradoxes. The first of them is that β-blocking agents are contraindicated in a large proportion of the patients at high risk. The second paradox is that all the trials cite as a criterion for exclusion the indication for β-blocker treatment (it would have been unethical to randomize these patients with placebo). For this reason, the measure in which the β-blockers would benefit the subgroup of patients who are the principal theoretical candidates for this treatment, for angina or hypertension due to other causes, has not been studied. Most authors coincide in considering patients with postinfarctional angina or hypertension as candidates for β-blocker treatment, even though there is no statistical evidence of great benefits.

In second place, the trials do not provide enough information to conclude which risk subgroups would benefit from treatment. In the Norwegian timolol trial, patients were randomly distributed into three risk groups; in all three, benefits were obtained from treatment. However, restrospective analysis of the BHAT seems to indicate that there were more benefits in patients with electrical complications that in patients with mechanical complications and almost no effect in uncomplicated patients. In any case, the main problem is that when these trials were designed, prospective evaluation of infarction risk was not done with the techniques presently considered fundamental (ergometry, catherization, isotopes, Holter). As such, the spontaneous mortality of the subgroup with the lowest risk in the timolol trial is greater than that of the low risk subgroup that can be constituted by patients with uncomplicated first infarction and negative effort test. For example, we can deduce nothing of the protection offered by these drugs in patients with ischemic effort test response. Likewise, the benefits that patients with initial uncomplicated infarction and negative effort test, who have a very good prognosis, would receive from treatment are not evident, although probable.

Future perspectives

From the above, it can be understood that the clinical trials have left some unanswered questions. We will analyze possible areas of future study, often refered to in the literature. There is a question that may seem trivial, but we think it is still legitimate: *Should more clinical β-blocker trials be realized?* These trials are extremely expensive because they require a large number of patients, hospitals and specialized personnel. Other strategies for treating infarction are under study and now that we know that the β-blocking agents are globally useful, the findings of new studies are not likely to compensate the effort involved in their realization. It may be perfectly legitimate to give these drugs without further investigation to patients who are assumed to be high risk. It certainly does not seem to be justifiable, even ethically, to continue making global trials that 'repeat' earlier ones. It is probable that trials of partial aspects would be justified. This type of trial could follow one of the following three lines of research:

1. Continuation of classic studies. For example, analysis of the value of different β-blocking agents at varying dosages. It is improbable that extensive studies of this type will be undertaken, since this means 'repeating' large scale studies with all the difficulties this entails.
2. Evaluation of the efficacy of β-blocker treatment in subgroups of patients with determined risk levels, according to present stratification criteria. This possibility is suggested in various studies. However, in spite of the potential interest of these studies, they are not easy to realize and require a large number of patients. Of the numerous studies that analyze the value of some examination parameter to predict evolution, a study made in the Hospital Clinico of Barcelona by Sanz et al. [18] can be taken as a hypothesis. It was based on a subgroup of 45 patients with intermediate mortality (22% at 3 years), with three-vessel disease and 30–50% ejection fraction. The authors consider this group to be the most susceptible to prophylactic measures. We have roughly calculated that if we wish to demonstrate in a clinical trial that the β-blocking agents reduce mortality by 25% in this group, we would have to have 400 patients in the treated group and the same number in the placebo group to obtain a significance of $p < 0.05$. If we take into account that this subgroup represents only 17% of the infarctions in the series, the original population from which the subgroup would be drawn has to be very large. This approximate and hypothetical calculation illustrates the difficulties that can be encountered in designing studies of this type. Although it is probable that trials in high risk patient subgroups did not choose only this type of patients (or higher mortality subgroups were identified), meaning that the original population may have been smaller in both cases, the number of patients needed would always be elevated and the group would be complex in constitution.

3. A third possibility for future studies is to part from the assumption that the β-blocking agents have effects and analyze more precisely *how* these substances act, freeing the clinician from administering these drugs empirically. This type of study would be a search for indirect evidence of the effects of these drugs by examining the mechanism by which they exercise their protection. In reality, not much is known about the global effects of β-blockers in patients who have suffered infarction.

There are numerous effects that can be studied. For example, the antiarrhythmic effects, either direct or mediated by reduction of ischemia, are poorly known and diverse studies have produced discordant results. A recent metoprolol study could serve as an example for this type of trial. A sustained reduction was confirmed in the ventricular arrhythmias of the postinfarctional group treated with metoprolol in comparison with the placebo group [19].

The effect of β-blocking agents on ventricular function in postinfarctional patients is not clear. A recent study has shown that the ventricular function of patients with ischemic heart disease can increment normally with exercise; with propranolol, this increase was somewhat depressed, although not significantly. On the contrary, in ischemic patients with depressed ventricular function during exercise, propranolol significantly attentuated this depression, even in the postexertional phase, which is an improvement in ventricular function [20]. Could a phenomenon of this type be involved in the protection conferred by β-blockers, or is this phenomenon an expression of a protective effect of these drugs at another level? Or perhaps, this type of phenomenon is unrelated to reduction in mortality? Would analysis of postexertional ventricular function identify the candidates to benefit from treatment? We do not have responses to these questions, but they illustrate possible areas for future research.

Conclusions

To summarize, it can be concluded that the β-blocking agents produce a significant reduction in mortality after myocardial infarction. We do not know in what circumstances this protection is greatest, but we can assume that it is scant in subgroups with a low risk evolution. We are also unaware of the exact mechanism responsible. We know that there is a reduction in mortality with drug administration in the first-second year after infarction, but we do not know if the effect continues. Future research can clarify some of these points, although it will be difficult, and determine the role of β-blocking agents in the strategies for treating post myocardial infarction.

662

References

1. The Norwegian Multicenter Study Group: Timolol-induced reduction in mortality and rein-farction in patients surviving acute myocardial infarction. *N Engl J Med* 1981; 304: 801–807.
2. Beta-blocker Heart Attack Trial Research Group: A randomized trial of propanolol in patients with acute myocardial infarction. I. Mortality results. *JAMA* 1982; 247: 1707–1714.
3. Improvement in prognosis of myocardial infarction by long-term β-adrenoreceptor blockade using practolol. A multicenter international study. *Br Med J* 1975; 3: 735–740.
4. Taylor SH, Silke B, Ebbut A, Sutton GC, Prout BJ, Burley DM: Long-term prevention study with oxprenolol in coronary heart disease. *N Engl J Med* 1982; 307: 1293–1301.
5. Wilhelmsson C, Vedin JA, Wilhelmsen L, Tibblin G, Werko L: Reduction of sudden deaths after myocardial infarction by treatment with alprenolol. Preliminary results. *Lancet,* 1974; 2: 1157–1160.
6. Australian and Swedish Pindolol Study Group: The effect of pindolol on the two years mortality after complicated myocardial infarction. *Eur Heart J,* 1983; 4: 367–375.
7. Julian DG, Prescott RJ, Jackson FS, Szekely P: Controlled trial of sotalol for one year after myocardial infarction. *Lancet,* 1982; 1: 1142–1147.
8. Hjamarson A, Elmfeldt D, Herlitz J, Holberg S, Malek I, Nyberg G, et al.: Effect on mortality of metoprolol in acute myocardial infarction. A double-blind randomised trial. *Lancet,* 1981; 2: 823–827.
9. Frishman HW, Furberg CD, Friedewald WT: β-adrenergic blockade for survivors of acute myocardial infarction. *N Engl J Med,* 1984; 310: 830–837.
10. Singh BN, Phil D, Venkatesh N: Prevention of myocardial reinfarction and of sudden death in survivors of acute myocardial infarction: role of prophylactic βφadrenoreceptor blockade. *Am Heart J,* 1984; 107: 189–200.
11. Hampton JR: The use of β-blockers for the reduction of mortality after myocardial infarction. *Eur Heart J,* 1981; 2: 259–268.
12. Lewis JA: β-blockade after myocardial infarction. A statistical view. *Br J Clin Pharmac,* 1982; 14: 15S-21S.
13. Breckenridge A: Should every survivor of a heart attack be given a βφblocker? Part II. Evidence from a clinical pharmacological standpoint. *Br Med J,* 1982; 285: 37–39.
14. Prichard BNC: Mechanisms of myocardial infarct prevention with β-adrenoreceptor blocking drugs. *Drugs,* 1983; 25 (Suppl 2): 295–302.
15. Wilhelmsson C, Vedin A: Principles and practice of treatment with β-blockers in myocardial infarction. *Drugs,* 1983; 25 (Suppl 2): 308–313.
16. Moss AJ: Postinfarction therapy with β-blockers: who should be treated? *Int J Cardiol,* 1982; 1: 343–349.
17. Griggs TR, Wagner GS, Gettes LS: β-adrenergic blocking agents after myocardial infarction: an undocumented need in patients at lowest risk. *J Am Coll Cardiol,* 1983; 1: 1530–1533.
18. Sanz G, Castañer A, Betriu A, Magrina J, Roig E et al: Determinants of prognosis in survivors of myocardial infarction. A prospective clinical angiographic study. *N Engl J Med,* 1982; 306: 1065–1070.
19. Olsson G, Rehnqvist N: Ventricular arrhythmias during the first year after acute myocardial infarction: influence of long-term treatment with metoprolol. *Circulation,* 1984; 69: 1129–1134.
20. Marshall RCM, Wisenberg G, Schelbert HR, Henze E: Effect of oral propanolol on rest, exercise and postexercise left ventricular performance in normal subjects and patients with coronary artery disease. *Circulation,* 1981; 63: 572–583.

13.4 Criticism of Long-term Preventive Treatment after Myocardial Infarction

A. CASTAÑER MUÑOZ and A. SERRA PEÑARANDA

Ischemic heart disease is a health problem of capital importance in industrialized countries, in many of which it is the principle cause of death.

In recent decades, many studies have been realized with the object of modifying the natural history of myocardial infarction [1–4]. The first controlled studies with randomization of patients were initiated in the sixties and since then around 50,000 survivors of acute myocardial infarction have been included in more than 40 clinical trials. In spite of the enormous amount of work and expense this has supposed, the results obtained have not been very promising. Only recently, three studies involving β-blocking agents (metoprolol, timolol and propranolol) have demonstrated a significant reduction in mortality after myocardial infarction. The results of prospective long-term studies are undoubtedly influenced by three factors:

a) size of the study sample assigned to each group by randomization;
b) mortality rate in the study population because the lower mortality is, the larger the sample required; and
c) knowledge of the natural history of myocardial infarction and of the factors that condition its prognosis.

These may vary in the course of different phases of evolution of the infarction and can respond to different types of therapy.

Fig. 1 illustrates the first point. The upper curve represents the number of patients needed to detect a 20% reduction in the mortality of a control group with a 95% limit of confidence and a beta error of 0.1. For instance, if the mortality of the population studied is 5%, more than 9,000 patients are required in each randomized group for the sample to be statistically valid. If mortality were 45%, less than 1,000 patients in each group would be sufficient [10].

A similar mortality rate is observed in the control groups of different clinical trials and in studies of the natural history of myocardial infarction, there being a direct relation between the years of follow-up and mortality rate, which is 13–14% at 4–5 years (Fig. 2). The annual mortality is obtained by dividing the

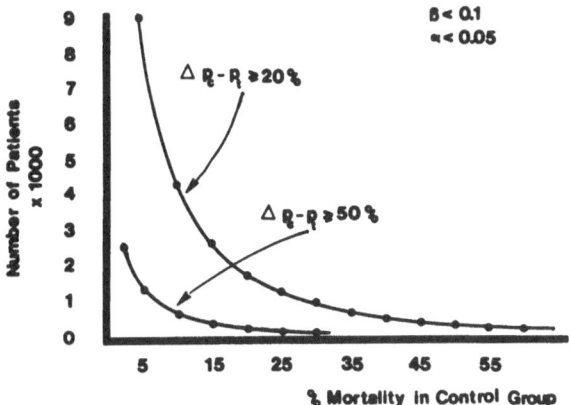

Fig. 1.

mortality rate by years of follow-up; the mortality rate of myocardial infarction is 2–5% per year in most studies (Fig. 3). There are studies in which annual mortality is surprisingly high. This is because the incidence of death in the first year of infarction is much greater than in later years and these studies have short follow-up periods, less than 18 months. Fig. 4 shows the mortality figures

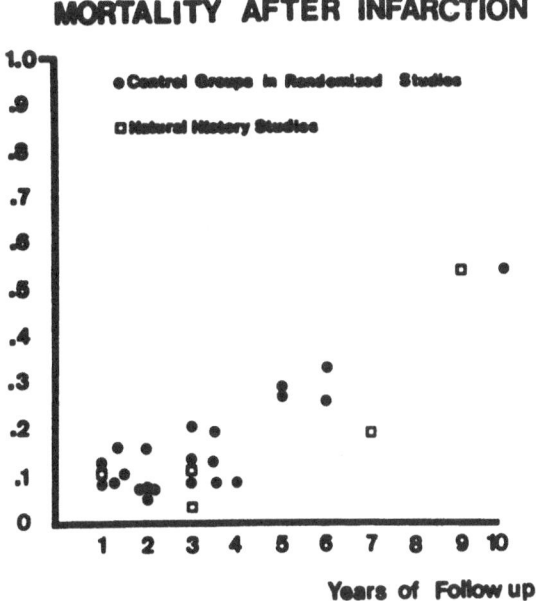

Fig. 2.

665

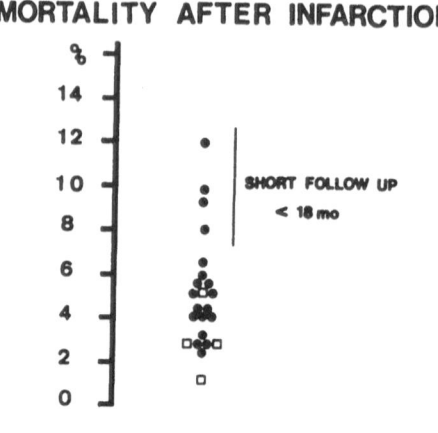

Fig. 3.

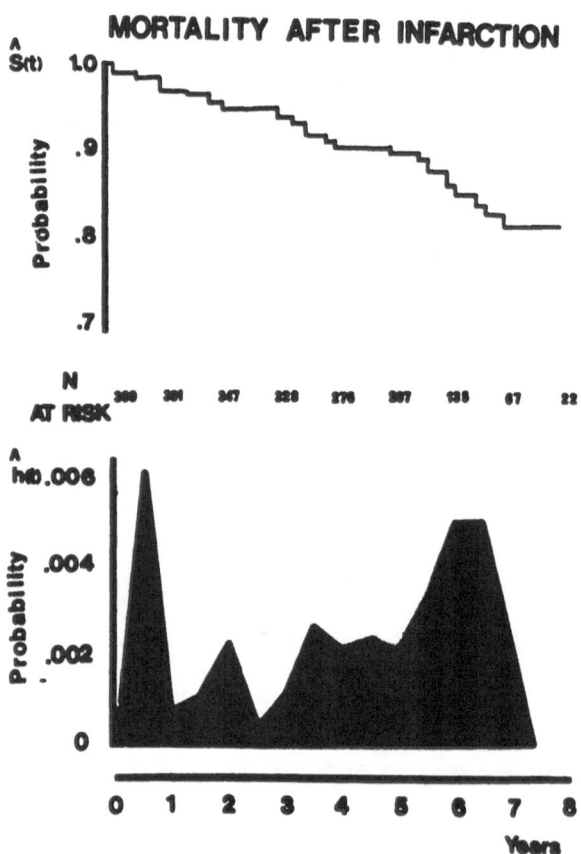

Fig. 4.

666

MORTALITY AFTER INFARCTION

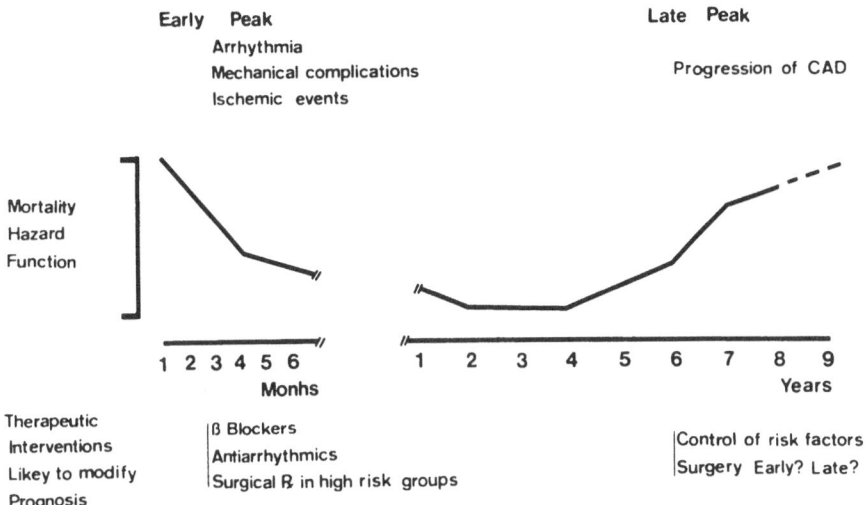

Fig. 5.

for our population of myocardial infarction patients in the Hospital Clínico of Barcelona [5] expressed two ways. The upper curve is a survival function showing the cumulative mortality of the population, 20% at 7 years, which concurs with most studies. Since the annual mortality of patients who survive myocardial infarction is not high, large samples must be used for secondary prevention studies to reach definitive conclusions. The lower graph in Fig. 4 is a risk function showing the probability of death within a fixed interval of time after myocardial infarction. Analysis of these mortality data allow separation of different periods with greater probability of postinfarctional death. There is an early peak of risk of death in the first 6 months, followed by stabilization at lower levels between the first and fifth years. After the sixth year, we have found a late rise in risk of death (Fig. 5). The factors that determine this late elevation in mortality have not been studied, but they may differ from those responsible for the first mortality peak. In the first peak, arrhythmias, me-chanical complications and new coronary accidents caused by the coronary lesions present at infarction probably determine this initial risk. It is logical to suppose that the positive effect that antiarrhythmic drugs, β-blocking agents or myocardial revascularization in high risk patients have on the first mortality peak is due to their effect on these factors. However, any study of the efficacy of therapeutic measures taken after the first year of infarction would require a large series of patients to reach definitive conclusions. The late mortality peak is probably due to progression of the coronary heart disease; as such, to modify

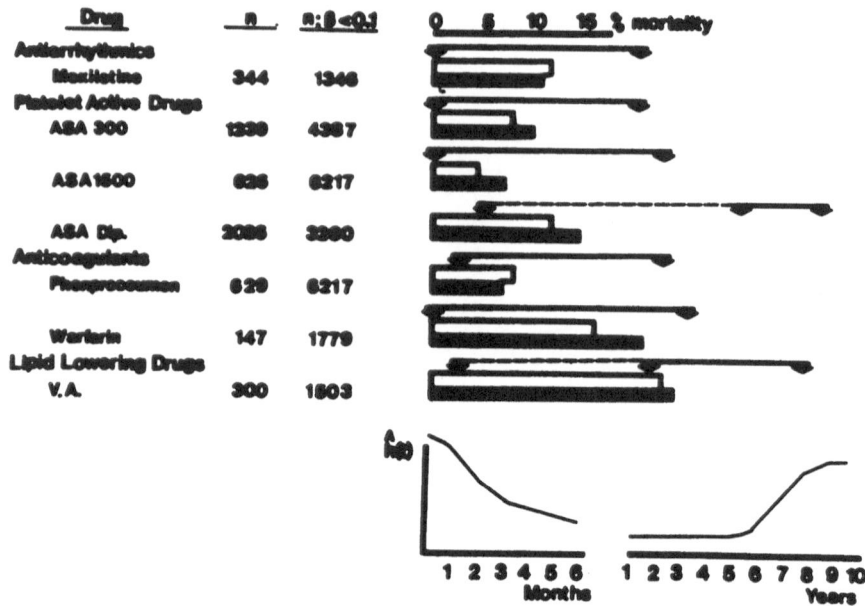

Fig. 6.

this peak, the factors conditioning the disease's advance should be controlled (coronary risk factors).

Fig. 6 shows the results of some clinical trials [6]. The antiarrhythmic drugs have not been found to have a beneficial effect on mortality. An important defect of these trials is the small sample size. The mexiletine study contained only 344 patients, when the minimum required sample was 1,300 for each group. The same defect and results are observed in other therapeutic trials which likewise did not provide definitive results, such as those realized with platelet antiaggregants, anticoagulants and lipid reducing agents.

Fig. 7 shows the results of clinical β-blocker trials. It can be seen that there is a significant reduction in postinfarctional mortality in the studies of practolol, propranolol, timolol and metoprolol. It is interesting that these studies have a better general design, with a more adequate number of patients and treatment beginning soon after infarction, which probably contributes to reducing the initial peak in risk of mortality. The oxprenolol study demonstrates the importance of early treatment. In the patients in whom treatment began within 4 months of infarction, there was a marked reduction in mortality. When treatment was initiated between 5 months and one year, there were no differences between the treated and control groups. When therapy began after the first year, mortality was higher in the treated group. These findings suggest that the reduction in mortality that takes place in earlier phases of myocardial in-

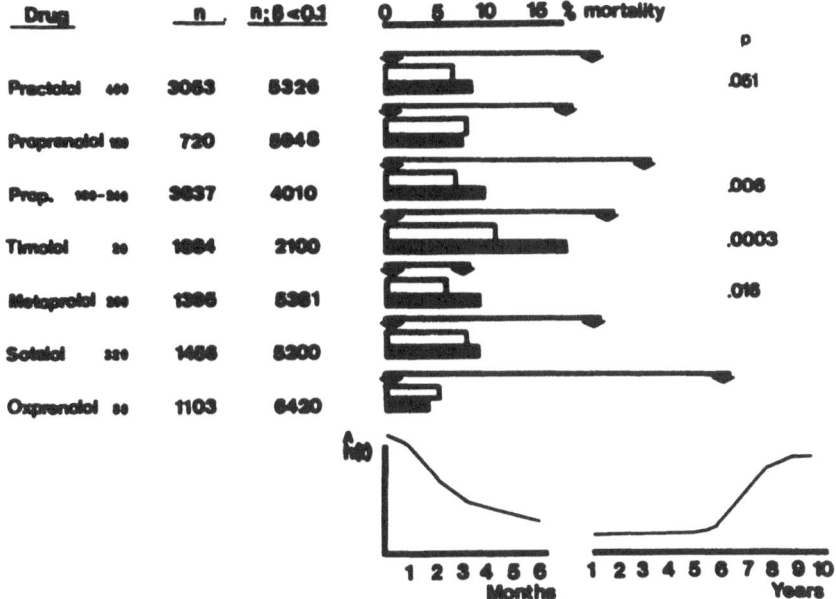

Fig. 7.

farction is probably due to a decrease in the incidence of arrhythmias and improvement in myocardial ischemia.

Among survivors of the acute phase of myocardial infarction, prospective epidemiological studies like those of the Multicenter Postinfarction Research Group [7], Perth Registry [8] and others identify patient subgroups with high, medium and low mortality risk. The high risk subgroup represents 15% of the postinfarctional population and has a mortality of about 20–40% in the first year. The low risk subgroup constitutes 25–30% of the population and has a mortality of about 2% in the first year. In this group it would be difficult to propose any therapy for reducing mortality, which is already very low. Fig. 8 shows the findings of our study in the Hospital Clínico of Barcelona. In the group of patients with moderate to severe left ventricular dysfunction (21–49% ejection fraction), mortality rises to almost 25% at 6–7 years. The risk function shows early and late peaks of mortality risk. However, in patients who have an ejection fraction superior to 50% after infarction, approximately 25% of the population, global mortality is much lower and there is no initial peak of mortality risk. These findings indicate that low risk patients do not benefit from β-blocking agents, the only drugs demonstrated to be effective in reducing mortality. The fact that there are no benefits is because the β-blockers act on the initial peak of mortality, which is absent in low risk patients.

To summarize, clinical trials oriented toward improving postinfarctional

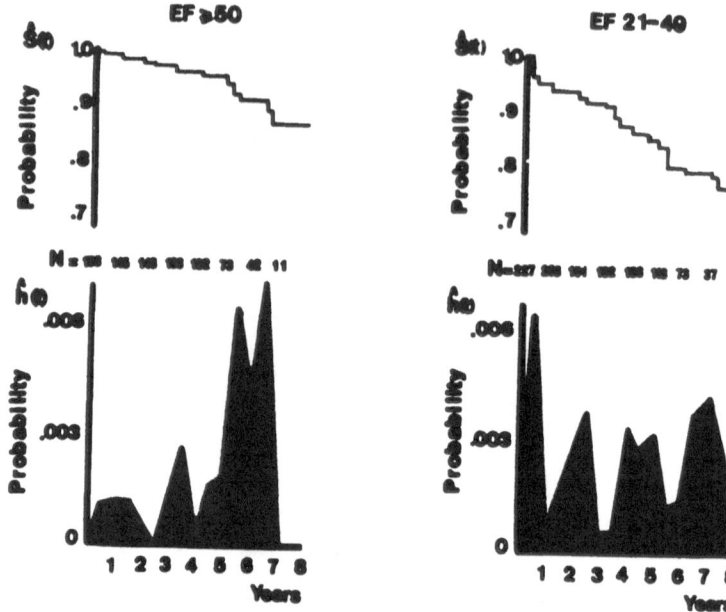

Fig. 8.

prognosis provide no conclusive results. Most of these trials have methodologic defects, such as insufficient sample size, inclusion of an elevated percentage of low risk patients and late initiation of therapy in some cases. With all these trials, only the β-blockers were demonstrated to be effective [9]. However, generalized use of these drugs after myocardial infarction is questioned because of their secondary effects. Moreover, it would be necessary to treat 100 patients with propanolol for 2 years to prolong the lives of 2 of them. Anticoagulants, antiarrhythmic drugs, lipid reducing agents and myocardial revascularization surgery should be reserved for specific indications.

References

1. Beta-blocker Heart Attack Trial Research Group: A randomized trial of propanolol in patients with acute myocardial infarction. I. Mortality results. *JAMA* 1982; 12: 1707–1714.
2. The Norwegian Multicenter Study Group: Timolol-induced reduction in mortality and reinfarction in patients surviving acute myocardial infarction. *N Engl J Med*, 1981; 304: 801–807.
3. Hjalmarson A, Elmfeldt D, Herlitz J, et al: Effect on mortality of metoprolol in active myocardial infarction. *Lancet*, 1981; 2: 823–826.
4. Taylor SH, Silke B, Ebbutt A, et al: A long-term prevention study with oxprenolol in coronary heart disease. *N Eng J Med*, 1982; 307: 1293–1300.
5. Sanz G, Castañer A, Betriu A et al: Determinants of prognosis in survivors of myocardial

infarction. A prospective angiographic study. *N Engl J Med* 1982; 306: 1065–1070.

6. May GS, Eberlein KA, Furberg CD, et al: Secondary prevention after myocardial infarction: a review of long-term trials. *Prog Cardiovasc Dis,* 1983; 24: 331–352.

7. The Multicenter Postinfarction Research Group: Risk stratification and survival after myocardial infarction. *N Engl J Med,* 1983; 309: 331–335.

8. Martin CA, Thomson PL, Armstrong BK, et al: Long-term prognosis after recovery from myocardial infarction: a nine year follow-up of The Perth Coronary Register. *Circulation,* 1983; 68: 961–969.

9. Frihman WH, Furberg CD, Friedewald WT: β-adrenergic blockade for survivors of acute myocardial infarction. *N Engl J Med,* 1984; 310: 830–836.

10. Halperin M, Rogot E, Gurian J, et al: Sample sizes for medical trials with special reference to long-term therapy. *J Chron Dis,* 1968; 21: 13.

13.5 Strategies for Postinfarction Treatment

G. SANZ and G. OLLER

The term 'strategy' is defined as a set of rules for assuring optimal decision-making at every moment. If we accept this definition, it is obvious that there is no strategy for treating patients who have survived the acute phase of myocardial infarction. The main reason for this is that there are still large gaps in our knowledge of this disease.

For many years, postinfarctional treatment has been based on correction of coronary risk factors and treatment of symptoms when they appear.

Multiple studies have demonstrated that the prognosis of patients treated this way varies, but as a group they have an elevated morbimortality rate [1–3].

One of the first and probably best known of these studies is the Framingham study [1], which demonstrated that 5 years after acute infarction 36% of males and 54% of females had died; 13% and 40% respectively had suffered another infarction. A more recent study, the Perth Coronary Register [3], confirmed these figures, showing an even higher 5-year mortality, 67%.

It is thus not surprising that in recent years considerable effort has been dedicated to studying other therapeutic regimens that would reduce the incidence of new coronary accidents after infarction [4]. None of them is universally accepted and many questions on how and in whom to apply them remain unanswered, such as: Is there a treatment that reduces the incidence of death and reinfarction? On the basis of the natural history of AMI, when should prophylactic treatment be initiated and interrupted? How can high risk patients be detected? The first of these questions has been extensively dealt with and apparently only β-blockers, of all treatments tested, prevent new coronary accidents. The two earlier papers coincided in the opinion that in spite of this, prophylactic therapy should ideally be applied only in high risk patients. We would add that coronary surgery improves survival and possibly the incidence of infarction in patients with severe coronary vascular disease [5]. β-blockers and surgery can thus be used prophylactically in certain cases.

672

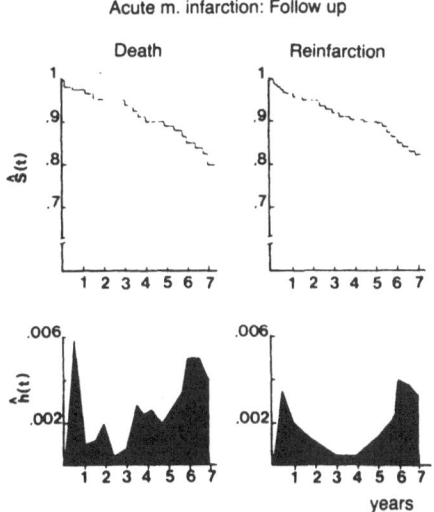

Acute m. infarction: Follow up

Fig. 1 Probability of survival and reinfarction (upper graphs) and risk function for the same coronary accidents at different time intervals after myocardial infarction.

Natural history of myocardial infarction

In the two graphs on the left of Fig. 1, the probability of survival and risk of death after infarction are shown, using the data previously presented by A. Castañer. On the right is the probability of survival without infarction (above) and the risk of infarction for different time intervals (below). When we speak of postinfarctional prevention, the possibility of a new infarction should be taken into account because, in contrast with angina, reinfarction definitively marks the patient's evolution. Like the risk of death, the risk of infarction can be studied and it has been found to be maximum in the first months, descending in the next 2 or 3 years and again rising after the fifth year. This brings out two points:
a) the need for early risk evaluation and treatment in survivors; and
b) the need for considering prevention of these late accidents in any treatment strategy.
Unfortunately, very little is known about the factors that determine long-term evolution and how to detect patients at risk for late death. Thus, except for control of risk factors, present therapeutic regimens refer only to the initial phase.

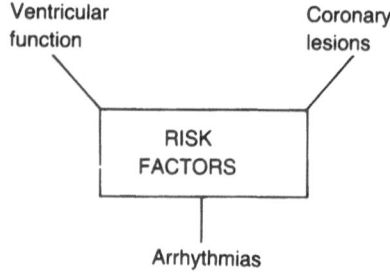

Fig. 2 Factors that determine post myocardial infarction prognosis.

Identification of high risk patients

Although there are many clinical, laboratory and hemodynamic parameters that correlate with mortality [6], it seems well established that the factors that really mark postinfarction prognosis are (Fig. 2) degree of ventricular dysfunction, severity of coronary affection and presence of certain ventricular arrhythmias. Various studies, including those of the Multicenter Postinfarction Group (MPRG) [7], Taylor [8], Norris [9] and our own [10], have demonstrated that these three factors have independent predictive values and that high risk groups can be identified with them. For example, in Norris' [9] study, patients with EF<40% had a 5-year mortality of 23%; in our protocol [10], this was superior to 50% for patients with EF under 20%. Since very few studies have made routine coronariography after infarction, data on the degree of coronary involvement are less common. In our series, patients with 3-vessel disease had a significantly higher mortality and reinfarction rate than the rest, although most of these new accidents occurred in patients who also had depressed ventricular function. The severity of coronary affection was the only factor with an independent predictive value for reinfarction.

Finally, the MRPG [7] findings show that patients with more than 10 ventricular extrasystoles (VE) per hour have a two-year mortality of 20%, although only half of these deaths were sudden and thus attributable to rhythm disorders. The incidence of Hinkle [11] type I death, from arrhythmias, is practically the same in all groups with more than 1 VE/hr. To prevent them, 40% of the population would have to be treated with antiarrhythmic drugs. This fact, and the absence of studies demonstrating the efficacy of antiarrhythmics in these patients invalidate this strategy to some degree. In a recent series, the predictive value of complex arrhythmias was 25% [12].

674

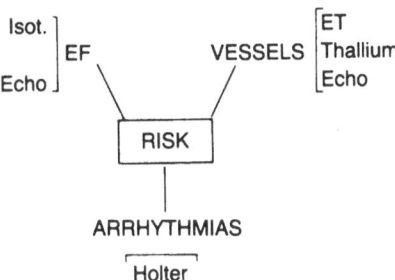

Fig. 3 Prognostic factors and noninvasive diagnostic methods.

Noninvasive techniques

Fig. 3 lists different noninvasive techniques used to study each of these parameters. To determine the EF, we have isotopic ventriculography and bidimensional echocardiography. The results of the exercise test, Te-201 isotopic studies and ECG correlated with the severity of coronary disease. Of all the methods proposed for detecting arrhythmias, Holter electrography seems to be the best. Nonetheless, for the reasons indicated above, I will not refer to this technique.

Fig. 4 shows the preliminary results of a study initiated in our service to evaluate noninvasive methods for detection of high risk post-AMI patients. On the left is a regression analysis between EF results obtained by isotopic ventriculography (ordenate) and those corresponding to cardiac catheter-

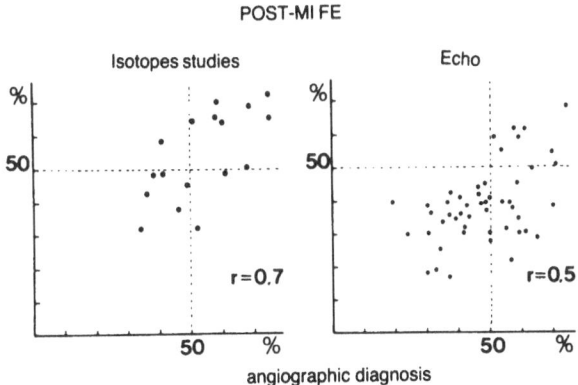

Fig. 4 Correlation between isotopic ventriculography (left) and echocardiography (right) with contrast ventriculography (abscissas).

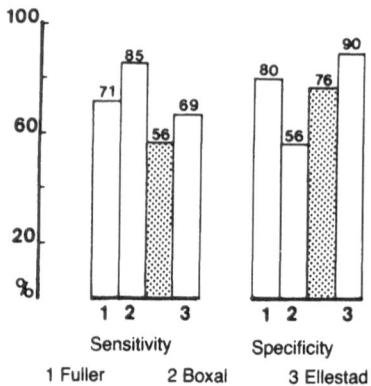

POST-MI EFFORT TEST

Fig. 5 Sensitivity and specificity of the effort test in detecting three-vessel disease after infarction, in three published series and the experience of the HCP (shaded column).

ization. On the right is the same analysis with bidimensional echocardiography. There is a good correlation between both techniques, isotopes and radioopaque contrast, and what is more important, were they used to discriminate between patients with normal or abnormal function, practically all patients would be well classified.

Correlation is not as good for the 2D ECHO, although it is statistically significant. In our hands it underestimates EF in many patients, leading to

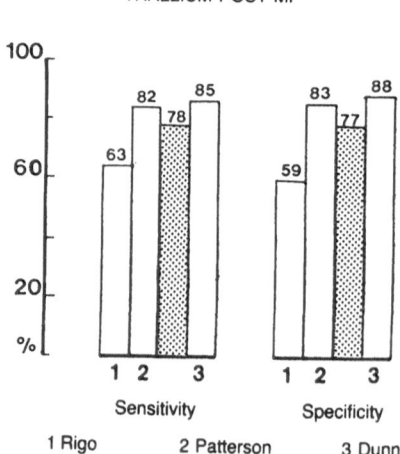

THALLIUM POST-MI

Fig. 6 Sensitivity and specificity of thallium gammagraphy for detecting three-vessel disease. Shade column: HCP data.

POST-MI 2D ECHO

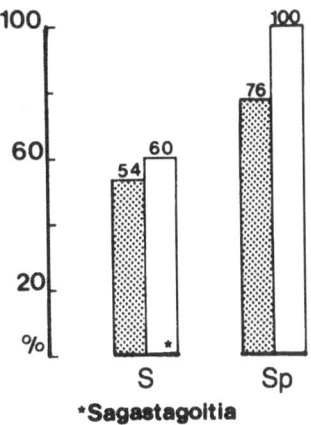

Fig. 7 Sensitivity (S) and specificity (Sp) of 2D ECHO for detecting three-vessel disease. Shaded column: HCP data.

erroneous high risk classifications. Unfortunately, isotopic ventriculography is still an expensive exploration.

Fig. 5, 6 and 7 show the sensitivity and specificity of the exercise test, Ta-201 studies and bidimensional echocardiography in detecting three-vessel disease in survivors of acute infarction. In each figure, the results of our series (shaded columns) are compared with others in the literature [13–19]. Altogether, the sensitivity and specificity are better for Ta-201 studies (63–85% and 59–88%, respectively) and very low for bidimensional echocardiography.

Fig. 8 compares these three techniques wit Ta-201 studies and coronary angiography, considering the cost of analyzing 100 patients and the percentage

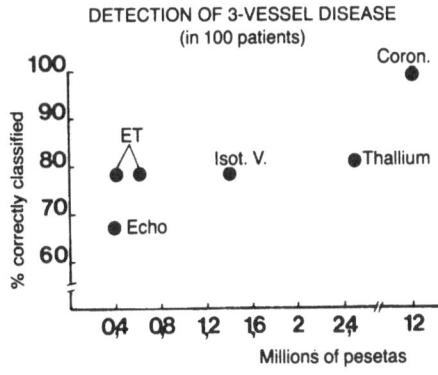

Fig. 8 Cost/effectiveness ratio (% of patients correctly classified) of different diagnostic methods.

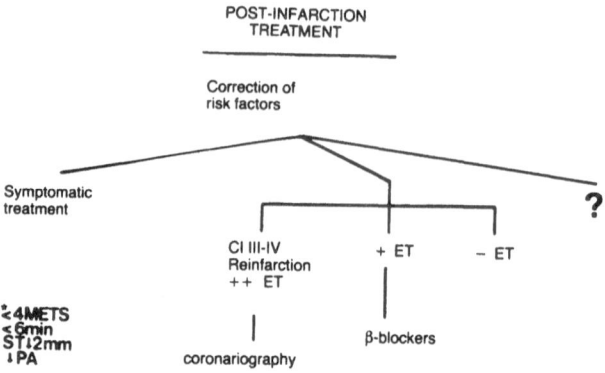

POST-INFARCTION
TREATMENT

Correction of
risk factors

Symptomatic
treatment

?

CI III-IV
Reinfarction
++ ET

+ ET   − ET

≦4METS
≤6min
ST↓2mm
↓PA

coronariography

β-blockers

Fig. 9 Algorithm of treatments after myocardial infarction.

of correct classifications. Naturally, coronary angiography would detect all patients with three-vessel disease, but its cost would reach a prohibitive 12 million pesetas. Among the noninvasive techniques, Ta-201 studies is slightly superior to the others, but it is also more expensive. The conventional exercise test seems to be a good compromise between cost and effectiveness.

On the basis of the above, it seems clear that there is no single treatment strategy for these patients and that selection of one or another will depend on economic considerations, experience and availability of equipment, etc. Fig. 9 shows two of the most widely used regimens: correction of risk factors is common to both, especially restriction of smoking, and control of hypertension and dyslipemia. On the left is shown a very conservative approach, consistent in treating only patients who are symptomatic after infarction, especially those with angina, who can benefit from beta-bockers.

At present, the most accepted tendency is to select high risk patients on the basis of exercise test response and certain data in the clinical history. Patients with severe heart failure in the coronary unit, history of previous infarction and very positive effort test (reduced effort tolerance, severe ST depression or abnormal blood pressure response), are considered high risk patients and candidates for coronary arteriography to detect lesions susceptible to surgical treatment. In patients with a moderate or slightly positive exercise test and no contraindications, β-blocking agents can be given prophylactically. Finally, a negative exercise test indicates a good prognosis, excluding the need for further studies.

As was mentioned above, this treatment strategy is not the only option. When facilities are available for routine isotopic ventriculography, high risk patients can be indentified by the ejection fraction, those with moderate or severe depression of ventricular function being candidates for coronariography. Nonetheless, as occurs with any other present regimen, this is incomplete and does not identify all high risk patients.

References

1. Kannel WB, Sorlie P, McNamara PM: Prognosis after initial myocardial infarction: the Framingham study. *Am J Cardiol* 1979; 44: 53–58.
2. Moss AJ: Prognosis after myocardial infarction. *Am J Cardiol,* 1983; 52: 667–668.
3. Martin CA, Thomson PL, Armstrong BK, et al: Long-term prognosis after recovery from myocardial infarction: a nine year follow-up of the Perth Coronary Register. *Circulation,* 1983; 68: 961–969.
4. May GS, Eberlein KA, Furbery CD, et al: Secondary prevention after myocardial infarction: a review of long-term trials. *Prog Cardiovasc Dis,* 1982; 24: 331–351.
5. European Coronary Surgery Study Group: Prospective randomized study of coronary artery by-pass surgery in stable angina pectoris. *Lancet,* 1980; 2: 491–495.
6. Gilpin EA, Karliner JS, Ross J Jr: Risk assessment after acute myocardial infarction. In: Karliner JS, Gregoratos G (eds) *Coronary care.* Churchill Livingstone, New York, 1981; 1041–1066.
7. Multicenter Postinfarction Research Group: Risk stratification and survival after myocardial infarction. *N Engl J Med,* 1983; 309: 331–336.
8. Taylor GJ, Humphiries JO, Mellits ED, et al: Predictors of clinical course, coronary anatomy and left ventricular function after recovery from acute myocardial infarction. *Circulation,* 1980; 62: 960–969.
9. Norris RM, Barnaby PF, Brandt PWT, et al: Prognosis after recovery from first acute myocardial infarction: determinants of reinfarction and sudden death. *Am J Cardiol,* 1984; 53: 408–413.
10. Sanz G, Castañer A, Betriu A, et al: Determinants of prognosis in survivors of myocardial infarction. *New Engl J Med,* 1982; 306: 1065–1070.
11. Hinkle L, Thaler H: Clinical classification of cardiac deaths. *Circulation,* 1982; 65: 457–464.
12. Higginson LAJ, Williams WL, Bairol MG, et al: Prediction of outcome following acute myocardial infarction using noninvasive techniques. In: Hurst W (ed) *Clinical essays on the heart.* McGraw-Hill, New York, 1984.
13. Fuller CM, Raizner AE, Verani MS, et al: Early post myocardial infarction treadmill stress testing. *Ann Intern Med,* 1981; 94: 734–739.
14. Boxal J, Ho B, Saltips A: Is routine coronary arteriography justified after myocardial infarction? *Circulation,* 1983; 68 (III): 411.
15. Ellestad MH: *Stress testing,* 2nd ed. Davis, Philadelphia, 1980.
16. Rigo P, Bailey IK, Griffith LSC, et al: Stress thallium 201 myocardial scintigraphy for the detection of individual coronary artery lesions in patients with and without previous myocardial infarction. *Am J Cardiol,* 1981; 28: 209.
17. Patterson RE, Horowitz SF, Eng C, et al: Can noninvasive exercise indentify patients with left main or 3-vessel coronary disease after a first myocardial infarction? *Am J Cardiol,* 1983; 51: 362–372.
18. Dunn RF, Freedman B, Bailey IK, et al: Noninvasive prediction of multivessel disease after myocardial infarction. *Circulation,* 19; 62: 726–734.
19. Sagastagoistia JD, Etxebeste J, Molinero E, et al: Valor de la prueba de esfuerzo y del echocardiograma para determinar la afeccion multivaso en el IAM inferior no complicado. *Rev Esp Cardiolog* 1983; 36 (Suppl 4): 53.

13.6 Conclusions

J. SOLER SOLER

The overall conclusion of this chapter is that there is no definitive strategy for preventing death and reinfarction in survivors of myocardial infarction. In the absence of this strategy, there are at least a few therapeutic measures that merit the benefit of a doubt as to their utility, justifying their use in daily practice.

The following aspects deserve particular attention:

1. Control of coronary risk factors continues to be very important in the management of these patients. Reduction of the cholesterol concentrations is particularly important, although it is not necessary or opportune to obtain levels under 220 mg/dl. The treatment of choice for hypercholesterolemia is diet. Drug treatment should be reserved for patients under 60 years who are resistant in spite of correct diet. There is no drug of choice and secondary effects are not infrequent.

2. Of the diverse treatments for preventing death and reinfarction, only β-blocking adrenergic drugs have provided substantial documented benefits in the first 1–2 years after myocardial infarction.

3. Considering the low mortality (2–3% per year for the first 5 years) of patients with low risk infarction (25–30% of survivors), systematic use of β-blocking agents in these patients is questionable since their prophylactic efficacy is situated at around 25%.

4. In the absence of clinical data indicative of high risk, the conventional exercise test, in spite of its limitations, has an adequate cost/benefit relation for indentifying high risk patients. It can be used to indicate β-blocking therapy, independent of whatever other information it provides.

5. Patients with postinfarctional angina and/or hypertension should be treated with β-blocking agents, although because of protocol design there is no firm evidence that this therapy improves the evolution of infarction in this patient subgroup.

Index of subjects

DEVELOPMENTS IN
CARDIOVASCULAR MEDICINE

Recent volumes